WU 100

D0184438

Medical Problems in Dentistry

Medical Problems in Dentistry

Third edition

Crispian Scully PhD, MD, MDS, FDSRCPS(Glas), RCSEng, FRCPath
*Professor, Consultant and Head of University Department of Oral Medicine,
Pathology and Microbiology, University of Bristol*

Roderick A Cawson MD, BDS, FDS, RCSEng, RCPS(Glas), FRCPath
*Emeritus Professor of Oral Medicine and Oral Pathology, University of
London: Visiting Professor, Baylor Dental College and University Medical
Center, Dallas, Texas*

WRIGHT

Wright
An imprint of Butterworth-Heinemann Ltd
Linacre House, Jordan Hill, Oxford OX2 8DP

A member of the Reed Elsevier plc group

OXFORD   LONDON   BOSTON
MUNICH   NEW DELHI   SINGAPORE   SYDNEY
TOKYO   TORONTO   WELLINGTON

First published 1982
Second edition 1987
Third edition 1993
Reprinted 1993, 1994 (twice), 1995

British Library Cataloguing in Publication Data
Scully, Crispian
    Medical Problems in Dentistry. – 3Rev.ed
    I. Title   II. Cawson, Roderick A.
    616.00246176

ISBN 0 7236 0999 3

Library of Congress Cataloguing in Publication Data
Scully, Crispian
    Medical problems in dentistry/Crispian Scully, Roderick A.
    Cawson – 3rd ed.
    p.   cm.
    Includes bibliographical references and index.
    ISBN 0 7236 0999 3
    1. Sick – Dental care.   2. Oral manifestations of general diseases.
    I. Cawson, R. A.   II. title
    [DNLM: 1. Dentistry.   2. Medicine.   WB 100 S437m]
    RK55.S53S38   92-49862
    617.6–dc20   CIP

Composition by Scribe Design, Gillingham, Kent
Printed and bound in Great Britain by
Hartnolls Limited, Bodmin, Cornwall

Contents

Preface to the Third Edition

When this text was first written, HIV infection had not been recognized. Within a mere decade the epidemic of AIDS has spread worldwide with explosive rapidity. As a consequence, of this infection particularly, dental clinicians have been forced to review their practices. Another consequence has been that the public has become increasingly concerned about medical problems in dentistry, especially after media publicity given to the transmission of AIDS in an American dental practice.

This third edition cannot therefore avoid considerable emphasis on HIV infection as well as the risks from the different types of viral hepatitis and other infections such as endocarditis. All of these problems create health hazards for patients or dental workers but increasingly are having medico-legal implications. With such considerations in mind, the whole of this text has been updated and we hope that any errors or ambiguities in the previous editions have been eliminated. We welcome any comments but hope that the very few thus far received – less than a handful in ten years – truly reflect the accuracy of the contents.

C. S.
R. A. C.

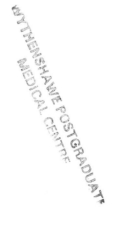

Preface to the Second Edition

In the relatively short time since the first edition of this book there has been a substantial increase in the awareness among dental surgeons of the importance of medical problems in dentistry. A second edition is therefore long overdue, especially now that the Acquired Immune Deficiency Syndrome (AIDS) has appeared since the preparation of the previous edition.

Although reviews of the first edition were very generous and we have received virtually no suggestions for improvements we have not only included new systemic diseases, particularly AIDS, recent diseases of increasing importance such as delta agent infection, new oral complications of disease and therapy such as cyclosporin-induced gingival hyperplasia, and relevant newly recognized diseases such as the MAGIC syndrome, Legionnaire's disease and Lyme disease, but also some aspects omitted from the first edition, such as some causes of bleeding tendency, myelodysplastic syndromes, antral and nasopharyngeal carcinoma, premature infants, and points relevant to anaesthesia. We have tried to avoid too great an increase in size by eliminating much excess verbiage, especially in the chapters on Cardiovascular disease and on Neurological disease, and by eliminating the lists of drug names. We have updated the whole text, added new figures and tables and, hopefully, corrected the few printing errors.

This text is not designed to cover all aspects of *oral disease* but rather to highlight systemic diseases that influence dental care or treatment. Standard oral medicine texts should be consulted for fuller details of oral diseases.

In relation to this edition we are grateful to Mrs M. Seward, Editor of the *British Dental Journal,* for permission to include material from the *Hospital Dental Surgeon's Guide* (Scully C., *Br. Dent. J.,* 1985) and from papers we have published in the Journal. We are also most grateful to Stephen Porter, Karen Porter and Stephen Flint for stimulating discussions and for their help in reading the proofs.

C. S.
R. A. C.

Preface to the First Edition

Unless he is quite unusually oblivious to potential consequences, the dentist who discovers that a patient has a disease of any of the major organ systems is likely to be made anxious by the possibility that complications might result from dental treatment. It is often worse when the patient has some uncommon syndrome with a bizarre name. Such anxiety may well be justified, and may be increased by doubt as to which aspects of dental treatment may be hazardous for such a patient.

There are three basic problems regarding the dental treatment of patients with significant systemic disease. The first is to detect such patients. This is a difficult task but an attempt at medical assessment of the patient must always be made, especially when a general anaesthetic has to be given—even if that anaesthetic is euphemistically termed sedation with methohexitone, Very often, however, there are severe limitations on what can be discovered about a patient who may have no significant symptoms or, if under medical treatment, may have only the haziest of ideas of what it is all about. The problem is even greater with patients who speak poor or little English and with those of low intelligence or who are unable to give a clear history for any other reason.

It has to be accepted that, largely as a result of current drug treatment, the days are past when it was reasonable to assume that a patient walking in from the street was as fit as he appeared. There is no doubt therefore that it is the dentist's responsibility at least to attempt to make a medical assessment of his patients. Apart from the fate of the patient, neglect of the medical history can result in unpleasant medico-legal complications.

Secondly, if a patient is found to have a systemic disease, it then becomes necessary to determine what implications the disease or its treatment have for dental management. Finally, once this has been decided, it then remains necessary to discover how best to deal with the problem.

It is easy to exaggerate the frequency with which systemic disease can seriously complicate dental treatment. The very rarity of such an emergency as cardiac arrest makes it likely that at some time it may catch the dentist by surprise and sometimes, as a consequence, powerless to do anything to help the patient significantly. Nevertheless, the fact is that cardiovascular disease, the most frequent underlying cause of cardiac arrest and other emergencies, is very common.

These considerations aside, hospital dental staff can find themselves in the difficult position of having to manage the total initial care of patients with maxillofacial injuries who may also be comatose for one or more of a variety of reasons.

Unfortunately it is difficult to discover, from any one of the standard texts, the great variety of dental implications of systemic diseases and how any such problems should be managed. The aim of this book was therefore to try to ease this task for the dentist, but the writing of this text made it only too apparent how wildly ambitious we had been in setting our sights on such a target.

Some areas of medicine are particularly difficult. Many dentists have a mental block about the subject of immunology. We thought it worth while therefore to review briefly the working of the immune system before considering how disorders of this system are related to disease. In practice, however, few immunologically mediated diseases, apart from Sjogren's syndrome, are of major relevance for dentistry. By contrast, treatment of many such diseases with immunosuppressive drugs, particularly corticosteroids, is relatively common and can cause serious complications in dental practice.

Another traditionally difficult area of medicine is neurology, and unfortunately the neurology of the head and neck region is by no means the easiest part of this subject. Some trouble has therefore been taken to delineate the disorders affecting the cranial nerves and the clinical features that help to differentiate them. This aspect is particularly important in the case of maxillofacial injuries where cranial nerve lesions can be extracranial or the result of brain damage.

Perhaps most difficult of all is the subject of psychiatric disease. Nevertheless, dentists are perhaps insufficiently aware of how frequently psychiatric disease can cause difficulties with their patients. In addition, oral symptoms probably have a psychiatric basis more frequently than is generally realized.

Overall, therefore, this book is intended for hospital dental staff, for those studying for the Fellowship and for interested general practitioners.

The structure of this book is as follows. First, we have tried to provide sufficient background information about systemic diseases and their management to make their effects understandable. Secondly, we have outlined the relevance of these diseases and their treatment for dentistry. Thirdly, we have tried to suggest, wherever possible, how these problems should be dealt with. In some cases, as indicated in the text, the only satisfactory solution is to refer the patient for specialist care.

Our original intention was to be very brief, but there are few conditions that do not have *some* dental implications, however slight. Moreover, though rare diseases are unlikely to be encountered in routine dental practice, it is typically these, or unusual aspects of common diseases, which can cause most difficulties. Moreover, the rarity of a disease in statistical terms does not mean that it cannot be a source of trouble. It is of no comfort to tell someone who has been struck by lightning that it shouldn't have happened! Therefore, to avoid overloading the main body of the text even further, many of these rare syndromes have been summarized in tabular form as appendices. Tropical diseases are not included, neither is detailed coverage of oral diseases.

We have unavoidably had to be dogmatic about many things. However, it is impossible to cater exactly for all the variables in dental practice, such as the facilities provided and the calibre or availability of medical advice and assistance, let alone the different types of patient encountered at different clinics. Inevitably also, there is no general agreement as to how best to manage some problems.

All we can hope therefore—whether too much or too little information has been provided—is that this book will help to answer some of the many questions that have been put to us over the years.

C. S.
R. A. C.

Note on Drug Names and Use

Information on the correct writing of prescriptions is available in the *British National Formulary* and the *Dental Practitioners' Formulary*.

The Appendix to Chapter 19 tabulates possible drug contraindications, interactions and effects. These are not necessarily absolute and often depend on severity of the disease state, drug dosage, etc. It cannot be stressed too strongly that all drug doses, particularly for children and the elderly, and possible contraindications to drug use should be checked in the most recent edition of the *BNF* or the *DPF*. Untoward adverse reactions to drugs should be reported to the Committee for Safety of Medicines (1 Nine Elms Lane, London SW8 SNQ).

Drug information may be obtained from Poisons Centres in cases of poisoning or adverse reactions (*see* Appendix to Chapter 18).

Chapter 1

Assessment of the Patient and Anaesthetic Considerations

Provided that the patient is fit and local anaesthesia is used, dentistry is a safe procedure. Risks arise when these conditions do not apply and the dentist attempts anything overambitious in terms of his skill or knowledge.

It has been said that 'Dentists are now concerned not with the treatment of teeth in patients but the treatment of patients who have teeth' (Morris, 1967); we hope very much that this is true. At one time any patient who could climb a flight of stairs without distress was judged fit for dental general anaesthesia. Today, many patients with life-threatening diseases survive as a result of advances in surgical and medical care. One result of this is that an apparently fit patient, coming for dental treatment, can have a serious systemic disease and be under drug treatment. Either or both can significantly affect the dental management or even the fate of the patient, particularly when general anaesthesia or sedation is going to be given. These problems may be compounded by the fact that patients are seen briefly and that medical support is lacking in the dental surgery. The report of the Department of Health Working Party on General Anaesthesia Sedation and Resuscitation in Dentistry, shows the concern at official levels for improvement in patient assessment and management in these fields (DH, 1990).

Communication between doctors and dentists is sometimes also poor and both patients and dentists often fail fully to appreciate the relevance of the medical history. Some patients may even resent being questioned. Some patients may have particular language or communication difficulties in giving their medical history.

The object of the medical history and patient assessment is first, to determine whether the patient is fit to undergo dental treatment and whether any drugs or general anaesthesia are contraindicated and second, to exclude oral disease. No patient should suffer any deterioration of health as a result of dental treatment.

The prevalence of medical disorders that might affect dental treatment is relatively high. McLundie, Watson and Kennedy (1969), for example, found that of 2500 patients attending the conservation and prosthetics departments of a dental hospital or general practice, 3.4 per cent gave a history of prolonged bleeding and 48 per cent had respiratory disorders. Another UK study (Rothwell and Wragg, 1972) found relevant medical problems in 38 per cent of patients in general dental practice. Among 4785 dental patients, 8 per cent were known to be hypertensive, but measurement of the blood pressure at the dental clinic showed that a further 7 per cent were hypertensive (Halpern, 1975). More than 50 per cent of patients have more than one medical disorder (Cottone and Kafrawy, 1979) of which drug reactions and cardiovascular and psychiatric disorders appear to be most frequent (Sonis et al., 1983). Blood and urine glucose levels may be abnormal in 5 per cent or more of dental patients (Falace, 1978) and screening may detect unsuspected diabetes mellitus. The prevalence of systemic disease is much higher in certain groups, particularly the elderly, the handicapped and inpatients.

The magnitude of the problem of drug interactions in dental practice is unknown but, in view of the relatively limited prescribing habits of dentists, it must fall well below that experienced in medical practice. However, Oksas (1978) reported that 30 per cent of a group of 2418 dental hospital patients had a history of chronic systemic disorders that could contraindicate the use of some drugs used in dentistry. Of these patients, 23 per cent also admitted to having drug-related reactions, many of which involved drugs commonly used in dentistry. In the hospital under study, adverse drug reactions were possible in about one in every 24 prescriptions given.

It is therefore essential to establish as clearly as possible, within the practical limitations of dental practice, the presence and significance of medical problems likely to affect dental management and particularly, whether general anaesthesia or sedation may be particularly hazardous. Good preoperative assessment endeavours to anticipate and prevent trouble. Morbidity and mortality following dental operations is even less excusable than when it follows more serious surgery. Morbidity or mortality are significantly less when local anaesthesia is used than in any other technique. By contrast, with intravenous or inhalational general anaesthesia, control of vital functions is impaired or lost to the anaesthetist.

PRACTICAL ASPECTS OF ASSESSMENT

Adequate assessment is essential if the patient is to have general anaesthesia or even sedation. The criteria of 'fitness' are not absolute but depend on the health of the patient, the degree of urgency of the procedure and the skill and experience of the anaesthetist and operator. Overall, sedation is considerably safer than general anaesthesia, but even so, must be carried out by adequately trained personnel and with due consideration of the possible risks as indicated by the General Dental Council's Notes for Dentists (1989). Further details of perioperative care have been provided by Carter (1988).

Since medical examination of the patient is neither generally feasible nor appropriate, the most useful aspect of assessment is the medical history. This must be accurate but also concise and systematically applied to ensure that the maximum information is obtained. Many systems are available but each should have a preamble to explain why the questions are being asked and, in particular, to make it clear that the purpose of the questions is to ensure the patient's safety. In one such system the history is reduced to 12 routine questions (A to L) as follows:

1. Anaemia.
2. Bleeding disorders.
3. Cardiorespiratory disorders.
4. Drug treatment and allergies.
5. Endocrine disorders.
6. Fits or faints.
7. Gastrointestinal disorders.
8. Hospital admissions and attendances.
9. Infections.
10. Jaundice or liver disease.
11. Kidney disease.
12. Likelihood of pregnancy or pregnancy itself.

Further enquiry should be made about any positive answers. Each answer should be recorded as Yes or No to ensure accuracy. Some centres use a questionnaire that the patient answers in the waiting room. This saves time and allows the patient to write about things they might not wish to speak openly about. It also provides documentary evidence that proper enquiries have been made, if any complications lead to medicolegal complications. Answers from such a questionnaire should always be confirmed by the dental surgeon, as quite serious disease is sometimes neglected by both the patient and the dentist (Scully and Boyle, 1983; Dunne and Clark, 1985). Indeed, only 68 per cent of patients provided valid data in one study (Brady and Martinoff 1980); by contrast some overestimated their problems (Mohammad and Ruprecht, 1983).

One limitation of such questionnaires is the delicate matter of sexually transmitted diseases and in particular, that of AIDS. There is no easy answer. If direct questions are asked, the patient is likely to be offended; there also is no guarantee that answers are honest or even that the patient is aware of having been infected. However, it is worthwhile to have a final section headed 'Please add anything else about your health or medication which may be relevant'. In the writers' experience, a very conventional-looking young business man admitted, in this last section, that he had or had had an impressive list of sexually transmitted diseases and was currently under investigation for AIDS. In fact he was already infected with HIV.

A few patients bring a list of their medical complaints and histories with them. Whilst these may sometimes be accurate and helpful, they are occasionally a sign of neuroticism (Chapter 14).

Clinical assessment—the face and general appearance in diagnosis

Much can sometimes be learned simply by looking at the patient. Conditions which may suggest an immediate diagnosis include:

Pallor (anaemia or an imminent faint), cyanosis (cardiac or respiratory disease), jaundice (liver disease), prominent cervical lymph nodes (HIV and other infections particularly), hyper- or hypothyroidism, prognathism and thickened facies (acromegaly), Cushing's disease or cushingoid facies due to corticosteroid treatment, emaciation (possibly due to anorexia, malignant disease or AIDS), Parkinson's disease, myotonia, tardive dykinesia, myasthenia gravis, pupil abnormalities, facial and other cranial nerve palsies, Down's or Turner's syndromes, congenital syphilis, hereditary haemorrhagic telangiectasia, pigmentation (Addison's disease and other causes), systemic sclerosis, lupus erythematosus, dermatomyositis, hypertrichosis, bullous erythema multiforme, salivary gland swellings and other swollen faces, eye disorders (such as uveitis or Sjögren's syndrome), osteogenesis imperfecta, dyspnoea, herpes, candidosis (angular stomatitis in AIDS and other diseases), pregnancy, finger clubbing (cardiorespiratory disease) and neurotic or psychotic behaviour. Oral manifestations of systemic disease such as thrush secondary to HIV infection should also be looked for.

Speech may be defective as a result of severe xerostomia, neurological or muscle diseases such as myasthenia gravis, or drug intoxication.

The value and limitations of routine blood pictures and their interpretation

It is useless to ask for 'full blood counts' unless the clinician is aware of the value of a routine haematological print-out. The interpretation of haematological results is summarized in the Appendix to Chapter 4, but it is essential to appreciate that routine print-outs are mainly of value in the diagnosis of anaemias, leukaemias and some immunodeficiency states. For example, otherwise unexplained lymphopenia may suggest the possibility of HIV infection.

Routine blood pictures are of no value in assessing bleeding tendencies, unless platelets are severely decreased. They also do not provide information relating to blood grouping. Haemostatic function and blood grouping therefore require specific tests.

Anaemia

Anaemia is often a contraindication to general anaesthesia, particularly if the haemoglobin is less than 10 g/dl. Lassitude, weakness, pallor, breathlessness or swelling of the ankles are signs of severe anaemia. Racial origins may be important, especially in the case of haemolytic anaemias such as sickle cell disease or thalassaemia (Chapter 4).

Bleeding disorders

Though the history is of paramount importance in assessing bleeding disorders, inquiries about abnormal bleeding produce more vague answers than do most other questions. Specific questions should therefore be asked, as suggested in Chapter 3. Bleeding disorders are a significant hazard and any such possibility must always be taken seriously. A history of involvement of other members of the family or of admission to hospital for control of bleeding is particularly important.

Cardiorespiratory disorders

Cardiac disease is often a contraindication to general anaesthesia or it may necessitate antibiotic cover as prophylaxis against infective endocarditis, or both. Inquiry must be made about a history of rheumatic or congenital heart disease, ischaemic heart disease, cardiac operations and previous attacks of infective endocarditis.

Respiratory disorders also significantly influence the choice of anaesthesia. Asthma, bronchitis and emphysema are the most common problems (Chapter 6) but even the common cold can be a contraindication to general anaesthesia.

Chest pain, dyspnoea, swelling of the ankles, palpitations and hypertension are all significant features suggesting cardiovascular disease. Wheeze, cough or dyspnoea are common symptoms of respiratory disease.

Drug treatment and allergies

Drugs may not only influence dental disease or treatment but their nature may be the only indication of serious underlying disease. Corticosteroids, antihypertensives, anticonvulsants, anticoagulants, antibiotics and antidiabetics are all important drugs in this respect. In order to get useful answers about drug treatment it is often necessary to phrase the question 'Do you ever take any injections, drugs, pills, tablets or medicines of any kind?' Many patients neglect to mention such drugs as analgesics, hypnotics or contraceptives (*Fig.* 1.1). Smoking and drinking habits must also be asked about and in some cases the possibility of drug abuse must be considered. Drug allergies or atopic disease (which may be associated with an increased tendency to drug allergies) should be carefully noted. All drugs taken by the patient should be checked in the current *British National Formulary* (BNF) or a recent copy of the *Monthly Index of Medical Specialities* (MIMS). The type of drug, potential side-effects, and possible interactions should then be established (*see* Appendix to Chapter 19). If, as is often the case, the patient does not know or cannot recall the name of medicines, treatment should be deferred until the drug is identified by checking the drug itself, by consulting the patient's doctor or in hospital, the Drugs Information Unit or Pharmacy.

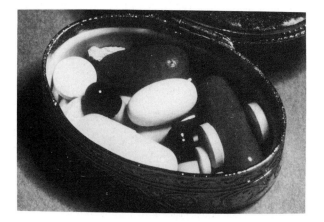

Fig. 1.1. Pill box presented by an outpatient who proved to be taking eight different medications, including a corticosteroid, daily.

The most serious drug interactions in dentistry are with general anaesthetic agents (intravenous or inhalational), monoamine oxidase inhibitors and anti-hypertensive agents. Aspirin may be a hazard in anticoagulated or diabetic patients. Suxamethonium may interfere with the action of digoxin and may itself be potentiated by ecothiopate eye drops (*see* Appendix to Chapter 19).

Endocrine disorders

Diabetes mellitus is a relatively common disease. Hypothyroidism is less common and hypoadrenocorticism is rare but both are also important (Chapter 10).

Fits or faints

Epilepsy and other causes of loss of consciousness can disrupt dental treatment and may result in injury to the patient. The type and severity of epilepsy should be noted; treatment is best carried out during a stable phase (Chapter 12).

Gastrointestinal disorders

Some gastrointestinal disorders such as Crohn's disease or coeliac disease may lead to oral complications, and gastric disorders may increase the risk of vomiting during general anaesthesia. Questioning should be directed towards the presence of abdominal pain, frequency and type of stool, bleeding and weight loss (Chapter 7).

Hospital admissions and attendances

Operations are good indicators of the possible reactions to general anaesthesia and surgery. A patient who has had a tonsillectomy for example, without complications is most unlikely to have a congenital bleeding disorder. Hospital admissions may also indicate underlying disease, and past operations may suggest the possibility of future complications that can influence dental treatment.

Infections

The possibility of transmissible infections and their sequelae must be considered, particularly in at-risk groups. Infection with human immune deficiency viruses (HIV), for example, is an increasing problem, especially in male homosexuals and abusers of intravenous drugs. Patients who have attended sexually transmitted disease clinics are more likely to have a history of infection with HIV, hepatitis viruses, herpes simplex, syphilis, gonorrhoea and many other infections (*Fig.* 1.2 and Chapters 8, 16 and 17).

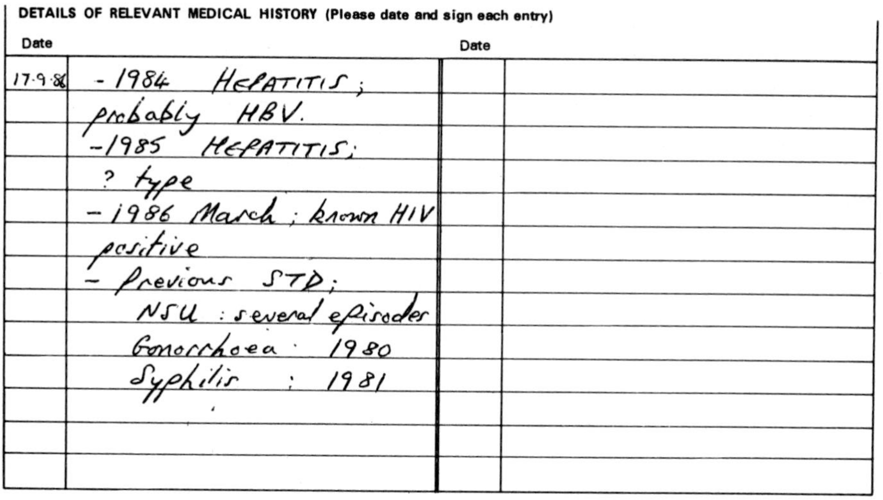

DETAILS OF RELEVANT MEDICAL HISTORY (Please date and sign each entry)

Date		Date	
17.9.8	- 1984 HEPATITIS; probably HBV. -1985 HEPATITIS; ? type - 1986 March : known HIV positive - previous STD: NSU : several episodes Gonorrhoea · 1980 Syphilis : 1981		

Fig. 1.2. Medical history from a male promiscuous homosexual.

Jaundice and liver disorders

A history of jaundice may imply carriage of hepatitis viruses, although jaundice is by no means always infective. A prolonged bleeding state and impaired drug metabolism can result from liver disease (Chapter 8). Jaundice after an operation may have resulted from halothane hepatitis and if this is suspected, a different anaesthetic, such as isoflurane, should be given.

Kidney disorders

Renal disorders can affect dental management, mainly because excretion of some drugs is impaired. Nocturia and hypertension are early manifestations of renal failure, while polyuria, anorexia, vomiting, lassitude and weight loss are late features. Rarely, renal failure or complications of renal transplantation can give rise to oral signs or affect dental management.

Pregnancy

It is important to know whether a woman is pregnant, since any dental procedure involving drugs, radiography or general anaesthesia is best left until the middle trimester (Chapter 10). Though there is no known risk of teratogenic effects from most drugs used in dentistry, drug administration should be kept to an absolute minimum.

These questions cover most of the important conditions that may influence, or be influenced by, dental treatment. However, it is essential that the history be updated before each course of treatment, every sedation session and especially before a general anaesthetic, as it may radically change. Ellinger et al. (1973) followed a small group of middle-aged and elderly dental patients and reported that nearly 20 per cent developed significant medical disorders (mostly cardiovascular) over a period of 5 years.

Patients should be asked if they carry a medical warning card and careful note should be taken of it, particularly in respect of corticosteroid use, a bleeding disorder or diabetes. Similar attention should be given to any medical warning medallion such as Medic-Alert (*Figs* 1.3, 1.4).

It is important to emphasize again that the history is of prime importance in dentistry where physical examination is usually inappropriate. However, as mentioned earlier, it is important to look at the patient for such readily visible signs such as pallor, cyanosis, or jaundice and dyspnoea or wheezing, and not merely examine the mouth.

Although every care should be taken to identify the unfit patient, it must be appreciated that the means to do so are limited and by no means always successful. It is impossible to legislate for all possibilities and there have been many cases where apparently fit people have dropped dead within a short time of having passed a medical examination. This fact that serious disease can fail to

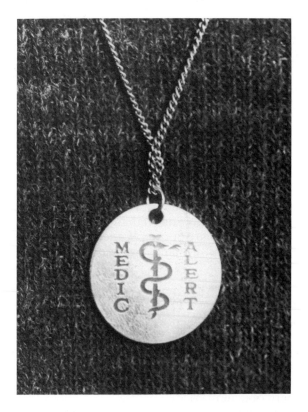

Fig. 1.3. Medic–Alert warning emblem: the patient's main diagnosis or drug treatment is engraved on the reverse, together with the telephone number of the company which holds details of the medical history.

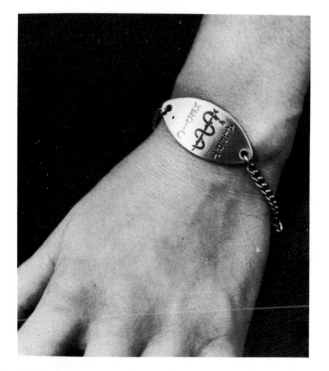

Fig. 1.4. Medic–Alert bracelet.

reveal itself during medical examination should act as a deterrent to the use of general anaesthesia or so-called sedation with intravenous barbiturates, which are a significant cause of morbidity or even mortality. Local anaesthesia, with conscious sedation if necessary, should therefore be used wherever possible for outpatient dentistry.

SPECIAL HAZARDS OF OUTPATIENT GENERAL ANAESTHESIA

Five aspects of general anaesthesia for ambulant dental patients deserve special consideration (Young, 1975).

1. The patient is ambulant, is in the premises for a short period and is observed for only a brief time postoperatively.

2. The operation site is close to the airway—any inflammatory oedema, haemorrhage or foreign bodies can endanger respiration.

3. Equipment, facilities and technical assistance are rarely of the standard found in a modern operating theatre.

4. Fewer than one in four general anaesthetics in dental practice are given by anaesthetists who have had postgraduate training.

5. Patients may have pre-existing medical disorders.

Mark each item with a tick or N/A for *every* sedation given	Patient label					
STAFF CHECK DATE:						
Experienced qualified DSA present?						
Another dentist/doctor/nurse/DSA is within easy call?						
Operator and assistants know emergency procedures?						
EQUIPMENT CHECK						
Site of emergency equipment known?						
Have the following been checked by the operator? Oxygen						
Suction – dental unit						
Suction – mobile/back-up						
Positive pressure ventilating bag						
Sphygmomanometer						
Pulse oximeter						
Other automatic monitor (BP/ECG)						
Emergency drugs (Flumazenil)						
Sedation equipment						
Have the following been checked? Dental equipment						
Dental unit						
PATIENT CHECK						
Patient, parent or guardian know what is planned?						
Written consent has been obtained?						
Written pre + postoperative instruction issued?						
Medical and dental history checked?						
Routine medication taken?						
Last meal or drink checked?						
Fasting patient?						
If Yes – has glucose been given?						
Patient has consumed alcohol today?						
If Yes – advise to postpone session?						
Responsible escort present?						
Weight recorded?						
BP recorded?						
OPERATOR'S NAME IN CAPITALS:						

Fig. 1.5. Checklist for operator before giving sedation (see also pp. 42–43). (Courtesy Miss A. M. Skelly.)

It has been reported that, following outpatient general anaesthesia, despite instructions to the contrary (Ogg, 1980):

1. Thirty-one per cent of patients returned home unaccompanied by a responsible person.

2. Thirty per cent of car owners drove within 12 hours of general anaesthesia and 9 per cent even drove themselves home from the surgery.

Patients should therefore be asked to agree (Appendix 1):

1. To bring an accompanying responsible adult who will supervise them after discharge from the surgery.

2. Not to attempt to drive a vehicle, ride a bicycle or pillion on a motorcycle, work with unguarded machinery, or make important decisions, until the day after having had a general anaesthetic.

3. Not to drink alcohol or take drugs, particularly sleeping tablets, the night before or until the day after having had a general anaesthetic.

Obviously it is impossible to control the behaviour of irresponsible patients, but it is essential to point out the dangers in the clearest possible terms. Patients may also fail to take in or forget verbal instructions, particularly after benzodiazepine sedation. To protect both the patient and operator the patient and escort should be given written instructions (pp. 42–43), and every other item should be checked (Fig. 1.5).

PREOPERATIVE ASSESSMENT FOR GENERAL ANAESTHESIA

Deaths related to dental treatment are rare (*Table 1.1*), but most of them have been as a result of general anaesthesia, as discussed later.

Table 1.1 Deaths associated with dental treatment:
England and Wales

Year	Total	Number including general anaesthesia	Place of operation	
			Dentists	Hospital
1979	11	9	4	5
1980	5	4	1	2
1981	5	4	4	0
1982	8(1)	7(1)	3(1)	4(0)
1983	5(1)	5(1)	4(1)	1(0)
1984	3(1)	3(1)	2(1)	1(0)
1985	4(4)	4(4)	1(1)	3(3)
1986	4(2)	3(2)	3(2)	1(0)
1987	5(2)	4(2)	2(1)	3(1)
1988	3	1	0	1

Figures in brackets relate to children under the age of 16 years

Adequate preoperative assessment is crucial to the safety of the patient and many diseases are relative or absolute contraindications to general anaesthesia in the dental surgery, as discussed in subsequent chapters. However, the first consideration is that a dentist should *never* act as both operator and anaesthetist (Appendix to this chapter). Quite apart from the risk to the patient, any accident involving an operator-anaesthetist is certain to provoke disciplinary action by the General Dental Council. If a death results, a charge of manslaughter may have to be faced. By contrast, local anaesthesia is remarkably safe and, in competent hands, even minor complications are uncommon. In those few cases where general anaesthesia is unavoidable, it is wiser to refer patients to hospital or a suitably equipped and staffed clinic for this purpose.

The following comments apply mainly to anaesthesia in the dental surgery, as inpatients should be assessed by the anaesthetist who can also ensure that any supplementary investigations are carried out. The reader should also refer to the report of the Working Party (DH, 1990) mentioned earlier.

Though every precaution must be taken to assess fitness for anaesthesia, and especially to make sure that all details of a patient's medication are known, it must be accepted that diseases such as some congenital cardiac defects may cause no symptoms and remain completely unsuspected until complications develop. More common still is unsuspected hypertension or coronary artery disease which is one of the main causes of death under anaesthesia. Under the circumstances, it is obviously essential that general anaesthesia should only be given in the dental surgery if absolutely essential. If, however, this has to be done, then it is the responsibility of the dentist to tell the anaesthetist all he knows about the patient's medical state, particularly about the presence of any of the following:

1. Respiratory disease.
2. Cardiovascular disease or hypertension.
3. Diabetes mellitus.
4. Neuromuscular disorders.
5. Medication and allergies, including details of smoking and alcohol intake.
6. Previous anaesthetic complications and any recent general anaesthetics (see halothane hepatitis, Chapter 8).
7. Pregnancy.
8. Symptoms or signs such as productive cough, dyspnoea, palpitations, chest pain, ankle oedema, raised blood pressure, dysrhythmias.
9. Any airway obstruction or threat to the airway or possible intubation difficulty (Table 1.2).
10. Infections, particularly hepatitis or by HIV.

Special investigations that may be needed preoperatively should be checked with the anaesthetist. The following may be required (see Appendix 1 for normal values and interpretation of abnormalities):

1. Haemoglobin estimation and blood picture.
2. Sickle test in Afro-Caribbeans

▶

Fig. 1.6. Simplified protocol for preoperative investigation.

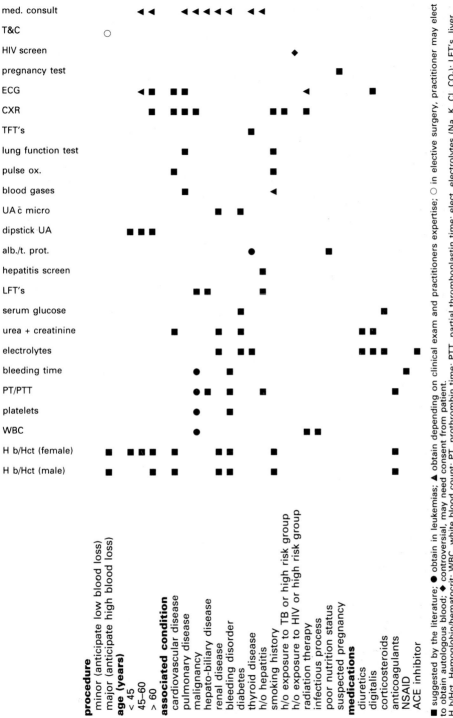

3. Blood pressure estimation.

4. Chest radiograph.

5. Electrocardiogram (ECG), particularly for patients over 60.

6. Urinalysis.

7. Urea and electrolytes if an intravenous infusion is to be used, or patient is on diuretic therapy.

8. Liver function tests

The question of routine screening has been discussed elsewhere particularly in respect of the possible cost/benefit ratio. A suggested protocol for preoperative investivation is suggested in Fig. 1.6.

If there is any doubt about fitness for general anaesthesia a specialist medical opinion should be obtained; indeed the proper person to check the preoperative assessment is the anaesthetist.

The relative indications and contraindications for general and local anaesthesia and sedation are shown in *Table 1.2.*

In the case of anaesthetics or more frequently, sedation given in the dental surgery it is also important to give the patient a questionnaire to make sure that nothing has been forgotten and in the event of any mishap, to provide documentary evidence that this assessment has been carried out.

Table 1.2. Relative indications and contraindications of general anaesthesia (GA), local anaesthesia (LA) and sedation

Indications	*Contraindications*
GA	
Major surgery	Severe respiratory disease
Multiple extractions	Severe cardiac disease
Acute infections (but not Ludwig's angina)	Severe anaemia (especially sickle cell anaemia)
Allergy to LA	Severe infections in floor of mouth
Handicapped or anxious	Unescorted patient
LA	
Minor surgery	Sepsis in field
Poor-risk patient for GA	Uncooperative patient
No anaesthesia available	Major surgery
Inadequate facilities for GA	Bleeding tendency
Recent meal	Haemangioma in field
SEDATION	
Patient too anxious to accept treatment under local anaesthesia Many prolonged operations such as removal of third molars or preparation for implants for which GA would otherwise be needed	Chronic obstructive pulmonary disease (intravenous benzodiazepines especially) Airways obstruction or respiratory infections Disabling severe heart disease Psychotic personalities

Note: For epileptics or those with asthma, relative analgesia is preferable to intravenous sedation because it provides better control of the patient.

PRECAUTIONS BEFORE GA OR SEDATION
(*see also* Appendix to this chapter)

Patients quickly forget or fail to take in what they are told. As mentioned earlier therefore, it is important not merely to give verbal instructions as suggested below, but also give these same instructions in written form when it has been decided that either anaesthesia or sedation is necessary.

Identification of the patient and operation site

The patient's name and the reason for having general anaesthesia must be confirmed. This apparently obvious precaution avoids embarrassing confusion between patients coming from a crowded waiting room.

Informed consent

Written consent to general anaesthesia must be obtained before each operation. Parental or guardian's consent is needed for those under 16 years of age and for the mentally handicapped.

Suitable consent forms are supplied by the medical defence societies. It is also helpful and there is increasing pressure to provide patients with written information relevant to their treatment (Appendix to this chapter).

No food, drink or oral medication for 4 hours preoperatively

Food or drink present in the stomach may be vomited and inhaled during anaesthesia. Clear instructions must be given that no food or drink (including tea or alcohol) should be taken for 4 hours preoperatively (Appendix 1). Vomiting is more likely in a patient who is pregnant or has gastric disease or a head injury, or has taken alcohol or a drug such as erythromycin which may precipitate vomiting. The bladder should be emptied preoperatively.

Psychological preparation and premedication

Most people are apprehensive of general anaesthesia; some are terrified. Dental treatment in general, and oral surgery in particular, are stressful for many patients, and may induce a rise in blood pressure and pulse rate, and ECG changes. Apart from poor cooperation as a result of anxiety, autonomic overactivity can precipitate cardiac dysrhythmias, swings in blood pressure and vomiting.

One of the most effective methods of reducing anxiety is by sympathetic reassurance and brief discussion of a patient's particular anxieties. However, if this fails, premedication with a benzodiazepine may be necessary, though this is not usually feasible in general dental practice as it delays recovery. Benzodiazepines may also be ineffective in children.

Anaesthetists vary widely in their requirements for premedication. This aspect must be discussed with the anaesthetist. The main purpose of premedication is to lessen anxiety and it is typically given 30–35 minutes preoperatively. For inpatients, opioids (pethidine, morphine or omnopon) are traditional premedicants because of their sedative action. However, they increase nausea, vomiting and respiratory depression. Promethazine or trimeprazine may be used for its sedative and anti-emetic effect, for premedication of children, but it has a prolonged action and is often ineffective. It also increases blood sugar levels – a consideration when treating diabetics. Children may be given oral trimeprazine or triclofos, or rectal barbiturates such as thiopentone.

Benzodiazepines are useful because of their anxiolytic and amnesic action. Their relative freedom from side-effects and wide safety margin have caused diazepam, lorazepam or temazepam to be increasingly widely used. Beta-blockers may also be used and may help to prevent dysrhythmias induced by surgery.

Atropinics such as atropine or hyoscine are anti-emetics and may reduce the parasympathomimetic effects and dysrhythmias sometimes associated with suxamethonium but are unlikely to be needed for outpatients. However the effectiveness of atropinics in preventing dysrhythmias other than vagal overactivity is controversial. Glaucoma is a specific contraindication to the use of atropinics and diazepam. Since the maximal effect of atropine is apparent 30–60 minutes after injection, some anaesthetists now give the drug during induction of anaesthesia, thus achieving the desired parasympatholytic effect during the operation while sparing the patient the unpleasant dry mouth and thirst during the preoperative period. Hyoscine is best avoided in the elderly, in whom it may cause confusion. Atropinics should not be given to febrile patients.

Cardiac dysrhythmias are common during oral surgical procedures, presumably because afferent impulses via the trigeminal nerve stimulate sympathetic nerve centres; regional anaesthesia (such as with bupivacaine) reduces such dysrhythmias, and also postoperative pain.

Removal of dentures

Dentures should be removed preoperatively. The anaesthetist must be warned of the presence of crowned, fragile or loose teeth, or bridges which could be damaged during intubation.

GENERAL ANAESTHETIC AGENTS AND INTRAOPERATIVE CARE

It is beyond the remit of this book to discuss anaesthetic agents or intraoperative care in detail, but the main features of anaesthetic agents are summarized in *Tables 1.3* and *1.4*. Many of the available general anaesthetic agents are less than ideal for outpatients. Enflurane and isoflurane are useful alternatives for patients at risk from halothane hepatitis (Chapter 8) and cardiac rhythm is more stable. However they cause greater respiratory depression than halothane and induction is less pleasant. Immediate recovery is also slower after isoflurane and there may be some coughing.

An essential aspect of operative care is constant monitoring of the patient's state by:

1. Clinical observation of colour, respiration and pulse.
2. Use of:
    a. a blood pressure monitor
    b. pulse oximeter.

A stethoscope and suitable resuscitative equipment must be available.

Ideally, there should also be an electrocardiograph monitor, but this is rarely practicable in the absence of expert interpretation of the tracing. However, the DH Working Party regard it as desirable to have an ECG and, in addition, a capnograph for measurement of end tidal carbon dioxide when endotracheal anaesthesia is practised. The Working Party also recommend that the resuscitative equipment should include a defibrillator.

Nevertheless, a survey by postal questionnaire (Allen, Dinsdale and Reilly, 1990) of 95 practitioners showed that though 6 of them were still using methohexitone and 11 were using methohexitone with halothane, none had a pulse oximeter. Fewer than 1 in 5 had a pulse monitor but variable numbers had other emergency equipment such as oral airways, endotracheal tubes or a laryngoscope and the majority had an emergency drug kit.

Pulse oximeters. These instruments provide a measure of the degree of haemoglobin oxygen saturation by means of spectrophotometry. They are usually very accurate and are a valuable safety measure. However they are expensive (currently £1500–£4000) and under certain circumstances can give misleading readings (Severinghaus and Spellman 1990 and Editorial, *Lancet* 1990 **ii**, 1130–1131).

Table 1.3. Local anaesthetic agents*

Agents	Available as	Comments	Maximum safe dose for fit adults
Lignocaine 2% plain	Lignostab Neo-Lidocaton Xylocaine Xylotox	Poor and brief analgesia	200 mg (5 × 2 ml cartridges)
Lignocaine 2% plus adrenaline† 1 in 80 000		Effective analgesia for >90 min	500 mg (12 × 2 ml cartridges)
Prilocaine 4% plain	Citanest	Poor and brief analgesia Methaemoglobinaemia	400 mg (6 × 2 ml cartridges)
Prilocaine 3% plus felypressin 0.03 i.u./ml	Citanest with Octapressin	Usually effective analgesia for 90 min‡ Methaemoglobinaemia	600 mg (10 × 2 ml cartridges)
Bupivacaine 0.25% plain	Marcain	Used only for prolonged nerve block (up to 8 h)	

*Allergy to local anaesthetic agents, if it exists, is *very* rare (supposed 'allergies' are common however).
†The total dose of adrenaline must never exceed 500 µg, i.e. not more than 40 ml of LA containing adrenaline in a 1 in 80 000 solution.
‡No evidence that it is safer than lignocaine with adrenaline for patients on MAOI or tricyclic antidepressants.

Table 1.4. Agents for general anaesthesia and sedation

Drug	Proprietary names	Adult dose	Comments
Drugs for intravenous anaesthesia			
Etomidate	Hypnomidate	0.2 mg/kg	Good for outpatient anaesthesia. Pain on injection: use large vein and give fentanyl 200µg first. After operation give naloxone 0.1-0.2 mg and oxygen. Little cardiovascular effect. Often involuntary movements, cough and hiccup. Hepatic metabolism. Avoid in repeated doses on traumatized patient—may suppress adrenal steroid production
Ketamine	Ketalar	0.5-2 mg/kg	Rise in BP, cardiac rate, intraocular pressure. Little respiratory depression. Often hallucinations Contraindicated in hypertension, psychiatric, cerebrovascular or ocular disorders. Rarely used in dentistry
Methohexitone	Brietal	1.5 mg/kg 1 % solution (10 mg/ml)	Ultra short-acting barbiturate . The most commonly used i.v. anaesthetic in dentistry. No analgesia. Mild hyperventilation or apnoea if given rapidly. Dose-dependent cardiovascular depression. Relatively non-irritant to tissues. Hepatic metabolism. Contraindicated in epilepsy, cardio-respiratory disease, porphyria, barbiturate sensitivity. Rarely: acute allergy, cough, hiccups, sneeze
Propofol	Diprivan	2 mg/kg	May cause pain on injection. Occasional fits or anaphylaxis. Contraindicated in children.
Thiopentone	Intraval	2.5 mg/kg (2.5% solution)	Ultra short-acting barbiturate. No analgesia. Danger of laryngospasm. Rapid injection may cause apnoea. Irritant if injected into artery or extravascularly. Contraindications as for methohexitone
Drugs for intravenous sedation*			
Diazepam	Valium	Up to 20 mg	Benzodiazepine: gives sedation with amnesia but no analgesia Give slowly i.v. in 2.5 mg increments until ptosis begins i.e . eyelids begin to droop (Verril's sign). Rapid injection may cause respiratory depression. Then give local analgesia Disadvantages: (1) May cause pain or thrombophlebitis (2) Drowsiness returns transiently 4–6 h postoperatively due to metabolism to oxazepam and desmethyldiazepam and enterohepatic recirculation (3) May produce mild hypotension and respiratory depression

Table 1.4. (Continued)

Drug	Proprietary names	Adult dose	Comments
	Diazemuls	Up to 20 mg	Preferred to Valium since, although it has most of the actions above, it causes less thrombophlebitis and therefore can be given into veins on dorsum of hand. Expensive. Do not give intramuscularly
Midazolam	Hypnovel	0.07 mg/kg (up to 7.5 mg total dose)	Benzodiazepine. Compared to diazepam: (1) Onset of action is quicker (30 s) (2) Amnesia is more profound, starting 2–5 min after administration and lasting up to 40 min (with no retrograde amnesia) (3) Recovery is more rapid. Midazolam is virtually completely eliminated within 5 h, without the recurrence of drowsiness that may follow the use of diazepam (4) Incidence of venous thrombosis is less than with Valium (5) At least twice as potent. Signs of sedation less predictable – very slow injection required. Occasional deaths in elderly.
Inhalational agents†			
Nitrous oxide	–		Analgesic, but weak anaesthetic. Non-explosive. No cardiorespiratory effects . Mainly used as a vehicle for other anaesthetic agents, or for sedation.
Halothane‡	Fluothane		The most widely used anaesthetic agent. Non-explosive. Anaesthetic but weak analgesic. Causes fall in B.P., cardiac dysrhythmias and bradycardia. Hepatotoxic on repeated administration. Post-anaesthetic shivering is common, vomiting rare
Enflurane	Ethrane Alyrane		Less potent anaesthetic than halothane. Non-explosive. Less likely to produce dysrhythmias or affect liver than halothane. Powerful cardiorespiratory depressant
Isoflurane	Forane Aerrane		Isomer of enflurane, which causes less cardiac but more respiratory depression than halothane. Induction and recovery are slower than with halothane
Trichloroethylene	Trilene		Analgesic and anaesthetic. Non-explosive. Bradycardia and dysrhythmias are common as are tachypnoea, nausea and vomiting

*Particular caution in pregnancy, the elderly, children and those with liver or respiratory disease. Do *not* give pentazocine with a benzodiazepine. Midalozam is the preferred preparation.
†Gas scavenging should be used.
‡Do not give halothane if patient has had halothane within the previous 6 weeks or has previously had an adverse reaction to halothane.

CHOICE OF AGENTS FOR SEDATION

The main factors are the administrator's experience and facilities, but some consideration should be given to the relative safety of the different agents available. Nitrous oxide and oxygen is overall the safest combination because of its lack of respiratory or cardiodepressant effects, and rapid reversibility.

The benzodiazepines are mild respiratory depressants with minimal risk to healthy persons but potentially dangerous to those with cardiorespiratory disease and particularly chronic obstructive pulmonary disease. Moreover, midazolam is considerably ($\times$ 2 or 3) more potent than diazepam and the onset of signs of sedation are less reliable. As a consequence there have been a few deaths after administration of midazolam alone in elderly patients. More dangerous still is the combination of a benzodiazepine with an opioid such as pentazocine. These are both respiratory depressants and deaths have resulted from their combined use.

In conducting sedation, the requirements of the General Dental Council's Notice (1989) to dentists must be fulfilled.

POSTOPERATIVE CARE AFTER GENERAL ANAESTHESIA OR SEDATION

The immediate postoperative period is a particularly dangerous time and is mainly the responsibility of the anaesthetist. However, merely because the operative procedure has been completed, the dental surgeon must not neglect his patient. The patient must be closely supervised until conscious, by the dental surgeon and then by the nurse or other responsible adult, until alert and able to stand without dizziness or ataxia.

During recovery the patient should be laid in the semi-prone (tonsillar) position and the airway must be protected. Hardeman et al. (1990) have reported that 20 per cent of patients may become hypoxic after intravenous sedation and have suggested that supplemental oxygen should be given during the recovery period.

Postoperatively, analgesics and anti-emetics should be given as necessary, but the anaesthetist should be consulted first. Patients on monoamine oxidase inhibitors must not be given pethidine or other opioids.

Most patients have a relatively smooth postoperative recovery, especially after short procedures. However, nearly 45 per cent develop symptoms attributable to the anaesthetic, especially drowsiness (30 per cent) or headache (13 per cent). Headache seems more common in women, especially if halothane has been used. Sore throat, if the patient was intubated, and muscle pains if suxamethonium has been given, are common. After prolonged anaesthesia, especially in the elderly there are dangers of postoperative complications such as atelectasis (Chapter 6). The patient should therefore be strongly encouraged to undertake breathing exercises and to cough up any sputum. A transient rise in temperature is common after general anaesthesia and is usually caused by localized pulmonary infection which may not be clinically detectable. Persistent fever for several days postoperatively, especially if spiking, may indicate haematoma, wound infection, deep vein thrombosis or more serious pulmonary infection.

Postoperative haemorrhage usually has a local cause (*see* Chapter 3) and patients should have written as well as verbal guidance on how to care for their wounds (Appendix to this chapter).

Postoperative collapse is shown by signs of shock, loss of consciousness, hypotension, weakness, sweating and rapid pulse with pallor. The causes can be difficult to find but include:

1. Haemorrhage.
2. Pulmonary embolism.
3. Cardiac arrest (usually myocardial infarction).
4. Adrenal insufficiency.

Another hazard is amnesia which persists for at least 5 hours after sedation with diazepam or midazolam. As a result, patients are likely to forget post-sedation instructions, or worse, have an accident as a result of forgetting to take normal precautions when using power tools or other dangerous equipment. Bizarre behaviour has also been described even 24 hours after sedation.

It is also important to make sure that the patient is not anticipating going abroad immediately after the anaesthetic or sedation. Complications might develop on board an aircraft or at a destination where medical care is limited. That aside, it is difficult enough for most people to have to deal with the problems of getting through an airport without having their faculties blunted by the after-effects of a benzodiazepine.

As mentioned earlier therefore it is essential to give the patient written instructions to cover the necessary precautions of the post-anaesthetic or sedation period.

ADVERSE REACTIONS TO GENERAL ANAESTHETIC AGENTS

These are outlined in Chapter 19.

POST-ANAESTHETIC MORBIDITY

Post-anaesthetic symptoms in ambulant patients include drowsiness, headache (particularly with halothane) and vomiting. Most of these symptoms are more common in females, and well over 60 per cent of patients having outpatient general anaesthesia return home with significant symptoms.

POSTOPERATIVE COMPLICATIONS

Complications after operations under general anaesthesia can be immediate or delayed. They can be only briefly discussed here. Important immediate complications include the following:

1. Cardiorespiratory complications.
2. Delayed recovery of consciousness.
3. Pain.
4. Nausea and vomiting.

Delayed complications include the following:

1. Respiratory disorders.
2. Cardiac disease.
3. Jaundice.
4. Wound infection.

Cardiorespiratory Complications

In essence, many post-anaesthetic complications result from or lead to hypoxia and therefore include both impaired respiratory function and cardiac disease. Important causes therefore include the following:

1. *Upper airway obstruction.* This is particularly important in dental surgery because of operating around the airway and the risk of inhaling foreign material. Facilities, such as suction must always be immediately available for locating and clearing any blockage. The recovery period is the most dangerous time and great care must be taken to keep the airway clear.

2. *Lower airways obstruction.* Accumulation of secretions is a frequent cause and this can be particularly severe in patients with chronic bronchitis (Chapter 6). In dentistry, inhalation of a tooth or fragments of materials is another possible cause of collapse of a lobe or lobule (atelectasis) and subsequent lung abscess.

Occasionally, bronchospasm can result from a hypersensitivity reaction to an intravenous anaesthetic agent or other drug used during the operation.

3. *Respiratory weakness.* Reversal of the action of neuromuscular blocking drugs (muscle relaxants) depends on many factors but if delayed, results in weak respiratory movements which cannot be made stronger by the patient's conscious efforts. Suxamethonium apnoea is discussed in Chapter 10.

4. *Impaired chest movements.* Damage to the chest is a common accompaniment of maxillofacial injuries, particularly when they result from road traffic accidents (*see* Chapter 13).

5. *Respiratory depression.* This can result from the effects of the anaesthetic and ancillary drugs. Methohexitone and pentazocine for example form a potent combination of respiratory depressants, which can be aggravated by hypoxia, often from a similar cause, during the operation.

6. *Cardiac complications.* Myocardial infarction, cardiac failure or severe dysrhythmias can follow anaesthesia and are the chief risk in those with pre-existing cardiac disease (*see* Chapter 2).

7. *Peripheral circulatory failure.* Shock syndrome is more likely to be a complication of major surgery. Contributory factors are pre-existing heart disease, dehydration, haemorrhage, sepsis or anaphylactic reactions. However, neurogenic circulatory failure is a possible consequence of anaesthesia in a pathologically anxious patient (*see* Chapter 2).

Delayed Recovery of Consciousness

Important causes are overdose of anaesthetic agents or the use of long-acting opioids for premedication, diabetic coma or hypoglycaemia, cardiac complications mentioned earlier, or cerebrovascular accidents. The last may be either in susceptible patients (elderly hypertensives) or as a result of emboli (*see* Chapter 12). Occasionally hysterical patients may feign persistent unconsciousness.

Pain

Pain after oral surgery usually starts after anaesthetic drugs have worn off and may result from unavoidable operative trauma. Alternatively it may result from a complication such as a fractured jaw.

Nausea and Vomiting

Postoperative vomiting is both unpleasant for the patient and dangerous if protective laryngeal reflexes have not returned, allowing inhalation of vomit. Nausea and vomiting are usually the result of opioids used for premedication rather than modern anaesthetic agents and are less likely to follow oral surgery than some other types of operation unless a considerable amount of blood has been swallowed. In many cases the cause of postoperative nausea is unclear but some patients seem to be particularly susceptible. An anti-emetic such as metoclopramide (Maxolon) or prochlorperazine (Stemetil) is usually effective.

Delayed Complications

Occasionally pneumonia or a lung abscess can be precipitated especially in those with chronic respiratory disease, if foreign material is inhaled or if an emergency operation has had to be carried out in spite of the presence of an acute upper respiratory tract infection (*see* Chapter 6).

Pre-existing cardiac disease may be aggravated or myocardial infarction can follow at an unpredictable interval after the anaesthetic, especially in those with ischaemic heart disease (*see* Chapter 2). Myocardial infarction is the chief cause of deaths associated with anaesthesia.

Jaundice

Postoperative jaundice can result from many causes including the following:

1. Viral hepatitis (usually hepatitis C if blood has been given).
2. Halothane hepatitis and hepatotoxic effects of other drugs (Chapter 8).
3. Alcoholic hepatitis.
4. Aggravation of pre-existing liver disease.
5. Hepatic necrosis secondary to circulatory failure.
6. Transfusion reactions.

These conditions are discussed more fully in Chapter 8 and it is only necessary to emphasize here that liver damage should not be a consequence of anaesthesia for oral surgery if care is taken to exclude the high-risk groups listed above. However, it must be appreciated that anaesthesia for high-risk patients cannot be avoided for emergencies such as maxillofacial injuries, and this group of patients includes an unduly high proportion of alcoholics.

Halothane should be avoided if the patient has been exposed to it within the previous 6 months or has had a previous episode of halothane hepatitis. In a series of 300 patients who had been given halothane on more than one occasion within a month and who subsequently developed hepatitis, no fewer than 46 per cent died. Isoflurane is an appropriate alternative; in some hospitals it has replaced halothane but its cost is causing concern.

Wound infection

Wound infection is managed by drainage and the use of antimicrobials as indicated (*see* Appendix to this chapter).

Fantasies of sexual assault during benzodiazepine sedation

It is essential that a dental surgeon does not administer sedation in the absence of a second trained person. The latter is required not merely to assist and help deal with any mishaps but also to act as a chaperone. If the patient makes unjustified allegations that sexual improprieties had been committed as a result of fantasies induced by the sedating agent, these can be effectively dispelled by the assistant.

DEATHS UNDER GENERAL ANAESTHESIA

The mortality rate for general anaesthetics carried out in the dental surgery is small, as mentioned earlier, but had been estimated to have been about 10 deaths for every million anaesthetics administered (Lewis, 1983). Nevertheless, any deaths related to dental treatment are unacceptable. The true mortality rate cannot be determined since the total number of administrations is unknown. However, the number of deaths in dental practices has fallen from 4 in 1979 to zero in 1988, probably as a result of the declining use of general anaesthesia in dentistry. Deaths under general anaesthesia for more major surgery have, also, incidentally, steadily declined in the same period, in spite of the great number of high-risk patients now undergoing surgery and the adventurous nature of modern operations, particularly cardiovascular surgery.

Of even more concern is the fact that, unlike deaths during major surgery, those who have died under dental anaesthesia have frequently been fit young people. The average age range for those who have died during conservative dentistry appears to have been between 8 and 28 years (average age 17) and between 4 and 72 (average age 26) for extractions. It must not be assumed that all these deaths have been at the hands of dentists; specialist anaesthetists have been involved in some cases. In the period 1979 to 1988 there was a total of 40 deaths associated with dental treatment in dental practice and 20 deaths associated with dental treatment in hospitals in England and Wales. Between 1982 and 1987 in England and Wales, 15 died in dental practices and of these 7 were under the age of 16.

The information about deaths under dental anaesthesia is of limited value since (a) the numbers are small, (b) information about factors relating to the causes of death is often scanty and (c) even when information is available, the causes of death sometimes remain obscure. Nevertheless, such information as there is strongly suggests that there is a highly unpredictable element involved in dental anaesthesia and, in view of the kind of patients who die under such circumstances, it must be assumed that unsuspected systemic disease has escaped recognition or that anaesthetic mishaps are more common than they should be. This excess of deaths of young apparently fit patients during dental anaesthesia, reinforces the need for taking a careful history and for referring patients with any suspicion of systemic disease to hospital. The last consideration is particularly important in view of the fact that many practitioners do not possess resuscitation equipment adequate for use in an emergency (Allen et al. 1990). However the increased popularity of sedation as well as the restrictions imposed by the GDC guidelines has greatly reduced the use of anaesthesia in the dental surgery and it is to be hoped that deaths under dental anaesthesia will cease to happen.

HAZARDS OF GENERAL ANAESTHESIA TO DENTAL PERSONNEL

Nitrous oxide and halothane can accumulate in appreciable concentrations in operating areas and particularly around the patient's face, close to where the operator is working. As a consequence, there has been much concern about the possible teratogenicity or carcinogenicity that might result from continual exposure to anaesthetic agents. The consensus of data from animal experiments at subanaesthetic concentrations has, however, not yielded convincing evidence of toxicity.

Epidemiological studies also suggest that there is no convincing evidence of any effect of chronic exposure to anaesthetic agents on mental performance, cancer, or fetal disorders such as low birth weight, stillbirth or malformation.

By contrast, megaloblastosis and a neurological disorder resembling subacute combined degeneration of the cord has been reported in dentists *abusing* nitrous oxide as a result of its interference, in the long term, with vitamin B_{12} metabolism (*see* Chapter 19).

These considerations are discussed elsewhere (Scully, Cawson and Griffiths, 1990). Nevertheless, the following precautions should be taken where general anaesthesia or relative analgesia is used.

1. Every effort should be made to reduce contamination of the surgery atmosphere by anaesthetic gases by avoiding over-usage of general anaesthesia or relative analgesia, by careful use of the anaesthetic machine, adequate surgery ventilation and, most important, by using a scavenger system.

2. Pregnant staff, or staff likely to become pregnant, should not work in a contaminated environment unless there is an effective scavenging system.

Bibliography

Allen N. A., Dinsdale R. C. W., Reilly C. S. (1990) *Br. Dent. J.* **169**, 168–72
Barker I., Butchart D. G. M., Gibson I. et al. (1986) IV, Sedation for conservative dentistry. *Br. J. Anaesth.* **58**, 371–7.

Becker L.C. (1987) Is isofluorane dangerous for the patient with coronary artery disease? *Anesthesiology* **66**, 259–62.

Bedi R. and Crawford A. N. (1982) Assessment of the medical status of Asian immigrant children undergoing dental care. *J. Dent.* **10**, 144–8.

Beeby C. and Thurlow A.C. (1986) Pulse oximetry during general anesthesia for dental extractions. *Br. Dent. J.* **160**, 123–5.

Brady W. F. and Martinoff I. T. (1980) Validity of health history data collected from dental patients and patient perception of health status. *J. Am. Dent. Assoc.* **101**, 642–5.

Brahams D. (1989) Benzodiazepine sedation and allegations of sexual assault. *Lancet* **i**, 1339–40.

Carter D.C. (ed) (1988) Perioperative care. *Br. Med. Bull.* **617**, 235–514.

Cattermole R. W., Verghese C., Blair I. J. et al. (1986) Isoflurane and halothane for outpatient dental anaesthesia in children. *Br. J. Anaesth.* **58**, 385–9.

Cawson R. A. (1969) The problem of the newer drugs in dentistry. *Br. Dent. J.* **120**, 109–10.

Cawson R. A., Curson I. and Whittington D. R. (1983) The hazards of dental local anaesthetics. *Br. Dent. J.* **154**, 253–7.

Cawson R.A. and Spector R.G. (1989) *Clinical Pharmacology in Dentistry*. 5th ed. Edinburgh, Churchill Livingstone.

Coplans M. P. and Curson I. (1982) Deaths associated with dentistry. *Br. Dent. J.* **153**, 357–62.

Cottone J. A. and Kafrawy A. H. (1979) Medications and health histories: a survey of 4365 dental patients. *J. Am. Dent. Assoc.* **98**, 713–18.

Dinsdale R.C.W. and Dixon R.A. (1976) Anaesthetic service to dental patients: England and Wales. *Br. Dent. J.* **144**, 271–9.

Dunne S. M. and Clark C. G. (1985) The identification of the medically compromised patient in dental practice. *J. Dent.* **13**, 45–51.

Ellinger C. W., Kanner I., Wesley R. et al. (1973) Are your patients as healthy as you think they are, doctor? *J. Am. Soc. Prev. Dent.* **3**, 36–8.

Evans B. E. (1978) Dental care for patients with systemic health problems. *NY J. Dent.* **48**, 313–19.

Fahy A. and Marshall M. (1969) Postanaesthetic morbidity in outpatients. *Br. J. Anaesth.* **41**, 433–8.

Falace D. A. (1978) An evaluation of the clinical laboratory as an adjunct to dental practice. *J. Am. Dent. Assoc.* **96**, 261–5.

Fraser C. G. (1985) Urine analysis. *Br. Med. J.* **291**, 321–5.

Gold B. D. and Wolfersberger W. H. (1980) Findings from routine urinalysis and hematocrit on ambulatory oral and maxillofacial surgery patients. *J. Oral Surg.* **38**, 677–8.

Halpern I. L. (1975) Patient's medical status—a factor in dental treatment. *Oral Surg.* **39**, 216–26.

Hampton J. R., Harrison M. J. G., Mitchell J. R. A. et al. (1975) Relative contributions of history-taking, physical examination and laboratory investigation to diagnosis and management of medical outpatients. *Br. Med. J.* **2**, 486–9

Harrison G. G. (1978) Death attributable to anaesthesia: a 10-year survey (1967–76). *Br. J. Anaesth.* **50**, 1041–6.

Kaplan E.B., Sheiner L.B., Boeckman A.J. et al. (1985) The usefulness of preoperative laboratory screening. *JAMA* **253**, 3576–81.

Kaufman L. and Sumner E. (1979) *Medical Problems and the Anaesthetist*. London, Arnold.

Leading Article (1975) Fitness for anaesthesia. *Lancet* **1**, 25–26.

Leading Article (1989) Nausea and vomiting after general anaesthesia. *Lancet* **i**, 651–2.

Lewis B. (1983) Deaths and dental anaesthetics. *Br. Med. J.* **286**, 3–4.

Lindsay S. J. E. and Yates J. A. (1985) The effectiveness of oral diazepam in anxious child dental patients. *Br. Dent. J.* **159**, 149–53.

Lunn J. N. and Mushin W. W. (1982) *Mortality Associated with Anaesthesia*. London, Nuffield Provincial Hospitals Trust.

McAteer P. M., Carter I. A., Cooper G. M., Prys-Roberts C. (1986) Comparison of isoflurane and halothane in outpatient paediatric dental anaesthesia. *Br. J. Anaesth.* **58**, 390–3.

McGimpsie J. G. et al. (1983) Midazolam in dentistry. *Br. Dent. J.* **155**, 47–50.

McLundie A. C.,Watson W. C. and Kennedy G. D. C. (1969) Medical status of patients undergoing dental care. *Br. Dent. J.* **127**, 265–71.

Matthews R. W.. Scully C. and Levers B. G. H. (1984) The efficacy of diclofenac sodium with and without paracetamol in the control of postsurgical dental pain. *Br. Dent. J.* **157**, 357–9.

Mohammad A. R. and Ruprecht A. (1983) Assessment of dental patients' comprehension of health questionnaire. *J. Oral Med.* **38**, 74–75.

Morris A. L. (1967) The medical history in dental practice. *J. Am. Dent. Assoc.* **74**, 129–37.

Norman J. (1980) Use of anaesthesia. Preoperative assessment of patients. *Br. Med. J.* **1**, 1507–8.

O'Boyle C. A., Harris D. and Barry H. (1986) Sedation in outpatient oral surgery. *Br. J. Anaesth.* **58**, 378–84.

Ogg T. W. (1976) Assessment of preoperative cases. *Br. Med. J.* **1**, 82–83.

Ogg T. W. (1980) Use of anaesthesia: implications of day-case surgery and anaesthesia. *Br. Med. J.* **2**, 212–13.

Ogg T. W., MacDonald I. A., Jennings R. A. et al. (1983) Day case dental anaesthesia. *Br. Dent. J.* **155**, 14–17.

Oksas R. M. (1978) Epidemiologic study of potential adverse drug reactions in dentistry. *Oral Surg.* **45**, 707–13.

Osman F., Scully C.. Dowell T. B. et al. (1986) Use of panoramic radiographs in general dental practice in England. *Comm. Dent. Oral Epidemiol.* **14**, 8–9.

Osman F., Scully C., Dowell T. B. et al. (1986) The reasons for taking radiographs in general dental practice. *Comm. Dent. Oral Epidemiol.* **14**, 146–7.

Padfield A. (1989) The future of general anaesthesia in the dental surgery: a discussion papaer. *J. Roy. Soc. Med.* **82**, 30–2.

Parbrook, G.D. (1986) Death for anaesthesia in the general and community dental services. *Br. J. Anaesth.* **58**, 369–70.

Porter S. R., Scully C., Welsby, P., Gleeson, M. (1992) *Colour Guide to Medicine and Surgery for Dentistry.* Edinburgh, Churchill–Livingstone

Rothwell P. S. and Wragg K. A. (1972) Assessment of the medical status of patients in general dental practice. *Br. Dent. J.* **133**, 252–4.

Scully C. (1979) Orofacial manifestations of disease. 1: Normal appearances. *Hospital Update* **5**, 817. *Dental Update* **6**, 443.

Scully C. (1980) Examination of the head and neck—Part I. *Student Update* **2**, 159

Scully C. (1980) Examination of the head and neck—Part II. *Student Update* **2**, 197

Scully C. (1980) Examination of the head and neck—Part III. *Student Update* **2**, 228.

Scully C. (1985) *Hospital Dental Surgeon's Guide.* London, British Dental Association.

Scully C. and Boyle P. (1983) Reliability of a self-administered questionnaire for screening medical problems in dentistry. *Comm. Dent. Oral Epidemiol.* **11**, 105.

Scully C., Cawson R.A. and Griffiths M.J. (1990) *Occupational Hazards to Dental Staff.* British Dental Journal, London.

Scully C. and Prime S. (1980) Acute dental problems in medical practice. *Update* **21**, 1239.

Scully C. and Prime S. (1980) Acute dental problems in medical practice. *Update* **21**, 1511.

Seymour R. A. (1985) Prescribing analgesics. *Br. Dent. J.* **159**, 177-81.

Shirlaw P. J., Scully C., Griffiths M. J. et al. (1986) General anaesthesia, parenteral sedation and emergency drugs and equipment in general dental practice. *J. Dent.* **14**, 247–50.

Smiddy F. G. (1976) *The Medical Management of the Surgical Patient.* London, Arnold.

Smith B. L. and Young P. N. (1976) Day stay anaesthesia. *Anaesthesia* **31**, 181–9.

Sonis S. T., Fazio R., Setkowicz A. et al. (1983) Comparison of the nature and frequency of medical problems among patients in general speciality and hospital dental practices. *J. Oral Med.* **38**, 58–61.

Summers L. (1981) An investigation into the effects of surgical stress on the fit and poor-risk patient including the modifying effects of relative analgesia and B blockade. *Br. J. Oral Surg.* **19**, 3–12.

Suomi J. D., Horowitz H. S. and Barbano J. P. (1975) Self-reported systemic conditions in an adult study population. *J. Dent. Res.* **54**, 1092.

Sykes P. (1980) Should dental practitioners give anaesthetics? *SAAD Digest* **28**, 101–9.

Vessey M. P. and Nunn J. F. (1980) Occupational hazards of anaesthesia. *Br. Med. J.* **281**, 696–8.

Wessberg G. (1978) Role in screening for hypertension in patient management. *J. Am. Dent. Assoc.* **96**, 1040–4.

Wilson I. H., Richmond M. N. and Strike P. W. (1986) Regional analgesia with bupivacaine in dental anaesthesia. *Br. J. Anaesth.* **58**, 401–5.

Young I. V.I. (1975) General anaesthesia for ambulant dental patients. *Br. J. Hosp. Med.* **13**, 441–8.

Appendix to Chapter 1

PROCEDURES FOR SUBMITTING SPECIMENS FOR LABORATORY INVESTIGATIONS

1. Haematology Specimens

Blood for film and red cell indices must be collected into a tube containing potassium EDTA (4 ml into an EDTA; or sequestrene tube). The blood must be gently mixed to ensure that the anticoagulant is well distributed, clotted samples are useless. Blood for assay of corrected whole blood folate levels is also collected in an EDTA tube. Most other necessary investigations are performed on serum.

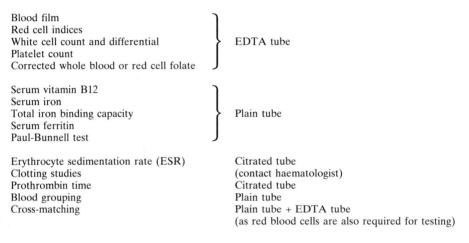

Blood film Red cell indices White cell count and differential Platelet count Corrected whole blood or red cell folate	EDTA tube
Serum vitamin B12 Serum iron Total iron binding capacity Serum ferritin Paul-Bunnell test	Plain tube
Erythrocyte sedimentation rate (ESR)	Citrated tube (contact haematologist)
Clotting studies	
Prothrombin time	Citrated tube
Blood grouping	Plain tube
Cross-matching	Plain tube + EDTA tube (as red blood cells are also required for testing)

2. Biochemistry Specimens

There is currently some variation as to whether serum or plasma are needed for certain biochemical tests depending on the laboratory involved. Special containers may be required for automated multi-channel analysers which give a full biochemical profile on a single blood specimen. However, most biochemical estimations can be carried out on serum (collect blood in a plain container), although plasma (collect in a lithium heparin tube) may be needed for estimation of electrolytes, cortisol and proteins. Blood glucose assays are carried out on a sample in fluoride bottle.

3. Immunology Specimens

Most tests of humoral immunity and complement components are carried out on serum (plain tube). Autoantibodies are determined on serum. In order to prevent the rapid decay of complement components the serum should be separated as soon as possible and frozen at least at –20 °C and preferably at –70 °C. Serum for immune complexes and cryoglobulins may need special handling, details of which can be obtained from the relevant laboratory.

Tests of cell-mediated immunity are expensive and can often only be carried out once special preparations have been made (consult the laboratory).

See *below* for direct immunofluorescence specimens.

4. Histopathology Specimens

A biopsy of adequate size and representative of the lesion should be taken, placed in a fixative such as formol saline, and sent to the pathology laboratory carefully labelled and with the appropriate form of request for histopathological examination.

1. Specimens for routine histological examination: these should be fixed in a 10 per cent formol saline; at least 10 times the volume of the biopsy is needed for adequate fixation.

2. Specimens for immuno fluorescent investigations: these are not usually carried out on formol saline fixed tissue but should be sent for immediate freezing at –70°C and direct immunofluorescence. Serum should also be sent for indirect immunofluorescence.

If tuberculosis or a deep mycosis is suspected a tissue specimen should be sent for culture.

5. Microbiology Specimens

Specimens should be collected before antimicrobials are started. If pus is present a sample should be sent in a sterile container, in preference to a swab. Requests for culture and antibiotic sensitivity should indicate possible aetiology, present antimicrobial therapy and any drug allergies. If tuberculosis is suspected this must be clearly indicated on the request form.

If the microbiological specimen cannot be dealt with within 2 hours, the swab should be placed in transport medium and kept in the refrigerator at 4 °C (not a freezer) until dealt with by the microbiology department.

Actinomycosis: Preferably send pus for culture but in the absence of adequate pus send a dressing that has been for several hours in contact with the wound.

Candidosis: Swabs from the lesions and from the fitting surface of the denture should be sent for culture.

Viral hepatitis or HIV infection: Many centres have defined protocols for the collection of specimens from patients with suspected hepatitis or HIV infection. Particular care must be taken to avoid needlestick injuries and contaminating the outside of the containers and to indicate the hazard of the infection. Special coloured plastic bags (usually red) to indicate this hazard should be used for transporting the specimen.

Other viral infections: Swabs must be sent in viral transport medium: dry swabs are no use. Acute and convalescent serum samples (10 ml blood in plain container) should be taken. The convalescent serum is collected 2–3 weeks after the acute illness.

Syphilis: Oral lesions should be cleaned with saline to remove oral treponemes before a smear is made for dark ground examination: 10 ml of serum should be sent for VDRL testing (Chapter 17) .

GENERAL DENTAL COUNCIL ADDENDUM TO NOTICE FOR THE GUIDANCE OF DENTISTS DATED NOVEMBER 1989

Amendment to the Notice for the Guidance of Dentists approved by the Council at its meeting on 9 May 1989, to replace paragraphs 12 to 16 of the Notice dated May 1988.

General Anaesthesia and Sedation

(1) Where a general anaesthetic is administered, the Council considers that it should be by a person other than the dentist treating the patient, who should remain with the patient throughout the anaesthetic procedure and until the patient's protective reflexes have returned.

(2) This second person should be a dental or medical practitioner appropriately trained and experienced in the use of anaesthetic drugs for dental purposes. As part of a programme of training in anaesthesia, the general anaesthetic may be administered by a dental or medical practitioner under the direct supervision of the said second person.

(3) Where intravenous or inhalational sedation techniques are employed, a suitably experienced practitioner may assume the responsibility of sedating the patient, as well as operating, provided that as a minimum requirement a second appropriate person is present through the procedure. Such an appropriate person might be a suitably trained dental surgery assistant or dental auxillary, whose experience and training enables that person to be an efficient member of the dental team and who is capable of monitoring the clinical condition of the patient. Should the occasion arise he or she should also be capable of assisting the dentist in case of emergency.

(4) For these purposes, the following definition of simple should be understood to apply: ' A technique in which the use of a drug or drugs produces a state of depression of the central nervous system enabling treatment to be carried out, but during which communication is maintained such that the patient will respond to command throughout the period of sedation. The drugs and techniques used should carry a margin of safety wide enough to render unintended loss of consciousness unlikely'.

(5) Neither general anaesthesia nor sedation should be employed unless proper equipment for their administration is used and adequate facilities for the resuscitation of the patient are readily available, with both dentist and staff trained in their use. Resuscitation is very much a matter of skill and timing and dentists must ensure that all those assisting them know precisely what is required of them, should an emergency arise, and that they regularly practise their routine in a simulated emergency against the clock. The Council considers it essential that the equipment necessary for basic life support, including suction apparatus to clear the airway, oral airways to maintain it and positive pressure equipment with appropriate attachments to inflate the lungs with oxygen, must be immediately to hand and ready for use in the operating room.

(6) A dentist who carried out treatment under general anaesthesia or sedation without fulfilling these conditions would almost certainly be considered to have acted in a manner which constitutes serious professional misconduct.

May 1989

Recommendations from the Poswillo Report

(i)   The use of general anaesthesia should be avoided wherever posssible.

(Para 3.8)

(ii)   The same general standards in respect of personnel, premises and equipment must apply irrespective of where the general anaesthetic is administered.

(Para 3.11)

(iii)   Dental anaesthesia must be regarded as a postgraduate subject.

(Para 3.13)

(iv)   All anaesthetics should be administered by accredited anaesthetists who must recognise their responsibility for providing dental anaesthetic services.

(Para 3.14)

(v)   Anaesthetic training should include specific experience in dental anaesthesia.

(Para 3.14)

(vi)   Health authorities should review the provision of Consultant dental anaesthetic sessions to ensure they are sufficient to meet local needs.

(Para 3.16)

(vii)   Doctors and dentists with knowledge, experience and competence sufficient to satisfy the College of Anaesthetists and the Faculty of Dental Surgery be under no detriment.

(Para 3.17)

(viii)   The no detriment arrangements must have been implemented within two years of the publication of this report.

(Para 3.17)

(ix)   The administration of general anaesthesia, in dental surgeries and clinics equipped to the recommended standards of monitoring necessary for patient safety shall continue,

(Paras 3.16 and 3.19)

(x)   An electrocardiogram, a pulse oximeter and a non-invasive blood pressure device are essential for the non-invasive monitoring of a patient under general anaesthesia.

(Para 3.20)

(xi)   A capnograph be used where tracheal anaesthesia is practised.

(Para 3.20)

(xii)   A defibrillator must be available.

(Para 3.21)

(xiii)   Equipment conforming to recognised standards should be purchased and installed, regularly serviced and maintained in accordance with manufacturer's instructions.

(Para 3.21)

(xiv)   General anaesthetic surgeries be subject to inspection and registration.

(Para 3.22)

(xv)   Intravenous agents should be administered via an indwelling needle or cannula which should not be removed until the patient has fully recovered.

(Para 3.25) and (4.15)

(xvi)   Appropriate training must be provided for those assisting the anaesthetist and the dentist.

(Para 3.26)

(xvii)   At no time should the recovering patient be left unattended.

(Para 3.26)

(xviii) Adequate recovery facilities should be available.

(Para 3.26)

(xix) Good contemporaneous records of all treatments and procedures be kept.

(Para 3.30)

(xx) Written consent be obtained on each occasion prior to the administration of a general anaesthetic.

(Para 3.31)

(xxi) Consideration be given to developing a national general anaesthetic/sedation consent form for general dental practitioners.

(Para 3.31)

(xxii) Patients be provided with comprehensive pre and post treatment instructions and advice.

(Para 3.31)

ANTIMICROBIALS*

Erythromycin	Similar antibacterial spectrum to penicillin. Often used for penicillin-allergic patients. Avoid erythromycin estolate which may cause liver disturbance
Erythromycin stearate	Given by mouth, but absorption erratic and unpredictable Useful in those hypersensitive to penicillin Effective against some staphylococci and most streptococci May cause nausea or hearing loss in large doses Rapid development of resistance Reduced dose indicated in liver disease
Clindamycin	Mainly reserved, *as a single dose* for prophylaxis of infective endocarditis in patients allergic to penicillin Given by mouth, very reliably absorbed Mild diarrhoea common Repeated doses may cause pseudomembranous colitis, especially in the elderly and in combination with other drugs
Gentamicin	Reserved for serious infections and prophylaxis of endocarditis Can cause vestibular and renal damage Contraindicated in pregnancy and myasthenia gravis
Metronidazole	Given by mouth Effective only against anaerobes Use only for 7 days (or peripheral neuropathy may develop, particularly in patients with liver disease) Avoid alcohol (disulfiram-type reaction) May increase warfarin effect i.v. preparation available but expensive Avoid in pregnancy
Penicillins Amoxycillin	Given by mouth (absorption better than ampicillin) Broad spectrum (effective against many gram negative bacilli) *Staphylococcus aureus* often resistant Not resistant to penicillinase Contraindicated in penicillin allergy Rashes particularly in infectious mononucleosis, lymphoid leukaemia, or during allopurinol treatment May cause diarrhoea
Augmentin	Mixture of amoxycillin and potassium clavulanate: inhibits some penicillinases and therefore active against most *S. aureus*; also active against some gram-negative bacilli Contraindicated in penicillin allergy

Ampicillin	Less good absorption than amoxycillin otherwise similar. (Many analogues but few advantages) Contraindicated in penicillin allergy
Benzylpenicillin	Given i.m. or i.v. Most effective penicillin when organism sensitive. Not resistant to penicillinase. Contraindicated in penicillin allergy. Large doses may cause K+ to fall. Na+ to rise
Flucloxacillin	Given by mouth Effective against most penicilin-resistant staphylococci Contraindicated in penicillin allergy
Phenoxymethyl penicillin (penicillin V)	Given by mouth Not resistant to penicillinase Contraindicated in penicillin allgery
Procaine penicillin	Depot penicillin Not resistant to penicillinase Contraindicated in penicillin allergy Rarely, psychotic reaction due to procaine
Triplopen	Depot penicillin (benzyl penicillin 300 mg, procaine penicillin 250 mg, and benethamine penicillin (475 mg) Not resistant to penicillinase Contraindicated in pencillin allergy
Rifampicin	Reserved mainly for treatment of tuberculosis May be used in prophylaxis of meningitis after head injury since *N. meningitidis* and *S. aureus* frequently resistant to sulphonamides. Safe and effective but resistance rapidly develops. Body secretions turn red May interfere with oral contraception Occasional rashes, jaundice or blood dyscrasias
Sulphonamides	Main indication is for prophylaxis of post-traumatic meningitis but meningococci increasingly resistant Contraindicated in pregnancy and in renal disease Adequate hydration essential to prevent (rare) crystalluria. Other adverse reactions include rashes, erythema multiforme and blood dyscrasias
Co-trimoxazole (trimethoprim with sulphamethoxazole)	Given by mouth Broad spectrum May be used for sinusitis Occasional rashes or blood dyscrasias Contraindicated in pregnancy or liver disease May increase effect of protein-bound drugs
Teicoplanin	Reserved mainly for endocarditis prophylaxis. Occasional rashes, nausea, fever, anaphylaxis. May cause hearing loss or tinnitus. Reduce dose in renal failure and elderly.
Tetracyclines	Very broad antibacterial spectrum. Little to choose between the many preparations, but doxycycline and minocycline (*see below*) are safer for patients with renal failure. In children, tetracyclines cause dental discoloration. Absorption impaired by iron, antacids, milk, etc. Use of tetracyclines may predispose to candidosis

Tetracycline	Given by mouth Many bacteria now resistant Contraindicated in pregnancy and children up to at least 7 years (tooth discoloration) Reduce dose in renal failure, liver disease and elderly Frequent mild gastrointestinal upsets
Doxycycline	Given by moth in a single daily dose Contraindicated in pregnancy and children up to at least 7 years (tooth discoloration) Safer than other tetracyclines in renal failure Reduce dose in liver disease and elderly Mild gastrointestinal effects
Minocycline	Given by mouth Active against some meningococci Safer than tetracycline in renal disease May cause dizziness and vertigo Absorption not reduced by milk Contraindicated in pregnancy and children up to at least 7 years (tooth discoloration). May also cause mucosal pigmentation
Vancomycin	Reserved for serious infections or prophylaxis of endocarditis, given by slow (60 minutes) i.v. infusion. Extravenous extravasation causes necrosis and phlebitis Effective by mouth for pseudomembranous colitis May cause nausea, rashes, tinnitus, deafness when given i.v. Contraindicated in renal disease or deafness

*Warn patients on the oral contraceptive to use additional precautions if on antimicrobials for more than a single dose.

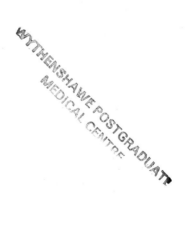

ANALGESICS

Analgesic	Comments	Tablet contains	Route	Adult dose
Aspirin[a]	Mild analgesic Causes gastric irritation Interferes with haemostasis Contraindicated in bleeding disorders, peptic ulcers, children, asthma, late pregnancy, renal disease	300 mg	O	300–600 mg up to 6 times a day after meals (use *soluble* aspirin) with fulid (maximum 4 g daily)
Mefenamic acid[a]	Mild analgesic May be contraindicated in asthma, gastro-intestinal, renal and liver disease, and pregnancy May cause diarrhoea or haemolytic anaemia	250 mg *or* 500 mg	O	250–500 mg up to 3 times a day
Paracetamol	Mild analgesic Hepatotoxic in overdose or prolonged use Contraindicated in liver or renal disease	500 mg	O	500–1000 mg up to 6 times a day (maximum 4 g daily)
Diflunisal[a]	Analgesic for mild to moderate pain Long action Effective against pain from bone or joints Contraindicated in pregnancy, peptic ulcer, allergies, renal and liver disease	250 mg *or* 500 mg	O	250–500 mg twice a day
Ibuprofen[a]	Analgesic for mild to moderate pain Fewer side-effects than other NSAIDs Contraindicated in peptic ulcers, elderly asthmatics, pregnancy, renal and liver disease	200 mg	O	200–400 mg up to 4 times a day after meals
Dihydrocodeine tartrate	Analgesic for moderate pain May cause drowsiness and constipation Contraindicated in children, hypothyroidism, asthma, renal disease	30 mg	O	30 mg up to 4 times a day (*or* 50 mg i.m.)

Drug	Notes		Route	Dose
Buprenophine*	Potent analgesic More potent analgesic than pentazocine, longer action than morphine No hallucinations May cause salivation, sweating, dizziness and vomiting Respiratory depression in overdose. Can cause dependence Contraindicated in children, pregnancy, MAOI†, liver disease or respiratory disease	0.2 mg	Sublingual	0.2–0.4 mg up to 4 times a day (or 0.3 mg i.m.)
Meptazinol	Potent analgesic Claimed to have a low incidence of respiratory depression. Side-effects as buprenorphine	No tablet	i.m. or i.v.	75–100 mg up to 6 times a day
Pentazocine*	Potent analgesic May produce dependence May produce hallucinations May provoke withdrawal symptoms in narcotic addicts Contraindicated in pregnancy, children, hypertension, myocardial infarction, respiratory depression, head injuries or raised intracranial pressure.	25 mg	O	50 mg up to 4 times a day (or 30 mg i.m. or i.v.)
Pethidine*	Potent analgesic Used as alternative to morphine Risk of dependence Contraindicated in head injuries, MAOI†	25 mg	O or i.m. or i.v.	50–100 mg up to 6 times daily

* Controlled drugs
† MAOI = Monoamine oxidase inhibitors
a = NSAID

URINALYSIS: INTERPRETATION OF RESULTS

	Protein	Glucose[†]	Ketones	Bilirubin[‡]	Urobilinogen	Blood[§]
Health	Usually no protein but a trace can be normal in young people	Usually no glucose, but a trace can be normal in 'renal glycosuria' and pregnancy	Usually no ketones, but may be present in vomiting, fasting or starved patient	Usually no bilirubin	Usually present in normal healthy patients, particularly in concentrated urine	Usually no blood
False positives	Alkaline urine Container contaminated with disinfectant, e.g. chlorhexidine. Blood or pus in urine. Polyvinyl pyrrolidone infusions	Cephamandole Container contaminated with hypochlorite	Patients on levodopa or any phthalein compound	Chlorpromazine and other phenothiazines	Infected urine Patients taking ascorbic acid, sulphonamides or paramino-salicylate	Menstruation Container contaminated with some detergents
Diseases	Renal diseases Also cardiac failure, diabetes, endocarditis, myeloma, amyloid, some drugs, some chemicals	Diabetes mellitus[¶] Also in pancreatitis, hyperthyroidism, Fanconi syndrome, sometimes after a head injury, other endocrino-pathies	Diabetes mellitus Also in febrile or traumatized patients on low carbohydrate diets	Jaundice-hepatocellular and obstructive	Jaundice-haemolytic, hepatocellular and obstructive. Prolonged antibiotic therapy	Genitourinary diseases. Also in bleeding tendency, some drugs, endocarditis

*Using test strips, e.g. Ames Reagent Strips or BM-Test-5L. Normal or non-fresh urine may be alkaline; normal urine may be acid. *See also* Zilva J.F. (1985) Br. Med. J. **291**, 323.

†Dopa, ascorbate or salicylates may give false negatives.
‡May be false negative if urine is stale.
§Ascorbic acid may give false negative.
¶A negative result does not exclude diabetes.

INTERPRETATION OF SERUM AND PLASMA BIOCHEMICAL RESULTS

Biochemistry*	Normal range†	Level ↑	Level ↓	Comments on collection‡
Acid phosphatase	0-13 I.U./l	Prostatic malignancy; renal disease; acute myeloid leukaemia	—	Plain tube. Separate serum immediately. Haemolysed blood unsuitable
Alanine transaminase (ALT)	3-60 I.U./l	Liver disease; infectious mononucleosis	—	Plain tube
Alkaline phosphatase	30-116 I.U./l (3-13 KA units)	Puberty; pregnancy; Paget's disease; osteomalacia; fibrous dysplasia; malignancy in bone; liver disease; hyperparathyroidism	Hypothyroidism; hypophosphatasia	Plain tube
Alpha-1-antitrypsin	200-400 mg%	Cirrhosis	Congenital emphysema	Plain tube
Alpha fetoprotein	<12 µg/litre	Pregnancy; gonadal tumour; liver disease. Hepatoma. Neural tube defect in pregnancy	Drop in pregnancy indicates fetal distress	Plain tube
Amylase	70-300 I.U./l	Pancreatic disease; mumps; some other salivary diseases	—	Plain tube
Antistreptolysin 0 titre (ASOT)	0-300 Todd units/ml	Streptococcal infections; rheumatic fever	—	Plain tube
Aspartate transaminase (AST)	30 I.U./l	Liver disease; biliary disease; myocardial infarct; trauma	—	Plain tube
Bilirubin (total)	1-17 µmol/l	Liver disease; biliary disease; haemolysis	—	Plain tube
Caeruloplasmin	1.3-3.0 µmol/l	Pregnancy;cirrhosis; hyperthyroidism; leukaemia	Wilson's disease	Plain tube
Calcium	2.3-2.6 mmol/l (Total calcium)	Hyperparathyroidism; malignancy in bone; renal tubular acidosis; sarcoidosis; thiazides	Hypoparathyroidism; renal failure; rickets; nephrotic syndrome	Plain tube. Collect with tourniquet off. Repeat several times for reliability. Assay albumin as well

INTERPRETATION OF SERUM AND PLASMA BIOCHEMICAL RESULTS (continued)

Biochemistry*	Normal range†	Level ↑	Level ↓	Comments on collection
Cholesterol	3.9–7.8mmol/l	Hypercholesterolaemia; hypothyroidism; diabetes; nephrotic syndrome; liver disease	Malnutrition; hyperthyroidism	Plain tube. Collect fasting sample
Complement (C3)	0.79–1.60 g/l	Trauma; surgery; infection	Liver disease; immune complex diseases, e.g. lupus erythematosus	Plain tube
Complement (C4)	0.2–0.4 g/l	—	Liver disease; immune complex diseases; hereditary angioedema	Plain tube
Cortisol (see steroids)				
Creatine phosphokinase (CPK)	50–100 I.U./l (< 130)	Myocardial infarct; trauma muscle diseases	—	Plain tube. Serum must be separated immediately
Creatinine	0.06–0.11 mmol/l	Renal failure; urinary obstruction	Pregnancy	Plain tube
C reactive protein (CRP)	< 10 µg/ml	Inflammation; trauma; myocardial infarct; malignant disease	—	Plain tube
Cl esterase inhibitor	0.1–0.3 g/l	—	Hereditary angioedema	Plain tube
Ferritin	Adult male 25–190 ng/ml Adult female 15–99 ng/ml Child mean 21 ng/ml	Liver disease; haemochromatosis; leukaemia; lymphoma; other malignancies; thalassaemia	Iron deficiency	Plain tube. Better than assay of serum iron
Fibrinogen	200–400 mg%	Pulmonary embolism; nephrotic syndrome; lymphoma	Disseminated intravascular coagulopathy (DIC)	Plain tube
Folic acid	3–20 µg/litre (red cell folate 120–650 µg/litre)	Folic acid therapy	Alcoholism; dietary deficiency; haemolytic anaemias; malabsorption; phenytoin	EDTA tube
Free thyroxine index (FTI = serum T4 × T3 uptake)	1.3–5.1 U	Hyperthyroidism	Hypothyroidism	Plain tube

Test	Reference range	Raised in	Lowered in	Specimen
Gammaglutamyl transpeptidase (GGT)	15–42 I.U./l	Liver disease; myocardial infarct; pancreatitis, diabetes, renal diseases; tricyclics; alcoholism	—	Plain tube
Globulins (total) (see also under protein)	22–36 g/l	Liver disease; myelomatosis; autoimmune disease; chronic infections	Chronic lymphatic leukaemia; malnutrition; protein-losing states; hereditary immunodeficiency; nephrotic syndrome	Plain tube
Glucose	2.8–5.0 mmol/l	Diabetes mellitus; hyperthyroidism; hyperpituitarism; Cushing's disease; liver disease	Hypoglycaemic drugs; Addison's disease hypopituitarism; hyperinsulinism	Collecting fasting or at least 2 h after meal: special fluoride bottle Yellow top
Hydroxybutyrate dehydrogenase (HBD)	100–250 I.U./l	Myocardial infarct	—	Plain tube
Immunoglobulins Total	7–22 g/l	Liver disease; infection; sarcoidosis; connective tissue disease	Immunodeficiency; nephrotic syndrome; enteropathy	Plain tube
IgG	5–16 g/l	Myelomatosis; connective tissue diseases	Immunodeficiency; nephrotic syndrome	Plain tube
IgA	1.25–4.25 g/l	Alcoholic cirrhosis; Buerger's disease	Immunodeficiency	Plain tube
IgM	0.5–1.75 g/l	Primary biliary cirrhosis; nephrotic syndrome; parasites; infections	Immunodeficiency	Plain tube
IgE	<0.007 mg%	Allergies; parasites	—	Plain tube
Lactic dehydrogenase (LDH)	90–300 I.U./l	Myocardial infarct; trauma; liver disease	—	Plain tube. Unsuitable if blood haemolysed
Lipase	0.2–1.51 I.U./l	Pancreatitis	—	Plain tube
Lipids	50–150 mg% (triglycerides) See also Cholesterol	Hyperlipidaemia; diabetes mellitus; hypothyroidism	—	Plain tube. Collect fasting sample

INTERPRETATION OF SERUM AND PLASMA BIOCHEMICAL RESULTS (continued)

Biochemisry*	Normal range†	Level ↑	Level ↓	Comments on collection
Magnesium	0.7–0.9 mmol/l	Renal failure	Cirrhosis; malabsorption; diuretics; Conn's syndrome; renal tubular defects	Plain tube
5'-Nucleotidase	1–15 I.U./l	Liver disease	—	Plain tube
Phosphate	0.8–1.5 mmol/l	Renal failure; hypoparathyroidism; hypervitaminosis D	Hyperparathyroidism; rickets;malabsorption syndrome;insulin	Plain tube. Collect fasting sample. Separate serum promptly
Potassium	3.5–5.0 mmol/l	Renal failure; Addison's disease Acidosis	Vomiting; diabetes; diarrhoea; Conn's syndrome; diuretics; Cushing's disease; malabsorption	Plain tube. Fresh blood should be sent to laboratory. Haemolysis causes abnormal results
Protein (total)	62–80 g/l	Liver disease; myelomatosis	Nephrotic syndrome; enteropathy; renal failure	Plain tube. Collect fasting sample
Albumin	35–55 g/l	Dehydration	Liver disease; malabsorption; nephrotic syndrome	Plain tube
Alpha 1 globulin	2–4 g/l	Oestrogens	Nephrotic syndrome	Plain tube
Alpha 2 globulin	4–8 g/l	Infections; trauma	Nephrotic syndrome	Plain tube
Beta globulin	6–10g/l	Hypercholesterolaemia; liver disease; pregnancy	Chronic disease	Plain tube
Gamma globulin	6–15 g/l	(see Immunoglobulins)	Nephrotic syndrome; immunodeficiency	Plain tube
Sodium	130–145 mmol/l	Dehydration; Cushing's disease	Oedema; renal failure; Addison's disease	Plain tube
Steroids (corticosteroids)	110–525 nmol/l (14±6 μg%)	Cushing's disease, some tumours	Addison's disease, hypopituitarism	Plain tube. Collect at 0800–0900 h
Thyroxine (T4)	50–138 nmol/l	Hyperthyroidism; pregnancy; contraceptive pill	Hypothyroidism; nephrotic syndrome; phenytoin	Plain tube

Urea	3.3–6.7 mmol/l	Renal failure; dehydration	Liver disease; nephrotic syndrome; pregnancy	Plain tube
Uric acid	0.15–0.48 mmol/l	Gout; leukaemia; renal failure; myelomatosis .	Liver disease; probenecid; allopurinol	Plain tube. Serum must be separated immediately
Vitamin B_{12}	150–800 ng/l	Liver disease; leukaemia	Pernicious anaemia; post-gastrectomy; Crohn's disease; vegans	Plain tube

Note: Values may differ from laboratory to laboratory. For further information – consult Eastham R.D. (1975) *Biochemical Values in Clinical Medicine.* Wright, Bristol. There are many other causes of abnormal results than outlined here.
*See Appendix 4 for haematology.
†Adult levels; always consult your own laboratory.
‡Vacuum tubes.
SI values: 10^{-1} = deci (d); 10^{-2} = centi (c); 10^{-3} = milli (m); 10^{-6} = micro (μ); 10^{-9} = nano (n); 10^{-12} = pico (p); 10^{-15} = femto (f).

ROUTINE CHECKS BEFORE GENERAL ANAESTHESIA OR INTRAVENOUS SEDATION FOR DENTAL TREATMENT

Always check:

1. Patient's name (and hospital number).
2. Nature, side and site of operation.
3. Medical history, *particularly* of cardiorespiratory disease or bleeding tendency.
4. That consent has been obtained in writing from patient or, in a person under 16 years of age, from parent or guardian, and that patient adequately understands the nature of the operation and sequelae.
5. That necessary oral investigations, e.g. radiographs, are available.
6. That patient has had *nothing by mouth, including drugs* for *at least* the previous 4 hours.
7. That patient has emptied the bladder.
8. That patient's dentures have been removed and bridges, crowns and loose teeth have been noted by anaesthetist.
9. That any premedication (and, where indicated, regular medication such as the contraceptive pill, anticonvulsants or antidepressants) has been given but not usually within the previous 4 hours.
10. That anaesthetic and suction apparatus are working satisfactorily and that emergency drugs are available and not date-expired (see Fig. 1.5).
11. That patient is escorted by a responsible adult.
12. That patient has been warned not to drive, operate unguarded machinery, drink alcohol or make important decisions for 24 hours postoperatively.

INSTRUCTIONS TO PATIENTS BEFORE GENERAL ANAESTHETIC OR INTRAVENOUS SEDATION (PREFERABLY IN WRITING)

1. Do not take food or liquids after midnight before a morning appointment, or after a light breakfast at 8 a.m. before an afternoon appointment. In any event a general anaesthetic will NOT be given until at least 4 hours have elapsed since the taking of food or liquid.
2. You must be accompanied by a responsible adult, over the age of 18 years, who will undertake to escort the patient home and remain with them 24 hours after treatment. Such a person must not be accompanied by children under 14 years of age.
3. Do not wear nail varnish or make-up.
4. After a general anaesthetic or sedation *you must not* on the same day:
   – drive a motor vehicle
   – ride a bicycle or motorcycle, even as passenger
   – cook or use unguarded machinery
   – take alcohol
   – take sedative drugs without medical advice
   – make important decisions or sign any documents
5. If you develop a cold before your appointment, please telephone the hospital or dental surgery for advice.

PATIENTS WHO FAIL TO COMPLY WITH THESE SIMPLE SAFETY PRECAUTIONS WILL NOT BE GIVEN A GENERAL ANAESTHETIC OR SEDATION

INSTRUCTIONS TO PATIENTS AFTER TOOTH EXTRACTION (PREFERABLY IN WRITING)

After a tooth has been extracted the socket will usually bleed for a short time. This bleeding stops because a healthy blood clot forms in the tooth socket. These clots are easily disturbed and if this happens bleeding will recur. To avoid disturbance of the clot please follow these instructions:

1. After leaving the hospital or dental surgery do not rinse out your mouth for 24 hours, unless you have been told otherwise by the dentist.
2. Do not disturb the clot in the socket with your tongue or fingers.
3. For the rest of the day take only soft foods.
4. Try not to chew on the affected side for at least 3 days.

5. Avoid unnecessary talking, excitement or exercise for the rest of the day.
6. Do not take alcoholic or very hot drinks for the rest of the day.

If the tooth socket continues to bleed after you have left the surgery, do not be alarmed – much of the liquid which appears to be blood, is saliva. If bleeding persists make a small pad from a clean handkerchief or cotton wool, place over the socket and close the teeth firmly on it. Keep up the pressure for 15–30 minutes. If the bleeding still does not stop, seek dental or medical advice.

SUGGESTIONS FOR THE CARE OF THE MOUTH AFTER TOOTH EXTRACTION

Your tooth socket may heal more quickly if you keep it clean and use hot salt mouth baths, but not until 24 hours after the extraction. Dissolve a teaspoonful of table salt in a tumbler of hot water (about the same temperature as a hot cup of tea). Take a mouthful and tilt your head so that the hot salt water bathes the affected area. After about 15 seconds, spit out and repeat the bathing until you have used the whole tumblerful. If possible, the hot salt water mouth baths should be used three times daily for three days, after meals.

Brush your teeth in the normal way. The affected area can be cleaned by wiping with cotton wool moistened with the hot salt water if it is tender.

Discomfort or mild pain after tooth extraction may be relieved by the pain-killer you would normally use. Paracetamol tablets, one or two every 4 hours, are recommended for adults. Children may take paracetamol syrup, the dose depending on their age (follow instructions on the container).

You should seek the advice of your dentist if you have pain which is severe or persists for more than 24 hours.

Chapter 2

Cardiovascular Disease

Cardiovascular diseases, particularly hypertension and ischaemic heart disease, are the most common causes of death in Britain, the USA and many other countries. There are some millions of ambulant patients with some form of heart disease, treated or untreated. Dental procedures or drugs used in dentistry can aggravate heart disease or possibly even provoke a heart attack. Moreover, a dental procedure can occasionally be the main factor precipitating a potentially lethal form of heart disease, namely infective endocarditis. Myocardial infarction is one of the most serious emergencies that can happen in the dental surgery and is one where the dental surgeon may be able to help save the patient's life.

Heart failure is present when the heart is unable to supply the circulatory demands of the body. Any increase in these demands as a result of tachycardia worsens the problem. At one extreme the person with a failing heart can manage fairly well if exertion is limited but, at the other extreme, established failure causes severe breathlessness even at rest. Failure is usually the result of disease of the heart, but an otherwise normal heart can fail as a consequence of overwork caused by hyperthyroidism or the attempt to oxygenate the tissues in severe anaemia.

Failure is usually progressive but, if adequately treated, may cause few symptoms. Activity is, however, always limited to some degree. Cyanosis and dependent oedema (usually swollen ankles) are prominent signs.

Cardiac arrest is a sudden event in which the heart stops beating. Immediate collapse and (if untreated) death follow within a few minutes. Arrest may follow ventricular fibrillation but the two conditions are not clinically distinguishable.

Patients with heart disease, particularly ischaemic heart disease, are at greatest risk from cardiac arrest. This is important to bear in mind, since awareness of the possibility of arrest may make it possible to start resuscitation immediately.

Shock (peripheral circulatory failure) is the clinical term for hypotension, coldness, pallor and sweating as a result of severe reduction in the circulating volume, because of haemorrhage or other causes. In severe shock, if the circulatory volume is not maintained by, for example, blood transfusion, the heart fails. Shock can also be caused by acute heart failure, typically the result of myocardial infarction, or can occasionally result from anaphylaxis

Ischaemia is a local interruption or reduction of blood supply to a single part. It is especially important when it affects the heart or brain. Ischaemic heart

44

disease is due to occlusion of the coronary arteries (usually by atheroma) and leads to angina pectoris or myocardial infarction, which, if severe, causes acute failure of the whole circulation, loss of cerebral blood supply and often death.

CLINICAL ASPECTS OF CARDIOVASCULAR DISEASE

Common Signs and Symptoms

Serious heart disease is frequently asymptomatic and patients can die suddenly from myocardial infarction in particular, despite never having experienced chest pain or any other symptoms. However, in many cases signs and symptoms can be effectively controlled so that most patients with cardiac disease coming to the dental surgery appear well. Only the drug history may give a clue as to the nature of their illness.

Breathlessness (dyspnoea) or *chest pain* are typical symptoms of cardiovascular disease. Dyspnoea is particularly caused by left-sided heart failure. *Chest pain* is the typical symptom of ischaemic heart disease. Palpitations may be a symptom of dysrhythmia and sudden loss of consciousness can be a sign of a defect in conduction (heart block).

Cyanosis: central cyanosis (seen in the lips or within the mouth) is usually an indication either of cardiac failure or of respiratory disease, or both together in cor pulmonale. It is an indication of gross hypoxia and such patients must not therefore be given a general anaesthetic or sedation in the dental surgery, but should be treated in hospital.

Palpation of the pulse enables a clinician to assess the heart rate, force of contraction and rhythm, disturbances of which may be informative when, for example, a patient loses consciousness or appears to be having a heart attack.

The *blood pressure* measured on only a single occasion can be misleading as it is frequently raised by anxiety. However, a check-up in the surgery may not raise the pressure and the finding of either normal levels (less than 160/95 for a male of 45 or over) or grossly raised levels is informative. In an injured patient a falling blood pressure is also a danger sign which must not be ignored, since it implies a serious complication such as haemorrhage or shock.

The stethoscope is mainly of use to those with experience; even to the cardiologist the differentiation between functional (harmless) murmurs and those caused by cardiac disease may occasionally be difficult. However, absence of heart sounds, a cardinal feature of cardiac arrest, should be instantly detectable with a stethoscope, but absence of pulse is more quickly detected by palpation.

Enlargement of the heart, for example in cardiac failure or hypertension, can be reliably seen in a chest radiograph, while electrocardiography is invaluable for the diagnosis of dysrhythmias and of damage to the myocardium.

TYPES OF CARDIOVASCULAR DISEASE

Organic disease can affect the myocardium, endocardium or pericardium in any combination. Myocardial disease secondary to hypertension or coronary artery

Table 2.1. Causes of heart disease

Organic disease of the heart
1. Myocardial
    (*a*)   Myocardial overload secondary to hypertension or valve disease*
    (*b*)   Coronary (ischaemic) heart disease*
    (*c*)   Cardiomyopathies
2. Endocardial
    (*a*)   Rheumatic heart disease
    (*b*)   Congenital anomalies*
    (*c*)   Infective endocarditis
3. Pericardial
    (*a*)   Pericarditis
    (*b*)   Pericardial effusion
Functional disorders
1. Hypertensive heart disease*
2. Disorders of cardiac control
    (*a*)   Tachycardia
    (*b*)   Bradycardia
    (*c*)   Other dysrhythmias
3. Changes in circulatory volume
    (*a*)   Hypovolaemia (shock syndrome)
    (*b*)   Hypervolaemia (circulatory overload)
    (*c*)   Others
Extra-cardiac disease
1. Anaemia
2. Respiratory disease—cor pulmonale*
3. Hyperthyroidism

---

*Common causes of heart failure.

disease is the most common and important cardiac disease. Functional disorders, where there is no organic disease of the heart itself, can also cause circulatory failure, as in shock (*Table 2.1*).

A variety of common extracardiac diseases can aggravate heart disease, particularly if there is impaired oxygenation, as in severe anaemia.

HEART FAILURE

Heart failure is not a single disease but an effect of many disorders. The common causes are ischaemic heart disease, hypertension, valve disease and chronic obstructive pulmonary disease (*Table 2.1*). Failure can predominantly affect either the left or right side of the heart, but failure of one side usually leads to failure of the other. Heart failure is a common cause of death and patients are poor risks for general anaesthesia.

Left-sided heart failure

Left-sided heart failure is more common than right-sided failure. Causes of left-sided heart failure include:

1. Ischaemic heart disease.
2. Aortic and mitral valvular disease (left-side valves).
3. Hypertension.

Clinically, left-sided failure causes congestion and oedema primarily of the lungs, but function of the brain and kidneys is also impaired. As the left ventricle fails, blood is dammed back in the pulmonary circulation where the venous pressure rises, causing oedema. Pulmonary oedema causes difficulty in breathing (dyspnoea), the most troublesome symptom of left-sided heart failure. Initially, dyspnoea mainly follows effort, but later is present at rest and persists or worsens when lying down (orthopnoea). Coughing is another typical consequence of pulmonary oedema. The sputum is frothy and, in severe cases, pink with blood. Paroxysmal nocturnal dyspnoea (cardiac asthma) is a sudden attack of severe dyspnoea due to pulmonary oedema which wakes the patient from sleep with a terrifying sensation of suffocation. Lying down increases pulmonary congestion and oedema and also makes respiration less efficient, because the abominal viscera move the diaphragm higher and reduce the vital capacity of the lungs. It is obviously dangerous, therefore, to lay a patient with left-sided failure supine during dental treatment.

In the more advanced stages of left-sided heart failure there is inadequate cerebral oxygenation leading to symptoms such as loss of concentration, restlessness and irritability or, in the elderly, disorientation.

Right-sided heart failure

Right-sided failure is often a sequel to left-sided failure, particularly when there is mitral stenosis: the resulting condition is known as congestive cardiac failure. Failure of the right side of the heart alone is uncommon and is most often secondary to chronic obstructive lung disease (cor pulmonale).

In contrast to left-sided failure, pulmonary congestion in right-sided failure is minimal, but congestion of the systemic and portal venous systems predominantly affects the liver, gastrointestinal tract, kidneys and subcutaneous tissues. The liver is usually enlarged due to passive congestion and in severe cardiac failure, increased portal venous pressure also leads to escape of large amounts of fluid into the peritoneal cavity (ascites). Subcutaneous oedema gravitates to dependent parts; ankle oedema is therefore seen in ambulant patients and sacral oedema in patients in bed.

Clinical Aspects of Heart Failure

Obvious signs and symptoms of established cardiac failure include:

1. Breathlessness (dyspnoea).
2. Oedema, particularly of the lower limbs or sacrum, if in bed.
3. Distension of neck veins.
4. Cyanosis.
5. Fatigue.

The pulse may be rapid and irregular, particularly if there is atrial fibrillation, and in extreme cases patients are cyanotic, polycythaemic, dyspnoeic at rest and oedematous as a result of advanced failure beyond the control of drugs.

General Management

The medical treatment typically includes diuretics or drugs to increase cardiac efficiency and treat dysrhythmias and often, a vasodilator.

Dental aspects of heart failure

Elective surgery under general anaesthesia is contraindicated until cardiac failure is under control, but even then should be in hospital. In the controlled patient, treatment under local anaesthesia can safely be carried out providing that consideration is given to the underlying cause of the cardiac failure (*Table 2.1*). Placing the patient supine may increase dyspnoea and should therefore be avoided. Care should be taken after general anaesthesia especially, since there is a predisposition to venous thrombosis and pulmonary embolism. Some of the drugs that may complicate treatment include digitalis (vomiting), procainamide (leucopenia or a lupus-like reaction) or acetazolamide (facial paraesthesia).

HYPERTENSION

Hypertension is a persistently raised blood pressure resulting from increased peripheral arteriolar resistance. Dental management can be complicated, since any procedure causing stress can further raise the blood pressure and may precipitate acute complications such as a cardiac arrest or a cerebrovascular accident. Chronic complications of hypertension, especially impaired renal function, can affect dental management.

The blood pressure is easily measured (by convention in the right arm) with a sphygmomanometer (*Table 2.2*). Since the blood pressure increases with anxiety, measurements should be made with the patient relaxed and fully at rest. In practice, the diagnosis of hypertension is made at an arbitrary point when the blood pressure at rest exceeds 160/95 mmHg (systolic/diastolic), and by this criterion probably over 10 per cent of the population are hypertensive.

Hypertension is secondary to defined diseases, particularly renal or endocrine disorders, in only about 10—20 per cent of cases (*Table 2.3*) and occasionally to the oral contraceptive. The cause is unknown in most cases and the condition is then termed *essential hypertension.*

Table 2.2. Manual technique for recording the blood pressure

1. Seat the patient and allow to rest for as long as possible.
2. Place sphygmomanometer cuff on right upper arm with about 3 cm of skin visible at the antecubital fossa.
3. Palpate radial pulse.
4. Inflate cuff to about 200–250 mmHg, or until the radial pulse is no longer palpable.
5. Deflate cuff slowly while listening with stethoscope over the brachial artery over skin on inside of arm below cuff.
6. Record the systolic pressure as the pressure when the first tapping sounds appear.
7. Deflate cuff further until the tapping sounds become muffled (diastolic pressure).
8. Repeat. Record blood pressure as systolic/diastolic pressures.

Table 2.3. Causes of hypertension

Idiopathic (essential) *hypertension*

Secondary hypertension
1. Renal disease
        Renal artery disease
        Pyelonephritis
        Glomerulonephritis
        Polycystic disease
        Post-transplant
2. Endocrine disease
        Cushing's syndrome
        Hypoaldosteronism
        Phaeochromocytoma
        Acromegaly
3. Cerebral disease
        Cerebral oedema (mainly strokes, head injuries or tumours)
4. Coarctation of aorta (hypertension in upper half of body only)

Essential hypertension becomes more frequent as age advances and genetic influences, obesity, and a variety of other factors can contribute.

About 40 per cent of hypertensive patients have raised levels of circulating catecholamines (adrenaline or noradrenaline) and may therefore have abnormal sympathetic activity. Acute emotion, particularly anger and anxiety, can cause great increases in catecholamine output and transient rises in blood pressure.

Uncomplicated hypertension causes no symptoms and is one of the few diseases in which the diagnosis can be entirely mechanical and quantitative, that is, by means of a sphygmomanometer. Some may live out their lives with a persistently raised blood pressure which has no overt effects but common and important complications are as follows.

Heart disease

Persistent hypertension causes the heart to hypertrophy until it outgrows its blood supply and heart failure may thus result without any other significant complications. However, atheroma (atherosclerosis) of the coronary arteries frequently also develops and this reduces the heart's blood supply even further. A very common result is angina pectoris or myocardial infarction.

Blood vessel disease

In addition to contributing to development of atherosclerosis, hypertension causes thickening of the walls of the arterioles of the kidney and this may lead ultimately to renal failure. Epistaxes may result from the combined effect of the raised blood pressure and weakening of the nasal vessel wall.

Brain damage

Hypertension, particularly when associated with atheroma, is a major cause of strokes, either as a result of haemorrhage into the brain from rupture of an artery or as a result of thrombosis complicating an atheromatous plaque.

Malignant (Accelerated) Hypertension

Malignant hypertension is uncommon: it can have an acute onset or can develop in pre-existing essential hypertension.

Malignant hypertension typically affects young adults and, like essential hypertension, causes no symptoms until complications develop. The chief complication is a severe form of nephrosclerosis with resulting ischaemic damage to the kidneys and renal failure. Facial palsy is an occasional complication.

Rapid deterioration in renal function was a common cause of death which, in the absence of treatment, often followed within a year of diagnosis. However, vigorous treatment , if started before renal damage is too far advanced can greatly improve the expectation of life. About 50 per cent of such patients can now expect to live for at least 5 years.

Other causes of death are cardiac failure or cerebrovascular accidents.

General management

Lifelong treatment is usually necessary, even for mild hypertension. Weight loss, a reduction in salt intake and increased exercise are beneficial. Smoking should be stopped as it increases the risks of ischaemic heart disease, and alcohol consumption should be limited. Diuretics are usually the first line of drug treatment, but may occasionally cause hypokalaemia in the elderly. A beta–blocker is the usual first choice of additional drugs if these measures fail. Antihypertensive agents currently used are shown in *Table 2.4*. Side-effects can be sometimes be troublesome and antihypertensive treatment has to be tailored to each patient's response and the optimal result, in terms of lowering blood pressure with the least adverse effects, may require a combination of drugs.

Dental aspects

There are no recognized oral manifestations of hypertension but antihypertensive drugs can sometimes cause side-effects (*Table 2.4*), such as xerostomia, salivary gland swelling or pain, lichenoid reactions, gingival hyperplasia, sore mouth or paraesthesiae.

Blood pressure tends to rise during oral surgery under local anaesthesia, but this is usually of little practical importance. By contrast, dangerous *hypotension* can result from potentiation of hypotensive drugs by general anaesthetic agents. However, antihypertensive drugs should not be stopped, as rebound hypertension can result. The management of such patients should therefore be in the hands of specialist anaesthetists in hospital.

Table 2.4. Important antihypertensive drugs (apart from diuretics)

	Possible oral effects	Other comments snd side effects
BETA ADRENO-RECEPTOR BLOCKERS		
Propranolol	Dry mouth	May cause bronchospasm
Acebutolol	Lichenoid	Contraindicated in asthma
Atenolol	lesions	Avoid in heart failure
Bextaxolol	Paraesthesiae	or heart block
Bisoprolol	with labetalol	Muscle weakness
Labetalol		Lassitude
Metoprolol		Disturbed sleep
Nadolol		
Oxprenolol		
Pembutolol		
Pindolol		
Sotalolol		
Timolol		
VASODILATORS		
Hydralazine		Headache
		May cause hypertrichosis
Minoxidil		Oedema
ANGIOTENSIN-CONVERTING ENZYME INHIBITORS		
Captopril	Sinusitis with quinapril. Loss	1st dose may cause sudden fall in blood pressure
Enalapril	of taste with	May impair renal
Lisinopril	enalapril. Burning	function especially if NSAIDs
Perindopril	sensation or ulceration	also given
Quinapril	or loss of taste	Cough
Ramipril	with captopril	
CALCIUM CHANNEL BLOCKERS		
Amlodipine	Salivation with	Headache and flushing
Diltiazem	nicardipine.	fairly common.
Isradipine	Gingival hyperplasia	Swollen legs
Nicardipine	possible with	
Nifedipine	diltiazem,	
Nomodipine	nifedipine,	
Verapamil	verapamil	

Postural hypotension. An important side-effect of some antihypertensive drugs is a tendency to produce acute postural hypotension. Raising the patient suddenly from the supine position may therefore cause loss of consciousness.

General anaesthesia. All antihypertensive drugs are potentiated by general anaesthetic agents, especially barbiturates, and by opioids for premedication; severe hypotension can result. A severely reduced blood supply to vital organs can be dangerous even in a normal person, but in the chronically hypertensive patient the tissues have become adapted to the raised blood pressure which becomes essential (hence the term 'essential hypertension') to overcome the resistance of the vessels and maintain adequate perfusion. A fall in blood pressure below the critical level needed for adequate perfusion of vital organs, particularly kidneys, can therefore be fatal.

Though mild hypertension is not a contraindication to general anaesthesia, the latter may be hazardous if there are any of the following:

1. Severe hypertension.
2. Cardiac failure.
3. Coronary or cerebral artery insufficiency.
4. Renal insufficiency.

When a general anaesthetic is given, the risks of cerebrovascular accidents and cardiovascular instability that result from withdrawal of antihypertensive medication and rebound hypertension, outweigh the dangers of drug interactions which to some extent are predictable and manageable by an expert anaesthetist. Antihypertensive treatment is usually therefore maintained, but the management of such patients is a matter for the specialist anaesthetist.

Intravenous barbiturates in particular can be dangerous in patients on antihypertensive therapy, but halothane, enflurane and isoflurane may also cause hypotension in patients on beta-blockers. In practice, therefore, the severe (BP over 200/150) or elderly hypertensive, whether on hypotensive treatment or not, should not be given a general anaesthetic in the dental surgery. Patients with hypertension are best treated under local anaesthesia. Local anaesthetics with adrenaline (up to four cartridges) are safe and unlikely to cause trouble.

Chronic administration of some diuretics such as frusemide may lead to potassium deficiency and thereby predispose to dysrhythmias and increased sensitivity to muscle relaxants such as curare, gallamine and pancuronium. Frusemide should therefore be discontinued a few days before a general anaesthetic is given.

Dental management. The anxiety associated with dental treatment typically causes a rise in blood pressure and may rarely precipitate cardiac arrest or a cerebrovascular accident. Preoperative reassurance is therefore important and sedation may be helpful. Patients are best treated in the morning and given short appointments only. Though its benefits are unproven, an aspirating syringe may be used to give a local anaesthetic, since adrenaline given intravenously may (theoretically) increase hypertension and precipitate dysrhythmias. The management of hypertensive patients may also be complicated by the underlying disease (*Table 2.3*) or others such as cardiac or renal failure. Systemic corticosteroids may raise the blood pressure and antihypertensive treatment may have to be adjusted accordingly.

CORONARY (ISCHAEMIC) HEART DISEASE

Ischaemic heart disease (IHD) is the result of progressive myocardial ischaemia due to persistently reduced coronary blood flow, usually because of atherosclerosis (atheroma). Hypertension is a major contributory factor.

Coronary heart disease affects at least 20 per cent of adult males under 60 years and increasingly thereafter. In Western populations atheroma may affect up to 45 per cent of young adult males and ischaemic heart disease accounts for about 35 per cent of total mortality in Britain and the United States. It is a disease predominantly of males particularly of affluent societies. There is a genetic component in some but more commonly, smoking, hypertension, lack of exercise and possibly consumption of too much saturated (animal and dairy) fat are contributory. Nevertheless immigrants from the Indian subcontinent have a higher than average morbidity and mortality from coronary heart disease despite a lower fat diet and cigarette consumption than the rest of the population.

There is an increased incidence of IHD in the hyperlipoproteinaemias, diabetes mellitus and hypothyroidism.

IHD itself causes no symptoms but impaired coronary blood flow causes progressive damage to the heart, can go on to cardiac failure and can cause dysrhythmias. Usually the first signs of IHD are its dramatic complications, namely angina pectoris or myocardial infarction without warning or history of heart disease. Angina pectoris and myocardial infarction, the main acute manifestations of IHD, have many features in common but there are also important differences.

First, both diseases are the result of ischaemia and are common. The blood supply to the myocardium is chronically reduced but additional factors are involved in precipitating the acute attack. Second, chest pain is more severe and persistent in myocardial infarction. Third, angina (unlike myocardial infarction) is reversible and the pain is typically controlled by rest. Nevertheless, angina is typically followed sooner or later by myocardial infarction. Fourth, myocardial infarction leads to irreversible cardiac damage or sudden death.

Angina Pectoris

Angina pectoris is the name given to paroxysms of severe ischaemic chest pain which are typically precipitated by effort and relieved by rest. The usual cause of angina is coronary atherosclerosis. Arterial spasm or reduced filling of the coronary arteries can contribute or, occasionally, are responsible alone.

The most common precipitating cause of angina is physical exertion, particularly in cold weather. Emotion, especially anger or anxiety, can also induce attacks and some patients who can tolerate moderate exercise are vulnerable to angina when emotionally stressed.

The pain of angina is often unmistakable and described as a sense of strangling or choking. Tightness, heaviness, compression or constriction of the chest may be complaints but the pain is rarely of the unbearable, crushing and persistent nature of myocardial infarction. The typical site is behind the sternum radiating to the left particularly, sometimes to the left upper arm and occasionally to the left mandible or rarely to the teeth, tongue or palate.

Although the pain of angina can be relieved by rest it is more quickly relieved by giving nitrates, such as glyceryl trinitrate, which lower peripheral resistance and reduce the oxygen demands of the heart.

Patients who develop angina often have no history of heart disease. They may then have repeated attacks of angina over a long period or have a myocardial infarct soon after the first one or two attacks. The mortality rate in angina is about 4 per cent per year. The prognosis depends on the degree of coronary artery narrowing and is therefore highly variable and unpredictable. Angina occasionally remits spontaneously, but most patients need treatment with beta-blockers or glyceryl trinitrate. Artery or vein bypass grafts may be used to increase the coronary flow when angina fails to respond to drugs.

Although the typical picture of angina has been described, there are many patients who have painless acute myocardial ischaemia as shown by arteriography and the ECG changes in response to exercise.

In an experiment to assess whether those who had painless myocardial ischaemia were hyposensitive to pain, electrical pulp stimulation was used as an objective measure of response to pain. In a study on 108 patients with proven coronary artery disease, 71 per cent of those who had painless exercise–induced ischaemia had no discomfort from maximal stimulation. By contrast, over 80 per cent of patients who had exercise–induced angina had intense pain from maximal electrical pulp stimulation.

These findings suggest that the majority of those who suffer acute but painless myocardial ischaemia have hyposensitivity to pain.

Dental aspects

A study in Finland found that patients with IHD had more severe dental caries and periodontal disease than the general population, but whether these infections bear any causative relationship to the heart disease or whether they share some aetiological factor remains speculative.

Angina is a rare cause of pain in the mandible, teeth or other oral tissues, as mentioned earlier. Before dental treatment, patients with angina should be reassured and possibly sedated with oral diazepam but prophylactic administration of glyceryl trinitrate may be more effective. If angina follows dental attention, the patient should be given his usual medication (usually glyceryl trinitrate) before treatment is started. In any event the vasodilator should be readily available for use as required. Other medication, such as propranolol, should not be interfered with.

If a patient experiences chest pain, dental treatment must be stopped and if there is a history of angina, he should be given glyceryl trinitrate 0.5 mg sublingually and oxygen, and be kept sitting upright. The pain should be relieved in 2–3 minutes; the patient should then rest and be accompanied home. If chest pain is not relieved within about 2 minutes, myocardial infarction is the probable cause (*see below*).

For anything but minor treatment under local anaesthesia, the physician should be consulted and consideration should be given to any other complicating factors such as beta-blocker therapy, hypertension or cardiac failure.

General anaesthesia should be deferred for at least 3 months in patients with recent onset angina, unstable angina or recent development of bundle branch block, and in any case, it should be given in hospital. Intravenous barbiturates are particularly dangerous.

Patients with bypass grafts do not require antibiotic cover against infective endocarditis.

Myocardial Infarction

Myocardial infarction (often called a coronary thrombosis or heart attack) is the most severe and lethal form of coronary heart disease. Between 30 and 50 per cent of patients die within the first hour after the attack and a further 10–20 per cent within the next few days.

Fewer than 50 per cent of patients have any premonitory symptoms, but over 30 per cent may have warnings such as a change in the character of anginal pain or indigestion-like pain.

The pain may start either at rest or during activity, is typically unbearably severe and terrifying in character, is unrelieved by rest or nitrates, and can persist for hours if death does not supervene. Vomiting, facial pallor, sweating, restlessness and apprehension are common. Other features may include breathlessness, cough and loss of consciousness, but the clinical picture is variable. A significant number of patients have silent (painless) infarctions and as discussed earlier, this may be due to hyposensitivity to pain, including dental pain.

The pain is felt in the chest but can radiate to the same sites as angina. On rare occasions pain is felt in the left mandible alone. In about 10 per cent of cases pain is slight or even absent and the first signs of a myocardial infarct may then be the sudden onset of left ventricular failure, shock, loss of consciousness, or death. Characteristic electrocardiographic (EGG) changes and the release of heart muscle enzymes into the blood confirm the diagnosis.Severe disorders of rhythm are common and may be fatal.

Sudden cardiac death

Death soon after the onset of chest pain is common: less often there is sudden cardiac death characterized by immediate collapse without premonitory symptoms and loss of pulses. In such cases the precipitating event is a severe dysrhythmia such as ventricular fibrillation. Nevertheless, immediate cardiopulmonary resuscitation can be life-saving. The fact that at least 50 per cent of survivors of such attacks have no evidence (from the EGG or serum creatinine phosphokinase, lactic dehydrogenase and aspartate transaminase levels) of damage to the myocardium, suggests that sudden cardiac death is not the same as a myocardial infarct.

Diagnosis and management

The onset of myocardial infarction is usually obvious from the clinical features (*Table 2.5*). Nausea and vomiting are common.

The patient should be kept at rest, reassured as well as possible and given oxygen by a face mask. Morphine, 10 mg, preferably by slow intravenous injection (2 mg/min) or up to 15 mg i.m. according to the size of the patient, alternatively, nitrous oxide with at least 28 per cent oxygen, should be given to relieve pain. Pentazocine is contraindicated as it can cause dysphoria and raises pulmonary arterial pressure. An ambulance should be called. Ventricular fibrillation is an important cause of death, but controllable by defibrillation. Nearly 50 per cent of deaths are in the first hour. If there is cardiac arrest the patient

Table 2.5. Myocardial infarction—diagnosis

1. Changes in heart rate
2. Dysrhythmias
3. Hypotension
4. Shock
5. Fever and leucocytosis
6. ECG changes
7. Rise in serum enzymes

must be given external cardiac massage and oxygen or mouth-to-mouth ventilation (Chapter 18). Thrombolytic agents may be indicated.

Prevention or reducing the risks from myocardial infarction include stopping smoking, low fat intake, more exercise and aspirin 75 mg daily or 300 mg on alternate days. Such are the complexities of prostaglandin metabolism and the difficulties in interpreting clinical trials, that though the antiplatelet effect of aspirin is agreed to be valuable, there is, as yet, no consensus as the optimal dose. The smaller dose may be less likely to cause gastric upset and *may* be more effective. Beta–blockers, particularly atenolol or metoprolol given intravenously in the acute phase can lessen mortality and oral propranolol or timolol, in the convalescent stage can reduce the risk of recurrence after a myocardial infarct, but such drugs are contraindicated for patients with asthma or in heart failure.

Dental aspects

The severity of a myocardial infarct is suggested by the resulting disability, by the length of the acute illness and whether or not the patient was hospitalized. Nevertheless it is important to consult the patient's physician before undertaking operative treatment. General anaesthesia is contraindicated after a recent myocardial infarct, but the risk decreases with time. The incidence of myocardial infarction after general anaesthesia in patients with documented preoperative infarcts is up to eight times that of patients with no previous history. Nearly 30 per cent of patients having a general anaesthetic within 3 months of an infarct have another in the first postoperative week and at least 50 per cent die. The prognosis of recurrent infarction is also influenced by the time after the first attack; elective surgery under general anaesthesia should therefore be postponed for at least 3 months and preferably a year. General anaesthesia should not be administered in the general dental surgery but, if essential, must be given by a specialist anaesthetist in hospital.

Simple emergency dental treatment under local anaesthesia may be given during the first 3 months after a myocardial infarct. Treatment under local anaesthesia should be carried out with care to avoid excess dosage and intravenous injection, and anything that might cause undue anxiety. Prilocaine with felypressin is frequently advocated but there is no evidence that it is safer than lignocaine with adrenaline which is a more effective local anaesthetic. Thrombolytic agents can produce a bleeding tendency (Chapter 3).

The management of myocardial infarction as an emergency in the dental surgery is along the lines mentioned in the previous section and summarized in

Chapter 18. Pentazocine is less effective than morphine even when given by injection but, worse, does not relieve or may even increase anxiety. Pentazocine can also increase the load on the heart to an undesirable degree: it is also now a Controlled Drug and is therefore no easier to obtain or store than morphine.

Heart block resulting from damage to the conduction tissues by an infarct may necessitate insertion of a cardiac pacemaker and result in other complications, as discussed later.

Other Causes of Chest Pain

Angina or myocardial infarction are the main possible causes to bear in mind, but other causes are listed in *Table 2.6*.

Kawasaki's disease

Kawasaki's disease (mucocutaneous lymph node syndrome) is now a considerably more common cause of severe childhood heart disease in Britain than rheumatic fever. Though considerably more prevalent in Japan, over 100 cases a year are recognized in the UK. The most important complication is cardiac involvement and the overall mortality is 5–10 per cent. The cause is unknown and though an infection is suspected no agent has been consistently isolated.

The ages affected range from 7 weeks to 8 years and males preponderate in a ratio of more than 2 to 1. The main clinical features are (i) fever lasting at least 5 days, (ii) erythema and oedema of the extremities, (iii) a polymorphous rash, (iv) mucosal erythema, (v) cervical lymphadenopathy, and (iv) conjunctival injection. There are cardiac complications in approximately 25 per cent of cases.

Cardiac damage is the result of vasculitis which may result in coronary artery aneurysm formation and myocardial infarction. Other complications include 'extreme misery' in many cases or, less commonly, aseptic meningitis or encephalopathy, arthritis or arthralgia, abdominal pain, diarrhoea or vomiting, and hepatosplenomegaly. The majority have leucocytosis and thrombocytosis but a few have normochromic normocytic anaemia, leucopenia or thrombocytopenia.

Table 2.6. Causes of acute chest pain

Cause	Features	Predisposing factors
Myocardial infarction	Severe persistent crushing retrosternal pain possibly radiating to left arm. Unrelieved by glyceryl trinitrate. May be nausea or vomiting	Coronary heart disease Hypertension
Angina pectoris	Retrosternal pain possibly radiating to left arm. Often previously experienced. Relieved in 3 minutes by glyceryl trinitrate	Coronary heart disease Hypertension
Oesophagitis	Low retrosternal pain on lying down or stooping. Improved by antacids	Hiatus hernia
Anxiety (Hyperventilation syndrome)	Anxious patients with precordial pain Overbreathing, panic and precordial pain	Stress

Diagnosis and management

Echocardiography should be carried out on suspicion and repeated at least at 14–21 days, 60 days and 12 months after the onset.

Aspirin (80–100 mg/kg daily) should be started within 10 days of onset and supplemented with intravenous gammaglobulin, 400 mg/kg daily for 4 days. In the convalescent stage (after the 14th day if the child is afebrile), aspirin 3–5 mg/kg daily should be continued for 6–8 weeks then stopped if there is no coronary artery disease on echocardiography.

Dental aspects

Characteristic oral changes are a strawberry tongue, labial oedema or cracking of the lips, pharyngitis and oropharyngeal erythema. Cervical lymphadenopathy is also common and usually unilateral but occasionally massive. Facial palsy is sometimes seen. It is self–limiting but usually associated with cardiovascular involvement.

Any infant or young child with these features and particularly if there is also a desquamating rash on the extremities should be immediately referred to a paediatric cardiologist for investigation.

THE CARDIOMYOPATHIES

Cardiomyopathy is disease of the myocardium other than that caused by hypertension, ischaemia, valve disease or cor pulmonale. There are many causes of cardiomyopathy, but all except alcoholic heart muscle disease are uncommon.

Alcoholic Heart Muscle Disease

Chronic overindulgence in alcohol can damage both skeletal and cardiac muscle. The incidence of alcoholic heart disease appears to be higher still in those with sickle cell trait.

The clinical effects of alcoholism on the heart are variable but may cause precordial pain and palpitations, dysrhythmias or pulmonary hypertension and right ventricular failure. Sudden unexpected death (probably caused by ventricular fibrillation) appears to be relatively common among young alcoholics.

Moderate social drinking (1 or 2 glasses of wine a day), by contrast, may be associated with a lower than average mortality from myocardial infarction.

Dental aspects (*see* Chapter 19)

Hypertrophic Cardiomyopathy (Idiopathic Hypertrophic Subaortic Stenosis: IHSS)

This is regarded as a rare disease but may frequently pass unrecognized. Hypertrophic cardiomyopathy is characterized by hypertrophy of the septum and wall of the left ventricle causing progressive obstruction to its filling and outflow. Congestive cardiac failure with atrial fibrillation can result or alternatively, there may be angina, sudden death or infective endocarditis.

Congestive Cardiomyopathy

This is probably the most common form of idiopathic cardiomyopathy in Britain but is even more difficult to recognize than the hypertrophic type.

The essential features are weakening and distension of the left ventricle, valvular regurgitation and progress to failure of both ventricles.

Dental aspects of idiopathic cardiomyopathies

Patients are at risk from infective endocarditis and are a poor risk for general anaesthesia because of dysrhythmias, cardiac failure, or myocardial ischaemia. Frequently, however, a patient is unaware of a cardiomyopathy until complications develop.

Infantile supravalvular subaortic stenosis may be associated with hypercalcaemia and a characteristic elfin facies (Chapter 11).

DYSRHYTHMIAS (ARRHYTHMIAS)

Disturbances of heart rhythm or gross disturbances of heart rate are usually caused by lesions of the sino-atrial or atrioventricular nodes, or of the conducting tissues. Most dysrhythmias reduce cardiac efficiency and cardiac output. Atrial fibrillation is the most common cardiac dysrhythmia.

Tachycardia: Tachycardia (abnormally rapid heart rate) increases the load on, and oxygen consumption of the heart. It can cause serious complications, especially if associated with IHD, and can be fatal. Sinus tachycardia is a normal response to exercise or fear but can also result from diseases such as hyperthyroidism.

Atrial tachycardia is often paroxysmal, of unknown cause and produces no more than palpitations in a normal person. If severe, atrial tachycardia can impair ventricular filling and breathlessness or fainting. In the presence of heart disease, it can cause ischaemic pain or cardiac failure.

Ventricular tachycardia—a rate above about 140 per minute is usually the result of IHD or digitalis overdosage. Myocardial pain or cardiac failure are typical consequences, but ventricular fibrillation may follow.

Bradycardia: A slow heart rate may be unimportant in a young person and is often found in athletes. A rate below about 60 per minute in an elderly person, especially when associated with heart disease, can cause sudden loss of consciousness (syncope).

In *sick sinus syndrome* the pacemaking function of the sino-atrial node becomes severely disturbed, with a variety of possible effects such as bradycardia, sino-atrial block, atrial tachycardia or atrial fibrillation. If there is sino-atrial block there is also dysrhythmia and in severe cases, consciousness can be lost.

Atrial fibrillation: Atrial fibrillation is characterized by totally uncoordinated and ineffectual contractions. Common causes of atrial fibrillation are congestive cardiac failure, ischaemic or rheumatic heart disease, or thyrotoxicosis. The effects of atrial fibrillation are impaired ventricular filling and an irregular, but usually rapid, ventricular rate. Thrombi may form in the atrium and can release emboli, for example to the brain. Anticoagulants may therefore be needed. Atrial fibrillation can also cause heart failure.

Ventricular fibrillation: Ventricular fibrillation results in complete failure of cardiac output and is typically fatal within a few minutes. It is the most serious type of dysrhythmia and the most common cause of sudden death. Ventricular fibrillation is often a consequence of myocardial infarction or, occasionally, thyrotoxicosis, halothane anaesthesia, or adrenaline or digitalis overdosage and is a cause of sudden death in cocaine addicts.

Disorders of conduction (heart block): These result from blocking of the cardiac impulse anywhere in the conduction system. Among the more common causes of conduction defects are IHD, drugs, especially digitalis and in the past, rheumatic fever.

Mild heart block may only be detectable on an EGG. In complete heart block the ventricle contracts at its intrinsic rate of about 30–40 per minute. The result is severely reduced cardiac output with pallor or cyanosis and syncopal attacks (Stokes–Adams attacks).

Extrasystoles: These are the most common type of intermittent dysrhythmia and give rise to the well-known sensation of a missed heart beat. Extrasystoles are usually of no significance and are abolished by exercise in normal persons.

General management

Many extraventricular tachycardias can be managed with beta-blockers, digitalis or other anti-dysrhythmic drugs. Patients with atrial fibrillation may also be given anticoagulants to reduce the risk of embolic complications. Patients with heart block may need to have a pacemaker inserted.

Dental aspects

The probability of developing dangerous dysrhythmias with general anaesthesia is increased if there is a significant preoperative dysrhythmia.

Dysrhythmias can be induced by anaesthetic agents, especially halothane (isoflurane is safer); by manipulation of the neck, carotid sinus or eyes (vagal-reflex); and by preoperative digitalization. The risk is greater in the elderly and those with coronary artery disease or aortic stenosis.

Syncope may be the result of bradycardia, heart block or atrial tachycardia, and may be recognized by the slowness or irregularity of the pulse. It may need to be distinguished from a simple fainting attack by these means. Otherwise the initial treatment is the same.

Ventricular fibrillation is clinically indistinguishable from asystole and is one of the most serious emergencies that may have to be managed in the dental surgery (*see* Chapter 18).

Several anti–dysrhythmic drugs can cause oral lesions. Verapamil, enalapril and diltiazem may cause gingival hyperplasia, some beta-blockers may rarely cause lichenoid ulceration and procainamide can cause a lupus–like reaction.

Cardiac pacemakers. Pacemakers generate impulses to regulate the cardiac rhythm when there is absence of spontaneous cardiac rhythm. They operate either at a fixed rate (asynchronous mode) or only on demand (synchronous). High frequency, external electromagnetic radiation can interfere with the sensing function of the pacemaker and may induce fibrillation in these patients. The chief hazards are electrosurgery and diathermy. Ultrasonic scalers, pulp testers, dental induction casting machines, belt-driven motors in dental chairs, microwave ovens and even television transmitters and faulty or badly earthed equipment *may* cause interference, but the risk is very small. The leakage of current when an instrument is in the patient's mouth may be so small as to be imperceptible to the operator but nevertheless can affect the pacemaker. Equipment emitting high frequency radiation may induce fibrillation in such patients.

The only safe procedure under such circumstances is to avoid the use of all such equipment whenever a patient with a pacemaker is being treated, as it is difficult to assess the level of risk in any individual patient. Patients should be treated in the supine position; electrical equipment kept over 30 cm away; and repetitive switching of electrical instruments avoided.

If a pacemaker shuts off, all possible sources of interference should be switched off and the patient given cardiopulmonary resuscitation in the supine position. Artificial respiration should force the heart to resume its rhythm and the pacemaker to start up again.

Unless a cardiac valve lesion is also present, patients with pacemakers do not need antibiotic cover to prevent endocarditis.

THYROID-RELATED HEART DISEASE

Hyperthyroidism raises the metabolic rate and activity of the heart, and sensitizes the myocardium to sympathetic activity. The heart has also to meet the increased demands resulting from the raised metabolic activity of the rest of the body.

Untreated thyrotoxicosis causes tachycardia and a tendency to dysrhythmias which can lead to cardiac failure or myocardial infarction, especially in the elderly. Beta-blockers are particularly useful.

Hypothyroidism slows the metabolic rate and activity of the heart and other tissues. In myxoedema, however, patients have hypercholesterolaemia associated with atherosclerosis. IHD (angina or myocardial infarction) often develops but is unusual in that it predominantly affects women.

Dental aspects

The same reservations about general anaesthesia apply to patients with uncontrolled hyperthyroid heart disease as to those with other dangerous heart diseases but sedation with diazepam should be beneficial. It has also been said that local anaesthetics containing adrenaline should be avoided because of the possible risk of dangerous dysrhythmias. There seems, however, scant confirmatory clinical evidence and the risk is probably only theoretical if overdose of local anaesthetics is avoided. However, some prefer to use prilocaine with felypressin but there is no evidence that it is any safer.

Patients with uncontrolled hyperthyroidism can sometimes be difficult to manage, as a result of heightened anxiety, hyperexcitability and increased sympathetic activity. Sedation may therefore be particularly desirable.

Hypothyroid patients may be at risk in the dental surgery if they have IHD. Sjögren's syndrome is rarely associated with hypothyroidism in spite of the fact that antithyroid auto-antibodies are relatively commonly found in the former.

In severe myxoedema, diazepam and other CNS depressants can precipitate coma.

COR PULMONALE

Cor pulmonale is the term given to heart disease resulting from the excessive load imposed on the right ventricle by chronic obstructive airways disease (Chapter 6). The essential features are right ventricular hypertrophy leading to right-sided failure, systemic venous congestion and persistent hypoxia. In the early stages there is dyspnoea, a chronic cough, wheezing and often cyanosis. Right-sided cardiac failure, which may be precipitated by intercurrent respiratory infection, causes more severe dyspnoea and cyanosis, together with oedema of the ankles and ascites.

Dental aspects

Under no circumstances should patients with cor pulmonale be given a general anaesthetic other than in hospital. Intravenous barbiturates are completely contraindicated and even diazepam is dangerous because of its respiratory depressant effect in these hypoxic patients.

ACUTE RHEUMATIC FEVER

Rheumatic fever is a disease which sometimes follows a sore throat caused by certain strains of beta–haemolytic streptococci (*S. pyogenes*). The inflammatory changes appear to result from cross-reactivity with some of the streptococcal antigens and immunologically-mediated tissue damage.

The chief importance of rheumatic fever was that, particularly in the past, it could lead, after the lapse of years, to chronic rheumatic heart disease as a result of fibrosis and distortion of the valves.

Rheumatic fever is now a very rare disease in the Western world and even among the few that are attacked, permanent cardiac damage hardly ever follows. In recent years, a few cases have appeared in the US and Britain, but there appears to be no major resurgence of the disease. It also appears to have

Table 2.7. Criteria of diagnosis of rheumatic fever

Major	Minor
Carditis	Pyrexia
Polyarthritis	Arthralgia
Chorea	Previous rheumatic fever
Erythema marginatum	ESR$\uparrow$ C-reactive protein$\uparrow$
Subcutaneous nodules	Characteristic ECG changes

changed in character. By contrast, in countries such as the Indian subcontinent and some of the Caribbean islands, rheumatic fever is common and is relatively quickly followed by permanent heart disease.

Children between 5 and 15 years are predominantly affected. In typical cases a sore throat is followed after about 3 weeks (2–26 weeks) by an acute febrile illness with pain flitting from one joint to another. The clinical manifestations are so variable, however, that the diagnosis should not be made unless at least two of the major criteria (*Table 2.7*) are fulfilled.

Preceding streptococcal infection is confirmed by a high or rising titre of antistreptolysin O (ASOT), and is suggestive, but not diagnostic of rheumatic fever and a low ASOT virtually excludes the diagnosis.

The duration of the disease is usually from 6 to 12 weeks and in the great majority of cases there is resolution without apparent after-effects.

Any cardiac tissue can be affected but the most serious feature is subendocardial inflammation, particularly along the lines of closure of the valve cusps, resulting in the formation of minute fibrinous vegetations. The mitral and aortic valves are particularly affected. There is usually little detectable effect on cardiac function in the acute phase of the disease but, in unusually severe cases, myocarditis can cause death from cardiac failure.

Pain in the large joints (which gives rheumatic fever its name) is conspicuous, but heals without permanent damage in about 3 weeks.

Other features are cerebral involvement causing spasmodic involuntary movements (Sydenham's chorea, St Vitus' dance), a characteristic rash (erythema marginatum), lung involvement and subcutaneous nodules, usually forming around the elbows.

General management

Treatment consists principally of the use of salicylates for arthritis and penicillin if streptococcal infection is still active. Complications such as cardiac failure are treated along conventional lines.

Prompt antimicrobial treatment (within 24 hours of onset) of a streptococcal sore throat prevents the development of rheumatic fever in most cases. After an attack, there is a risk of recurrence and continuous antibiotic prophylaxis becomes necessary to lessen the risk of permanent cardiac damage. The drug of choice in Britain is oral phenoxymethyl penicillin (500 mg daily) until the age of 20. For those allergic to penicillin, sulphadimidine (500 mg daily) by mouth should be given. These doses are insufficient for prophylaxis against infective endocarditis and the oral bacteria are likely to be penicillin–resistant if long term penicillin has been given. Chorea may recur during pregnancy or in patients taking the contraceptive pill, but does not indicate recurrent carditis.

Dental aspects

Patients are unlikely to be seen during an attack but emergency dental treatment may be necessary to relieve toothache for example. This can be done under local anaesthesia in consultation with the physician. General anaesthesia should be avoided because of the possibility of myocarditis but no other special precautions should be necessary as there appears to be little risk of infective endocarditis at this stage.

CHRONIC RHEUMATIC HEART DISEASE

In the past, approximately 60 per cent of children who survived acute rheumatic fever developed a cardiac lesion detectable after 10 years, but heart failure may take a further 10 or more years to develop. However, such complications have become increasingly rare and chronic rheumatic heart disease is only likely to be seen now in the middle–aged and some immigrants.

The essential features of rheumatic heart disease are fibrotic stiffening and distortion of the heart valves. The mitral valve is affected in most cases, either alone (60–70 per cent), or with the aortic valve in a further 20 per cent. The aortic valve alone is affected in only 10 per cent. Valve narrowing (stenosis) and regurgitation (incompetence) are associated in varying degrees.

Chronic rheumatic heart disease is essentially therefore a mechanical, haemodynamic disorder, in which the defective valves cause cardiac failure if function cannot be improved by surgery. Infective endocarditis may supervene at any time but is relatively rare.

The earliest sign of valve damage is a murmur. Later effects, particularly enlargement of the heart, may be detected clinically, radiographically and by ECG changes.

Dental aspects

The chief risk is of infective endocarditis which may follow dental surgery without antibiotic cover. Evaluation of a history of rheumatic fever is difficult. The only way to be certain is to refer the patient to a cardiologist to decide whether there has been any valve damage. The simpler alternative is to give antibiotic cover on the assumption that the history is valid, but this means that at least 70 per cent of such patients will receive the antibiotic unnecessarily (see below). It must be emphasized that all rheumatic heart lesions are at risk from infective endocarditis but the level of risk is not related to the severity of the defect. Asymptomatic lesions are often a greater risk than those which are severely disabling.

CONGENITAL HEART DISEASE

Congenital anomalies are now the most common type of heart disease among children and are now considerably more prevalent than rheumatic heart disease (*Fig.* 2.1). Congenital heart disease is present in about 1 per cent of live births, and, in the absence of treatment, possibly 40 per cent of those affected would die within the first 5 years. The prognosis has been enormously improved by cardiac surgery.

Congenital defects can involve the heart or adjacent great vessels. Dental management can be complicated by the hazard to some of these patients of general anaesthesia if the heart is failing, or of infective endocarditis. Cardiac defects can be associated in different combinations and some 20 per cent have other congenital anomalies. Midline defects are often multiple: ventricular septal defect, for example, may be associated with cleft palate and imperforate anus.

The causes of congenital heart disease are unknown in most cases but the best known acquired cause is congenital rubella or cytomegalovirus infection (Chapter 17). The best known genetic cause is Down's syndrome (Chapter 15).

The most striking feature of some types of congenital heart disease is cyanosis (more than 5 g reduced haemoglobin per dl) caused by shunting of deoxygenated blood from the right ventricle directly into the systemic circulation (right to left shunt). In severe cases, cyanosis is obvious at birth, particularly in Fallot's tetralogy. Chronic hypoxaemia causes severely impaired development and often gross finger and toe clubbing (*Fig.* 2.2). Where the shunt is in the opposite direction (left to right) some of the output of the left ventricle is recirculated through the lungs. There is then pulmonary hypertension and eventually, right ventricular hypertrophy. The direction of the shunt may then reverse

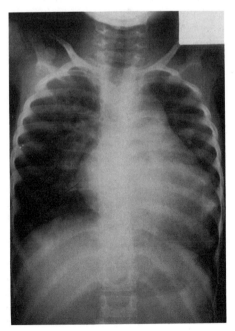

Fig. 2.1. Chest radiograph of a child with congenital heart disease showing gross cardiac enlargement (the heart width normally occupies less than half the width of the chest).

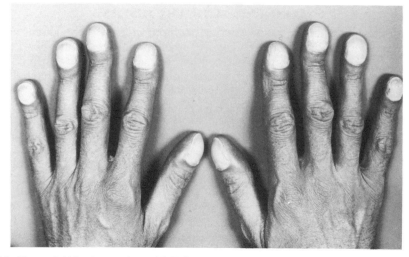

Fig. 2.2. Finger clubbing in a patient with Fallot's tetralogy. Finger clubbing can be found in several different disorders, particularly cyanotic heart disease, chronic respiratory disease, lung cancer, Crohn's disease etc., but is sometimes benign and hereditary.

and cyanosis develops later. Chronic hypoxaemia eventually results in polycythaemia which can cause haemorrhagic or thrombotic tendencies (Chapter 3).

Congenital heart lesions are susceptible to infective endocarditis, *irrespective of the severity of the defect.* It is well recognized that congenital defects have occasionally been discovered only as a result of the development of infective endocarditis. Different types of congenital heart lesion vary in their vulnerability to infection, but this is only of statistical significance and antimicrobial prophylaxis is needed before dental surgery in all such patients (*see below*).

Only the main types of congenital heart disease can be briefly considered here.

Ventricular septal defects (VSD): These range from mere pinholes which are compatible with survival at least into middle age, to defects so large as to cause death in infancy if untreated. As described earlier, there may eventually be right ventricular hypertrophy, reversal of the shunt and late onset cyanosis. Right ventricular failure may develop.

Another effect of the left to right shunt is that the jet of blood hitting the endocardium of the right ventricle causes an area of endocardial thickening (jet lesion) to form. This lesion, or the margins of the defect, can be the site of infective endocarditis. Ninety per cent of patients have an additional cardiac defect.

Atrial septal defect (ASD): This, the most common congenital heart defect, has little effect on cardiac function and is initially acyanotic. Survival into middle age is usual, even in uncorrected cases. However, right ventricular failure usually develops eventually in the absence of surgical correction. Another complication of ASD is that an embolus from a vein can pass from the right ventricle into the left and therefore directly into the systemic circulation and can occasionally be fatal (paradoxical embolism).

The risk of infective endocarditis in ASD appears to be very small, but antibiotic cover should be given for dental operations unless the defect has been repaired by direct suture more than 6 months previously.

Patent ductus arteriosus (PDA): PDA is a persistent opening (normally closed by the third month of life) between the aorta and pulmonary artery. This abnormal communication causes characteristically loud and continuous sawing, systolic and diastolic murmurs. Since the shunt is from left to right, it is initially acyanotic and the typical complication is right ventricular failure. Occasionally infective endocarditis supervenes. Antibiotic cover should therefore be given for dental operations unless the defect has been closed. If patency of the ductus is not necessary to maintain the systemic circulation, its closure can be promoted in early infancy by giving intravenous indomethacin, a prostaglandin inhibitor.

Coarctation of the aorta: This is an aortic narrowing usually sited beyond the origin of the subclavian arteries. The blood to the head, neck and upper body is not therefore obstructed and only the supply to the lower part of the body is restricted. The effect of the narrowing is to cause severe hypertension in the upper part of the body and a low blood pressure below. There are thus strong radial pulses at the wrists but weak or absent femoral pulses in the groins.

Secondary changes are enlargement of collateral arteries (such as the intercostal) and degenerative changes in the aorta which can lead to a fatal aneurysm. A bicuspid aortic valve is associated in 50 per cent of patients.

Infective endocarditis or left ventricular failure are other possible causes of death.

Pulmonary stenosis: The main symptoms are breathlessness and right ventricular failure, often in childhood. Reversal of the origins of the pulmonary artery and aorta causes cyanosis and breathlessness from birth, and early congestive failure. Death in infancy is common unless there are associated defects such as a patent interventricular septum or patent ductus arteriosus, which provide sufficient collateral circulation for oxygenation of the blood to maintain life a little longer.

Tetralogy of Fallot: The four defects which give the condition its name comprise

1. Ventricular septal defect.
2. Pulmonary stenosis.
3. Straddling of the interventricular septum by the aorta, into which blood flows from both ventricles—'overriding aorta'.
4. Compensatory right ventricular hypertrophy.

Among the most obvious clinical features are severe cyanosis and loud cardiac murmurs. Paroxysms of cyanosis and breathlessness, which typically cause cerebral anoxia and syncope, often supervene for no apparent reason. Another characteristic is that these children tend to squat, particularly after exertion, to get some relief from breathlessness.

The usual results of the persistent hypoxia are poor physical development, clubbing of the fingers and toes, and compensatory polycythaemia. In the absence of treatment there is typically heart failure, respiratory infection or, less often, infective endocarditis.

Floppy mitral valve (mitral valve prolapse): This common condition is said to affect 4 per cent of the population. It is an autosomal dominant trait frequently present in otherwise normal persons, but is also a characteristic feature of Ehlers–Danlos and Marfan's syndromes (Chapter 11). Up to 50 per cent of patients with panic disorder have been reported to have mitral valve prolapse.

A prolapsed mitral valve is typically asymptomatic, but if it causes a systolic murmur, can predispose to infective endocarditis, particularly in older persons.

Bicuspid aortic valve: This is usually asymptomatic, even in athletes, but is a high risk for infective endocarditis. The latter may be the first indication of the presence of the defect.

General management

Many of the congenital cardiovascular defects can be improved by cardiac surgery. Medical treatment is needed for patients with cardiac failure, polycythaemia, infective complications or emotional disturbances.

Dental aspects

Oral abnormalities associated with cyanotic congenital heart disease include delayed eruption of both dentitions, with an increased frequency of positional anomalies and enamel hypoplasia. The teeth often have a bluish-white or skimmed milk appearance and there is gross vasodilatation in the pulps. There appears to be greater caries and periodontal disease activity, probably because of poor oral hygiene and lack of dental attention. After cardiotomy, small white, non-ulcerated mucosal lesions of unknown aetiology may be seen.

In the case of the rare idiopathic hypercalcaemia, subaortic stenosis syndrome (Chapter 11) a characteristic facial appearance (elfin facies) is associated.

A special hazard in some types of congenital heart disease is the development of cerebral abscess: this has very occasionally been reported as a consequence of dental sepsis or even to follow endodontic treatment.

Far more important are the risks of general anaesthesia, infective endocarditis and bleeding tendencies. The last is caused by defective platelet function and increased fibrinolytic activity in cyanotic congenital heart disease. The dental management of these patients and prevention of infective endocarditis are discussed later, but general anaesthesia in the dental surgery is contraindicated and specialist referral is needed. Associated problems such as cleft palate, or syndromes such as Down's syndrome, Turner's syndrome, or idiopathic hypercalcaemia may also affect dental management (Appendix 2).

HEART SURGERY

Heart surgery is now frequently carried out for congenital cardiovascular disease, or other valve lesions. Correction of some congenital valve defects is only palliative but in many, such as patent ductus arteriosus, the results are excellent.

Heart valve defects may be corrected by valvotomy, grafts or prosthetic valves. The latter are susceptible to infective endocarditis and there is then a high mortality. However, such infection is not usually of dental origin and replacement of the diseased valve while the infection is still active, together with vigorous antimicrobial treatment, frequently eradicates the disease.

Dental management

Dental sepsis may be a threat to patients having cardiac surgery, as infective endocarditis can nullify any benefits from the operation and sometimes costs the patient's life. There may therefore be justification for preoperative clearance if the dental state is poor. However, the prospect of cardiac surgery is a great emotional stress and a source of severe anxiety to many patients. The idea of dental clearance at this time may therefore be too much for them to bear. It is desirable, however, if the opportunity is available, to reduce dental sepsis to the minimum before operation.

Candidal endocarditis is another threat and, though there is no evidence that these micro-organisms come from the patient's own mouth, it is an obvious precaution to eliminate any oral candidal infection with topical antifungal drugs before operation.

Management problems in patients after cardiac surgery include:

1. Residual cardiovascular disease.
2. Regular dental care.
3. Infective endocarditis.
4. Anticoagulation (Chapter 3).
5. Immunosuppression (heart transplant patients) (Chapter 16).
6. Psychiatric or psychological disturbances.

CARDIAC TRANSPLANTATION

Heart transplantation is increasingly used to treat patients with otherwise uncontrollable cardiac disease, especially severe IHD and idiopathic cardiomyopathy. Although postoperative mortality and morbidity are falling, the one-year survival is variable (20–80 per cent). Following transplantation, patients are immunosuppressed, usually with cyclosporin or azathioprine, corticosteroids and antithymocyte globulin, and are anticoagulated. To minimize the development of atherosclerosis in the transplanted heart, patients are often placed on a low cholesterol diet and given aspirin and dipyridamole to reduce platelet adhesion and prolong the bleeding time.

Dental aspects

A meticulous pre-transplant oral assessment is required and dental treatment undertaken with particular attention to establishing optimal oral hygiene and eradicating sources of potential infection. Dental treatment should be completed before transplantation since there will be complications afterwards, related to:

1. Bleeding tendencies (Chapter 3).
2. Corticosteroid treatment (Chapter 10).
3. Immunosuppression (Chapter 16).
4. A risk of infective endocarditis in some cases.
5. There may rarely be viral hepatitis or HIV infection (Chapters 8 and 16).

Post-transplant patients may develop oral complications such as cyclosporin-induced gingival hyperplasia, or candidosis, herpetic or other infections or rarely hairy leukoplakia because of the immunosuppression (Chapter 16).

INFECTIVE (BACTERIAL) ENDOCARDITIS

Infective endocarditis is an uncommon but dangerous infection predominantly affecting the heart valves but also capable of involving coarctation of the aorta or ductus arteriosus. The earlier name 'subacute bacterial endocarditis' is misleading – cases range from fulminatingly acute to chronic. Arteriovenous shunts for haemodialysis in chronic renal failure (Chapter 9) can also become infected and comparable diseases result.

The main effects of endocarditis are progressive cardiac damage and infection or embolic damage of many organs, especially the kidneys. Infective endocarditis is fatal in about 30 per cent of patients overall, and there is also a high morbidity.

Infective endocarditis results from two main predisposing factors. First, a cardiac lesion such as congenital heart disease may allow endocardial infection to become established and second, bacteraemia (caused by medical, surgical or dental procedures) may initiate the infection. Nevertheless, even an apparently normal heart can become infected and many factors in the pathogenesis of the disease remain unidentified.

Invasive medical procedures, such as instrumentation of the urinary tract and the increasing prevalence of intravenous drug abuse provide many portals of entry for microbes. Highly virulent bacteria such as staphylococci can be introduced into the bloodstream with the addict's needle or by open heart surgery and can cause particularly severe endocarditis. By contrast, micro-organisms which are harmless to the normal person can colonize the endocardium of a host with impaired defences.

The single most common type of microbial isolate from patients with infective endocarditis are viridans streptococci, particularly *S.mutans* and *S. sanguis*. These account for nearly 50 per cent of the many different causative organisms. A possible reason for the importance of viridans streptococci in dentally–related endocarditis is first, that they are present in enormous numbers in the mouth and second, are released into the bloodstream in large numbers during extractions particularly. They also have complex attachment mechanisms which may enable them to adhere to the endocardium. By comparison, other oral bacteria are only rarely incriminated.

The main local host factor is typically a defective or damaged heart valve. Prosthetic valves also provide the site for a severe form of endocarditis, but this

Table 2.8. Aetiological factors for infective endocarditis

Bacterial factors
Bacteraemia
    Causes: Extractions and some other dental procedures
        Cardiac surgery, particularly insertion of prosthetic valves
        Intravenous medication
        Intracardiac or venous catheters
        Obstetric and gynaecological procedures
        Intravenous drug addiction
        Other unknown sources
    Number of bacteria entering the blood
    Bacterial virulence
    Ability to adhere to endocardium

Host factors increasing susceptibility
Local lesions
    Congenital or rheumatic heart disease
    Prosthetic heart valves
    Other cardiac disease
Underlying disease
    Immunosuppressive treatment
    Cytotoxic agents
    Alcoholism

Protective factors
    Antimicrobial chemotherapy

---

is infrequently due to oral bacteria. Surgical correction of some congenital heart defects has made some of these patients less susceptible to infection. By contrast, patients who have had a previous attack of infective endocarditis are particularly vulnerable.

Despite the varied factors affecting aetiology (*Table 2.8*), the peak prevalence of infective endocarditis is now in the sixth or seventh decade and the disease is very uncommon in children.

Clinical features and mortality. The signs and symptoms are highly variable. In the previously healthy patient who acquires endocarditis due to viridans streptococci, the picture is likely to be that, 3 or 4 weeks after a dental operation, low fever and mild malaise develop and persist. Pallor (anaemia) or light (café-au-lait) pigmentation of the skin are typical. Later, increasing disability is associated with changing cardiac murmurs indicative of progressive heart damage, while release of emboli can have effects ranging from loss of a peripheral pulse to (rarely) sudden death from a stroke. Embolic phenomena include haematuria, which is common, cerebrovascular occlusion, petechiae or purpura of skin and mucous membranes, and splinter haemorrhages under the finger nails. Osler's nodes are small, tender vasculitic lesions in the skin. Endocarditis, if not punctuated by some dramatic episode, can progress unsuspected for months.

The mortality of approximately 30 per cent overall has not changed significantly since the introduction of penicillin. This results from the different risk factors that now operate. Thus, the increased age of the patients, the virulence of some infecting organisms and the presence of prosthetic heart valves or underlying disease all reduce the chances of survival. By contrast, the mortality from infective endocarditis caused by viridans streptococci (i.e. of oral origin) has fallen to between 5 and 15 per cent.

Diagnosis and management

If a patient with known heart disease develops a febrile illness, especially with changing heart murmurs, after some surgical procedure, then there is little doubt as to the diagnosis. Whether or not the diagnosis is obvious, blood culture is essential and must be carried out before antimicrobial treatment is started. At least three 20 ml samples of blood should be taken aseptically, at half-hourly intervals to increase the chances of obtaining a positive culture. The bacteriological findings determine the choice of antibiotics, but if viridans streptococci are the cause, then the usual treatment is with penicillin and gentamicin by injection for 2 or more weeks. Early treatment is needed to minimize cardiac damage. In severe cases such as prosthetic valve or candidal endocarditis, early removal of the infected valves and insertion of a sterile replacement can be highly effective.

The main cause of death is heart failure or, less frequently, uncontrollable infection. Cerebral or coronary embolism is relatively rare. The prognosis is poor in the elderly, the immunosuppressed, chronic alcoholics, in fungal or unusually virulent bacterial infections, or if the diagnosis is delayed. Further, some 5 per cent of those who develop infective endocarditis have a further episode with increased heart damage or death.

Dental disease and treatment as a cause of infective endocarditis

From the purely dental viewpoint it is obligatory to try to prevent the onset of infective endocarditis in view of the high morbidity and mortality. Although cardiologists sometimes state dogmatically that dental operations are the most common cause of infective endocarditis, this only illustrates outdated ideas. Indeed, cardiologists may be so vague about the dental history as to ascribe the disease to `poor dental repair', `gingivitis' or `dental problems'. By contrast, large surveys have shown that dental treatment precedes only 5–10 per cent of cases. There has also been a steady decline in the frequency of a history of dentally–related cases, since before the penicillin era. Moreover, the facts that (a) many of the patients are edentulous, that (b) the majority of patients are elderly and that (c) there is an increasing variety of non–dental causes of bacteraemia, indicate that few healthy ambulant patients acquire infective endocarditis as a result of dental treatment.

Experience in the pre-penicillin era showed that, even in patients with established rheumatic heart disease, infective endocarditis rarely followed dental extractions. Furthermore, it is clear that bacteria are released into the blood from the mouth (and other sites) on innumerable occasions unrelated to operative intervention, but cause no harm. The variables which determine whether micro-organisms will infect the heart are unclear, but the number released into the bloodstream is probably a deciding factor. Infective endocarditis can only be induced in animals under highly artificial conditions and with the use of huge inocula of bacteria.

The widespread but simplistic idea that bacteraemia is virtually synonymous with infective endocarditis is gross misapprehension. If that were so, it would be necessary to give antibiotic cover even for brushing the teeth.

In simple terms, therefore, bacteria from the teeth and elsewhere can enter the bloodstream on many occasions, but only rarely infect the heart. In statistical terms, the chance of dental extractions causing infective endocarditis, even in a patient with valvular disease, may (it is suggested) be as low as one in three thousand. Nevertheless, antibiotic prophylaxis is still essential, where appropriate (*see below*).

Prevention of infective endocarditis in dental patients depends in principle on:

1. Identification of patients at risk.
2. Planned preventive dental care.
3. Deciding which treatments require antimicrobial cover.
4. Giving the appropriate antibiotic(s) at the appropriate time.

1. Identification of patients at risk from infective endocarditis (*Table 2.9*)

Identification of all patients at risk is not possible but an attempt should be made to elicit a relevant history. Almost any type of heart lesion is susceptible to infection. Patients should therefore be asked if they have or have had:

(i) Valve defects, acquired or congenital (mitral valve prolapse is common and usually asymptomatic; cover is required for it only when it gives rise to a murmur).

(ii) Heart surgery (and its nature).

Table 2.9. Cardiac valvular disease (patients at risk from infective endocarditis)

Congenital heart disease
Prosthetic valves
Previous infective endocarditis
Degenerative (calcific) aortic valve disease
Hypertrophic cardiomyopathy
Mitral valve prolapse with systolic murmur
Rheumatic heart disease
Others
   Surgically constructed systemic-pulmonary shunts
   Syphilitic heart disease
   Systemic lupus erythematosus
   Carcinoid syndrome
   Ankylosing spondylitis
   Marfan's syndrome
   Ehlers–Danlos syndrome
   Osteogenesis imperfecta
   Hurler's syndrome

Note: The level of risk of infective endocarditis is very low in some of these diseases, such as some types of congenital heart disease

(iii) A heart murmur.

(iv) A previous attack of infective endocarditis.

(v) Any other heart disease and its nature.

As mentioned earlier, the alternatives are to give antibiotic cover to all patients giving positive answers to any of these questions, or to refer the patient for a cardiologist's assessment of the need for prophylaxis. However, most patients will not need such cover and antibiotic treatment has its own risks.

On the other hand, patients do not always remember the advice to tell their dentist about heart disease. There is also a large group who do not know that they have either a congenital defect or acquired valve disease, particularly calcific aortic degeneration. Overall, over 40 per cent of patients who suffer from infective endocarditis have a normal heart or an unsuspected defect.

Even the most careful dental surgeon has therefore to accept the possible embarrassment of a patient developing infective endocarditis in spite of a completely 'safe' history. This has happened in several dental practices in the writers' experience, as a result of totally unsuspected heart lesions. Nevertheless, the chances of this happening in any individual practice are very small.

At the other extreme, children with Down's syndrome have a high frequency of congenital heart defects such as mitral valve prolapse, immunodeficiencies and also a tendency to gross plaque accumulation and periodontal disease, yet despite these three factors which should favour it, do not appear to be particularly susceptible to infective endocarditis. Nevertheless, they should of course be given antibiotic cover like other children with heart defects.

There is a negligible risk of infective endocarditis after dental treatment following myocardial infarction or in patients who have had coronary artery bypass grafts.

2. Planned preventive care

All patients, particularly those with congenital or rheumatic heart disease, who have prosthetic heart valves or who have already had infective endocarditis, need meticulous preventive care. The aim is to keep periodontal infection at its lowest possible level, to obviate the need for extractions or, if extractions are unavoidable, to lessen the severity of the bacteraemia by keeping the gingiva healthy. However, it must be appreciated that scaling also requires antibiotic cover. Unfortunately, this aspect of care is frequently neglected.

3. Dental procedures for which prophylaxis should be given

Bacteraemia can follow virtually any dental procedure, even brushing teeth with clinically healthy gingivae, but mere bacteraemia should not be confused with infective endocarditis—many bacteraemias are so slight as to present no significant risk. However, there are such vast numbers of bacteria at the gingival margins and in the periodontal pockets that any operation disturbing these bacteria provides a good chance of precipitating infective endocarditis in a susceptible

Table 12.10. Procedures requiring antimicrobial prophylaxis

Tooth extraction
Oral surgery involving the periodontal tissues
Periodontal surgery
Subgingival procedures
Re-implantation of avulsed teeth
Repositioning of teeth following trauma

patient. In a survey of nearly 5000 cases of infective endocarditis attributable to dental treatment, it was found to have followed dental extractions in 95 per cent of cases. The current recommendations are therefore that antibiotic prophylaxis is mandatory only for the following types of dental treatment:

(i) Extractions. (ii) Scaling and subgingival procedures. (iii) Periodontal surgery or raising mucogingival flaps for any other purpose (Table 12.10).

Intraligamentary injections may also introduce large numbers of periodontal bacteria into the bloodstream. Though there appears to be no evidence as yet of these injections leading to infective endocarditis, they should be avoided in patients who are at risk. This is not to say that infective endocarditis *cannot* follow other forms of dental treatment but it does so rarely as not to present a significant risk. The dentist who falls over backward in trying to give antibiotic protection against every kind of procedure, quickly runs out of antibiotics effective against the resistant bacteria that such measures produce. Any theoretical benefits are outweighed by the risks, as no antibiotic is without side-effects and the more frequently these drugs are used, the greater the risk of toxic effects and the greater the numbers of resistant bacteria that may need to be controlled.

There seems to be persistent anxiety about the need for antibiotic cover for endodontic treatment even though it is hard to find an authenticated case of it having caused endocarditis. It must be appreciated that in comparison with the gingival margins there are few bacteria in periapical lesions and that quite unusual violence is likely to be needed to send them into the bloodstream. If endocarditis follows root canal therapy it is likely therefore to be mere coincidence or incompetence on the part of the operator.

Theoretically antibiotics might be given for almost any other dental procedure but, since both the necessity and efficacy of prophylaxis is unproven, the stage can be reached when the side-effects from these drugs could outweigh any protection they might give. A study in the USA even suggests that the mortality from penicillin anaphylaxis far exceeds that of infective endocarditis. There is no evidence for the need for antibiotic prophylaxis for local anaesthetic injections, non-surgical orthodontic, prosthetic or restorative procedures (*Table 2.10*) and the risks from antibiotic prophylaxis are likely to far exceed any benefits.

Choice of prophylactic antibiotic regimen

The 1990 recommendations are as follows:

1. *Patients not requiring a general anaesthetic and with no history of infective endocarditis*

(i) Not allergic to nor have received a penicillin more than once in the past month. Adults—3 g amoxycillin orally 1 h before the operation, taken in the presence of the dentist or DSA. For children under 10 one-half the adult dose; for children under 5, a quarter of the adult dose.

Note: Three grams of amoxycillin can be given on not more than two occasions in a month as this dose is sufficient to destroy the relatively resistant streptococci that have emerged.

(ii) Patients allergic to or who have received a penicillin more than once in the previous month. Adults—a *single* oral dose of clindamycin—600 mg for an adult, can be given one hour before the dental procedure. Children under 10 should have one-half the adult dose (300 mg) and children under 5 should have a quarter of the adult dose (150 mg). Clindamycin is is now preferred to erythromycin as it is less likely to cause nausea and is better absorbed. In a single dose it is not known to cause pseudomembranous colitis.

Alternatively, 1.5 g erythromycin stearate can be given orally under supervision 1–2 h before the dental procedure, followed by a second dose of 0.5 g 6 h later. For children under 10, one-half the adult dose; for children under 5, a quarter of the adult dose.

2. *Treatment under general anaesthesia. Patients with natural valve disease and no history of infective endocarditis, but not allergic to nor have had a penicillin more than once within the past month*

Amoxycillin 1 g intramuscularly in 2.5 ml of 1 per cent lignocaine before induction plus 0.5 g of amoxycillin orally 6 h later. Alternatively, 3 g of amoxycillin may be given by mouth 4 hours before induction and repeated as soon as possible after induction, if the anaesthetist agrees.

3. *Treatment under general anaesthesia. Patients with prosthetic valves not allergic to nor have had a penicillin more than once within the past month*

Amoxycillin 1 g intramuscularly in 2.5 ml of 1 per cent lignocaine plus gentamicin 120 mg intramuscularly immediately before induction. A further 0.5 g of amoxycillin should be given orally 6 h later.

If allergic to or have had penicillin more than once in the past month

Vancomycin 1 g by intravenous infusion over 60 min followed by 120 mg of gentamicin intravenously before induction. Vancomycin, if given too rapidly, can cause facial or widespread erythema (red man syndrome) among other toxic effects.

4. *Patients who have had a previous attack of infective endocarditis (irrespective of the type of anaesthetic) but not allergic to the penicillins and have not had a penicillin more than once in the previous month*

Amoxycillin 1 g intramuscularly in 2.5 ml of 1 per cent lignocaine plus gentamicin 120 mg intramuscularly immediately before induction. A further 0.5 g of amoxycillin should be given orally 6 h later.

If allergic to or have had penicillin more than once in the past month

Vancomycin 1 g by intravenous infusion over 60 min followed by 120 mg of gentamicin intravenously.

The reason that different cover is given for those who are going to have a general anaesthetic are that (i) parenteral administration removes the risk of vomiting, (ii) it is not feasible to give such large doses (3 g) of amoxycillin (for example) by injection, hence it has to be supplemented with gentamicin. In the case of patients allergic to penicillin there is no potent, convenient, injectable alternative to vancomycin. However the latter is likely to be replaced by teicoplanin, which is a similar drug, but does not need to be given by slow infusion.

Additional Measures

1. Application of an antiseptic such as 0.5 per cent chlorhexidine or tincture of iodine to the gingival crevice before the dental procedure may reduce the severity of any resulting bacteraemia and may usefully supplement antibiotic prophylaxis in those at risk.

2. Good dental health should reduce the frequency and severity of any bacteraemias and also reduce the need for extractions.

3. It is essential that, even when antibiotic cover has been given, patients at risk should be instructed to report any unexplained illness. Infective endocarditis is often exceedingly insidious in origin and can develop 2 or more months after the operation which might have precipitated it. Late diagnosis considerably increases both the mortality or disability among survivors.

4. Patients at risk should carry a warning card (obtainable from Dr N. E. Simmons, Department of Clinical Bacteriology, Guy's Hospital, London, SE1 9RT) to be shown to their dentist at each visit to indicate the danger of infective endocarditis and the need for antibiotic prophylaxis.

In summary therefore, it must be accepted that, although neither the need nor the efficacy of antibiotic prophylaxis can be established in any given case, antibiotics must be given before extractions, scaling and surgery involving the periodontal tissues to patients with a recognized predisposing cardiac disorder (*Tables 2.9, 2.10*). *In addition, it is essential to warn patients (whether or not antimicrobial prophylaxis has been given) to report back if even a minor febrile illness develops after dental treatment.*

It must also be remembered that patients at risk from infective endocarditis may also have a heart lesion that makes them a poor risk for general anaesthesia and a few are on anticoagulant treatment or on other drugs.

VENOUS THROMBOSIS AND PULMONARY EMBOLISM

Venous thrombosis and subsequent pulmonary embolism are important causes of death or significant morbidity, especially in elderly, bed-ridden and postoperative patients. Dental surgeons involved in the care of hospitalized or geriatric patients should be aware of these common problems.

Venous thrombosis usually affects the deep calf veins as a consequence of immobility. Pressure on the calf (from lying in bed) and increased blood coagulability follow general anaesthesia and surgery. Several other factors contribute, including sometimes, oral contraceptives.

Deep vein thrombosis can occasionally lead to pulmonary embolism. Superficial vein thrombosis may complicate intravenous injections, particularly of diazepam, but does not lead to pulmonary embolism.

Management of deep vein thrombosis

Prophylaxis against venous thromboembolism is important but not reliablyeffective. The calves must not rest on hard objects during surgery and stasis may be eliminated by calf contractions stimulated electrically, or by pneumatic compression. Early mobilization and leg movements postoperatively, must be encouraged.

Anticoagulant therapy with heparin is the most effective method of preventing thromboembolism but must be balanced against the risks of haemorrhage.

Pulmonary Embolism

Pulmonary embolism secondary to venous thrombosis may be fatal as a result of sudden circulatory collapse, may cause minor pulmonary infarcts with haemoptysis or pleurisy, or may gradually cause pulmonary hypertension and right-sided heart failure.

Management of pulmonary embolism

In massive pulmonary embolism with collapse and cardiac arrest, external cardiac massage may break up the embolus. Oxygen and intravenous heparin should also be given or streptokinase or urokinase. Minor pulmonary embolism usually resolves spontaneously but anticoagulants are given.

DENTAL MANAGEMENT OF PATIENTS WITH HEART DISEASE: SUMMARY

1. The chief hazards are likely to be:

(i)   Anxiety and pain which cause enhanced sympathetic activity. This increases the load on the heart and the risk of dysrhythmias.
(ii) General anaesthesia is particularly hazardous for many of these patients and is contraindicated in the general dental surgery.
(iii) Infective endocarditis, particularly after extractions or periodontal treatment, is a hazard for some.

2. Routine dentistry is safe for most patients with heart disease unless they are over-anxious.
3. Sedation with nitrous oxide is pleasant and usually acceptable. It is probably safer than intravenous sedation, because of the virtual absence of adverse cardiorespiratory effects and because of its rapid reversibility. If diazepam or midazolam is given, *very slow* injection is necessary.
4. Extractions under local anaesthesia can usually be carried out one or two at a time but the trauma and blood loss of multiple extractions should be avoided.
5. Local anaesthesia is generally safe and should always be used in preference to general anaesthesia. The hazard of adrenaline in local anaesthetic solutions used in sensible doses (up to four cartridges) is little more than theoretical. Lignocaine 2 per cent with adrenaline

1:80 000 has an outstanding record of safety during its use over more than a quarter of a century and it is invaluable for its reliably effective, total control of pain. Despite its claimed advantages, there is no evidence whatsoever that prilocaine with or without felypressin is any safer. Indeed it may confer a false sense of security in that, if it fails to achieve complete pain control, it could have worse effects by inducing endogenous adrenaline release and dysrhythmias.

Local anaesthetics containing noradrenaline are totally contraindicated as even in normal persons they have caused fatal hypertensive attacks.

General anaesthesia is contraindicated in the dental surgery and should only be considered if there is no other possible alternative. It is particularly hazardous for the following conditions:

(i)   After myocardial infarction, particularly if recent.
(ii) Angina pectoris, especially of recent origin or unstable.
(iii) Severe hypertension.
(iv) Intractable dysrhythmias (particularly digitalis toxicity).
(v)   Some congenital heart diseases.

General anaesthesia is a hazard to these patients because it may *(a)* depress myocardial activity and aggravate or possibly precipitate cardiac failure; *(b)* cause dysrhythmias (particularly halothane); *(c)* dilate the vascular bed causing a fall in blood pressure; *(d)* depress respiration and oxygenation (particularly the barbiturates).

Not least of the difficulties for the dental surgeon is that of assessing the level of risk for a particular patient, especially now that even severe forms of heart disease can be disguised by treatment. This is yet another reason why, if a general anaesthetic is unavoidable, it should be given by a specialist anaesthetist in a properly equipped hospital.

Methohexitone should not, under any circumstances, be used even for so-called sedation—it is a potent general anaesthetic agent which is a respiratory depressant with cardiovascular effects which can also be harmful.

In addition to the hazards conferred by general anaesthesia, surgery itself imposes stresses on the body and has important metabolic effects.

6. Myocardial infarction is a common enough tragedy and can happen anywhere, including the dental surgery. Dental treatment may possibly evencontribute to precipitating such an event—or may be blamed by the patient or relatives for it. Recognition and a quick and appropriate response by the dental surgeon may help to save the patient's life. The initial management of this emergency is discussed in Chapter 18.

Bibliography

Abraham-Inpijn L., Borgmeijer-Hoelen A. and Gortzak, R.A. (1988) Changes in blood pressure, heart rate and electrocardiogram during dental treatment with use of local anesthesia. *JADA* **116**, 531–6.

Barnett M.L., Friedman D. and Kastner T. (1988) The prevalence of mitral valve prolapse in patients with Down's syndrome: implications for dental management. *Oral Surg.* **66**, 445–7.

Cawson R.A. (1981) Infective endocarditis as a complication of dental treatment. *Br. Dent. J.* **151**, 409–414.

Cawson R.A. (1991) Essentials of Dental Surgery and Pathology 5th ed. Edinburgh, Churchill Livingstone.

Cawson R.A. and Spector R.G. (1989) Clinical Pharmacology in Dentistry. 5th ed. Edinburgh, Churchill Livingstone.

Dajani A.S. Bisno, A.L., Chung, K.J. et al. (1990) Prevention of bacterial endocarditis. Recommendations by the American Heart Association. *JAMA* **264**, 2919–22.

Ehrmann E.H. (1986) Infective endocarditis and the dentist. *Aust. Dent. J.* **31**, 351–60.

Field E.A. and Martin M.V. (1990) Need for antibiotic prophylaxis for dental patients with a penile prosthesis. *Br. Dent. J.* **164**, 75.

Friedlander A.H. and Gorelick D.A. (1987) Panic disorder: its association with mitral valve prolapse and appropriate dental management. *Oral Surg.* **63**, 309–12.

Grace C.J., Levitz R.E., Katz-Pollak H. et al. (1988) *Actinobacillus actinomycetemcomitans* prosthetic valve endocarditis. *Rev. Infect. Dis.* **10**, 922–9.

Mattila K.J., Nieminen M.S. and Valtonen V.V. (1989) Association between dental health and acute myocardial infarction. *Br. Med. J.* **298**, 779–81.

Michel M.F. (1986) Review of the guidelines of the Dutch Heart Foundation for the prevention of endocarditis. *Ned. Tijdschr. Geneeskd.* **130**, 2211–12.

Schweizerischen Arbeitsgruppe fur Endokarditisprophylaxe. (1984) Prophylaxe der bakteriellen Endokarditis. *Schweiz. Med. Wochenschr.* **114**, 1146–52.

Simmons N.A., Cawson R.A. Eykyn S.J. et al. Endocarditis Working Party. British Society for Antimicrobial Chemotherapy (1990) Antibiotic prophylaxis of infective endocarditis. *Lancet* **335**, 88-89.

Van der Meer J.T.M., van Wilk W., Thompson J. et al (1992) Awareness of need and actual use of prophylaxis: lack of patient compliance in the prevention of bacterial endocarditis. *J. Antimicrob. Chemother.* **29**, 187–94.

Working Party of the British Society for Antimicrobial Chemotherapy. (1982) The antibiotic prophylaxis of infective endocarditis. *Lancet* **ii**, 187–94.

Working Party of the British Society for Antimicrobial Chemotherapy. (1986) Prophylaxis of endocarditis. *Lancer* **i**, 1267.

Working Party of the British Society for Antimicrobial Chemotherapy. (1992) Antibiotic prophylaxis of infective endocarditis. *Lancet* **339**, 1292–3.

Appendix to Chapter 2

GENETIC SYNDROMES WITH ASSOCIATED CARDIAC DEFECTS: MAIN FEATURES

Chromosomal disorders
Down's
Edward's
Patau
Turner
XXXY
XXXXX

} Appendix to Chapter 5

Mental handicap: hypogonadism
Mental handicap: small hands

Hereditary disorders
Ehlers–Danlos
Marfan
Osteogenesis imperfecta

} Chapter 11

The mucopolysaccharidoses (Hurler's
and related syndromes)

Appendix to Chapter 10

Ellis–van Creveld
T A R
Holt–Oram
Multiple lentigenes
Rubenstein–Taybi

Appendix to Chapter 11
*T*hrombocytopenia: *A*bsent *R*adius
Hypoplastic clavicles: upper limb defect
Basal cell naevi: rib defects
Broad thumbs and toes: hypoplastic maxilla

Chapter 3

Haemorrhagic Disorders

Prolonged bleeding after dental extraction, though usually of local cause, is one of the most common signs of haemorrhagic disease and causes of haemorrhagic emergencies. It is sometimes the way by which the disease is first recognized.

Haemorrhagic disease can be caused by disorders of platelets, or of the clotting mechanism, such as haemophilia, and only rarely by vascular diseases (*Table 3.1*).

Platelet and vascular defects give rise to purpura characterized by superficial (capillary) bleeding with the formation of petechiae or widespread ecchymoses into the skin or mucous membranes, and spontaneous gingival bleeding.

The coagulation disorders characteristically cause severe bleeding deep in the tissues and extensive haematoma formation after superficial injury, while bleeding after surgery or trauma can be so prolonged and severe as to be potentially lethal, if untreated.

Table 3.1. Causes of bleeding disorders

Platelet disorders
  Thrombocytopenia
    Idiopathic thrombocytopenic purpura (ITP)
    HIV-associated thrombocytopenic purpura
    Leukaemias
  von Willebrand's disease
  Drugs such as aspirin, cytotoxics β lactam antibiotics and valproate
  Thrombasthenia
  Others

Coagulation defects
  Haemophilia
  Anticoagulants and thrombolytic agents
  Liver disease, including obstructive jaundice
  von Willebrand's disease
  Others

Rare causes of bleeding diseases
  Aplastic anaemia (idiopathic, drug-associated and others)
  Chronic renal failure
  Dysproteinaemias, especially multiple myeloma
  Lupus erythematosus
  Bernard-Soulier syndrome
  Deficiencies of factors XII and XIII and others
  Disseminated intravascular coagulation

INVESTIGATION OF THE PATIENT WITH HAEMORRHAGIC DISEASE

Haemorrhage is alarming to the patient and may be an emergency. An adequate history *is the single most important part of the evaluation*; physical examination is also necessary but laboratory tests are needed to confirm the diagnosis. An accurate diagnosis is essential in order to provide replacement therapy where appropriate, and to enable other management procedures to be organized.

The History

Any suggestion of a haemorrhagic tendency *must* be taken seriously. Nevertheless, patients can be remarkably capricious as to the information they provide and, in any case, can hardly be expected to know when bleeding can legitimately be regarded as `abnormal'. Previous dental extractions provide a useful guide, but prolonged bleeding (up to 24–28 hours) as an isolated episode is usually the result of local factors, especially excessive trauma, *which is the most common cause of excessive bleeding*. By contrast, even patients who know that they have a serious haemorrhagic tendency can keep the fact to themselves unless specifically asked.

Special emphasis must therefore be placed on the following:

Features of previous episodes: Deep haemorrhage into muscles, joints or skin suggests a clotting defect. Bleeding from and into mucosae and skin ('bruising')

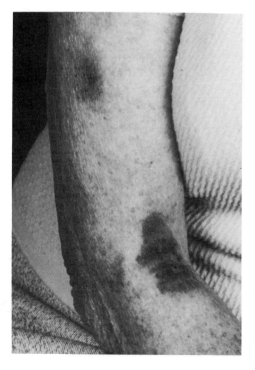

Fig. 3.1. Purpura in a patient with myeloid leukaemia.

suggests purpura (*Fig.* 3.1). Women with no bleeding disorder often state that they 'bruise easily', but any such bruises are usually insignificant and less than about 5 cm across. Excessive menstrual bleeding is most often the result of factors other than bleeding disorders.

Past history: Most congenital bleeding disorders become apparent in childhood but mild haemophiliacs can escape recognition until adult life if they manage to avoid injury or surgery.

Surgery: Patients who have had tonsillectomy or dental extractions without trouble are most unlikely to have severe congenital bleeding disorders. On the other hand, a mild haemophiliac can have oozing from an extraction socket for 2–3 weeks in spite of any local measures such as suturing.

Previous treatment: It is important to know how previous dental bleeding was controlled. If it responded to local measures then the patient is unlikely to have a serious haemorrhagic disease. On the other hand, admission to hospital and blood transfusion or comparable measures have obvious implications.

Family history: Haemorrhagic disease in another blood relative is strongly suggestive of a clotting defect.

Relevant medical history: Many drugs such as anticoagulants, or corticosteroids may cause bleeding tendencies, as may hepatic, renal, HIV and other disease. Patients may be aware of having haemorrhagic disease and carry an appropriate medical card (*Fig.* 3.2). Patients may be in high-risk groups for hepatitis B, delta or C viruses, or HIV and other infections (Chapters 8 and 16).

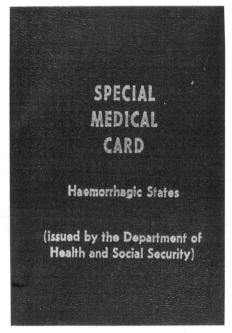

SPECIAL
MEDICAL
CARD

Haemorrhagic States

(issued by the Department of
Health and Social Security)

IN CASE OF INJURY, BLEEDING, OR SERIOUS ILLNESS, THIS PERSON MAY HAVE URGENT NEED OF CARE AT A SPECIAL CENTRE.

IN EMERGENCY, TELEPHONE THE CENTRE NAMED OPPOSITE.

NEITHER INTRA - MUSCULAR INJECTIONS NOR ASPIRIN PREPARATIONS SHOULD BE GIVEN.

a

b

Fig. 3.2. (a) Special Medical Card that should be carried at all times by patients with haemorrhagic states; (b) Special Medical Card showing warnings inside the cover.

Examination

Signs of purpura in the skin or mucosa such as spontaneous gingival bleeding, petechiae or ecchymoses are found mainly in platelet disorders (*Fig.* 3.1). Oral purpura is also seen in leukaemia and AIDS. Alternatively it may be localized to the mouth (sometimes grandiloquently termed angina bullosa haemorrhagica') and not associated with any abnormal bleeding tendencies. Joint deformities from haemarthroses, characteristic of haemophilia should also be looked for but are infrequently seen now. Signs of underlying disease such as anaemia and lymphadenopathy in leukaemia, for example, must also be looked for.

Laboratory Tests

It is important to consult the haematologist to ensure that appropriate blood samples are taken, but it is not necessary to specify individual tests on the request form. All that is needed is to say: 'History of abnormal bleeding. Would you please investigate haemostatic function?' and to give as much clinical detail as possible. A routine 'blood count' will not identify a clotting defect but may show platelet deficiency. The sample should be adequately labelled and sent immediately for testing together with relevant clinical information.

Essential tests include:

1. The bleeding time.
2. Full blood count, film, platelet count (EDTA sample).
3. Prothrombin, activated partial thromboplastin and thrombin times (citrated sample) (*see Tables 3.2–3.4, Fig.* 3.3), but normal results do *not* rule out all mild bleeding disorders.
4. Serum for blood grouping and cross-matching (clotted sample).

Table 3.2. Protocol for investigation of a bleeding disorder

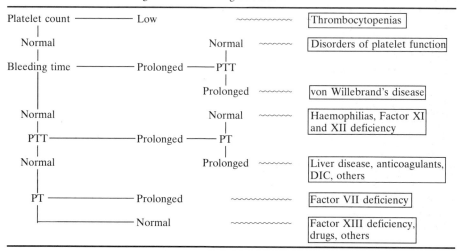

PTT, partial thromboplastin time (also APTT, activated PTT, and KPTT, kaolin PTT).
PT, prothrombin time, *See* text and Appendix.

Table 3.3. Laboratory findings in clotting disorders

Disorder	PTT	PTT	TT	FL	FDP
Haemophilia A Haemophilia B von Willebrand's disease Deficiency of Factors XI, XII	N	↑	N	N	N
Coumarin (Warfarin) therapy Obstructive jaundice—or other causes of vitamin K deficiency Deficiency of Factor V or X	↑	↑	N	N	N
Heparin therapy	↑	↑	↑	N	N
Disseminated intravascular coagulation Parenchymal liver disease	↑	↑	↑	↓	↑
Deficiency of Factor VII	↑	N	N	N	N

PT, Prothrombin time; APTT, activated partial thromboplastin time (or KPTT); TT, thrombin time; FL fibrinogen level; FDP, fibrin-degradation products.
Arrows indicate a value above or below normal (N).
Adapted from Nossel H. L. (1980) In: Isselbacher K.J. et al. (ed.) *Harrison's Principles of Internal Medicine.* Tokyo, McGraw-Hill Kogakusha.

Table 3.4. Typical findings in platelet disorders

Disorder	Bleeding time	Platelets count	Clot retraction	Platelet aggregation	Platelet FIII activity
Thrombocytopenia	↑	↓	↓	—	—
Thrombasthenia	↑	N	↓	↓	↓
Storage pool deficiency	↑	N	N	N or ↓	↓
Aspirin von Willebrand's disease	↑	N	N	↓ (only with ristocetin)	N
Thrombocythaemia	↑	↑	N or ↓	N or ↓	N or ↓

Arrows indicate a value above or below normal (N). FIII = factor 3.
Adapted from Nossel H. L. (1980) In: Isselbacher K. J. et al. (eds) *Harrison's Principles of Internal Medicine.* Tokyo, McGraw-Hill Kogakusha.

Coagulation defects. Precise characterization of a congenital clotting defect depends on assay of the individual factors and a wide range of other investigations may be indicated according to the type of case. For example, the assay usually used in diagnosis of haemophilia A is the Factor VIII coagulant activity (FVIIIC). The whole blood clotting time is uninformative and obsolete.

It is particularly important also to investigate patients for anaemia because: (a) anaemia is an expected consequence of repeated haemorrhages; (b) any further bleeding as a result of dental surgery will worsen the anaemia, or the anaemia may need to be treated before surgery can be carried out; and (c) anaemia may be an essential concomitant of the haemorrhagic tendency—as in acute leukaemia.

Patients may also need to be screened for HIV and hepatitis viruses.

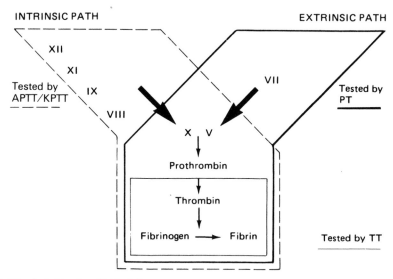

Fig 3.3. Blood clotting (*see* Table 3.3).

Platelet defects.   Aspirin should be avoided for at least 3 days before assessing platelet function.

In the Hess test (tourniquet test) more than a few petechiae on the forearm suggests a platelet or vascular defect but the test is not particularly specific.

A valuable test of platelet function is the bleeding time but normal values range from 2 to 9 minutes so that it is not completely reliable. *In vitro* tests of platelet adhesion and aggregation may be required to demonstrate abnormal function.

Table 3.5. Comparative features of haemorrhagic disorders

	*Platelet defects (the purpuras)**	*Coagulation defects*
Sex affected	Females more than males†	Males
Family history	Rarely	+
Nature of bleeding	Immediately after trauma	Delayed after trauma
	Relatively short lived	Persistent
Effect of locally applied pressure	May cause bleeding to cease	Bleeding recurs when pressure removed
Spontaneous bleeding into skin or mucosa or from mucosa	Common	Uncommon
Bleeding from minor superficial injuries, e.g. needle prick	Common	Uncommon
Deep haemorrhages or haemarthroses	Rare	Common
Bleeding time	Prolonged	Normal
Tourniquet test	+	−
Platelet count	Often reduced	Normal
Clotting function	Normal‡	Abnormal

*Purpura rarely vascular.
†Except in AIDS.
‡May be a prolonged prothrombin consumption test.

Platelet aggregation can also be measured using aggregating agents such as ristocetin. Unfortunately such tests are difficult to standardize and do not identify all platelet disorders; the clinical features are more important.

Table 3.5 shows comparative features of coagulation defects and platelet defects. It should be stressed again that a history of previous haemorrhagic episodes is the most important feature since screening tests of haemostasis do not always detect mild defects.

PLATELET DISORDERS

Impaired platelet function may be caused by many diseases or drugs (*Table 3.6*) but deficiencies of platelets (thrombocytopenias) are probably the most clinically important causes of purpura.

Table 3.6. Some drugs that may cause abnormal platelet function

NON-STEROIDAL ANTI-INFLAMMATORY DRUGS
  Aspirin
  Diclofenac
  Diflunisal
  Ibuprofen
  Mefenamic acid
β LACTAM ANTIBIOTICS
  Ampicillin and derivatives
  Methicillin
  Penicillin G (benzyl penicillin)
  Cephalosporins (some)
GENERAL ANAESTHETIC AGENTS
  Halothane
OTHERS
  Cytotoxic agents
  Asparaginase
  Carmustine
  Daunorubicin
  Vincristine
  Antihistamines (some)
  Tricyclic antidepressants
  Chlorpromazine
  Haloperidol

Adapted from George J. N. Shattil S.J. (1991) *New Engl. J. Med.* **324**, 27–39

Thrombocytopenias

Thrombocytopenia exists when the platelet count falls below 100 x 10^9/l and causes petechiae, ecchymoses and postoperative haemorrhage (*Table 3.7*). There are many causes of thrombocytopenia (*Table 3.1*).

Thrombocytopenic purpura is a relatively common feature of HIV infection and may be an early sign.

Table 3.7. Manifestations and management of surgery in thrombocytopenia

Platelet count ($\times 10^9/l$)	Severity of thrombocytopenia	Manifestations	Managment in relation to type of oral surgery Minor	Major
150–350	Normal	—	—	—
100–150	Mild	Mild purpura sometimes. Slight increase in postoperative bleeding	No platelet transfusion; observe	Consider platelet transfusion; observe
50–100	Moderate	Purpura, postoperative bleeding	Platelets needed	Platelets needed
25–50	Severe	Purpura, postoperative bleeding, and even from venepuncture	Platelets needed	Platelets needed; avoid surgery where possible
<25	Life-threatening	Purpura, spontaneous bleeding	Platelets needed; avoid surgery where possible	Platelet needed; avoid surgery where possible

Dental management

Drugs which affect platelet function, particularly aspirin should be avoided, as should other drugs rarely used in dentistry such as gentamicin, antihistamines, tricyclic antidepressants, phenothiazines, propranolol and frusemide. Regional anaesthetic block injections are also contra–indicated if the platelet levels are below $30 \times 10^9/l$.

Haemostasis after minor surgery is usually adequate if platelet levels are above $50 \times 10^9/l$; for major surgery, levels over $75 \times 10^9/l$ are desirable. Platelets can be replaced or supplemented by platelet transfusions, but sequestration of platelets is very rapid. Platelet transfusions are therefore best used for controlling already established bleeding caused by thrombocytopenia. When given prophylactically, platelets should be given either immediately before surgery to control capillary bleeding or immediately after operation to facilitate the placement of adequate sutures. Platelets should be used within 6–24 hours after collection and suitable preparations include platelet-rich plasma (PRP) which contains about 90 per cent of the platelets from a unit of fresh blood in about half this volume, and platelet-rich concentrate (PRC) which contains about 50 per cent of the platelets from a unit of fresh whole blood in a volume of only 25 ml. PRC is thus the best source of platelets. However, where there is immune destruction of platelets (e.g. in ITP) platelet infusions are less effective than corticosteroids and splenectomy may be necessary.

In such patients, the bleeding tendency is sometimes effectively controlled by corticosteroids and should not therefore be a problem. However, the corticosteroids can cause in the long term, well-recognized problems (Chapter 10) and 10–20 per cent of patients with ITP do not respond.

The need for platelet transfusions, which carry the risks of iso-immunization and of hepatitis and other infections, can be reduced by local haemostatic measures and the use of desmopressin or tranexamic acid (p. 95).

Absorbable haemostatic agents such as oxidized regenerated cellulose (Surgicel) or microcrystalline collagen (Avitene) may be put in the socket to assist clotting.

Other platelet disorders

Thrombasthenia (Glanzmann's syndrome)

Defective platelet aggregation is due to a defective membrane protein and causes a severe bleeding tendency. Platelet infusions are needed preoperatively.

Bernard–Soulier syndrome

Giant platelets characterize this heritable disorder, which in very many ways resembles von Willebrand's disease but is considerably more uncommon. The defect is in a platelet glycoprotein which acts as a receptor for von Willebrand factor.

Chronic renal failure (*see* Chapter 9)

Dysproteinaemias (*see* Chapter 16)

Storage pool deficiency

Platelets may lack the capacity to store serotonin and adenine nucleotides and consequently fail to aggregate. Usually this is congenital with autosomal inheritance, and may be associated with albinism (Hermansky–Pudlak syndrome). Platelet infusion or cryoprecipitate corrects the bleeding tendency.

Purpura in HIV infection

Purpura is a relatively common feature of HIV infection. It may be an autoimmune phenomenon but there appears also to be a platelet defect resulting from the infection. Oral purpura in HIV infection may closely mimic oral lesions of Kaposi's sarcoma (Chapter 16).

Thrombocythaemia

In many conditions a raised platelet count (thrombocytosis) may be found and predisposes to arterial thrombosis. Thrombocythaemia by contrast is a myeloproliferative disease and may be an isolated disorder or associated with myelofibrosis, polycythaemia or chronic granulocytic leukaemia. Thrombocythaemia can give rise to both thromboses and bleeding tendencies as the main effects.

Dental management. Patients are treated with ^{32}P-labelled phosphorus or cytotoxic agents (chlorambucil or busulphan), corticosteroids or aspirin. Anticoagulants are sometimes employed. The problems of dental management in thrombocythaemia can therefore be summarized as follows:

1. Haemorrhagic tendencies (Chapter 3).
2. Thromboses.
3. Complications of cytotoxic agents or corticosteroids (Chapter 10).

VASCULAR PURPURA

Serious bleeding is caused rarely by vascular disorders. Bleeding into mucous membranes or skin starts immediately after trauma but ceases within 24–28 hours.

Hereditary Haemorrhagic Telangiectasia

Hereditary haemorrhagic telangiectasia (HHT) is an autosomal dominant condition characterized by telangiectasia on the skin or any part of the oral, nasal, gastrointestinal or urogenital mucosa (*Fig.* 3.4). Fragility of the affected vessels leads to bleeding and consequently, sometimes, to iron deficiency anaemia or rarely even to cardiac failure. Cryosurgery is useful to treat oral telangiectases. Bleeding from oral surgery is unlikely to be troublesome but postoperative observation is advisable. There may be an associated IgA deficiency or, rarely, von Willebrand's disease (*see below*).

Localized oral purpura

Blood blisters, especially in the soft palate, are occasionally seen in the absence of generalized purpura, any other bleeding tendency or evidence of autoimmune disease. However a systemic cause of the blood blisters must be excluded before the diagnosis can be confidently made and the patient reassured.

These blood blisters may sometimes be a centimetre or more in diameter and after rupture may leave a sore area for a time. When a large blood blister of this type is in the pharynx it can cause an alarming choking sensation and was therefore originally termed 'angina bullosa haemorrhagica'. However, almost any site in the mouth can be affected.

Palatal purpura also may seen be in infectious mononucleosis HIV or rubella.

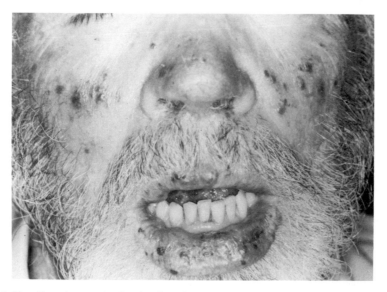

Fig. 3.4. Hereditary haemorrhagic telangiectasia.

CONGENITAL COAGULATION DEFECTS

The most important hereditary bleeding disorders in terms of prevalence and severity are haemophilia A and B (Christmas disease) and von Willebrand's disease. Less common disorders are summarized in Appendix 1.

Haemophilia A

Haemophilia A is the most common clotting defect, with a prevalence of about 5 per 100 000 of the population. It is about 10 times as common as haemophilia B except in Indians, where frequencies are almost equal. Inherited as a sex-linked recessive trait, haemophilia affects males. A family history can, however, be obtained in only about 65 per cent of cases. All daughters of an affected male are carriers but sons are normal. Sons of carriers have a 50:50 chance of developing haemophilia while daughters of carriers have a 50:50 chance of also being carriers.

Haemophilia typically becomes apparent in childhood when bleeding into muscles or joints (haemarthroses) follows injuries. Abdominal haemorrhage may simulate an acute abdomen. Haemarthroses can cause joint damage and cripple the patient, but bleeding after dental extractions is sometimes the first or only sign of mild disease. Bleeding into the cranium, bladder and other sites can cause severe or fatal complications. Haemorrhage in haemophiliacs is dangerous either because of loss of blood, or because there may be damage to joints, muscles and nerves, or pressure on vital organs if haemorrhage is internal. Thus compression of the larynx and pharynx following haematoma formation in the neck can be fatal. Dental extractions or deep lacerations are followed by persistent oozing for days or weeks and in the past have been fatal. The haemorrhage cannot be controlled by pressure and, although clots may form in the mouth, they fail to stop the bleeding. The characteristic feature of bleeding in haemophilia is that it seems to stop immediately after the injury (as a result of normal vascular and platelet response) but, after an hour or more, intractable oozing or rapid blood loss starts and persists.

The severity of the disease is variable but correlates well with the Factor VIII level of the plasma. Normal plasma contains 1 unit of Factor VIII per ml, a level defined as 100 per cent. If the Factor VIII level is above 25 per cent the disease is mild. Severe haemophiliacs have a Factor VIII (antihaemophilia factor, AHF) activity of less than 5 per cent (FVIII C level less than 1 I.U./dl) and typically less than 1 per cent.

The severity of bleeding is dependent on two main factors:

1. The level of Factor VIII C activity.
2. The severity of trauma.

In general, if the level of Factor VIII is above 25 per cent (FVIIIC over 5 I.U./dl), the patient can lead a relatively normal life and may remain undiagnosed, although there can be prolonged bleeding after trauma or surgery. With Factor VIII levels of between 5 and 25 per cent (FVIII C 1–5 I.U./dl) comparatively minor trauma can lead to persistent bleeding.

Some mild haemophiliacs may not bleed excessively even after a simple dental extraction, so that the absence of post-extraction haemorrhage cannot always be used to exclude haemophilia. Most will, however, bleed excessively after more traumatic surgery, such as tonsillectomy.

Diagnosis and management

The typical findings in haemophilia can be summarized as follows:

1. Prolonged activated partial thromboplastin time (APTT).
2. Normal prothrombin time (PT).
3. Normal bleeding time.
4. Reduced Factor VIII C but normal VIII R: Ag (von Willebrand factor) and R: RCo (ristocetin cofactor).

Factor VIII assay is required as even the APTT may be normal in mild haemophilia. If bleeding starts or is expected, treatment consists of replacement of the missing clotting factor, rest and often the use of antifibrinolytic agents.

Rarely, von Willebrand's disease may mimic haemophilia. The history may help to distinguish (*Table 3.8*) but laboratory testing is essential (*see below*).

Regular prophylactic replacement of Factor VIII (AHF) is used when possible but necessitates daily injections. AHF is also in short supply and expensive, and its use may be complicated by antibody formation or viral infections (Chapter 8), but heat treatment should inactivate HIV that might have been missed in the screening of donors. Increasing reliance is therefore placed on desmopressin and tranexamic acid.

Table 3.8. Important differences between haemophilia A and von Willebrand's disease

	Haemophilia A	von Willebrand's disease
Inheritance	Sex-linked recessive	Dominant
Haemarthroses/deep haematomas	Common	Rare
Epistaxes	Uncommon	Common
Gastrointestinal bleeding	Uncommon	Common
Haematuria	Common	Uncommon
Menorrhagia	None (males)	Common
Post-extraction bleeding	Starts 1–24 hours after trauma, lasts 3–40 days. Not controlled by pressure	Starts immediately Lasts 24–48 hours and is often controlled by pressure
Bleeding time	Normal	Prolonged
Factor VIII coagulant activity	Reduced	Reduced
Factor VIII R; RCo	Normal	Reduced

Note: von Willebrand's disease is occasionally identical to haemophilia.

Replacement therapy. Human freeze-dried Factor VIII concentrate (Factor VIII fraction, dried) is used when the deficiency is sufficiently severe. This preparation is stable for one year at 4° C but once reconstituted should be used without delay. In milder cases (factor VIII levels within 5–25 per cent of normal) desmopressin may be satisfactory and is increasingly used.

Dental management

Operative treatment can be lethal unless managed correctly. Dental extractions are a major problem and treatment must be planned from an early age in order to reduce dental disease and operative intervention to a minimum. Haemophiliacs require the care of specialists of many disciplines and should therefore be treated in Haemophilia Reference Centres, or associated units (*see* Department of Health memorandum FPN 105 HC (76)4). Haemophilia cards are issued to confirmed haemophiliacs and give details of the diagnosis and the Centre from which advice can be obtained (*Fig.* 3.2).

Difficulties in the management of haemophiliacs may include:

1. Dental neglect necessitating frequent dental extractions.
2. Trauma, surgery and subsequent haemorrhage.
3. Hazards of anaesthesia and intramuscular injections.
4. Risks of hepatitis, and liver disease.
5. HIV infection.
6. Aggravation of bleeding by drugs.
8. Anxiety.
8. Drug dependence as a result of chronic pain.

Preventive dental care. Education of patient or parents, and preventive dentistry, should be started as early as possible. Dental neglect is common and can lead to serious consequences. Bleeding after dental extractions is an important cause of emergencies.

The use of fluorides, fissure sealants, dietary advice on the need for sugar restriction and regular dental inspections from an early age are crucial to the long-term care of the teeth. Prevention of periodontal disease is also imperative. Comprehensive dental assessment is needed at the age of about 12–13, to plan for the future and to decide how best to forestall difficulties resulting from overcrowding or misplaced third molars or other teeth.

Surgery and postoperative haemorrhage. Dental extractions and surgery are dangerous for haemophiliacs. Surgery should therefore be carefully planned to avoid complications. Radiographs should be taken for any unsuspected disease and to assess whether further extractions might prevent future trouble.

Bleeding after extraction in an unprepared haemophilic responds quickly to antihaemophilia factor, but bleeding deep in the tissues from an inferior dental block can be life–threatening. Rarely, even submucosal infiltrations have caused widespread haematoma formation. Local anaesthesia should therefore be avoided in the absence of Factor VIII replacement, but intraligamentary injections may be safe.

Before major surgery the patient is assessed by haemostatic screening (APTT, PT, platelet count), Factor VIII assay, specific antibody test, fibrinogen estimation, hepatitis B and HIV tests and liver function tests.

The patient should be admitted to hospital and haemoglobin estimation carried out. Blood is also grouped and cross-matched for use in emergency. Surgery is best carried out on Thursdays and Fridays, since bleeding is most likely on the day of operation or from 4 to 10 days postoperatively. All surgical procedures must be covered with AHF which is given 1 hour preoperatively.

Table 3.9. Outline of managment of haemophiliacs requiring dental surgery

Operation	Factor VIII level required	Preoperatively give	Postoperative schedule
Dental extraction	Minimum of 50 per cent at operation	Factor VIII i.v.* Tranexamic acid 1 g.i.v. (or by mouth starting 24 h preop.)	Rest inpatient for 7 days unless resident close to Centre (then 3 days). Soft diet. For 10 days give tranexamic acid 1 g q..i.d. and penicillin V 250 mg q.i.d. If there is bleeding during this period give repeat dose of Factor VIII*
Maxillofacial surgery	100 per cent at operation; 50 per cent for 7 days postop.	Factor VIII i.v.†	Rest inpatient for 10 days. Soft diet. Twice daily i.v. Factor VIII* for 7–10 days

*Factor VIII dose in Units = weight in kg × 25 given 1 h preoperatively.
†Factor VIII dose in Units = weight in kg × 50 given 1 h preoperatively.

The dose of AHF given before operation depends both on the severity of haemophilia and the amount of trauma involved (*Table 3.9*). Factor VIII is effective only for about 12 hours and therefore must be given regularly at least twice-daily postoperatively for major surgery.

A Factor VIII level of between 50 and 75 per cent is required for dental extractions. AHF may also need to be given postoperatively but many patients can be managed with antifibrinolytic agents given during the subsequent 10 days. If oral bleeding recurs postoperatively, Factor VIII must be given: some advise the administration of a further single dose of Factor VIII as a routine on the fourth or fifth postoperative day. However, this should be unnecessary if adequate Factor VIII has been given preoperatively.

Antifibrinolytics significantly reduce Factor VIII requirements. Tranexamic acid (Cyklokapron) is used in a dose of 1 g (30 mg/kg) orally, four times daily starting 24 hours preoperatively. Antifibrinolytics must not be used where residual clots are present, for example in the urinary tract or intracranially. In haemophiliacs, the urine should therefore be examined preoperatively for haematuria.

Tranexamic acid used topically significantly reduces bleeding. Ten ml of a 5 per cent solution used as a mouthrinse for 2 minutes, four times daily for 7 days is recommended. This solution can be made up by diluting 10 per cent tranexamic acid solution for injection, with sterile water.

Desmopressin (deamino-8-D arginine vasopressin: DDAVP) given as an intravenous infusion (0.5 µg/kg, repeated 12 hourly if necessary) temporarily corrects the haemostatic defect in mild haemophilia by releasing Factor VIII C (endogenous procoagulant) and von Willebrand Factor into the blood. Desmopressin may be useful for patients with Factor VIII inhibitors and is also increasingly widely used, as mentioned earlier, for the management of mild haemophiliacs for such purposes as extractions. As desmopressin also causes release of plasminogen activator, tranexamic acid should also be given.

Desmopressin may cause facial flushing and slight tachycardia but the chief adverse effect is tachyphylaxis—decreasing response on repeated injection.

Local measures are also important to protect the operation area and minimize the risk of postoperative bleeding. Thus surgery should be carried out with minimal trauma to both bone and soft tissues, and careful mouth toilet postoperatively is also essential. Suturing (though theoretically unnecessary) is desirable to stabilize gum flaps and to prevent postoperative disturbance of wounds by eating. Non-resorbable sutures are preferred and should be removed at 4–7 days. Suturing carries with it the risk, if there is postoperative bleeding, of causing blood to track down towards the mediastinum with danger to the airway. However, such an eventuality is an indication of inadequate preoperative replacement therapy, although complications of this sort can result from the presence of Factor VIII inhibitors when postoperative haemostasis is less predictable.

Prevention of infection. Antimicrobials such as oral penicillin V 250 mg four times daily should be given postoperatively for a full course of 7 days to reduce the risk of secondary haemorrhage. Infection also appears to induce fibrinolysis.
   In the case of difficult extractions, when mucoperiosteal flaps must be raised, the lingual tissues in the lower molar regions should preferably be left undisturbed since trauma may open up planes into which haemorrhage can track and endanger the airway. The buccal approach to lower third molars is therefore safer. Minimal bone should be removed and the teeth should be sectioned for removal where possible.
   The packing of extraction sockets is unnecessary in haemophilia if replacement therapy has been adequate but some advise the packing of a small amount of oxidized cellulose soaked in tranexamic acid into the bases of the sockets. Acrylic protective splints are rarely used now, in view of their liability to cause mucosal trauma and to promote sepsis, but they may be needed in certain sites such as the palate.
   Postoperatively, care should be taken to watch for haematoma formation—which may manifest itself by swelling, dysphagia or hoarseness. The patency of the airway must always be ensured.

Hazards of anaesthesia and intramuscular injections. As mentioned earlier, local anaesthesia or surgery is hazardous in the absence of factor replacement. Conservative treatment of the primary dentition and sometimes of the permanent dentition may be carried out without anaesthesia. If conservative treatment is not tolerated without anaesthesia, papillary or intraligamentary infiltration may achieve sufficient analgesia and is unlikely to cause serious bleeding. Topical application of 10 per cent cocaine to the exposed pulp is the choice for vital pulp extirpation. Infiltration anaesthesia may be used with caution and is adequate for conservative work in children, but lingual infiltration must be avoided. Regional (inferior dental or posterior superior alveolar) blocks or injections in the floor of the mouth must not be used since they can cause haemorrhage, allowing blood to track down to cause airway obstruction, and even submucous injections can sometimes cause massive deep haematomas. If factor replacement therapy has been given, regional anaesthesia can be used, providing the Factor VIII level is maintained above 30 per cent, but infiltration is still preferable. Intravenous midazolam or relative analgesia can be used.
   Endotracheal intubation for general anaesthesia may cause bleeding and is dangerous in unprepared patients, but since replacement therapy has to

be given for the surgical procedure, intubation can be carried out. An oral latex cuffed endotracheal tube is recommended to minimize trauma to the nasal and tracheal lining. The possibility of anaemia (Chapter 4) due to earlier blood loss must also be remembered if general anaesthesia is contemplated.

Intramuscular injections should be avoided unless replacement therapy is being given, as they can cause large haematomas. Oral alternatives are in any case satisfactory in most instances.

Trauma to the head and neck. Haemophiliacs with head and neck injuries are at risk from bleeding into the cranial cavity or into the fascial spaces of the neck. They should, therefore, be given factor replacement to a level of 100 per cent prophylactically after a head or facial trauma. If there are lacerations that need suturing, a minimum level of Factor VIII of 50 per cent is required at the time, with further cover for 3 days.

Endodontics: Root canal treatment may obviate the need for extractions and can usually be carried out without special precautions other than care to avoid reaming through the apex. However, in severe haemophilia, bleeding from the pulp and periapical tissues can be persistent and troublesome .

Periodontal treatment: In all but severe haemophiliacs scaling can be carried out under antifibrinolytic cover. Periodontal surgery necessitates factor replacement. All necessary surgery (and other dental treatment) should of course be performed at one operation.

Conservative dentistry: Soft tissue trauma must be avoided and a matrix band may help prevent gingival laceration. However, care must be taken not to let the matrix band cut the periodontal tissues and start gingival bleeding. A rubber dam is also useful to protect the mucosa from trauma but the clamp must be carefully applied. High speed vacuum aspirators and saliva ejectors must be used with caution in order to avoid production of haematomas. Trauma from the saliva ejector can be minimized by resting it on a gauze swab placed in the floor of the mouth.

Orthodontics: There is no contraindication to the movement of teeth in haemophilia. However, there must be no sharp edges to appliances, wires etc., which might traumatize the mucosa.

Other problems. *Haemophiliacs with inhibitors:* Between 5 and 20 per cent of haemophiliacs who have had multiple transfusions develop inhibitory antibodies, which reduce the activity of Factor VIII. Occasionally other patients also develop Factor VIII antibodies. Bleeding episodes are not more frequent when inhibitors are present but are more difficult to control. Two types of inhibitor are known—high and low titre inhibitors.

In general, those with low titre inhibitors can have dental treatment in the same way as those who have no antibodies. However, in those with high titre inhibitors' surgery and other traumatic procedures must be avoided unless absolutely essential. If the concentration of inhibitors is low, Factor VIII may be effective for 4–5 days or longer if immunosuppressive therapy has been given. In those with higher concentrations of inhibitors, Human Factor VIII Inhibitor Bypassing Fraction is available. In many cases, desmopressin is an effective alternative.

Hepatitis, infection with HIV and liver disease: Haemophiliacs are at risk from viral hepatitis and infection with HIV. Older patients, treated before blood products were screened for hepatitis B or heat-treated against HIV are particularly at risk. Hepatitis C and delta infection, however, are increasingly prevalent (Chapter 8). It is essential therefore to treat all such patients as possibly infective and to take the precautions outlined in Chapters 8 and 16.

Bleeding aggravated by drugs: Aspirin or other nonsteroidal anti–inflammatory drugs such as indomethacin, should not be given to patients with haemophilia since they can cause gastric bleeding and worsen the haemorrhagic tendency by depressing platelet aggregation. Codeine and paracetamol are safer alternative analgesics for patients witha bleeding tendency.

Anxiety: Many haemophiliacs are acutely anxious about dental treatment. Emotional factors significantly influence fibrinolytic activity so that reassurance of the patient and use of sedatives may be helpful.

Drug dependence: The severe pain from haemarthroses may occasionally lead to drug dependence (Chapter 19) but this is uncommon.

Christmas Disease (Haemophilia B)

Christmas disease (Factor IX deficiency) is clinically identical to haemophilia A and inherited in the same way, but it is about one-tenth as common as haemophilia A and female carriers often have a bleeding tendency.

Dental management

The earlier comments on dental management in haemophilia A apply equally to patients with haemophilia B, but Factor IX replacement is needed before surgery. Human dried Factor IX concentrate is supplied as a powder to be reconstituted with distilled water for intravenous administration. A dose of 20 units Factor IX per kg body weight is used intravenously 1 hour preoperatively. The standard preparation may also contain Factors II, VII and X. Factor IX is more stable than Factor VIII. Its half-life is often up to 2 days, so that replacement therapy can sometimes be given at longer intervals than in haemophilia A.

Von Willebrand's Disease

Von Willebrand's disease (pseudohaemophilia) is a bleeding disorder caused by a deficiency of von Willebrand factor and Factor VIII. It is usually inherited as an autosomal dominant but a severe form of the disease may be inherited as a sex-linked recessive trait like true haemophilia. Von Willebrand's disease affects from 1 to 45 per 100 000 of the population and is thus as least as common as haemophilia A but usually presents considerably less severe problems of management. Von Willebrand's disease is characterized by a prolonged bleeding time, usually a prolonged APTT, low levels of von Willebrand's factor (Factor VIII R: Ag), and low Factor VIII C and VIII R: RCo (Ristocetin cofactor) levels. The low level of Factor VIII R results in poor platelet adhesion after trauma. Platelets usually fail to aggregate in the presence of ristocetin so that, unlike haemophilia, purpura is common and the bleeding time is prolonged.

Von Willebrand's disease not only affects females as well as males but the clinical presentation usually differs from haemophilia A (*Table 3.8*). The common bleeding pattern is purpura of mucous membranes and the skin. Gingival haemorrhage is more common than in haemophilia and haemarthroses are rare. Although the disorder is usually less severe than haemophilia A, postoperative haemorrhage can be troublesome. Symptoms appear to diminish with age.

The severity of von Willebrand's disease varies from patient to patient and from time to time; some patients have a clinically insignificant disorder, while others have Factor VIII levels low enough to cause severe clotting defects as well as a prolonged bleeding time. However, the severity does not correlate well with the Factor VIII level (*see* Appendix 3). Pregnancy and the contraceptive pill may cause transient amelioration.

Rarely, von Willebrand's disease may be acquired, particularly in patients with autoimmune or lymphoproliferative diseases

Dental management

In most patients with von Willebrand's disease, the haemostatic defect can be controlled with desmopressin. The chief exceptions are type IIB disease in which desmopressin is contraindicated because it stimulates release of dysfunctional von Willebrand Factor which leads, in turn, to platelet aggregation and severe but transient thrombocytopenia. It is also contraindicated in type III disease where so little von Willebrand factor is formed that essentially the same management is required as for haemophilia A. However, since Factor VIII has a prolonged half-life, less frequent infusions may be required.

Aspirin should be avoided.

Hereditary haemorrhagic telangiectasia, mitral valve prolapse, or Factor XII deficiency may be associated and may require to be considered in the management plan.

Other Congenital Coagulation Defects

Any of the other clotting factors can be deficient and all may be associated with a haemorrhagic tendency, except Factor XII deficiency (in spite of prolonged clotting time and prolonged APTT in this defect). Most are uncommon or rare defects. Factor XI deficiency (plasma thromboplastin antecedent deficiency) is one of the more common and is sometimes known as haemophilia C.

Fresh frozen plasma will usually correct most of these coagulation defects, but local haemostatic measures should also be applied. Further details are found in Appendix 1.

ACQUIRED COAGULATION DEFECTS

Acquired haemorrhagic disorders are much more prevalent than the congenital diseases but are usually less severe, except in anticoagulant therapy or liver disease.

Important causes include:

1. Anticoagulant therapy.
2. Vitamin K deficiency or malabsorption.
3. Aspirin and other nonsteroidal anti–inflammatory analgesics
4. Liver disease.
5. Disseminated intravascular coagulation.
6. Fibrinolytic states.

Nevertheless, some of those with clinical bleeding tendencies do not have a defect detectable by current laboratory methods.

Anticoagulant Treatment

The commonly used anticoagulants are coumarins, such as warfarin, for long-term, and heparin for short-term treatment. Anticoagulants are given for thromboembolic disease but their use varies widely (*Table 3.10*).

Table 3.10. Important conditions for which anticoagulants may be used

Deep vein thrombosis
Embolization secondary to myocardial infarction
Atrial fibrillation
Renal dialysis
Heart valve replacements
Cerebral thrombosis

Coumarins are given orally and antagonize the action of vitamin K so that the prothrombin and activated partial thromboplastin times are prolonged. The effects are delayed for 8–12 hours, are maximal at 36 hours, but persist for 72 hours. Coumarin anticoagulant therapy should maintain a prothrombin time of 2–2$^{1/2}$ times the control (control 11–15 seconds), or a thrombotest of 5–20 per cent. Prothrombin times are often now recorded as the international normalized ratio (INR), a ratio of 1.5–2.5 being the usual therapeutic range but up to 4.5 for recurrent deep vein thrombosis.

Heparin given by injection acts immediately, mainly by inhibiting the thrombin–fibrinogen reaction. The prothrombin, activated partial thromboplastin and thrombin times are therefore prolonged. This effect is usually lost within less than 6 hours of stopping heparin.

Reduction in anticoagulant dosage can lead to rebound thrombosis: therefore, there should be no interference with such treatment without the agreement of the clinician in charge. Neglect of this important point has led to thrombosis of prosthetic cardiac valves and even thrombotic deaths after dental surgery.

Dental management of patients on oral (coumarin) anticoagulation

The prothrombin time (PT) or the Thrombotest are the most useful laboratory tests for monitoring oral anticoagulant activity. Blood (citrated) for the

Table 3.11. Assessment of oral anticoagulant therapy

	Prothrombin time	*Thrombotest*
Normal level	<1.3	>70%
Therapeutic range	2–4.5	5–20%
Levels at which		
minor surgery can be carried out	<2.5	>15%

prothrombin time is tested as soon as possible (within a few hours of venepuncture.). Blood for the Thrombotest must be collected in special siliconized containers (*Table 3.11*).

In general, patients on coumarin anticoagulants should not have their medication stopped or changed. Minor surgery (simple extractions of two or three teeth) may be carried out safely with *no* change in anticoagulant treatment if the prothrombin time is within the normal therapeutic range ($1^{1/2}$–$2^{1/2}$ times normal: INR >1.5: Thrombotest 15 per cent or higher). Regional blocks should be avoided. Surgery should be as atraumatic as possible, and a small amount of haemostatic material (e.g. oxidized cellulose) may be sutured over the socket, but is not essential.

More major oral surgery is best done in hospital and with the agreement of the clinician in charge, anticoagulation may need to be modified. If anticoagulants are to be continued, vitamin K should preferably be avoided as it makes subsequent anticoagulation difficult. If the use of vitamin K cannot be avoided, only 10 mg should be given in these circumstances. In an emergency an antifibrinolytic agent (tranexamic acid) can be used to control haemorrhage.

Patients on oral anticoagulants are especially at risk from haemorrhage under the following circumstances.

1. Irregular tablet taking.
2. Liver disease or obstructive jaundice which impair vitamin K metabolism or absorption.
3. Prolonged broad spectrum antibiotic (tetracycline) therapy which reduces vitamin K synthesis (theoretically).
4. Liquid paraffin which leads to loss of vitamin K (theoretically).
5. Use of protein-binding drugs which displace the anticoagulant from plasma proteins and increase its effect, e.g. aspirin, phenylbutazone, sulphonamides. Co-trimoxazole, which contains a sulphonamide, is, therefore, contraindicated.
6. Use of aspirin and other non-steroidal anti-inflammatory agents which can cause gastric bleeding and also interfere with platelet function.
7. Withdrawal of barbiturates which decreases the breakdown of the anticoagulants.

Under such circumstances the Thrombotest should be repeated within 24 hours of surgery. It should be remembered that the condition for which anticoagulant therapy is being given, especially prosthetic heart valves, may also affect dental management (*Table 3.10* and Chapter 2).

Dental management of patients on heparin anticoagulation

The effect of heparin is best assessed by the thrombin time, which is usually maintained at 3–4 times normal (control 10–12 seconds). Low dose heparin therapy such as 'Minihep' (used to reduce postoperative complication of deep vein thrombosis) may have little effect on thethrombin time or on postoperative bleeding.

Heparin is given intravenously and its use is therefore restricted to inpatients. It has an immediate effect on blood clotting but acts for only 4–6 hours, so that no specific treatment is needed to reverse its effect. This can be achieved immediately during an emergency by intravenous protamine sulphate. Usually there is no need to interfere with anticoagulant treatment for simple extractions.

Surgery can safely be carried out after 6–8 hours, when the effects of heparinization have ceased. In renal dialysis patients surgery is best carried out on the day after dialysis as the effects of heparinization have then ceased and there is maximum benefit from dialysis (Chapter 9).

Vitamin K Deficiency and Malabsorption

Vitamin K is taken in with the diet and also synthesized by the gut flora. It is a fat-soluble vitamin and its absorption in the small gut depends on the presence of bile salts. After transport to the liver, vitamin K is used for the synthesis of Factors II (prothrombin), VII, IX and X.

Haemorrhagic disease may, therefore, result from inadequate amounts of vitamin K reaching the liver particularly as a result of obstructive jaundice or malabsorption. Alternatively, vitamin K metabolism may be impaired by anticoagulants or severe liver disease. In the last, many haemostatic functions are severely impaired and vitamin K is of little or no value (*Table 3.12*).

Table 3.12. Clotting defects involving vitamin K

1. Lack of synthesis in gut*
   Broad spectrum antibiotics used for prolonged periods or inpatients on parenteral feeding
2. Poor absorption*
   Malabsorption syndromes
   Obstructive jaundice
3. Failure of utilization
   Oral anticoagulant treatment
   Liver failure

*Responds to parenteral vitamin K.

Dental aspects

Dental management in vitamin K deficiency may be complicated by problems resulting from: (*a*) the clotting defect and (*b*) the underlying disorder, particularly obstructive jaundice (Chapter 8), which may be caused by gallstones, viral hepatitis or carcinoma of the head of the pancreas.

The underlying disorder should preferably be corrected, but vitamin K can be given if surgery is urgent. Phytomenadione (5–25 mg) is the most potent and rapidly acting form and should preferably be given intravenously to avoid intramuscular injection. The prothrombin time should be monitored after 48 hours, and, if the defect has not been corrected by then, this suggests parenchymal liver disease.

Liver Disease

Liver disease is an important cause of bleeding disorders. The haemostatic defects in liver failure include impaired vitamin K metabolism; increased fibrinolysis; failure of synthesis or increased consumption of normal clotting factors; synthesis of abnormal clotting factors and thrombocytopenia.

Haemorrhage can be severe and difficult to manage because of the complexity of these defects. Antifibrinolytic treatment and fresh-frozen plasma may sometimes be effective. If there is an obstructive element to the disease vitamin K may be effective but only if parenchymal disease is mild (Chapter 8).

Disseminated Intravascular Coagulation

Disseminated intravascular coagulation (DIC), also known as consumption coagulopathy or defibrination syndrome, is an uncommon, complex and not fully understood process in which the main effect is probably activation of the haemostasis-related mechanisms within the circulation. There is a variety of both precipitating causes including incompatible blood transfusions, severe sepsis, obstetric complications, severe trauma or burns, and cancers in various sites. In one series of head injuries some degree of DIC was found in 57 per cent.

Possible effects of disseminated intravascular coagulation include:

Haemorrhagic tendencies: These result from the consumption of platelets and clotting factors internally and from activation of the fibrinolytic system. Purpura and bleeding from sites such as the gastrointestinal tract can result. In the case of head injuries, DIC may lead to intracranial haemorrhage.

Thrombotic phenomena: Clotting in capillaries can damage any organ but the kidneys, liver, adrenals and brain are particularly vulnerable. Brain ischaemia by vascular occlusion may therefore result from DIC secondary to head injury.

Haemolysis: Red cells become damaged as a result of the changes in the capillaries (microangiopathic haemolysis).

Shock: Shock may be caused by adrenal damage or obstruction of the pulmonary circulation by fibrin deposition and other factors.

Management. The management of disseminated intravascular coagulation is controversial and must in any case depend on the cause and pathological changes taking place. In general the underlying cause and any hypoxia or acidosis should be corrected. In addition, heparinization, replacement of clotting factors and platelets, or antifibrinolytic therapy may be given as appropriate. No single programme of treatment is effective for all cases.

DIC is an acute emergency and dental treatment is highly unlikely to be considered—except afterwards in survivors.

Fibrinolytic States

Fibrinolytics, such as the drugs streptokinase, alteplase, anistreplase and urokinase, and local activation of plasmin by infection for example, may cause abnormal bleeding. Dental surgery should be deferred where possible in patients on fibrinolytic therapy.

Other Disorders Associated with Bleeding Tendencies

These include the following:

1. Polycythaemia vera (Chapter 5).
2. Myelofibrosis, leukaemia or lymphoma (Chapter 5).
3. Chronic renal failure (Chapter 9).
4. Cyanotic congenital heart disease (Chapter 2).
5. Gram-negative shock.
6. After massive transfusions.
7. Antibodies to clotting factors.
8. Head injuries (Chapter 13)

Blood Blisters in the Mouth

Causes of blood blisters in the mouth include:

1. Trauma.
2. Any cause of purpura.
3. Mucous membrane pemphigoid (Chapter 16).
4. Localized oral purpura (angina bullosa haemorrhagica. Chapter 16).
5. Amyloidosis (causing factor X deficiency. Chapter 5).

Tendency to Thrombosis (Appendix 2)

Bibliography

Abubaker A.O., Bontempo F.A. and Braun T. (1987) Use of deamino-8-D arginine vasopressin in a patient with moderate von Willebrand's disease. *J. Oral Maxillofac. Surg.* **45**, 728.
Bailey B. M. W. and Fordyce A. M. (1983) Complications of dental extractions in patients receiving Warfarin anticoagulant therapy. *Br. Dent.* **155**, 308–10.
Barnard N., and Scully C. (1992) *Epstein's Syndrome Implications for the Oral Surgeon* (in press).
Benoliel R., Leviner E., Katz S. et al. (1986) Dental treatment for the patient on anticoagulant therapy. Prothrombin-time value: what difference does it make? *Oral Surg.* **62**, 149–51.
Cameron C.B. and Kobrinsky N. (1990) Perioperative management of patients with von Willebrand's disease. *Can. J. Anaesth.* **37**, 341–7.
Campbell H. D. and Payne R. W. (1977) Dental extractions in a family with von Willebrand's disease. *Br. Dent. J.* **142**, 402.
Castaldi P. A. (1980) The patient with easy bruising and bleeding. *Medicine (UK)* **28**, 1416–20.
Cawson R.A. and Spector R.G. (1989) *Clinical Pharmacology in Dentistry*. 5th ed. Edinburgh, Churchill Livingstone.
Colin W. and Needleman H. L. (1985) Medical and dental management of apatient with congenital Factor XIII deficiency. *Pediatr. Dent.* **7**, 227–30.
Editorial (1983) DDAVP in haemophilia and von Willebrand's disease. *Lancet* **ii**, 774–5.
Evans B. E. (1989) Dental management. In: Hilgartner M. W., Pochedly, C. (eds) *Hemophilia in the Child and Adult*. 3rd ed. New York, Raven Press, pp. 89–119.
Eyster M. E. (1978) Hemophilia: a guide for the primary care physician. *Postgrad. Med.* **64**, 75–81.
Feffer S. E., Parray H. R. and Westring D. W. (1978) Seizure after infusion of aminocaproic acid. *JAMA* **240**, 2468.
Geffner I. and Porteous S. R. (1981) Haemorrhage and pain control in conservative dentistry for haemophiliacs. *Br. Dent. J.* **151**, 256–8.
Gilmore W. C. and Doku H. C. (1979) Factor IX deficiency resulting in severe postoperative haemorrhage after odontectomy. *J. Oral Surg.* **37**, 885-7.

Green D. (1980) Von Willebrand's disease. *Postgrad. Med. J.* **67**, 241–8.

Hobson P. (1981) Dental care of children with haemophilia and related conditions. *Br. Dent. J.* **151**, 249–53.

Johnson W.T. and Leary J.M. (1988) Management of dental patients withbleeding disorders: review and update. *Oral Surg.* **66**, 297–303.

Larson C. E., Chang J-L., Bleyaert A. L. et al. (1980) Anesthetic considerations for the oral surgery patient with hemophilia. *J. Oral Surg.* **38**, 516–19.

Leading Article (1983) DDAVP in haemophilia and von Willebrand's disease. *Lancet* **ii**, 774.

Levine P. H. (1985) The acquired immunodeficiency syndrome in persons with hemophilia. *Ann. Intern. Med.* **103**, 723–6.

Lowe G. D. O. and Forbes C. D. (1979) Laboratory diagnosis of congenital coagulation defects. *Clin. Haematol.* **8**, 79–94.

Lusher J. M. (1980) Efficacy of prothrombin-complex concentrates in hemophiliacs with antibodies to Factor VIII: a multicenter therapeutic trial. *N. Engl. J. Med.* **303**, 421–5.

Mannucci P. M., Ruggeri Z. M., Pareti F. I. et al. (1977) Deamino-8-D-arginine vasopressin: a new pharmacological approach to the management of haemophilia and von Willebrand's disease. *Lancet* **ii**, 869–72.

Marengo-Rowe A. J. and Leveson J. E. (1977) Evaluation of the bleeding patient. *Postgrad. Med.* **62**, 171–7.

Marshall W. G. and Colvin B. T. (1978) Maxillo-facial injury in severe haemophilia. *Br. J. Oral Surg.* **15**, 57–63.

McDonough R.J. and Nelson C.L. (1989) Clinical implications of factor XII deficiency. *Oral Surg.* **68**, 264–6.

Monsour P. A., Kruger B. J. and Harden P. A. (1986) Prevalence and detection of patients with bleeding disorders. *Aust. Dent. J.* **31**, 104–10.

Mulligan R. and Weitzel K.G. (1988) Pretreatment management of the patient receiving anticoagulant drugs. *J. Am. Dent. Assoc.* **117**, 479,83.

Needleman H. L., Kaban L. B. and Kevy S. V. (1976) The use of epsilon- aminocaproic acid for the management of hemophilia in dental and oral surgery patients. *J. Am. Dent. Assoc.* **93**, 586–90.

Peery W.H. (1987) Clinical spectrum of hereditary haemorrhage telangiectasia. *Am. J. Med.* **82**, 989–97.

Perkin R. F., White G. C. and Webster W. P. (1979) Glanzmann's thrombasthenia. *Oral Surg.* **47**, 36–9.

Poker I.D., Read, P.C. and Cook R.M. (1990) Factor XI deficiency disclosed following haemorrhage related to a dental extraction. *Aust. Dent. J.* **35**, 258–60.

Pollock A. (1977) The bleeding disorders. *Br. Dent. J.* **143**, 405–9.

Redding S. W. and Stiegler K. E. (1983) Dental management of the classic hemophiliac with inhibitors. *Oral Surg.* **56**, 145–8.

Richards A., Scully C., Eveson J. and Prime S.S. (1991) Epstein's syndrome: oral lesions in a patient with nephropathy, deafness and thrombocytopenia. *J. Oral Pathol. Med.* **20**, 512–13.

Royer J.W. and Bates W.S. (1988) Management of von Willebrand's disease with desmopressin. *J. Oral Maxillofac. Surg.* **46**, 313–4.

Sindet-Pedersen S.,Ingerslev J., Ramstrom G. et al. (1988) Management of oral bleeding in haemophilic patients. *Lancet* **ii**, 566.

Stephenson P., Lamey P.I., Scully C. et al. (1987) Angina bullosa haemorrhagica: clinical and laboratory features in 30 patients. *Oral Surg.* **36**, 25–9.

Stephenson P., Scully C., Prime S. S. et al. (1987) Angina bullosa haemorrhagica: lesional immunostaining and haematological findings. *Br. J. Oral Maxillofac. Surg.* **25**, 488–91.

Sugar A. W. (1979) The management of dental extractions in cases of thrombasthenia complicated by the development of isoantibodies to donor platelets. *Oral Surg.* **48**, 116–19.

Travis S., Wray R. and Harrison K. (1989) Perioperative anticoagulant control. *Br. J. Surg.* **76**, 1107–8.

Vinckier R. and Vermylen J. (1985) Dental extractions in hemophilia: reflections on ten years experience. *Oral Surg.* **59**, 6–9.

White G. C. and Lesesne H. R. (1983) Hemophilia, hepatitis and the acquired immunodeficiency syndrome. *Ann. Intern. Med.* **98**, 403–4.

Zakrzewska J. (1983) Gingival bleeding as a manifestation of von Willebrand's disease. *Br. Dent. J.* **155**, 157–60.

Appendix 1 to Chapter 3

RARE COAGULATION-RELATED FACTOR DEFECTS

Coagulation Factor Defect	Bleeding Tendency	APTT	PT	Basic Defect
V	+	↑	↑	Genetic: AR Streptomycin Liver disease, others
VII	+	—	↑	Genetic: AR Liver disease; anticoagulants many others
X Stuart-Prower factor	+ usually	↑	↑	Genetic: AR Primary amyloid; others
XI Plasma thromboplastin antecedent	+	↑	—	
XII Hageman factor	—	↑	—	Genetic: AR
XIII Fibrin stabilizing factor	+	—*	—*	Genetic: AR
α Antiplasmin (Miyasato disease)	+	—**	—**	Genetic: AR many others
Fibrinogen	+	↑	↑	Genetic: AR
Prekallikrein (Fletcher factor)	—	↑	—	Genetic: AR Nephrotic syndrome Liver disease

AR = autosomal recessive.
* = Assay by clot solubility.
** = Assay by α antiplasmin function.

Appendix 2 to Chapter 3

DISORDERS PREDISPOSING TO THROMBOSES

Factor Involved	Aetiology	Management
Platelets (Thrombocytosis and thrombo-cythaemia)*	Exercise; pregnancy; trauma; post-splenectomy; chronic inflammatory disease; malignancy	Treat underlying cause. Preoperative aspirin, dipyridamole or heparin
Antithrombin III deficiency	Genetic: AD Eclampsia, DIC Nephrotic syndrome	Superficial and deep vein thromboses with pulmonary embolism triggered by surgery, trauma, infection or pregnancy. Resistant to heparin anticoagulation—use oral anticoagulants ± fresh frozen plasma
Protein C deficiency or Protein S deficiency	Genetic: AD Liver disease DIC	Clinical features as for anti-thrombin III deficiency. In addition, skin necroses if oral anticoagulants given

* See Chapters 3 and 5.
AD = autosomal dominant; DIC = disseminated intravascular coagulopathy.

Appendix 3 to Chapter 3

SUB-TYPES OF VON WILLEBRAND'S DISEASE

	Type 1	*Type 11A*	*Type 11B*	*Type 11C*	*Type 111*
Inheritance	AD	AD	AD	AR	AR
Bleeding time	↑	↑	↑	↑	↑
Factor VIII C	↓	↓ or N	↓ or N	N	↓↓
Factor VIII R:Ag (von Willebrand factor)	↓	↓ or N	↓ or N	N	↓↓
Factor VIII R:RCo (ristocetin cofactor)	↓	↓↓	↓ or N	↓	↓↓
Platelet aggregation with ristocetin	↓ or N	↓	↑	↓	↓
Other comments	Mild bleeding tendency. Desmopressin restores haemostasis	—	May have thrombo-cytopenia	—	May be severe bleeding tendency

AD = autosomal dominant; AR = autosomal recessive.
N = normal; ↑ = increased; ↓ = decreased.

Chapter 4

Anaemia

The essential feature of anaemia is a haemoglobin level below the normal (less than approximately 12 g/dl) for the age and sex (Appendix to this chapter). Its effect, therefore, is to reduce the oxygen-carrying capacity of the blood. Anaemia, particularly sickle cell disease, can thus make general anaesthesia hazardous. Some anaemias can also cause oral lesions or sometimes affect dental management in other ways.

Anaemia is not a disease in itself and may be a feature of many diseases (*Table 4.1*), but the different types of anaemia have many clinical features in common (*Table 4.2*). In the early stages anaemia is frequently asymptomatic; skin colour is misleading but pallor of the oral mucosa suggests severe anaemia. Anaemia exacerbates or can cause heart failure and also aggravates the effects of pulmonary disease.

The most common cause of anaemia in Britain is chronic blood loss and consequent iron deficiency. Folate and vitamin B_{12} (cobalamin) deficiency are the next most common causes, but the precise nature of anaemia can only be established by clinical and laboratory investigation (*see* Appendices to this chapter and Chapter 1).

The main types of anaemia which have to be considered are iron deficiency (microcytic anaemia MCV below 78 fl); macrocytic anaemia (MCV more than 99 fl), usually caused by vitamin B_{12} or folate deficiency; and normocytic anaemia, which may result from leukaemia or other causes, particularly sickle cell disease, as discussed later.

Table 4.1. Causes of anaemia

1. Blood loss
   Menorrhagia
   Any gastrointestinal lesion (e.g. ulcer or carcinoma)
   Lesions of the urinary tract
   Trauma
2. Impaired absorption of haematinics
3. Increased demands for haematinics
   especially pregnancy
4. Poor intake of haematinics (uncommonly)
5. Aplastic anaemia and leukaemia
6. Haemolytic anaemias
7. Miscellaneous mechanisms, including drugs and chronic disease

Table 4.2. Clinical features of anaemia

1. Sometimes none
2. General lassitude
3. Cardiorespiratory
    Dyspnoea
    Congestive cardiac failure
    Murmurs
    Angina pectoris
4. Cutaneous
    Pallor
    Brittle nails
    Koilonychia (iron deficiency)
5. Oral
    Sore mouth
    Oral ulceration
    Angular cstomatitis
    Glossitis

Laboratory Investigations

The most basic, and in many ways most useful, investigations are haemoglobin estimation and examination of a stained blood film. Automated examination of blood provides a quick and reliable count of all the blood cells and important cytological features of red cells such as cell volume and haemoglobin content. For this purpose a 4 ml sample of EDTA anticoagulated blood should be sent, with as much clinical information as possible, to the haematologist. A blood film may also be required as a mixed macro– and microcytic picture may sometimes not be revealed by an automated counter. Special investigations are discussed with the specific diseases. The laboratory investigation of the common anaemias is summarized in *Fig.* 4.1 (*see also* Appendix to this chapter).

Dental Aspects of Anaemia–General Considerations

Specific treatment of the different types of anaemia is considered later. The main danger is when a general anaesthetic is given, as it is vital to ensure full oxygenation. Nevertheless, the myocardium may be unable to respond to the demands of anaesthesia (Chapter 2). Whenever possible therefore the cause of the anaemia should be corrected preoperatively, but at least the haemoglobin level must be raised, if necessary by transfusion.

Elective operations under general anaesthesia should not usually be carried-out when the haemoglobin is less than 10 g/dl (male). In an emergency, anaemia can be corrected by whole blood transfusion, but this should only be given to a young and otherwise fit patient. Transfusion risks include fluid overload, and viral infections such as hepatitis and HIV. Packed red cells avoid the risk of fluid overload and can be given in emergency to the elderly patient or those with incipient congestive cardiac failure. A diuretic given at the same time further reduces the risk of congestive cardiac failure. The patient should be stabilized at least 24 hours preoperatively and it should be noted that haemoglobin estimations are unreliable for 12 hours post-transfusion. Nitrous oxide is possibly contraindicated in vitamin B_{12} deficiency (*see below*).

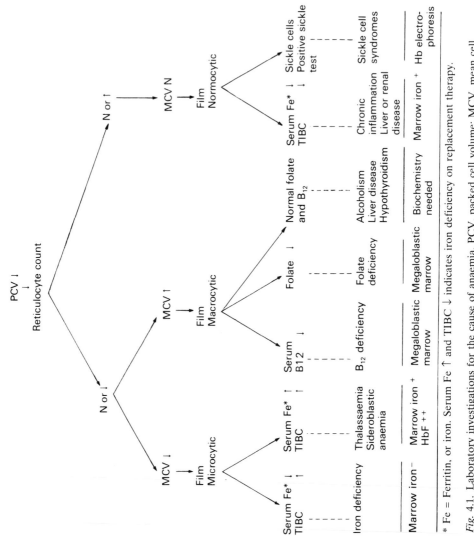

Fig. 4.1. Laboratory investigations for the cause of anaemia. PCV, packed cell volume; MCV, mean cell volume; TIBC, total iron binding capacity; HbF, fetal haemoglobin.

* Fe = Ferritin, or iron. Serum Fe ↑ and TIBC ↓ indicates iron deficiency on replacement therapy.

DEFICIENCY ANAEMIAS

Iron Deficiency Anaemia

The most common cause of anaemia worldwide is iron deficiency as a result of nutritional deficiencies in developing countries or chronic blood loss in the West. Women of child-bearing age and older are therefore mainly affected. In some studies, about 5 per cent of American women had mild iron deficiency anaemia and up to 25 per cent had low iron levels without anaemia. Excessive menstrual losses or gastrointestinal blood loss are the main causes. Very many children are mildly iron deficient because of the high demands for growth, especially during adolescence. By contrast, iron deficiency in an adult male almost invariably indicates blood loss, usually from the gastrointestinal or genitourinary tracts. The same holds true for post-menopausal women. The important features of iron deficiency anaemia are summarized in *Fig.* 4.1 and *Table 4.3.* In childhood, iron deficiency may predispose to developmental or behavioural disorders. However, symptoms ascribed to iron deficiency do not always respond to iron replacement. Serum ferritin levels are one of the most sensitive indices of iron deficiency but this test is not universally available. Transferrin saturation (serum iron/total iron binding capacity) is sometimes used: a value of less than 16 per cent indicates iron deficiency. An early feature is a reduction in the mean corpuscular volume (MCV), increasing variation in red cell size; later there is hypochromic microcytic anaemia with reduced marrow iron stores. Hypochromic microcytic anaemia with normal marrow iron stores is not caused directly by iron deficiency; it is uncommon but is a feature of thalassaemia and sideroblastic anaemia, as discussed later.

Table 4.3. Laboratory findings during the development of iron deficiency anaemia

	MCV	Hb	MCHC	Serum ferritin	Transferrin saturation*	Marrow iron stores
Normal	N	N	N	N	33%	N
Mild iron deficiency anaemia	↓	N or ↓	N	↓	>16%<33%	↓
Moderate iron deficiency anaemia	↓	↓	↓	↓	<16%	↓
Severe iron deficiency anaemia	↓↓	↓↓	↓↓	↓↓	<16%	↓↓

Arrows indicate a value above or below normal (N)
* Transferrin saturation = serum iron concentration/total iron binding capacity.
Note: It is now preferable to measure serum ferritin levels if this assay is available as it is more indicative of low iron stores than is the transferring saturation.

The best treatment of iron deficiency is an iron salt by mouth but the cause of the deficiency should first be found and eliminated. Ferrous gluconate 250 mg/day can be given if ferrous sulphate is not tolerated. Oral iron may need to be given for 3 months or more to replenish marrow iron stores. Parenteral iron has no advantages except, for example, when inflammatory bowel disease is aggravated by oral iron.

Vitamin B$_{12}$ Deficiency

Pernicious anaemia

Pernicious (Addisonian) anaemia is the most common type of macrocytic anaemia and typically affects women in the middle age or over, particularly of Northern European descent. It is caused by a specific defect of absorption of vitamin B$_{12}$, not by malnutrition. Autoantibodies against gastric parietal cells and/or intrinsic factor or both are found and the disease is sometimes seen with other autoimmune diseases, especially hypothyroidism, or less often, diabetes mellitus, vitiligo, Addison's disease or hypoparathyroidism (Chapter 10).

The underlying lesion is an atrophic gastritis causing failure of production of intrinsic factor by parietal cells and of gastric acid (achlorhydria). There may therefore be gastrointestinal symptoms and also an increased risk of stomach cancer.

Pernicious anaemia develops slowly because the liver stores of vitamin B$_{12}$ can last some 3 years, but ultimately there is macrocytic (megaloblastic) anaemia with depressed production of all blood cells (see Fig. 4.1).

In addition to the usual signs and symptoms of anaemia, neurological symptoms, particularly paraesthesiae of the extremities, develop in about 10 per cent. These are reversible with treatment but, in the past particularly, could lead to subacute combined degeneration of the spinal cord and, ultimately, paraplegia. Premature greying of the hair is another a well-recognized feature. Nitrous oxide can also interfere with vitamin B$_{12}$ metabolism and interfere with neurological function if administration continues for 12 or more hours or if it is used as a drug of abuse.

The diagnosis of pernicious anaemia depends on the clinical findings and low serum B$_{12}$ levels together with the auto antibodies. Vitamin B$_{12}$ absorption is impaired as shown by the Schilling test summarized in Table 4.4.

Serum B$_{12}$ levels may occasionally remain normal in patients who are cobalamin deficient. Conversely, macrocytosis may not be found in patients who have low vitamin B$_{12}$ levels: this is sometimes because there is concomitant iron deficiency which would otherwise cause microcytosis. In yet other circumstances, patients, such as those who abuse nitrous oxide, become vitamin B$_{12}$ deficient and develop neurological symptoms but not anaemia.

In a large study in the USA, 5 per cent of persons over 50 were found to have low serum cobalamin levels. This was previously thought to be of no

Table 4.4. Schilling test for B$_{12}$ deficiency

1. Radiolabelled vitamin B$_{12}$ (small dose) given orally
2. Unlabelled vitamin B$_{12}$ (large dose) given i.m. 2 hours later
3. Collect urine over 24 hours (or whole body counting)
4. Normal: excrete more than 15 per cent of radiolabelled B$_{12}$ in 24 hours
   B$_{12}$ deficiency; excrete less than 15 per cent of radiolabelled B$_{12}$ in 24 hours
5. Repeat with added oral intrinsic factor
   Pernicious anaemia; excretion of B$_{12}$ increases to normal
   Ileal disease: excretion of B$_{12}$ remains low

significance but the early finding that neurological damage could precede anaemia or even macrocytosis was confirmed. Absence of macrocytosis in some cases is due to concomitant iron deficiency, but in another study on 70 patients with very low (less than 100 ng/l) serum cobalamin levels, anaemia was absent in 19 per cent and macrocytosis was absent in 33 per cent. In some of these cases cobalamin deficiency was manifested first as cerebral abnormalities and what has been termed 'megaloblastic madness'.

Pernicious anaemia is treated with intramuscular hydroxycobalamin at about 2-monthly intervals for the rest of the patient's life.

Other causes of B_{12} deficiency

These are shown in *Table 4.5*, but pernicious anaemia is by far the most common in Britain.

Folate Deficiency

Red cell folate levels, when low, are unequivocal evidence of folate deficiency but may remain normal for a time in a few folate deficient patients until older erythrocytes are replaced. Serum folate assays are considerably less reliable. The main causes of folate deficiency are summarized in *Table 4.6*, but occasionally no cause can be discovered.

The effects of folate and B_{12} deficiency are very similar. Both cause megaloblastic changes in the marrow and macrocytic anaemia (*see Fig.* 4.1), defective DNA synthesis, impaired production of blood cells and, ultimately, of many other cells.

However, folate deficiency does not lead to subacute combined degeneration of the cord. It is also essential to distinguish it from pernicious anaemia, as treatment of the latter with folic acid will improve the haematological picture to some degree but aggravates the neurological damage.

In folate deficiency the red cell folate levels are low, serum B_{12} normal, and the B_{12} absorption (Schilling) test is normal; these tests enable the important

Table 4.5. Causes of vtamin B_{12} deficiency

1. Poor intake	Poverty
	Strict vegetarians (vegans, some Hindu Indians)
2. Malabsorption	*(a)* Defect in intrinsic factor production
	Congenital
	Autoimmune (pernicious anaemia)
	Gastrectomy
	(b) Ileal disease
	Coeliac disease
	Tropical sprue
	Crohn's disease (more frequently folate deficiency)
	Blind loop syndrome
	Resections
	Fish tapeworm (Finland, Asia)
	(c) Transcobalamin II deficiency
3. Drugs	Colchicine
	Neomycin
	Nitrous oxide (administration for more than 24 hours)

Table 4.6. Causes of folate deficiency

1. Poor intake	Poverty
	Old age
	Alcoholism
2. Malabsorption	Coeliac disease
	Crohn's disease
	Other malabsorption states
3. Increased demands	Infancy
	Pregnancy
	Chronic haemolysis
	Malignant disease
	Exfoliative skin lesions
	Chronic dialysis
4. Drugs	Alcohol
	Barbiturates
	Phenytoin
	Primidone
	Methotrexate
	Pyrimethamine
	Triamterene
	Co-trimoxazole
	Pentamidine
	Oral contraceptives

distinction to be made from B_{12} deficiency. Once the cause has been found and rectified, treatment with folic acid (5 mg daily by mouth) rapidly restores the normal blood picture.

Oral aspects of the deficiency anaemias

Oral mucosal lesions seem to be seen particularly frequently in the deficiency anaemias. For unknown reasons the tongue is especially affected, to the extent that soreness of the tongue can develop even before the haemoglobin falls below the lower limit of normal. Oral changes are of the following types.

The sore or burning, but otherwise normal tongue. Soreness of the tongue without depapillation or colour change can be caused by early deficiencies, often with normal haemoglobin levels. It is important to have haematological examination of these patients, especially as cobalamin deficiency can be the cause and as discussed earlier, anaemia or macrocytosis may be absent at this stage. It can, also at this early stage, occasionally also be associated with neurological disorders. Though sore tongue can be neurotic in origin (Chapter 14), it is important not to make this assumption without full investigation.

Atrophic glossitis. The red, glossy smooth sore tongue is the best known effect of severe anaemia but is much less frequently seen than in the past.

Moeller's glossitis and other colour changes In early B_{12} deficiency particularly, the tongue is sore and may also show a pattern of red lines without depapillation. In Moeller's glossitis a red line forms along the lateral margins and around the tip of the tongue, but this is rare. More commonly a less regular pattern of red lines forms on the dorsum. Alternatively, red sore patches may form. These may come and go but range from pin-head red spots to circular areas up to a centimetre across, which may resemble erythroplasia clinically and, though they resolve with treatment of the anaemia, may show dysplasia histologically.

Candidosis. Candidosis can be aggravated or precipitated by anaemia and may be the presenting feature. In a few cases adequate treatment of anaemia alone, without antifungal treatment, relieves the infection. The majority of patients with chronic mucocutaneous candidosis, particularly the familial and diffuse types, are also iron deficient and treatment with iron appears to improve the response to antifungal treatment. On the other hand, very many patients with mild candidosis, particularly denture-induced stomatitis, appear not to have haematological disease (Chapter 16),

Angular stomatitis (cheilitis). Angular stomatitis is also a well-known sign, particularly of iron deficiency anaemia, but it affects only a minority of cases. Nowadays it is more frequently caused by infection, mainly by *Candida albicans.* It is not known how frequently the angular stomatitis of anaemia is mediated by infection or whether this lesion can be caused by the anaemia itself. Angular stomatitis is an uncommon feature of pernicious anaemia.

Aphthous stomatitis. Aphthous stomatitis is sometimes associated with haematological deficiency, particularly of folate, which if remedied, can sometimes bring about a cure. Deficiencies should be suspected especially in patients of middle age or over who develop aphthae.

Paterson–Kelly syndrome. The Paterson–Kelly (Plummer–Vinson) syndrome of glossitis and dysphagia with hypochromic (iron deficient) anaemia is uncommon. Women are mainly affected and the prevalence appears to be highest in Northern Europe. There is a substantial risk of carcinoma in the post-cricoid region or in the mouth (*Fig.* 4.2). Rarely this syndrome is associated with a macrocytic anaemia.

Anaemia Associated with Systemic Disease
Anaemia of various types may be associated with systemic disorders which include:

1. Chronic inflammation (infections or connective tissue disease).
2. Neoplasms including leukaemia (Chapter 5). Acute leukaemia is an important cause of anaemia and should always be considered when anaemia is seen in a child.
3. Liver disease (Chapter 8).

Or very rarely:

4. Hypothyroidism (Chapter 10).
5. Hypopituitarism (Chapter 10).
6. Hypoadrenocorticism (Chapter 10).
7. Uraemia (Chapter 9).
8. HIV infection.

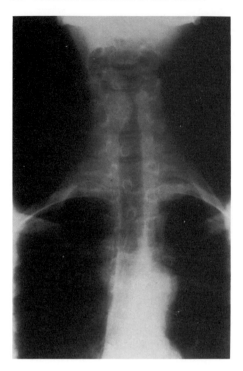

Fig. 4.2. Post-cricoid carcinoma in a patient with Paterson–Kelly (Plummer–Vinson) syndrome.

APLASTIC ANAEMIA

Bone-marrow aplasia is a rare disease causing refractory normochromic, normocytic anaemia, leucopenia and thrombocytopenia. Drugs are an important cause (*Table 4.7*) but many cases are idiopathic, though probably viral or immunologically mediated. The clinical manifestations are those of anaemia together with abnormal susceptibility to infection, a bleeding tendency and purpura, which is often the first manifestation.

The prognosis is poor and 50 per cent of patients die within 6 months usually from haemorrhage or infection.

The principles of management include the following:

1. Removal of the cause. Even when this is discoverable, as in the case of drugs, such as chloramphenicol, marrow damage may still be irreversible.

2. Isolation and antibiotics to control infection.

3. Androgenic steroids. (Corticosteroids are of questionable benefit.)

4. Bone marrow transplantation after intense immunosuppression. This in turn may cause graft-versus-host disease (GVHD) which is often lethal (*see below* and Chapter 16).

Tables 4.7. Causes of aplastic anaemia

---

1. Idiopathic (? autoimmune)
2. Genetic
    Fanconi's anaemia
    Dyskeratosis congenita
3. Drugs
    Phenylbutazone
    Chloramphenicol
    Sulphonamides
    Gold
    Penicillamine
    Anticonvulsants
    Cytotoxic agents
4. Chemicals
    Benzene
    Toluene
    Heavy metals
    Glue-sniffing
5. Viruses
    Hepatitis

Dental aspects

Oral manifestations of aplastic anaemia, and management, are somewhat similar to those of leukaemia, namely:

1. Anaemia.
2. Haemorrhagic tendencies (Chapter 3).
3. Susceptibility to infections.
4. Effects of corticosteroid therapy (Chapter 10).
5. Hepatitis B and other viral infections (Chapter 8).

Oral lichenoid lesions, or a Sjögren–like syndrome may develop if there is graft-versus-host disease if marrow transplantation has been carried out to relieve the anaemia (see below and Chapter 16). Gingival hyperplasia may develop if cyclosporin is used.

Fanconi's anaemia is a rare autosomal recessive syndrome characterized by skeletal defects, hyperpigmentation, pancytopenia and other congenital anomalies. It is associated with an increased susceptibility to oral or other head and neck carcinomas at an early age, as is dyskeratosis congenital.

Bone-marrow Transplantation

Bone-marrow transplantation is increasingly used, particularly in the treatment of aplastic anaemia, leukaemias and some immune deficiencies (Chapter 16). Patients are usually prepared for transplant with cyclophosphamide, with or without total body irradiation, such that they will accept donor bone-marrow with minimal chance of rejection. Recipients are then, after transplantation, treated with methotrexate or more usually cyclosporin for 6 months or more to prevent or ameliorate graft-versus-host disease (Chapter 16).

Dental aspects

Oral symptoms are the main complaint in patients after bone-marrow transplantation and consist of mucositis, dry mouth, sinusitis, parotitis and other infections, pain or bleeding. These develop usually within the first month of the transplant and are exacerbated by chemotherapy and immunosuppressive treatment. Cyclosporin may induce gingival hyperplasia.

Management problems can include:

1. Oral complications of cytotoxic treatment and radiotherapy (Chapter 5), particularly oral herpetic and fungal infections which are now recognized as the main causes of death.
2. Immunosuppressive therapy (Chapter 16).
3. Graft-versus-host disease (Chapter 16).

Pure Red Cell Aplasia

Pure red cell aplasia is a rare disease which may be congenital or acquired— the latter is often associated with a thymoma and sometimes chronic mucocutaneous candidosis (Chapter 16). These patients need regular blood transfusions and are therefore at risk from hepatitis virus and HIV infection.

Anaemia Caused by Marrow Infiltration

Replacement of haemopoietic marrow by abnormal cells (metastases, leukaemias, myeloma or myelofibrosis) causes normocytic anaemia and often leucopenia or thrombocytopenia with a leucoerythroblastic peripheral blood picture. There may be extramedullary haemopoiesis in other organs.

Dental care may be complicated by susceptibility to infections, haemorrhage (as in aplastic anaemia) or the underlying disease.

HAEMOLYTIC ANAEMIA

Worldwide, malaria is the most common cause of haemolytic anaemia but is rare in Britain. Haemolytic anaemia may also result from many other causes including:

1. Abnormal haemoglobin (the haemoglobinopathies).
2. Abnormal structure or function of the erythrocyte.
3. Damage to erythrocytes (autoimmune or infective).

The increased rate of erythrocyte destruction leads to bilirubin overproduction and sometimes jaundice. The spleen may enlarge and increased red cell turnover raises the reticulocyte count, plasma lactate dehydrogenase and uric acid levels. This increases the demand for folic acid and may in turn cause macrocytic changes.

Any of the haemolytic anaemias may be a contraindication to the use of general anaesthesia but, in practical terms, sickle cell disease is by far the most important cause of difficulties in dental management.

Congenital Haemolytic Anaemias

Haemoglobinopathies

The haemoglobinopathies are hereditary disorders characterized by abnormal haemoglobin production. Each of the haemoglobin peptide (globin) chains has a unique amino acid sequence which can be altered as a result of DNA mutations and lead to 'variant haemoglobins'. Quantitative rather than qualitative defects in the production of globins leads to the thalassaemias.

The diagnosis of haemoglobinopathy rests on the history, examination and laboratory investigations. A family history is especially important as many of these disorders have a racial distribution. Short stature, abnormal skeletal development, jaundice and splenomegaly are often found, in addition to signs and symptoms of anaemia. A full blood picture and red cell indices should be obtained and blood should also be sent for electrophoresis (4 ml of EDTA anticoagulated blood) and for assay of variant haemoglobins. Special tests such as the Sickledex may also be useful (*see below*).

The sickling disorders

Sickle cell disease can cause severe complications in general anaesthesia. Deoxygenation causes the erythrocytes to deform into sickle forms which have a reduced survival and also form stacks which impede blood flow in small vessels.

The sickling disorders include:

1. Heterozygous sickle cell trait (HbAS).
2. Homozygous sickle cell anaemia or disease (HbSS).
3. Heterozygous sickling trait associated with another haemoglobinopathy.

These diseases mainly affect Africans and Afro–Caribbeans but are also found in Asians and in those from the Mediterranean littoral. In West Africa some 2 per cent of the population have sickle cell disease and ten times as many have the trait.

Sickle cell trait (heterozygote) is many times more common than sickle cell anaemia (homozygote) in Britain and affects some 9 per cent of children of Afro–Caribbean descent, and 18 per cent of African descent in Britain.

Sickle cell trait (HbAS). The sickling trait is frequently asymptomatic, but sickle cell crises (*see below*) can be caused by reduced oxygen tension (general anaesthesia, high altitudes or unpressurized aircraft). At times such patients may have renal complications causing haematuria or splenic infarcts.

Sickle cell anaemia (HbSS). Sickle cell anaemia is relatively rare in Britain where there are approximately 5000 persons with the disease. It is usually a serious disease with widespread complications (*Table 4.8*). It frequently becomes apparent about the third month of life. The patient suffers chronic anaemia punctuated by intermittent crises.

Crises of sickle cell disease are of two types, painful and haematological.

Table 4.8 Features of sickle cell anaemia

Anaemia
Jaundice
Impaired growth
Dactylitis
Skeletal deformities
Painful crises
Aplastic crises
Susceptibility to infections
Infarcts of CNS, lungs, kidney, spleen
Skin ulcers
Gallstones

Painful crises.   These are usually due to infarction as a result of sickling brought on by infection, dehydration, hypoxia, acidosis or cold and cause severe bone pain and pyrexia. Infarcts in the jaws can cause pain which may be mistaken for toothache or osteomyelitis. Infarcts may cause abdominal, pulmonary, renal or neurological damage. Abdominal crises may mimic a surgical emergency. Pulmonary infarcts cause chest pain and eventually lead to pulmonary hypertension and right-sided cardiac failure. The kidneys may also be affected, with haematuria and a nephrotic syndrome. Neurological damage may cause ocular defects or a cerebrovascular accident–often with hemiplegia.

Haematological crises.   These are often caused by parvovirus infections and can be of three types, namely:

1. Haemolytic.
2. Aplastic.
3. Sequestration crises.

Anaemia and the results of infarctions may be incapacitating, but the main cause of death in sickle cell anaemia is infection, particularly by pneumococci, meningococci and salmonellae, because of an associated immune defect mainly as a result of splenic dysfunction.

Laboratory investigations in sickling disorders

In sickle cell disease there is anaemia and reticulocytosis: sickled erythrocytes are sometimes seen in a stained blood film. By contrast, haematological findings are often normal in sickle cell trait. Sickling may be demonstrated in both sickle cell anaemia and trait, by tests relying on the decreased solubility of HbS (Sickledex) or by the addition of a reducing agent (such as 10 per cent sodium metabisulphite or dithionite) to a blood sample. Haemoglobin electrophoresis shows HbS and up to 15 per cent HbF, but no HbA in sickle cell anaemia.

General management of the sickling disorders

Patients with sickle cell anaemia need regular monitoring of their haematological state and a comprehensive care programme. Blood transfusions are needed for cerebrovascular symptoms in early childhood or recurrent pulmonary thromboses. Many patients, however, remain with moderate degrees of anaemia for most of their lives and transfusions can and should usually be avoided, especially because of the risk of hepatitis C and HIV infection. Folic acid needs to be given regularly and infections must be treated early. Painful crises should be treated promptly with analgesics and hydration.

Nowadays an increasing number of patients with sickle cell disease survive into late middle age; infections and thromboses are the main causes of death.

Dental aspects of the sickling disorders

Sickling disorders should be suspected in those with a positive family history and in any patient of African, West Indian or (less frequently) Asian or Mediterranean descent. All those at risk should be investigated if general anaesthesia is to be given. If the sickle cell test is positive, haemoglobin electrophoresis is required to establish the diagnosis, but if the haemoglobin is less than 11 g/dl sickle cell anaemia is probable.

Sickle cell trait (HbAS). Patients with the common sickle cell trait cause few problems in management but if general anaesthesia is necessary full oxygenation must be maintained throughout. Respiratory infections must be treated vigorously as they can cause a crisis.

Sickle cell anaemia (HbSS). The oral mucosa may be pale or jaundiced and there may be a susceptibility to dental infection. Preventive dental care is therefore of great importance. Hard tissue changes are conspicuous: hypercementosis may develop and there is bone-marrow hyperplasia with apparent osteoporosis of the jaw. Skeletal but not dental maturation is delayed. The lamina dura is distinct and dense and the permanent teeth may be hypomineralized, though neither caries nor periodontal disease is more severe. The skull is thickened but osteoporotic with a 'hair on end' pattern to the trabeculae. The diploe are thickened, especially in the parietal regions, giving a 'tower skull' form. Lesions suggestive of bone infarction–dense radio-opacities–may be seen in the skull and/or jaws. Bone scans using technetium diphosphonate show increased uptake in these areas. Infarction may cause pain and predispose to osteomyelitis, especially in the mandible, or to cranial neuropathies, including labial anaesthesia.

Patients with sickle cell anaemia must be managed with the help of a haematologist. Preventive dental care is important to lessen the need for radical treatment requiring general anaesthesia. Routine conservation should be carried out under local or relative analgesia. Oral pain, if not of local dental origin, may be caused by infarction or osteomyelitis. On rare occasions severe bone pain can be felt in the mandible only and even the patient may not recognize it as a sickling crisis. Pulpal symptoms are common in the absence of any obvious dental disease. Acute infections should be treated immediately, since they may precipitate a sickling crisis. Surgical procedures should have antibiotic cover.

General anaesthesia is hazardous in sickle cell anaemia because of the severe anaemia and because a crisis may be precipitated. Where possible, anaemia should be corrected preoperatively and the haemoglobin brought up to at least 10 g/dl. For elective surgery a phase when haemolysis is minimal should be selected. Exchange transfusion is occasionally required for major surgery but only in selected patients. Oral administration of folic acid may also be valuable in correcting the anaemia.

General anaesthesia should only be carried out in hospital with full anaesthetic facilities and blood available for transfusion. Drugs that can cause respiratory depression, including sedative agents, should not be given as they may lead to hypoxia; acidosis and hypotension must also be avoided. Some infuse sodium bicarbonate.

At least 30 per cent oxygen is needed and, provided that there is no respiratory depression or obstruction, normal anaesthetic procedures can be used. If a crisis develops, oxygen is given and bicarbonate infused. A packed red cell transfusion may be required if the haemoglobin falls below 50 per cent. Heparinization may be needed for those with abdominal or limb pain during a crisis, to prevent pulmonary embolism. Wherever possible, therefore, dental treatment should be carried out under local anaesthesia.

Some patients have such severe pain during crises that they abuse analgesics and become addicts (Chapter 19). As a consequence of this or of multiple transfusions some patients become infected with blood–borne viruses. Pain should be controlled with paracetamol or codeine rather than aspirin which in large doses can upset the acid–base balance.

Sickle cell trait with another haemoglobinopathy. Double heterozygotes can have sickle cell trait accompanied by thalassaemia (Sβ thalassaemia) or have both sickle cell haemoglobin S and C (SC disease). These are usually milder than isolated sickle cell anaemia (*Table 4.9*). The degree of anaemia is variable but they are at about the same level of risk as are those with sickle cell disease from general anaesthesia. Patients with other combined defects should be managed in the same way as are those with sickle trait.

Table 4.9 The sckling disorders

Disorder	Haemoglobin type	Origins of predominant racial groups affected	Clinical features
Sickle cell trait	S-A	Africa, West Indies, Mediterranean, India	Usually asymptomatic
Sickle cell anaemia	S-S	Africa, West Indies, Mediterranean, India	Severe anaemia Jaundice Impaired growth Crises Infarcts Infections
Sickle cell - HbC disease	S-C	West Africa, South East Asia	Variable anaemia
Sickle cell - HbD disease	S-D	Africa, India, Pakistan	Moderately severe anaemia
Sickle cell - HbE disease	S-E	South East Asia	Moderately severe anaemia
Sickle cell - thalassaemia	S-A-F	Mediterranean, Africa, West Indies	Moderately severe anaemia

Other haemoglobin variants.   There are over 60 haemoglobin variants in which changes in the peptide chain cause chronic haemolytic anaemia. Splenomegaly is common and splenectomy is necessary for severe disease. The diagnosis is made by determining the heat-stability of the haemoglobin. Various drugs may increase haemolysis and the physician must therefore be contacted.

The Thalassaemias

The thalassaemias are characterized by depressed synthesis of one or more of the globin chains, leading to decreased haemoglobin production and hypochromic microcytic anaemia. The unaffected chains are, however, produced in excess and precipitate within the erythrocytes to cause increased erythrocyte fragility and haemolysis.

Thalassaemias are predominantly found in those of Mediterranean, Middle Eastern or Asian descent. Typical features in homozygotes are chronic anaemia, marrow hyperplasia and skeletal deformities, splenomegaly and gallstones. Heterozygotes for thalassaemia may be asymptomatic.

Alpha-thalassaemias.   Alpha-thalassaemias are mainly found in Asians. There are four main subtypes, of varying degrees of severity.

Beta-thalassaemias.   Beta-thalassaemias (Mediterranean anaemia) mainly affect peoples from the Mediterranean littoral and Afro–Caribbeans. Heterozygous beta-thalassaemia (thalassaemia minor or thalassaemia trait) is common and usually asymptomatic, except for mild hypochromic anaemia which may be aggravated by pregnancy or intercurrent illness.

Homozygous beta-thalassaemia (Cooley's anaemia: thalassaemia major) is the most serious type and is characterized by failure to thrive, increasingly severe anaemia, hepatosplenomegaly and skeletal abnormalities. Affected children are susceptible to folate deficiency (as in other chronic haemolytic states) and also to infection. In spite of the anaemia, patients with homozygous beta-thalassaemia become overloaded with iron and haemosiderosis damages the heart, liver, pancreas, skin and sometimes the salivary glands, causing a sicca syndrome. Most thalassaemic children develop cardiomyopathy and dysrhythmias and die in early adult life from cardiac haemosiderosis. Hepatic and pancreatic dysfunction are also common.

Diagnosis is confirmed by finding severe microcytic, hypochromic anaemia with gross aniso- and poikilocytosis, target cell formation and basophilic stippling of erythrocytes. In contrast to iron deficiency anaemia, serum iron and ferritin levels are normal or raised and total iron binding capacity (TIBC) is normal. There is a great increase in HbF (fetal haemoglobin) and some increase in HbA2.

Although homozygous beta-thalassaemia is usually lethal in adolescence, some survive: these patients are thought to have a milder variant, such as beta-thalassaemia with high levels of HbF (*see Fig. 4.1*).

General management of beta-thalassaemias.   The main measures in beta-thalassaemia are blood transfusions, iron chelating agents (desferrioxamine) and folic acid supplements. Splenectomy may be required if there is hypersplenism causing increased blood destruction but is avoided otherwise, as it leads to accumulation of iron elsewhere and other complications.

Dental aspects of beta-thalassaemias.   The major oral changes in thalassaemia are enlargement of the maxilla caused by bone-marrow expansion (chipmunk facies). Alveolar bone rarefaction produces a chicken-wire appearance on radiography. Pneumatization of the sinuses may be delayed. Expansion of the diploe of the skull causes a hair-on-end appearance that is frequently conspicuous on lateral skull radiographs. There is often spacing of the teeth and forward drift of the maxillary incisors, so that orthodontic treatment may be indicated.

Less common oral complications include painful swelling of the parotids and xerostomia caused by iron deposition, and a sore or burning tongue related to the folate deficiency.

Maxillary enlargement may cause difficulties in intubation for the induction of general anaesthesia but the chronic severe anaemia, and often cardiomyopathy, are in any event contraindications to general anaesthesia. Hepatitis B or C, or HIV carriage may be a complication in multiply transfused patients. Since splenectomy results in an immune defect, it may be prudent to cover surgical procedures with prophylactic antimicrobials.

Homozygous thalassaemia has a poor prognosis; hospitalization is frequently needed and there may as a consequence be psychological problems.

Erythrocyte Membrane Defects

Hereditary spherocytosis (acholuric jaundice) is the main form of congenital haemolytic anaemia in Caucasians. It is an autosomal dominant trait characterized by haemolytic anaemia, jaundice, splenomegaly, gallstones, haemochromatosis and skin ulcers. Episodes of haemolysis may be precipitated by infections. Splenectomy and folic acid treatment are almost invariably required.

Hereditary ellipsocytosis (ovalocytosis) and hereditary stomatocytosis are similar autosomal dominant disorders characterized by chronic haemolytic anaemia. Splenectomy is invariably needed.

Erythrocyte Metabolic Defects

The most common disorder of this type is glucose 6-phosphate dehydrogenase (G6PD) deficiency, which affects up to 15 per cent of American Black males. A variant of G6PD deficiency affects those of Mediterranean, Middle Eastern or Asian descent and is more serious. Haemolysis is caused by oxidant drugs (*Table 4.10*) or by intercurrent infection. The diagnosis is confirmed by enzyme assays carried out in a specialist laboratory. Haemolysis in G6PD is self-limiting and splenectomy is usually not needed.

Dental aspects of G6PD deficiency.   Apart from the problems of anaemia it is vital to avoid oxidant drugs such as the sulphonamides (including co-trimoxazole) or menadiol (water soluble vitamin K) which can precipitate haemolysis. Aspirin can be safely used in G6PD deficiency. Metabolic acidosis also causes haemolysis and must be avoided during general anaesthesia.

Table 4.10 Drugs Causing Haemolysis in Patients
with G6PD Deficiency

1. Analgesics
     Phenacetin*
2. Sulphonamides
3. Antimalarials
4. Dapsone
5. Chloramphenicol
6. Water-soluble vitamin K
7. Naladixic acid

*No longer available

Acquired Haemolytic Anaemia

Intravascular destruction of erythrocytes can be caused by factors such asgross trauma, complement-mediated lysis, toxins and malaria.

These diseases are rare but may occasionally have dental relevance because of anaemia, corticosteroid treatment or haemorrhagic tendencies.

Bibliography

Addy D.P. (1986) Happiness is iron. *Br. Med. J.* **292**, 969–70.

Barret A. P. (1986) Oral complications of bone marrow transplantation. *Aust. NZ. J. Med.* **16**, 239–40.

Brain M. C. (1980) The clinical assessment of the anaemic patient. *Medicine (UK)* **27**, 1395–7.

Carmel R. (1988) Pernicious anemia: the expected findings of very low serum cobalamin levels, anemia, and macrocytosis are often lacking. *Arch. Intern. Med.* **148**, 1712–4.

Carmel, R., Sinow R.M., Siegel M.E. et al. (1988) Food cobalamin malabsorption occurs frequently in patients with unexplained low serum cobalamin levels. *Arch. Intern. Med.* **148**, 1715–9.

Cawson R.A. and Spector R.G. (1989) *Clinical Pharmacology in Dentistry.* 5th ed. Edinburgh, Churchill Livingstone.

Challacombe S. J., Scully, C., Keevil B. et al. (1983) Serum ferritin in recurrent oral ulceration. *Oral Pathol* **12**, 290–99.

Cox G. (1984) A study of oral pain experience in sickle cell patients. *Oral Surg.* **58**, 39–41.

Crawford J.M. (1988) Periodontal disease in sickle cell disease subjects. *J. Periodontol.* **59**, 164–9.

Crosby W. H. (1977) Who needs iron? *N. Engl. J. Med.* **297**, 543–5.

Demas D.C., Cantin R.Y., Poole A. et al. (1988) Use of general anesthesia in dental care of the child with sickle cell anemia. *Oral Surg.* **66**, 190–3.

Donaldson R.M. (1978) Serum B_{12} and the diagnosis of cobalamin deficiency. *N. Engl. J. Med.* **299**, 827–8.

Goldfarb A., Nitzan D. W. and Marmary L. (1983) Changes in the parotid salivary gland of B-thalassemia patients due to hemosiderin deposits. *Int. J. Oral Surg.* **12**, 115–9.

Hammersley N. (1984) Mandibular infarction occurring during sickle cell crisis. *Br. J. Oral Maxillofac. Surg.* **22**, 103–14.

Jacobs A. and Bentley D. P. (1980) Clinical investigation and management of disorders of iron metabolism. *Medicine (UK)* **27**, 1398–1405.

Leading Article (1980) Preventing iron deficiency. *Lancet* **i**, 1117–18.

Locksley R. M. (1985) Infection with varicella-zoster virus after marrow transplantation. *J. Infect. Dis.* **152**, 1172–81.

Luker J., Scully C. and Oakhill A. (1991) Gingival swelling as a manifestation of aplastic anaemia. *Oral Surg.* **70**, 55–6.

McClure S., Custer E. and Bessman D. (1985) Improved detection of early iron deficiency in nonanaemic subjects. *JAMA* **253**, 1021–3.

Murtata L. N., Stroud C. E., Davis L. R. et al. (1981) Admissions to hospital of children with sickle cell anaemia: a study in south London. *Br. Med. J.* **282**, 1048.

O'Rourke C. and Mitropoulos C. (1990) Orofacial pain in patients with sickle cell disease. *Br. Dent. J.* **169**, 130–2.

Oski F.A. (1985) Iron deficiency - facts and fallacies. *Pediatr. Clin. North Am.* **32**, 493–7.

Peterson P. K. (1983) A prospective study of infectious diseases following bone marrow transplantation: emergence of aspergillus and cytomegalovirus as the major causes of mortality. *Infec. Control* **4**, 81–9.

Schilling R. F. (1986) Is nitrous oxide a dangerous anaesthetic for vitamin B_{12} deficient subjects? *JAMA* **255**, 1605–6.

Schubert M. M. (1986) Head and neck aspergillosis in patients undergoing bone-marrow transplantation. *Cancer* **57**, 1092–6.

Scully C. (1986) Testing for sickle cell anaemia. *Br. Dent. J.* **160**, 40.

Sears R. S., Nazif M. M. and Zullo T. (1981) The effects of sickle cell disease on dental and skeletal maturation. *J. Dent. Child.* **27**, 275–7.

Seto B. G. (1985) Oral mucositis in patients undergoing bone-marrow transplantation. *Oral Surg.* **60**, 493–7.

Smith D.B. and Gelbman J. (1986) Dental management of the sickle cell anaemia patient. *Clin. Prevent. Dent.* **8**, 21–3.

Smith H.B., McDonald D.K. and Miller R.I. (1987) Dental management of patients with sickle cell disorders. *JADA* **114**, 85–7.

Stockman J.A. (1987) Iron deficiency anaemia: have we come far enough? *JAMA* **258**, 1645–7.

Terezhalmy G. T. and Hall E. H. (1984) The asplenic patient: a consideration for antimicrobial prophylaxis. *Oral Surg.* **57**, 114–7.

Van Dis M. L. and Langlais R. P. (1986) The thalassemias: oral manifestations and complications. *Oral Surg.* **62**, 229–33.

Appendix to Chapter 4

INTERPRETATION OF HAEMATOLOGICAL RESULTS

Blood	Normal range*	Level ↑	Level ↓	Comments on collection†
Haemoglobin	Male 130–180 g/dl Female 115–165 g/dl	Polycythaemia (vera or physiological) myeloproliferative disease	Anaemia	EDTA tube
Haematocrit (packed cell volume or PCV)	Male 40–54% Females 37–47%	Polycythaemia; dehydration	Anaemia	EDTA tube
Mean cell volume	78–99 fl $MCV = \dfrac{PCV}{RBC}$	Macrocytosis in vitamin B12 or folate deficiency; liver disease; alcoholism; hypothyroidism	Microcytosis in iron deficiency; thalassaemia; chronic disease	EDTA tube
Mean cell haemoglobin (MCH)	27–31 pg $MCH = \dfrac{Hb}{RBC}$	"	"	EDTA tube
Mean cell haemoglobin concentration (MCHC)	32–36 g/dl $MCHC = \dfrac{Hb}{PCV}$	"	Iron deficiency; thalassaemia; sideroblastic anaemia; anaemia in chronic disease	EDTA tube
Red cell count (RBC)	Male 4.2–6.1 × 10^{12}/l Female 4.2–5.4 × 10^{12}/l	Polycythaemia Dehydration	Anaemia; fluid overload	EDTA tube

INTERPRETATION OF HAEMATOLOGICAL RESULTS

Blood	Normal range*	Level ↑	Level ↑	Comments on collection†
White cell count Total	$4–10 \times 10^9/l$	Pregnancy; exercise; infection; trauma; leukaemia	Early leukaemia; some infections; bone-marrow disease; drugs; idiopathic	EDTA tube
Neutrophils	average $3 \times 10^9/l$	Pregnancy; exercise; infection; bleeding; trauma; malignancy; leukaemia	Some infection; drugs; endocrinopathics; bone marrow disease; idiopathic	EDTA tube
Lymphocytes	average $2.5 \times 10^9/l$	Physiological; some infections; leukaemia; bowel disease	Some infection; some immune defects (e.g. AIDS)	EDTA tube
Eosinophils	average $0.15 \times 10^9/l$	Allergic disease; parasitic infestations; skin disease; lymphoma	Some immune defects	EDTA tube
Platelets	$150–400 \times 10^9/l$	Thrombocytosis in myelo-proliferative disease; trauma	Thrombocytopenia related to leukaemia; drugs; infections; idiopathic; autoimmune	EDTA tube
Reticulocytes	0.5–1.5% of RBC	Haemolytic states; during treatment of anaemia	—	EDTA tube
Erythrocyte sedimentation rate (ESR)	0–15 mm/h	Pregnancy; infections; anaemia; connective tissue disease; myelomatosis; malignancy; temporal arteritis	—	Citrated tube
Plasma viscosity	1.4–1.8 cp	As ESR	—	EDTA tube Relative viscosity of plasma cf. water

*Adults unless otherwise stated. Check values with your laboratory.
†Vacuum tubes.

Chapter 5

Leukaemia and other Malignant Disease

THE LEUKAEMIAS

Leukaemias are diseases in which there is neoplastic proliferation of white blood cells. They are usually fatal if untreated. In acute leukaemias primitive blast cells are released into the blood, whereas in chronic leukaemia the abnormal cells retain most of the morphological features of their normal counteparts. The neoplastic cells may be lymphoid, monocytic or myeloid stem cells and classification is essential since there are important differences in response to treatment of the various types of leukaemia.

Dental management in leukaemia can often be complicated by oral lesions, bleeding tendencies and susceptibility to infection.

ACUTE LEUKAEMIAS

The acute leukaemias account for less than 2 per cent of cancers overall, but represent nearly 50 per cent of all malignant disease and are the most common cause of non–accidental death in children.

Acute lymphoblastic and non-lymphoblastic (myeloblastic) leukaemias are clinically indistinguishable (*Table 5.1*). Anaemia, lymphadenopathy, splenomegaly, infections, fever, bruising and bleeding tendencies are the main

Table 5.1. Acute leukaemia—typical features

Age:	Children—acute lymphoblastic leukaemia
Onset:	Adults—acute myeloblastic leukaemia
Symptoms and signs:	Acute
	1. Pallor (anaemia)
	2. Infections
	3. Purpura (bruising)
	4. Bleeding from mucous membranes
	5. Enlarged lymph nodes
	6. Splenomegaly
	7. Weight loss
	8. Bone pain
	9. Weakness
	10. Anorexia

features. There is an increased number of circulating white blood cells but there may be phases when it is normal (aleukaemic leukaemia). Diagnosis of leukaemia is made by the blood picture and in particular, a stained blood film and bone-marrow biopsy. Cytochemistry, analysis of membrane markers and immunophenotyping are required for categorization of the cell type.

Acute Lymphoblastic Leukaemia

Acute lymphoblastic leukaemia (ALL), the most common leukaemia of childhood, has a peak incidence at 3–5 years but can affect any age group.

Malignant lymphoblasts proliferate and infiltrate the bone-marrow, viscera, skin and nervous system. Marrow infiltration causes granulocytopenia, anaemia and thrombocytopenia.

Common (non-B cell, non-T cell) ALL is the most frequent type affecting children; T-cell ALL affects males predominantly and has a poor prognosis, while B-cell ALL also has a poor prognosis and is refractory to chemotherapy.

General management

Treatment is with cytotoxic drugs such as doxorubicin or vincristine, crisantapase and prednisolone. These typically cause severe nausea and vomiting and various other toxic effects. Patients may need to be isolated during the induction of remission as they are highly susceptible to infection at this time. Supportive care includes control of infections, haemorrhagic tendencies, anaemia, hyperuricaemia (gout) and renal malfunction.

Over 90 per cent of patients have a remission within 6 weeks and the 5-year survival rate is now over 50 per cent. The risk of relapse is greatest in the first 18 months and maintenance therapy is therefore usually continued for 3 years.

Relapse is higher in males, partly because of occult testicular or CNS disease. Craniospinal irradiation is no longer routine in low risk ALL patients but intrathecal methotrexate may be given. Bone-marrow transplantation may give better control if chemotherapy fails to prevent relapse but there are usually difficulties in finding a compatible donor.

Adult Acute Lymphoblastic Leukaemia

Adult ALL has a worse prognosis than childhood ALL, but treatment schedules are similar.

Acute Non-lymphoblastic (myeloblastic) Leukaemia

Acute non–lymphoblastic leukaemia is less common than ALL in children. About 7 subtypes have been described. Acute myeloblastic leukaemia (AML) is the most common acute leukaemia of adults. The clinical features are similar to those of acute lymphoblastic leukaemia except that CNS involvement is rare. Nevertheless the disease occasionally causes cranial nerve palsies.

General management

Combination chemotherapy has greatly improved the prognosis in AML but is much less successful than in childhood ALL. Remission can be obtained in up to 85 per cent of patients but is rarely maintained. Whenever possible, bone-marrow transplantation is employed and 5-year survival rates of up to 60 per cent are reported.

Dental aspects of the acute leukaemias

Oral manifestations.   Oropharyngeal lesions can be the initial complaint in over 10 per cent of cases of acute leukaemia overall but develop in 65–90 per cent of cases of acute myelomonocytic leukaemia as a consequence of the disease or treatment or both. Oral bleeding and petechiae are typical manifestations, together with mucosal pallor and sometimes gingival swelling (localized or generalized), mucosal or gingival ulceration, pericoronitis and cervical lymphadenopathy. Other oral findings include tonsillar swelling, paraesthesiae (particularly of the lower lip), extrusion of teeth, painful swellings over the mandible and of the parotid (Mikulicz syndrome). Fungal and herpetic infections are common and may occasionally be fatal. Candidosis is particularly common in the oral cavity and the paranasal sinuses. Aspergillosis or mucormycosis can involve the maxillary antrum and be invasive. Pseudomonas and other Gram-negative species occasionally cause oral lesions. It is important to appreciate that the mouth is a major source of septicaemia or metastatic infections in leukaemic patients.

Radiographic findings may include destruction of the crypts of developing teeth, thinning or disappearance of the lamina dura, especially in the premolar and molar regions, and loss of the alveolar crestal bone. Bone destruction near the apices of mandibular posterior teeth may also be seen. These bone changes may be reversible with chemotherapy.

The different subtypes of acute leukaemia differ in their oral manifestations to some extent. Mucosal pallor, petechiae, tonsillar swelling and cervical lymphadenopathy are typical of acute lymphoblastic leukaemia but gingival swelling is uncommon. Acute myeloblastic leukaemia, however, is characterized by gingival swelling in 20–30 per cent of patients. Many of the drugs used in the treatment of leukaemia can also cause oral lesions (*Table 5.2*), and patients may have complications from bone-marrow transplantation (Chapter 4).

Dental treatment.   The main dental management problems in acute leukaemia are as follows:

1. Oral infections.
2. Bleeding (Chapter 3).
3. Anaemia (Chapter 4).
4. Hepatitis B or C (Chapter 8) and HIV infection (Chapter 16).
5. Corticosteroid treatment (Chapter 10).
6. Disseminated intravascular coagulopathy (Chapter 3).
7. Complications of bone-marrow transplantation (Chapter 4).

Table 5.2. Oral manifestations of leukaemia

Cervical lymph node enlargement	
Bleeding from gingivae	
Purpura	
Infections	
Gingival swelling	Candidosis and other fungal infections
Oral ulceration	Herpes virus infections
Tonsillar membrane	
Drug side-effects	Oral ulceration (many of the cytotoxics)
	Dry mouth (adriamycin)
	Pigmentation (busulphan)
	Candidosis (antimicrobials)
	(*See also* Appendix 19)

8. Abnormal susceptibility to infection. Antimicrobial cover is needed for any surgery, particularly for those with indwelling atrial catheters.

9. Interaction of methotrexate with nitrous oxide (theoretical).

Many of the oral lesions are aggravated or caused by local infection and chemotherapy. Oral lesions are readily infected by opportunistic microbes and such infections may have serious or fatal consequences. Isolation of the patient may therefore be needed. Lesions tend to become infected with Gram–negative bacteria including pseudomonas, serratia, klebsiella, enterobacter, proteus and escherichia, or with candida or aspergillus. In severely immunosuppressed patients over 50 per cent of a series of systemic infections resulted from oropharyngeal micro-organisms. Microbiological investigations with care to obtain specimens for anaerobic culture are essential to enable appropriate antimicrobial therapy to be given. Meticulous oral hygiene should be carefully maintained with regular frequent warm 0.2 per cent aqueous chlorhexidine mouthrinses and the use of a soft nylon toothbrush. Prophylactic antifungal therapy, nystatin mouthwashes (10 ml of 100 000 units of nystatin per ml, four times daily) or pastilles, or amphotericin lozenges are also indicated (*see* Appendix to Chapter 1).

Herpetic infections are a very common and troublesome cause of oral ulceration, as are varicella–zoster infections; they should be treated vigorously with acyclovir. Varicella-zoster (VZV) and measles viruses can also cause encephalitis or pneumonia. Prophylactic acyclovir has greatly reduced the incidence, morbidity and mortality from VZV infections, including those who have had bone-marrow transplants. Such patients may need VZV immune globulin in the event of contact. They must not be given live vaccines and infected persons should be kept away.

Many of the cytotoxic drugs (*see Table 5.7*) can precipitate oral ulceration. Methotrexate is a major cause, but ulceration may be prevented or ameliorated by concomitant intravenous administration of folinic acid ('leucovorin rescue'). Topical folinic acid (1.5 mg in 15 ml if water) used three times daily may also be useful. Established oral ulcers may improve with chlorhexidine or povidone-iodine mouthwashes, or appropriate antibiotics for specific infections.

Severe bleeding from the mouth, particularly from the gingival margin, may need treatment by desmopressin, or even platelet transfusion.

Dental treatment should only be carried out after consultation with the physician, as it may be affected by various aspects of management and the probable life expectation. Preventive treatment is essential and conservative treatment may be indicated where possible, but surgery (except for emergencies such as fractures, haemorrhage, potential airways obstruction or dangerous sepsis) should be deferred until a remission phase. Regional local anaesthetic injections may be contraindicated if there is a severe haemorrhagic tendency.

Extractions should be avoided because of the dangers of haemorrhage and infections such as osteomyelitis or septicaemia. Before surgery, desmopressin or platelet infusions or blood may be needed, and antibiotics given until the wound has healed. Penicillin is the antibiotic of choice. Sockets should not be packed as this appears to predispose to infection. Operative procedures must be performed with strict asepsis and as atraumatically as possible. Absorbable polyglycolic acid sutures (Dexon) or soft catgut are preferred. Aspirin should not be given, since it aggravates bleeding.

Other preoperative precautions include screening for hepatitis B and HIV. Anaemia may be a contraindication to general anaesthesia—intravenous sedation or relative analgesia may be used as alternatives. However nitrous oxide, which interferes with vitamin B_{12} and hence folate metabolism, is possibly contraindicated if the patient is being treated with methotrexate since the toxic effects of the latter may be exacerbated.

CHRONIC LEUKAEMIAS

Chronic Lymphocytic Leukaemia

Chronic lymphocytic leukaemia (CLL) is the most common type of chronic leukaemia (*Table 5.3*). Men are particularly affected. Some 15 per cent of patients are asymptomatic and life expectancy may not be affected. In others, the disease is insidiously progressive with fever, weight loss, anorexia, haemorrhage and infections. Other effects are anaemia and thrombocytopenia. Lymph

Table 5.3. Chronic lymphoid leukaemias*

Disorder	Particular features
Chronic lymphocytic leukaemia	Splenomegaly, skin lesions Prolonged survival
Sezary syndrome	Generalized lymph node enlargement; pruritus; exfoliating erythroderma Chemotherapy relatively ineffective
Hairy cell leukaemia	Splenomegaly; may be associated with HTLV-1 infection; predisposes to mycobacterial infection Relatively long survival Responds to alpha interferon
Prolymphocytic leukaemia	Splenomegaly; resistant to chemo- and radiotherapy
Adult T-cell leukaemia-lymphoma	Resembles lymphocytic leukaemia Poor prognosis

*Except for sezary syndrome, which involves T-cells, most involve B-cells mainly.

Table 5.4. Treatment of chronic lymphocytic leukaemia

---

1. Chemotherapy
   Chlorambucil (Leukeran) usually ± mustine or cyclophosphamide (Endozana)
   plus
   Corticosteroids if there is haemolytic anaemia, marrow failure or thrombocytopenia
   Interferon for hairy cell leukaemia
2. Radiotherapy
   May be used for treating large lymph node masses
3. Supportive care includes
   Antimicrobials
   Allopurinol

Treatment required only if there is progressive marrow failure or complications.

node enlargement is early. Leukaemic infiltration of the skin is more common than in chronic myeloid leukaemia and may be a major manifestation. The 5-year survival is over 50 per cent.

General management.   Asymptomatic patients may not need treatment. Those that are symptomatic can be treated with radiotherapy, cytotoxic drugs and corticosteroids (*Table 5.4*). B-cell CLL responds better to treatment than T-cell CLL.

Chronic Myeloid Leukaemia

Chronic myeloid leukaemia (CML) is characterized by proliferation of myeloid cells in the bone marrow, peripheral blood and other tissues. Most patients with CML suffer from chronic granulocytic leukaemia (CGL) but there are several other rare subgroups (*Table 5.5*).

Chronic granulocytic leukaemia (CGL) mainly affects those over 40 years of age. The clinical features are similar to those of other chronic leukaemias. Splenomegaly and hepatomegaly are common but lymphadenopathy is rare: anaemia, weight loss and joint pains are not uncommon.

Table 5.5.   Chronic myeloid leukaemia

Disorder	Particular features
Chronic granulocytic leukaemia	Splenomegaly
	Positive for Philadelphia chromosome
	Fairly responsive to chemotherapy
Atypical chronic granulocytic leukaemia	Negative for Philadelphia chromosome
	Less responsive to chemotherapy
Juvenile	Mainly young children; lymphadenopathy
	Poor response to chemotherapy
Chronic myelomonocytic leukaemia	Little response to chemotherapy
Chronic neutrophilic leukaemia	Difficult to differentiate from a benign leucocytosis
Eosinophilic leukaemia	Eventual cardiac damage

Table 5.6. Chronic myeloid leukaemia—treatment

1. Chemotherapy
   Busulphan (Myleran) ± 6-thioguanine
   In the proliferative phase it may be necessary to use hydroxyurea (Hydrea) or mitobronitol
   (Myelobromol) ± radiotherapy
2. Supportive care may include
   Antimicrobials
   Allopurinol

The prognosis of CGL is variable, but sooner or later there is transformation to an acute phase similar to AML (blast crisis). Fever, haemorrhage or bone pain are then common.

General management

Treatment is by means of cytotoxic drugs, and remission for over 12 months may follow a single course of chemotherapy. Radiotherapy may be useful later (*Table 5. 6*)

In blast transformation the same treatment is given as for AML, but the acute phase is usually refractory to treatment and the patient may die within a few months.

Dental aspects of chronic leukaemia

Reports of oral manifestations relate mainly to CLL. Gingival swelling may be seen but less frequently than in the acute leukaemias. Palatal swelling (submucosal leukaemic nodules), gingival bleeding, oral petechiae or oral ulceration may also be features. Ulceration may be aggravated by cytotoxic therapy. Herpes simplex or zoster, or candidosis are common (*Fig.* 5.1).

In CML oral haemorrhage may result from platelet deficiency. Leukaemic infiltration of lacrimal and salivary glands can cause Mikulicz's syndrome. Granulocytic sarcoma is a rare tumour-like lesion which can affect the jaws and may rarely precede other manifestations or herald a blast crisis. Drug treatment of chronic leukaemia can also cause oral complications (*Table 5.7*).

The prognosis of most chronic leukaemias is better than for the acute leukaemias and routine dental treatment is more likely to be required. Close cooperation with the haematologist is needed since (as in all leukaemias) there may be:

1. Bleeding tendencies.
2. Liability to infection.
3. Anaemia.
4. Susceptibility to hepatitis B, C and HIV infection.
5. Side-effects of treatment, such as pulmonary fibrosis as a result of busulphan.

Ampicillin and amoxycillin may cause irritating rashes similar to those seen in infectious mononucleosis and are unrelated to penicillin allergy (*see* Appendix to Chapter 1).

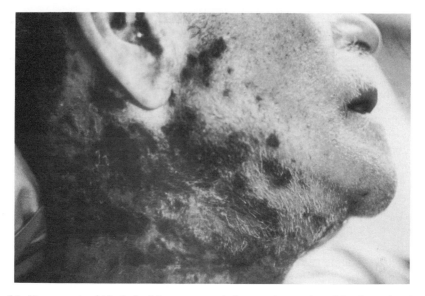

Fig. 5.1. Herpes zoster (shingles) of the upper cervical nerves in a patient dying from chronic leukaemia.

Table 5.7. Drugs used in cancer chemotherapy that frequently cause mouth ulcers*†

Group	Drug	Possible management problems
Antibiotics	Actinomycin	Vomiting
	Bleomycin	Lung fibrosis
	Daunorubicin	Cardiac damage
	Doxorubicin	Cardiac damage
	Mitozantrone	Cardiac damage
Antimetabolites	Cytosine arabinoside	
	5-Fluorouracil	
	Methotrexate	Liver and renal damage
Miscellaneous	Carboplatin	Neuropathy and renal damage
	Etoposide	Vomiting

*Most of these agents can depress the bone-marrow leading to a tendency to infection and a bleeding state: particular complications are noted here. *See also* Appendix 1.
†Oral ulceration can be a complication of virtually any cancer chemotherapeutic agent but is most common in these groups.

LEUCOPENIA AND AGRANULOCYTOSIS

Reduced numbers of circulating leucocytes—either in absolute numbers or as functionally effective cells—is a feature of many diseases (*Table 5.8*). Agranulocytosis, the name given to the clinical syndrome resulting from leucopenia, is characterized by abnormal susceptibility to infection.

Leucopenia can develop in isolation or be associated with other effects of depressed marrow function, notably anaemia and bleeding tendencies, as in

Table 5.8 Some causes of leucopenia

1. Leukaemia, other marrow infiltrations and myelofibrosis
2. Aplastic anaemia (Table 4.7)
3. Drugs
    Phenylbutazone
    Co-trimoxazole
    Sulphonamides
    Chloramphenicol
    Cephalothin
    Phenothiazines
    Anti-thyroid drugs
    Phenytoin
    Cytotoxic agents (Table 5.7)
4. Autoimmune
    Systemic lupus erythematosus
    Felty's syndrome
    Others
5. HIV infection
6. Cyclic neutropenia

acute leukaemia and aplastic anaemia. In Britain, phenylbutazone (the use of which is now restricted) was apparently the most common cause of aplastic anaemia and co-trimoxazole the most common cause of agranulocytosis, although overall these are uncommon complications in relation to the scale of use of these drugs. Marrow suppression, often irreversible, was an uncommon (but frequently lethal) complication of treatment with chloramphenicol, which should therefore only be given for life-threatening infections where no other antibiotic is effective.

Clinically, agranulocytosis is often sudden in onset and characterized by fever, weakness or prostration and sore throat. Gingival, oral and pharyngeal ulceration with pseudomembrane formation are common features but ulceration can affect any mucous membrane. Lymphadenopathy and sometimes rashes are also features. Later, haemorrhagic necrosis of mucous membranes and respiratory infection may go on to septicaemia as the terminal event. Although infections may be an early feature of acute leukaemia or aplastic anaemia, their clinical picture is more variable and bleeding as a result of thrombocytopenia may be the first manifestation.

The diagnosis is confirmed by blood examination and marrow biopsy and treatment depends on the underlying cause. In the case of drugs the triggering agent must be stopped and this may sometimes allow marrow function to recover. The main treatment measure is to control infections, particularly by Gram–negative bacteria, with antibiotics such as ticarcillin, mecillinam or one of the third generation cephalosporins such as cefotaxime.

Dental aspects of leucopenias

Infections and ulcers are the main oral manifestations of neutropenia and the management of such patients is similar to that of those with leukaemia.

Periodontal disease may be accelerated and minor oral infections may result in gangrenous stomatitis in severe cases.

Cyclic neutropenia is a very rare form of leucopenia which can cause oral manifestations, particularly recurrent oral ulcers (*see* Chapter 7). Lymphopenia may be an early sign of HIV infection (Chapter 16).

Septicaemia caused by various oral micro-organisms is a hazard of leucopenia. Surgical procedures should therefore be carried out under antibiotic cover.

MYELOPROLIFERATIVE DISORDERS

Proliferation of bone marrow cells, other than leucocyte stem cells, leads to myeloproliferative disorders (MPD). These are regarded as separate entities from leukaemias.

The main myeloproliferative disorders, which are all rare, are polycythaemia rubra vera, agnogenic myeloid metaplasia and essential thrombocythaemia. Chronic granulocytic leukaemia is sometimes also included in this group. Myeloproliferative disorders have several common features, transition between them is common, and any may terminate in acute leukaemia (*Table 5.9*).

Polycythaemia Rubra Vera

Polycythaemia rubra vera is an increase in red cell population which may be primary and idiopathic (PRV) or, more commonly, secondary. PRV is uncommon, mainly a disease of the elderly and has a slight male predominance. The clinical features result from the essential disturbances which are:

1. Increased numbers of red cells.
2. Bone replacement by erythropoietic tissue, and myeloid metaplasia in the liver and spleen.
3. Increased granulocyte and platelet production with platelet dysfunction.

The increased red cell mass leads to *hyperviscosity syndrome* . Increased cell turnover may lead to hyperuricaemia, gout and renal damage. Marrow expansion causes bone pain and there may eventually be myelofibrosis. Haemostatic defects due to platelet dysfunction may cause bruising, bleeding or thromboses.

Table 5.9. Important findings in myeloproliferative diseases

	RBC count	WBC count	Platelet count	Leucocyte alkaline phosphatase	Marrow fibrosis	Splenomegaly
Polycythaemia rubra vera	↑	↑	↑	↑	—	+
Agnogenic myeloid metaplasia	↓	↑	N or↑	↑	+	++
Essential thrombocythaemia	N	N	↑↑↑	N	—	+

Arrows indicate a value above or below normal (N).

General management

In the absence of treatment few patients with PRV survive more than 2 years. Repeated venesection reduces the red cell mass and extends survival to more than 10 years. Phosphorus-32 is also a simple and effective method of reducing erythropoiesis but may increase the risk of leukaemia. Cytotoxic agents (busulphan, chlorambucil or melphalan) may be given to suppress marrow activity, especially if there is thrombocytosis. Cyproheptadine to control pruritus and allopurinol for gout may also be needed.

Dental aspects

The main dental management problems are susceptibility to thrombosis and haemorrhage (Chapter 3). Venesection is especially important if surgery is indicated, since postoperative morbidity and mortality are greatly increased by thrombotic complications. There may also be oral complications from cytotoxic chemotherapy.

Myelofibrosis

Fibrosis of the bone-marrow gradually depresses cell proliferation and extends throughout the reticuloendothelial system. Myelofibrosis may be primary (agnogenic* myeloid metaplasia) or secondary (mainly to polycythaemia rubra vera, carcinomatosis or, rarely now, tuberculosis).

Most patients are elderly and have loss of weight, anaemia and thrombocytopenia. There may therefore be purpura and bleeding tendencies, weakness, bone pain, splenomegaly, hepatomegaly, gout and other features. The median survival time is about 5 years, but less in myelofibrosis secondary to carcinomatosis or polycythaemia.

General management

Most patients need correction of anaemia and thrombocytopenia by transfusion. Bone pains and hyperuricaemia also need to be controlled. Corticosteroids are used occasionally.

Dental aspects

Management problems may result from:

1. Anaemia.
2. Haemorrhage.
3. Possible hepatitis B, C or HIV carriage.
4. Corticosteroid treatment.

*Agnogenic = of unknown origin, idiopathic.

Essential Thrombocythaemia

Thrombocythaemia may be an isolated abnormality, or associated with other myeloproliferative disorders. The common effects are thromboses or haemorrhages. There is usually gross thrombocytosis with functionally defective, giant platelets.

Radioactive phosphorus is the treatment of choice but if this fails cytotoxic-drugs are used. Aspirin and dipyridamole are useful for preventing thrombosis, but heparin may be required. Surgery must be avoided until the disease is controlled, particularly because of the haemorrhagic tendencies.

MYELODYSPLASTIC SYNDROMES

The myelodysplastic syndromes are a group of stem cell disorders characterized by a reduction in one or more cell lines in the blood. Though the bone-marrow is initially active there is erythrodyspoiesis (*Table 5. 10*). Some patients succumb to marrow failure, others to acute leukaemia.

Table 5.10. The myelodysplastic syndromes

Type
1. Refractory anaemia alone
2. Refractory anaemia with ring sideroblasts
3. Refractory anaemia with excess blasts (RAEB)
4. Refractory anaemia with blasts in transformation
5. Chronic myelomonocytic leukaemia

Dental aspects

Gingival infiltration and oral ulceration have been reported in chronic myelomonocytic leukaemia but not in the other myelodysplastic syndromes.

Dental management may be complicated by:

1. Bleeding tendency due to thrombocytopenia (Chapter 3).
2. Anaemia (Chapter 4).
3. Neutropenia and a liability to infection including HBV and HIV (Chapter 16).

CRYOGLOBULINAEMIA

Cryoglobulins are immunoglobulins which precipitate when cooled below the normal body temperature. Cryoglobulins are of three main types. Type I is monoclonal and a typical feature of lymphoproliferative and related diseases; types II and III are typically associated with the connective tissue diseases and some infections, where the effects may result from immune complex formation.

In most cases the underlying disease is more important and cryoglobulins are an incidental finding. However, cryoglobulins can occasionally cause effects as a result of their physical properties, particularly Raynaud's phenomenon, or occasionally, peripheral thromboses and obstruction of small vessels. Purpura or bleeding tendencies may also result. Plasmapheresis may be beneficial.

PLASMA CELL DISEASES

Plasma cell diseases are an uncommon group of B-lymphocyte disorders (*Table 5.11*), each characterized by overproduction of a specific immunoglobulin detectable, and often dominating other proteins, on electrophoresis.

These homogeneous immunoglobulins (monoclonal immunoglobulins) are also defective, and the rates of production of immunoglobulin light or heavy chains may be unbalanced, leading to overproduction of light chains (Bence Jones protein) or heavy chains in the serum and urine (*Table 5.12*).

Table 5.11. Plasma cell diseases

1. Multiple myeloma
2. Solitary myeloma
3. Waldenström's macroglobulinaemia
4. Heavy chain disease
5. Idiopathic monoclonal gammopathy

Table 5.12. Paraprotein found in the plasma cell diseases

Disorder	Serum paraprotein	Bence Jones protemuria
Multiple myeloma	IgG (50%) IgA (25%) IgD or IgE rarely	+
Waldenström's macroglobulinaemia	IgM	— (rarely)
Heavy chain disease	α (or γ or μ)	—
Idiopathic monoclonal gammopathy	IgG (or IgA or IgM)	—

MULTIPLE MYELOMA (Myelomatosis)

Multiple myeloma is a disseminated plasma cell neoplasm. It is a disease mainly of the middle-aged and elderly, with a slight predilection for males.

The initial change is production of abnormal serum immunoglobulins alone, which are occasionally detectable by chance during routine haematological examination (by a raised ESR, rouleaux formation or high plasma viscosity) or serum protein investigations. Many years may elapse before symptoms appear. Neoplastic proliferation of plasma cells in the bone-marrow ultimately causes

Table 5.13. Multiple myeloma: clinical features and laboratory findings

Clinical features
1. Bone lesions
    Bone pain (especially spinal)
    Pathological fractures
2. Neurological lesions
    Paraesthesiae
    Weakness
3. Hyperviscosity syndrome
    Weakness
    Visual disturbances
    Bleeding tendencies
4. Anaemia
5. Renal failure
6. Hypercalcaemia

Laboratory findings
1. Haematological
    Normochromic anaemia
    Leucopenia
    Thrombocytopenia
    ESR very high
2. Biochemical
    Hypergammaglobulinaemia
    Monoclonal IgG (less often IgA, rarely IgD or IgE)
    Hypercalcaemia
    Hyperuricaemia (after treatment)
    Uraemia (in renal disease)
    Bence Jones proteinuria
3. Radiological
    Osteolytic lesions (skull, vertebrae, long bones)

marrow infiltration and suppression of haemopoiesis, bone destruction, hypercalcaemia, renal failure and many other secondary effects (*Table 5.13*).
Diagnosis depends on showing:

1. A monoclonal immunoglobulin peak on electrophoresis of serum.
2. Plasma cell neoplasia on marrow biopsy.
3. Osteolytic lesions in skeletal radiographs or by bone scanning.

General management

Anaemia, chronic renal failure, low serum albumin, and high levels of serum β2–microglobulin in the absence of renal disease, indicate a poor prognosis. Symptomatic patients or those with progressive bone lesions or increasing paraproteinaemia are treated by chemotherapy. The prognosis is variable, but the survival of treated patients averages 2 years. A few patients treated with cytotoxic chemotherapy develop acute myelomonocytic leukaemia.

An increasing number of asymptomatic patients are found to have myelomatosis by electrophoretic evidence of hypergammaglobulinaemia. Such patients must be followed and treatment started when appropriate.

Dental aspects

Oral manifestations. The skull, especially the calvarium, is ultimately affected in about 70 per cent of cases. Jaw lesions are seen less frequently and mainly involve the posterior part of the mandible. Small, rounded, discrete (punched-out) osteolytic lesions are typical and can simulate metastases. Root resorption, loosening of teeth, mental anaesthesia and, rarely, pathological fractures are other possible effects. Rare complications are gingival bleeding, oral petechiae, cranial nerve palsies and herpes simplex or zoster infections. Amyloid may be deposited in the oral soft tissues causing local or more widespread swellings, such as macroglossia, the nature of which can be confirmed by biopsy.

Dental treatment. Treatment may be complicated by:

1. Anaemia.
2. Infections.
3. Haemorrhagic tendencies.
4. Renal failure.
5. Corticosteroid therapy.

Solitary plasmacytoma (localized myeloma)

A solitary plasmacytoma occasionally forms in the jaws or soft tissues nearby. There is usually no abnormal immunoglobulin production but, even when present, the levels are low.

Soft tissue plasmacytomas are more likely than bone lesions to remain localized. Local radiotherapy may be useful, but cytotoxic chemotherapy is contraindicated. Patients should be kept under observation as multiple myeloma develops in many, even after 20 years.

WALDENSTRÖM'S MACROGLOBULINAEMIA

(Primary Macroglobulinaemia)

Macroglobulinaemia is a rare disease in which B-lymphocytes produce excessive amounts of monoclonal IgM. These large globulin molecules make the blood abnormally viscous and cause hyperviscosity syndrome (*see below*). There is usually also anaemia, recurrent infections and haemorrhagic tendencies and a wide variety of other possible manifestations, particularly lymphadenopathy and splenomegaly.

Despite the analogous pathogenesis to multiple myeloma, foci of bone destruction are not a feature of Waldenström's macroglobulinaemia. The prognosis of the latter is usually also slightly better than that of myeloma, but it may progress to lymphoma and a more rapid termination.

General management

The clinical course is very variable but nearly 25 per cent of patients need no treatment for long periods and there is a median survival of over 3 years.

Dental aspects

Oral manifestations.   Haemorrhagic tendencies may cause spontaneous gingival bleeding orpost-extraction haemorrhage. Deep punched-out ulcers of the tongue, buccal mucosa or palate have been reported, but are rare.

Dental treatment.   The major problems of dental treatment are:

1. Bleeding tendencies (Chapter 3).
2. Corticosteroid therapy (Chapter 10).
3. Anaemia (Chapter 4).

Benign Monoclonal Gammopathy and Secondary Macroglobulinaemia

Elderly patients who are otherwise healthy not infrequently produce excessive amounts of monoclonal immunoglobulin. It is essential not to interpret this finding as necessarily indicating myeloma. However, prolonged follow-up is essential to distinguish them from the 20 per cent who ultimately develop myeloma. Others die from amyloid renal disease.

Amyloidosis can result particularly from overproduction of immunoglobulin light chains. Macroglossia or deposits in other parts of the mouth may be the first clinical manifestation.

Many patients also produce large amounts of IgM secondary to connective tissue diseases, chronic liver disease or chronic lymphocytic leukaemia. This IgM is often polyclonal and not a precursor to myeloma or macroglobulinaemia.

HYPERVISCOSITY SYNDROME

Hyperviscosity syndrome is characterized by slowing of the peripheral circulation caused by excessive amounts of high molecular weight plasma proteins. Waldenström's macroglobulinaemia or myeloma account for most cases.

The large protein molecules adsorb platelets and erythrocytes causing increased platelet adhesiveness and erythrocyte rouleaux formation. They also activate clotting factors and complement, causing local thrombosis and inflammation.

General management

Plasmapheresis reduces the viscosity, but treatment should be aimed at the primary condition. Penicillamine is useful for a short period only, since the side-effects can be severe.

Dental aspects

Gingival haemorrhage or post-extraction haemorrhage, or oral ulceration due to penicillamine, may be.features.

Table 5.14. Diseases associated with amyloid formation

Disease	Amyloid fibril proteins
Idiopathic (primary) amyloidosis	AL proteins derived from immunoglobulin light chains
Myeloma-associated amyloidosis	AL proteins derived from immunoglobulin light chains
Secondary amyloidosis, e.g. to chronic infections, chronic inflammatory states, such as rheumatoid arthritis and ulcerative colitis	AA protein derived from serum amyloid A (SAA) protein, an acute phase protein released by the liver under influence of interleukin-1 from activated mononuclear phagocytes
Other forms of amyloidosis A heterogeneous group, some familial, others related to senility, medullary carcinoma of thyroid or calcifying epithelial odontogenic tumour and localized	A range of proteins, mainly like prealbumin

AMYLOID DISEASE

Amyloid disease is the deposition in the tissues of an eosinophilic hyaline material with a characteristic fibrillar structure on electron microscopy. Amyloid disease can result from deranged immunoglobulin synthesis as in benign monoclonal gammopathy (primary amyloidosis) or more commonly from excessive stimulation of the reticulo-endothelial system (secondary amyloidosis, *Table 5.14*) when the amyloid consists of AA proteins and is deposited mainly in and affects the function of the heart, skeletal muscle and gastrointestinal tract.

Other secondary amyloid is of uncertain origin but affects mainly the spleen, liver, kidney and adrenals.

The widespread lesions in amyloid disease make this disorder protean in its manifestations including a bleeding tendency related to a Factor X defect (*see* Appendix 1, chapter 3).

General management

Amyloidosis is a manifestation of several diseases, not a disease in itself. An underlying cause must therefore be sought after the diagnosis is established by biopsy. Combination therapy with corticosteroids, melphalan and fluoxymesterone may produce some improvement.

Dental aspects

Macroglossia, gingival swellings, oral petechiae, bullae or rarely, a sicca syndrome may result from amyloidosis, but virtually only in the primary type.

Dental management may be influenced by the underlying disorder, or by cardiac, renal, adrenal, corticosteroid complications or a bleeding tendency.

LYMPHOMAS

The lymphomas form a group of uncommon solid malignant tumours with a wide spectrum of clinical and pathological effects. Dental management may be complicated by anaemia, liability to infection, and corticosteroid or cytotoxic therapy.

Lymphomas originate in lymph nodes or extranodal tissue in any part of the body from any type of lymphocyte. Immunological characterization of the cell lineage and the extent of the disease determine the treatment and prognosis (*Table 5.15*).

Table 5.15. Simplified classification of lymphomas

1. Hodgkin's disease	
Lymphocyte predominant	
Nodular sclerotic	
Mixed cellular	
Lymphocyte depleted	
2. Non-Hodgkin's lymphoma	
Nodular	Indolent course
(i) Poorly differentiated lymphocytic	Most frequent; disseminated
(ii) Mixed cellular (lymphocytic and histiocytic)	Good response to chemotherapy
(iii) Histiocytic	Aggressive; behaves like a diffuse lymphoma
Diffuse	Aggressive course
(i) Lymphocytic	Chronic if well differentiated
	Others disseminated
(ii) Mixed cellular	Disseminated
(iii) Histiocytic	Formerly called reticulum cell sarcoma
(iv) Lymphoblastic	50% develop acute lymphoblastic leukaemia
(iv) Burkitt's lymphoma	Good response to chemotherapy

Note: Many other classifications.

HODGKIN'S DISEASE

About 40 per cent of all lymphomas are Hodgkin's disease, which can affect any age group but particularly males in their thirties.

Hodgkin's disease appears to originate in a cell of the monocyte-histiocyte series. There is progressive involvement of lymphoid tissue, often beginning in the neck (*Fig.* 5.2). The lymph nodes become enlarged, discrete and rubbery and can cause symptoms by pressure on other organs or ducts. Anaemia is common late in the disease.

Systemic symptoms including pain, remittent fever, night sweats, weight loss, malaise, bone pain and pruritus are common. Alcoholic drinks may cause pain in affected lymph nodes. Cellular immunity is impaired so that fungal and viral infections are common and may disseminate.

Treatment of Hodgkin's disease includes radiotherapy and chemotherapy (*Table 5.16*), depending on the staging of the disease. With such management the 5-year survival in the earlier stages is about 80 per cent and is over 60 per cent even in more advanced Hodgkin's disease. Those who relapse usually do so within the first 2 years.

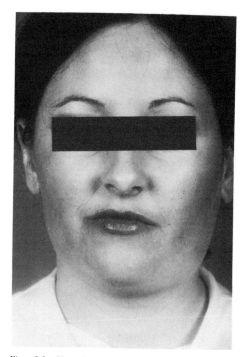

Fig. 5.2. Chronically enlarged cervical lymph nodes in a young patient raise the possibility of a lymphoma or HIV infection.

Table 5.16. Staging and treatment in Hodgkin's disease

Stage*	Definition	Treatment
I	Involvement of single lymph node or group of nodes	Radiotherapy
II	Involvement of two or more groups of lymph nodes on one side of diaphragm or Localized involvement of an extralymphatic organ or site and of one or more lymph nodes on the same side of diaphragm	Radiotherapy
III	Involvement of lymph nodes on both sides of diaphragm ± splenic or other sites	Radiotherapy (IIIA) or Quadruple therapy (IIIB)†
IV	Diffuse or disseminated disease of one or more extralymphatic organs or tissues ± associated lymph node involvement	Quadruple therapy†

*Stage is also qualified by a suffix A or B. B = presence of fever, night sweats or weight loss. A = absence of such systemic symptoms.
†Quadruple therapy is combined chemotherapy—either MOPP (*Mustine, Oncovin, Prednisolone and Procarbazine*) or ABVD (*Adriamycin, Vincristine and Dimethyltriazenoimidazole-carboxamide*).

Non-Hodgkin's lymphoma

Lymphomas other than Hodgkin's disease have a variable but generally poor prognosis. Most non-Hodgkin's lymphomas appear to be of B-cell origin and have a predilection for sites such as the gastrointestinal tract and CNS. They frequently involve the mesenteric lymph nodes and bone-marrow but often enlargement of cervical lymph nodes is the first sign. They can be a complication of AIDS, the connective tissue diseases or cytotoxic chemotherapy.

In general, non-Hodgkin's lymphomas are treated by multiple chemotherapy, since early dissemination is common, but radiotherapy may be useful in the initial stages.

Dental aspects of the lymphomas

Oral manifestations. Painless enlarged cervical lymph nodes are the initial complaint in 50 per cent of cases. A lymphoma may form in the oral cavity or oropharynx but this is rare except in association with HIV infection.

Involvement of Waldeyer's ring is more common in non-Hodgkin's lymphomas than in Hodgkin's disease. Lesions appear as erythematous swellings, often with surface ulceration as a result of trauma, and may involve the pharynx, palate, tongue, gingivae or lips, but lesions are frequently present elsewhere. The jaws may also rarely be involved. Herpes zoster, herpetic stomatitis and oral candidosis may be seen, especially in those on cytotoxic or radiation therapy. Zoster, secondary to immunodeficiency, may be the first overt sign of the disease. Though Hodgkin's disease frequently involves the cervical lymph nodes, it rarely affects the mouth, but when it does, is not clinically distinguishable from non–Hodgkin's lymphomas.

Oral lesions are only rarely the initial manifestation of lymphomas but an oral lymphoma may be the first sign of HIV infection. A lymphoma in the mouth of a young male particularly, should therefore lead to the suspicion of HIV infection.

In the perioral regions, non–Hodgkin's lymphomas are one of the most common type of non–epithelial tumour of salivary glands in adults, but account for only account for about 5 per cent of salivary gland tumours. Their diagnosis causes difficulties in this site because of possible confusion with benign lympho-epithelial lesions and Sjögren's syndrome, and the fact that either may progress to lymphoma in about 20 per cent of cases. By contrast Hodgkin's disease of salivary glands is rare. The high frequency shown in some series is due to inclusion of disease of the cervical lymph nodes, but even these remain discrete and rarely involve the adjacent submandibular or parotid gland parenchyma.

A rare type of T-cell lymphoma is the cause of some cases of midline granuloma syndrome in which there may be oral complications (Chapter 16).

Dental treatment. The main problems from lymphomas that may influence dental treatment are:

1. Oral infections, especially with viruses and fungi.
2. Oral ulceration caused by cytotoxic drugs.

3. Anaemia.
4. Corticosteroid therapy.
5. Bleeding tendencies.
6. Impaired respiratory function (pulmonary fibrosis due to irradiation).
7. Acute leukaemia (7 per cent of treated patients).

ORAL COMPLICATIONS OF CYTOTOXIC CHEMOTHERAPY

Many of the cytotoxic agents can cause oral complications, particularly if treatment is prolonged or in high dosage (*see Table 5.7* and Appendix 1). Some 90 per cent of children and approximately 50 per cent of adults develop oral lesions as in many cases, radiotherapy is also given. However the effects of these forms of treatment are described separately here.

Infections.　Cytotoxic agents predispose to oral infections with fungi, viruses, toxoplasma, or bacteria. Oral candidosis is common and is usually caused by *Candida albicans* or, less often, other candida species. Candidosis is promoted

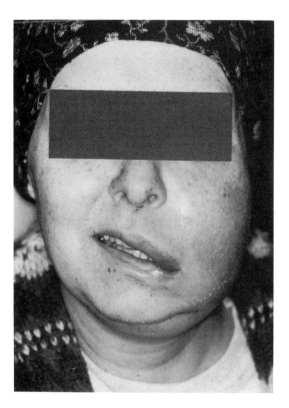

Fig. 5.3. Leukaemia with a dental abscess and spreading infection.

especially by severe leucopenia and the use of antibiotics. Oral mucormycosis (phycomycosis) or aspergillosis are rare. Herpetic infections (H. simplex or H. zoster) are common in patients on cancer chemotherapy and may cause chronic oral ulcers. Gram–positive bacterial infections (staphylococci) are less common as patients usually receive antibiotics prophylactically. Hospitalized patients on cytotoxic chemotherapy may, however, develop Gram-negative oral infections (with pseudomonas, klebsiella, escherichia, enterobacter, serratia or proteus) and dental infections may spread rapidly (*Fig. 5.3*).

Ulcers and mucositis. Oral ulceration is a common complication, especially in patients treated with antimetabolites and cytotoxic antibiotics (*Table 5.7;* Appendix to this chapter), and may be severe enough to preclude further chemotherapy. Ulceration often begins shortly after chemotherapy is started and may resolve within a few weeks of completion of treatment.

Oral ulceration most often complicates treatment with methotrexate, 5-fluorouracil, doxorubicin or bleomycin. It is often the first sign of methotrexate toxicity and can follow within 24 hours of a single dose of this agent. The ulcers are shallow and painful, affecting particularly the labial and faucial mucosa, but usually heal within 2 weeks of cessation of cytotoxic therapy.

Over 50 per cent of patients on methotrexate or 5-fluorouracil and 30 per cent of those on daunorubicin and 25 per cent of those on 6-mercaptopurine suffer from drug-induced oral ulceration.

Lip cracking. Lip cracking is common when there are febrile episodes.

Bleeding. Drug-induced thrombocytopenia may cause gingival bleeding, mucosal petechiae or ecchymoses.

Xerostomia. Cytotoxic agents (especially adriamycin) may cause xerostomia, similar to that resulting from radiation therapy, and can lead to caries and other oral infections.

When combined cytotoxic chemotherapy and radiotherapy were given Dreizen et al. (1986) found that the most common complications were infection (23 per cent), drug mucositis (6 per cent), bleeding (5 per cent), infection and mucositis (5 per cent) infection and haemorrhage (3 per cent), drug mucositis and bleeding (2 per cent), infection plus drug mucositis plus bleeding (3.5 per cent)

DENTAL MANAGEMENT OF PATIENTS ON CYTOTOXIC CHEMOTHERAPY

Before chemotherapy. A careful oral assessment should be carried out to enable extractions and any other surgery to be completed before cytotoxic treatment, as the latter can cause abnormal bleeding and susceptibility to infection (*Table 5.17*). Oral hygiene should be improved as far as possible.

Table 5.17. Dental treatment for patients on cytotoxic chemotherapy

Blood cell type	Peripheral blood count	Precautions
Platelets	>50 × 10⁹/l	Routine management though desmopressin or platelets are needed to cover surgery
	<50 × 10⁹/l	Platelets needed
Granulocytes	>2 × 10⁹/l	Routine management
	<2 × 10⁹/l	Prophylactic antimicrobials for surgery
Erythrocytes	>5 × 10¹²/l	Routine management
	<5 × 10¹²/l	Special care with general anaesthesia

During chemotherapy. It may be possible to avoid or reduce oral ulceration caused by methotrexate using systemic or topical folinic acid (leucovorin). A mouthwash of allopurinol (1 mg/ml) may lessen the stomatitis induced by 5–fluorouracil, but results of trials have been equivocal. Topical prostaglandin E2 may also be beneficial but this too remains to be confirmed. Established mucositis or oral ulceration is managed by maintaining good oral hygiene with a twice-daily 0.2 per cent aqueous chlorhexidine mouthrinses. Viscous 2 per cent lignocaine or benzydamine can be used to help reduce discomfort.

Many patients develop oral candidosis and this usually also implies oesophageal candidosis which may be a portal for haematogenous dissemination. Nystatin suspension (100 000 µ/ml) as a mouthwash or pastilles four to six times daily, may be given as a prophylactic antifungal but clotrimazole 25 mg three times a day is probably more effective. Some workers now therefore recommend ketoconazole or fluconazole for patients with candidosis who develop fever. Dentures should be carefully cleaned and stored overnight in 1 per cent hypochlorite to reduce candidal carriage. Oral herpetic infections should be treated with acyclovir suspension or systemic acyclovir (tablets or infusion). Prophylactic acyclovir is used in some centres and has reduced the incidence of and mortality from zoster. Zoster immune globulin may help ameliorate varicella or zoster. Although patients are frequently already on several antibiotics, Gram-negative infections may need treatment with gentamicin or carbenicillin as the oral lesions can be portals for systemic infection.

Aspirin should not be given to patients on methotrexate as it may enhance the toxicity of the latter (*see* Appendix to Chapter 19). Some cytotoxic drugs enhance the effects of suxamethonium (Chapter 10); others cause more serious complications that can influence dental management (*Table 5.7* and Appendix).

After chemotherapy. Most acute oral complications develop during chemotherapy but even afterwards there should still be close attention to oral hygiene and preventive dentistry, as many patients continue to have anaemia, bleeding tendencies and be susceptible to infection (*Table 5.17*).

OTHER ASPECTS OF MALIGNANT DISEASE

ORAL CANCER

Oral cancer is more fully discussed in specialist texts and only a brief synopsis is given here. Oral cancer is usually squamous cell carcinoma; common sites are the lips, lateral border of the tongue and floor of mouth. Cancer of the buccal mucosa and gingivae is less common and hard palate cancer is rare.

Oral cancer is mainly a disease of the elderly and there is a wide geographical variation in incidence, with very high rates particularly in India and Sri Lanka.

Predisposing causes are obscure. Despite widespread beliefs to the contrary, alcohol and cigarette consumption in Britain, does not correlate with the incidence of mouth cancer. Increased cigarette smoking, particularly since the 1940s, has been associated with a decline in oral cancer in males and no increase in females.

Premalignant lesions include erythroplasia (erythroplakia) and leucoplakia, particularly speckled leucoplakia or leucoplakias in the floor of the mouth. Syphilitic leucoplakia is now rare and the premalignant potential of candidal leucoplakia is uncertain. The hairy leucoplakia of HIV infection does not appear to be premalignant.

As a result of the AIDS epidemic, lymphomas and Kaposi's sarcoma of the oral cavity are now considerably more common than a decade ago.

The majority of salivary gland tumours are pleomorphic adenomas but there is a higher proportion of malignant tumours in the sublingual and minor oral salivary glands than in the parotids. Though uncommon there is also a higher relative frequency of malignant salivary gland tumours in children.

Patients with any cancer may have severe psychological disturbances in view of the nature of illness. These problems are compounded in oral cancer since there are additional handicaps, particularly interference with speech and swallowing, and disfigurement. Other problems are summarized in *Table 5.18.*

Table 5.18. Oral complications of treatment of cancer of the head and neck

1. Irradiation mucositis
2. Oral ulceration
3. Candidosis
4. Xerostomia
5. Radiation caries
6. Dental hypersensitivity
7. Periodontal disease
8. Loss of taste
9. Trismus
10. Osteoradionecrosis and irradiation-associated osteomyelitis

General management

Any lesion of dubious nature should be biopsied. Patients with established oral cancer are best managed by a team of specialists including the dental and maxillofacial surgeons as well as the oncologist. Opinion varies as to the value of radiotherapy or surgery: many early carcinomas can be treated by either method, while advanced cancer is in general, incurable by any technique. Palliation is then the most that can be offered. Combined treatment with cytotoxic chemotherapy has not proved to offer any better prognosis and, indeed there is a greater mortality as a consequence of the cytotoxic agents.

Lingual and labial cancers are often managed with radiotherapy, which may also provide the best palliation in patients with advanced disease. Cancer of the floor of the mouth presents considerable problems in surgery and may necessitate partial mandibulectomy.

In any incurable disease, management must include particular attention to the psychological problems of the patient. Patients may or may not know, or may not want to know, that they have malignant disease, and even if they are aware of it may not appreciate, or be willing to accept, the prognosis. Many different persons are involved in the care of these individuals and it is most important that there is good communication so that all are aware of (*a*) the prognosis; (*b*) how much the patient understands about his disease; (*c*) his psychological reactions to cancer; and (*d*) the side-effects of treatment. The quality of life is as important as or more important than its duration.

The type of dental care should to some extent be tailored to take account of the prognosis and must always be planned in relation to the interest that the patient has in his oral state. Just because patients are dying does not mean, however, that they should be allowed to suffer from dental pain, or that their appearance be neglected. Indeed, the provision of dental attention, for example the construction of a new denture, may help the patient's morale.

Potent analgesics such as narcotics, sedatives or antidepressants, may be needed in terminal cancer and can influence dental care.

Oral complications of radiotherapy involving the oral cavity or salivary glands

Mucositis. Mucositis is almost inevitable during radiotherapy where the field involves the oral mucosa. The degree of mucositis depends on the type of radiotherapy, dose and duration of treatment. The initial reaction is mucosal erythema followed by sloughing and considerable discomfort. Dysphagia and oral soreness become maximal 2–4 weeks after radiotherapy but usually subside in a further 2–3 weeks.

Loss of taste. Hypoguesia follows radiation damage to the taste buds but xerostomia alone can disturb taste sensation. Taste may start to recover within 2–4 months but, if more than 6000 CGy have been given, loss of taste is then usually permanent.

Xerostomia and infections. The fields of radiotherapy to cancers of the head and neck often involve the major salivary glands. Radiotherapy of tumours of the naso- and oropharynx is especially liable to damage the salivary glands.

Irradiation depresses salivary secretion and the saliva has a higher viscosity but lower pH. Salivary secretion diminishes within a week of radiotherapy in virtually all patients and the saliva becomes thick and tenacious. Some salivary function may return after many months.

Xerostomia predisposes to infections, particularly periodontal disease, caries, oral candidosis and acute ascending sialadenitis.

Radiation caries and dental hypersensitivity.   Patients frequently take a softer, more cariogenic diet because of dryness and soreness of the mouth and loss of taste. There is a change to a more cariogenic oral flora. Irradiation may also directly damage the teeth, which become hypersensitive, thus making oral hygiene difficult. These factors combine to cause rampant dental caries of any site, including areas such as incisal edges and cervical margins which are normally free from caries. Caries begins at any time between 2 and 10 months after radiotherapy, and may eventually result in the crown breaking off from the root. A complete dentition may be destroyed within a year of irradiation.

Osteoradionecrosis and osteomyelitis.   Death of bone of the jaw, particularly the mandible, is a potentially serious complication of irradiation endarteritis. If the soft tissues covering the bone are healthy and undisturbed, there may be no obvious consequences, but infection, often resulting from dental extractions carried out after radiotherapy, can lead to intractable osteomyelitis. In severe cases the whole of the body of the mandible may become infected, both the overlying mucosa and skin may be destroyed and the bone may become exposed internally and externally.

Irradiation-associated osteomyelitis may occasionally be precipitated by mucosal ulceration caused by a denture. As a consequence, some specialists refuse to permit patients to wear dentures, especially a full lower denture, after irradiation of the oral mucosa.

Osteoradionecrosis is, however, a less frequent problem now, as megavoltage radiotherapy has less effect on bone than did orthovoltage therapy. Osteoradionecrosis appears to develop mainly in patients receiving more than 6000 CGy, particularly to the floor of the mouth and mandible. Osteomyelitis may follow months or years after radiotherapy but about 30 per cent of cases develop within 6 months. Osteomyelitis is heralded by pain and swelling. The area of involved bone is often small (less than 2 cm diameter) and with antibiotics the signs and symptoms of inflammation may clear within a few weeks. Complete resolution can, however, take 2 or more years in spite of intensive treatment with antimicrobials.

Trismus.   Progressive endarteritis of affected tissues, with reduction in their blood supply, follows radiotherapy. The results may be replacement fibrosis of the masticatory muscles. Fibrosis becomes apparent 3–6 months after radiotherapy and can cause permanent limitation of opening.

Dental defects.   Irradiation of developing teeth can cause hypoplasia and retarded eruption.

Dental management of patients receiving radiotherapy to the head and neck

Treatment planning.   The complications of dental treatment after radiotherapy are such that planned treatment should be carried out before irradiation. Oral hygiene should be meticulous, preventive dental care instituted, and restorative procedures carried out at this stage. These measures can significantly reduce the caries incidence.

Extractions before radiotherapy.   It is not always necessary to extract all the teeth before radiotherapy. In any case, clearance before irradiation may not be practicable, because the patient is too old or ill, or the prognosis is too poor. Alternatively, the patient may have so healthy a dentition and such good oral hygiene, that dental complications after radiotherapy are unlikely.

Some patients may even refuse radiotherapy rather than lose their teeth. Furthermore, it is not easy to construct dentures if there is mucosal soreness, and dentures cannot always be worn after radiotherapy.

Most cancer patients are, however, of middle age or over and many have neglected dentitions. In such patients, teeth in the radiation path should be extracted or, if the patient has no objection, a total clearance may be preferable. The latter is essential where the teeth have been consistently neglected over many years.

The time interval permitted between extractions and radiotherapy is invariably a compromise because of the need to start radiotherapy as soon as possible. No bone should be left exposed in the mouth when radiotherapy begins since, once the blood supply is damaged by radiotherapy, wound healing is jeopardized. Many advise an interval of at least 2 weeks between extracting the teeth and starting radiotherapy but this is not always essential.

During radiotherapy.   Mucositis may be relieved by using warm normal saline mouthwashes and lignocaine viscous 2 per cent and it has been suggested, but not confirmed, that topical application of prostaglandin E2 may be helpful. Smoking and alcohol should be discouraged. A 0.2 per cent chlorhexidine mouthwash maintains oral hygiene and a benzydamine oral rinse or a saliva substitute such as carboxymethylcellulose may provide some symptomatic relief. Trismus may be reduced by instituting jaw-opening exercises with tongue spatulas or wedges used three times a day. Antifungal drugs such as nystatin suspension, 100 000 µ/ml, as a mouthwash or pastilles used four times daily may be required.

Recent studies suggest that elimination of Gram–negative bacteria by using a polymyxin and tobramycin lozenge four times a day, results in a significant reduction in mucositis.

After radiotherapy.   Oral hygiene and preventive dental care should be continued and mucositis managed as outlined above.

Dental extractions may precipitate osteomyelitis in the irradiated jaw but, if extractions are unavoidable, trauma should be kept to a minimum, raising the periosteum as little as possible and ensuring that sharp bone edges are removed. Careful suturing is needed and prophylactic antibiotics should be given in adequate doses and continued for 4 weeks at least.

However, some specialists may refuse to carry out extractions in the irradiated area because of the severity of radiation-associated osteomyelitis which can develop in spite of all precautions. Under these circumstances, dental infections are kept under control by means of antimicrobials.

Radiation caries and dental hypersensitivity can be controlled with daily topical fluoride applications (sodium fluoride mouthwash, stannous fluoride gel or acidulated fluoride phosphate gel). Occasionally full cover acrylic splints are used to protect the teeth (Coffin's caps). Unfortunately, only too many patients are told by their doctors to 'suck a sweet' to relieve the discomfort of their dry mouth. Clearly these patients must be disabused of such ideas and given practical guidance about diet. In essence all that should be necessary is avoidance of sweets and sweet confectionery and use of sugar substitutes such as saccharin or aspartame, wherever possible. Mouthwashes of sodium bicarbonate may help dissolve the stringy saliva that forms.

Mucosal trauma from dentures may predispose to osteomyelitis and some specialists therefore insist that dentures be abandoned. If dentures are required, they should be fitted at about 4–6 weeks after radiotherapy, when initial mucositis subsides and there is only early fibrosis.

Xerostomia: The dryness of the mouth is managed as for Sjögren's syndrome (Chapter 16) but palliation with liberal use of artificial saliva is usually the best that can be achieved.

HELP GROUPS FOR THOSE WHO HAVE HAD CANCER

Patients who have had oral cancer are not always advised adequately about the unpleasantness of the after-effects of treatment, and may need emotional support to overcome the anxiety caused by disfigurement. Help groups for these patients are listed in the Appendix to this chapter.

ANTRAL CARCINOMA

Antral carcinoma is a rare neoplasm of unknown aetiology but woodworking is a known occupational hazard. It is a disease of the elderly.

Antral carcinoma causes maxillary pain or effects from expansion and infiltration of adjacent tissues. It may cause an intra-oral swelling or ulcer in the palate or upper vestibule; a swelling in the cheek; unilateral nasal obstruction or epistaxis; obstruction of the nasolacrimal duct with consequent epiphora; infraorbital anaesthesia if the nerve is involved; or proptosis and ophthalmoplegia if the orbit is invaded.

Further details can be found in standard texts of ENT and oral surgery: treatment is usually by surgery.

NASOPHARYNGEAL CARCINOMA

Nasopharyngeal carcinoma (NPC) is a rare neoplasm which may be associated with Epstein–Barr virus and is especially common in Asia, particularly amongst the Southern Chinese, some Eskimo races and in parts of N. Africa such as Tunisia. A similar tumour, *undifferentiated carcinoma with lymphoid stroma,* may affect the salivary glands in susceptible races and is one of the most common types of salivary gland cancer in Eskimos and Southern Chinese.

Often asymptomatic in itself, since the neoplasm does not obstruct the nasopharynx, NPC can present in a variety of ways.

1. Isolated cervical lymph node enlargement.
2. Unilateral conductive deafness (from obstruction of the Eustachian tube).
3. Elevation and immobility of the soft palate.
4. Pain, sometimes with anaesthesia, in the ipsilateral tongue, lower teeth and lower lip (invasion of the mandibular division of the trigeminal nerve).

A combination of the above is Trotter's syndrome. Treatment is usually by radiotherapy.

CANCER IN OTHER SITES

Tumours involving other parts of the body are discussed in the appropriate chapters. Their most obvious oral importance is as a source of metastases, which can form in the jaws or occasionally as soft tissue lesions and can mimic a simple

Table 5.19. Oral manifestations of internal cancer

1. Metastases in jaws or (rarely) oral soft tissues, especially from cancer of
   Breast
   Lung
   Prostate
   Thyroid
   Kidney
   Stomach
2. Effects of tumour metabolites
   Facial flushing (carcinoid syndrome)
   Pigmentation (ectopic ACTH-secreting tumours)
   Amyloidosis (multiple myeloma)
   Oral erosions (glucagonoma)
3. Changes caused by other functional disturbances
   Purpura, anaemia, infections (leukaemia)
   Infections (lymphoma, especially Hodgkin's disease)
   Bleeding (liver cancer)
   Anaemia (bleeding from gastrointestinal tumours)
4. Mucocutaneous diseases
   Dermatomyositis (carcinoma in 15 per cent)
   Acanthosis nigricans (gastric carcinoma)
   Erythema multiforme (lymphoma, leukaemia or carcinoma, especially after radiotherapy)
   Pemphigus vulgaris
   Pemphigoid
   Dermatitis herpetiformis
5. Inherited disorders with predisposition to internal malignancy and oral lesions
   Cowden's syndrome
   Gardner's syndrome
   Multiple endocrine neoplasia type III
   Neurofibromatosis (von Recklinghausen's disease)
   Gorlin–Goltz syndrome
   Tylosis
   Tuberous sclerosis
   Maffuci syndrome

epulis clinically. Histological examination of all such swellings is therefore essential.

Other oral manifestations of internal malignancy are summarized in *Table 5.19.*

Less obviously it must be borne in mind that any patient who has had cancer, even if treatment has apparently been successful, often has a limited expectation of life. If, further, there are signs of spread of the tumour such as involvement of cervical or other lymph nodes, or the appearance of oral lesions, then the prognosis is very poor indeed. The dental care of such patients may therefore have to be modified accordingly. Though there is great individual variation, the overall 5-year survival rates are shown for important cancers in *Table 5.20,* as it is perhaps insufficiently widely appreciated how short survival may be in some cases. Thus in the case of carcinoma of the pancreas only 3–4 per cent (in round

Table 5.20. Five-year survival (per cent) of cases of malignant disease*

Site	Sex	No. of registrations	5-year survival rate*
Lip	M	1196	93.53
	F	194	84.01
Tongue	M	907	37.13
	F	628	45.93
Oesophagus	M	5033	6.27
	F	3983	7.88
Stomach	M	19619	7.38
	F	12938	7.25
Large intestine, except rectum	M	14564	29.63
	F	19703	29.35
Rectum and rectosigmoid junction	M	13003	30.79
	F	10537	32.94
Pancreas	M	7051	3.78
	F	6071	3.12
Larynx	M	3890	64.40
	F	725	56.85
Trachea, bronchus and lung	M	71710	7.80
	F	16461	7.02
Breast	M	472	59.57
	F	57232	56.81
Cervix, uteri, excluding *in situ*	F	11965	54.42
Prostate	M	17943	35.93
Bladder	M	16172	53.79
	F	5629	47.35
Brain	M	3717	14.81
	F	2620	16.12
Lymphosarcoma and reticulum cell sarcoma	M	2785	30.07
	F	2435	31.70
Hodgkin's disease	M	2546	55.81
	F	1581	57.28
Lymphatic leukaemia	M	2560	30.41
	F	1741	34.15
Myeloid leukaemia	M	2314	7.60
	F	2140	6.44
All leukaemias	M	5555	18.17
	F	4422	17.24

*1971–73 Registrations: some may have improved recently.
†Corrected for age, etc.

figures) survive for 5 or more years but even the 1-year survival rate is only 10 per cent. To put it another way, a patient who develops cancer of the pancreas has only a one in ten chance of surviving for more than a year.

LANGERHANS CELL HISTIOCYTOSIS (SOLITARY AND MULTIFOCAL EOSINOPHILIC GRANULOMA)

These diseases are tumours or tumour–like lesions of Langerhans cells—the cutaneous counterparts of macrophages. This cell is recognizable by electron microscopy by the presence of rod–shaped Birbeck granules.

The three main types of disease are solitary eosinophilic granuloma, multifocal eosinophilic granuloma (Hand–Schüller–Christian disease) and Letterer–Siwe disease.

Both eosinophilic granuloma and Hand–Schüller–Christian disease are relatively benign. Letterer–Siwe disease is disseminated and malignant (*Table 5.21*).

Solitary Eosinophilic Granuloma

Eosinophilic granuloma is an osteolytic lesion of bone with a predilection for the mandible. Adults are mainly affected and typical symptoms are pain, tenderness, swelling or bone destruction. Radiographs show a tumour-like area of rarefaction. The diagnosis is by biopsy and typically shows foamy histiocytes and many eosinophils with ill-defined, somewhat fibrillar background and areas of necrosis. A bone scan should be carried out to ensure that the disease is not multifocal.

Eosinophilic granuloma is relatively benign and responds to curettage or, if recurrent, to modest doses of irradiation, or chemotherapy with vinblastine, prednisolone or cyclosphosphamide.

Eosinophilic granuloma can also affect the oral soft tissues, but less frequently than the mandible. However, a histologically somewhat similar lesion can be traumatic in origin or reactionary without any history of trauma and there must be some doubt about the nature of eosinophilic granulomas of soft tissues reported in the past.

Multifocal Eosinophilic Granuloma and Hand–Schüller–Christian Syndrome

These lesions are the same histologically as the solitary eosinophilic granuloma and are sometimes referred to indifferently as Hand–Schüller–Christian disease. Hand–Schüller–Christian syndrome, strictly speaking, comprises osteolytic lesions of the skull, exophthalmos and diabetes insipidus and is a variant of multifocal eosinophilic granuloma. Multifocal eosinophilic granuloma most frequently develops before the age of 5 years.

Diagnosis is by biopsy which shows essentially the same features as solitary eosinophilic granuloma, and by skeletal radiography or bone scan to assess the extent of the disease.

Table 5.21. Langerhans' cell histiocytoses

	Age of onset	Bone lesions	Skin or mucosal lesions	Visceral lesions	Pituitary lesions	Treatment	Prognosis
Solitary eosinophilic granuloma	> 10 yr	+	±	−	−	Surgery Local radiotherapy	Good
Multifocal eosinophilic (Hand–Schüller–Christian disease)	< 5 yr	+	+	±	+	Chemotherapy	Variable
Letterer–Siwe disease	Infancy	+	+	+	+	Chemotherapy Steroids	Usually fatal

Flat bones including the mandible are the main sites and soft tissues also become involved, but the triad of features of the classic Hand–Schüller–Christian syndrome develops in only 25 per cent. Lymphadenopathy and hepatosplenomegaly may develop in up to 50 per cent.

Malaise, fever and infections of the ear, mastoid and respiratory tract are common. Nevertheless, in approximately 50 per cent of cases the lesions gradually resolve spontaneously over the course of years but can leave residual disabilities as a result of limb lesions or diabetes insipidus. To reduce such complications, or in refractory cases, chemotherapy in relatively modest doses may be used as for solitary lesions. The mortality may be 25–30 per cent. The younger the patient and the more widespread the disease, the worse the prognosis.

Dental aspects of eosinophilic granuloma

Eosinophilic granuloma is an occasional cause of tumour-like swelling and radiolucent lesions of the mandible but the diagnosis can only be made by biopsy. Bone scans may show that the disease is (or becomes) multifocal, but the multifocal eosinophilic granuloma of childhood or Hand–Schüller–Christian syndrome rarely has initial manifestations in the jaws. However, either type of disease can produce a characteristic form of periodontal destruction with gross gingival recession and alveolar bone loss, typically involving a small group of teeth and often exposing the roots of the teeth.

Otherwise, complications can arise as a result of treatment, either radiotherapy to the oral or para-oral regions, or chemotherapy with corticosteroids or cytotoxic agents.

In the case of solitary eosinophilic granuloma of soft tissues care must be taken to distinguish the lesion from the traumatic eosinophilic granuloma. However, this depends upon the histopathologist. 'Traumatic' eosinophilic granuloma eventually resolves spontaneously, though it may need to be excised for cosmetic reasons. Alternatively, the lesion may be excised because of its clinical resemblance to a tumour.

Letterer–Siwe Disease

Letterer–Siwe disease was previously thought to be a different disease from those just described. Nevertheless the Langerhans cell can be identified in the lesions.

Clinically, Letterer–Siwe disease typically affects children between the ages of 2 and 3 years and follows a rapidly fatal course. The main features are lymphadenopathy, hepatosplenomegaly, and bone and skin lesions. Fever, infections and bleeding tendencies are secondary to pancytopenia which results from marrow displacement by the histiocyte-like cells.

Diagnosis is by biopsy, showing infiltration of the tissues by proliferating histiocyte-like cells which, unlike those of eosinophilic granuloma, contain little or no lipid.

The disease is rapidly fatal in most cases and occasionally death follows within a week of diagnosis. Treatment with radiotherapy, corticosteroids and cytotoxic drugs is rarely successful, but rarely, the course of the disease is less acute and recoveries have been reported.

Dental aspects of Letterer–Siwe disease

In view of the age group mainly affected and the rapidity of the course, patients are unlikely to be seen by dentists. In the few older patients with a more chronic form of the disease, the features relevant to dentistry are essentially those of severe types of multifocal eosinophilic granuloma and indeed may be examples of that disease. Corticosteroid treatment may complicate dental management.

Bibliography

Alezanian R. (1977) Plasma cell neoplasms. *Medicine (UK)* **30**, 1700–12.

Barbas A. P. (1980) Surgical problems associated with polycythaemia. *Br. J. Hosp. Med.* **23**, 289–94.

Barrett A.P. (1987) A long-term prospective clinical study of oral complications during conventional chemotherapy for acute leukemia. *Oral Surg.* **63**, 313–16.

Bennett J. M. (1982) The French, American British (FAB) cooperative group proposals for the classification of myelodysplastic syndromes. *Br. J. Haematol.* **51**, 189–99.

Bergmann O.J. (1989) Oral infections and fever in immunocompromised patients with haematologic malignancies. *Eur. J. Clin. Microbiol. Infect. Dis.* **8**, 207–13.

Beumer J. et al. (1983) Preradiation dental extractions and the incidence of bone necrosis. *Head Neck Surg.* **5**, 514–21.

Binnie W. H., Cawson R. A.,Hill G. B.et al. (1972) *Oral Cancer in England and Wales.* OPCS Studies on Medical and Population Subjects, No. 23. London, HMSO.

Bloch S. (1980) Psychiatric management of the dying patient. *Medicine (UK)* **36**, 1837–41.

Bokkerink J. P. M. and de Vaan G. A. M. (1980) Histiocytosis X. *Eur.J. Pediatr.* **135**, 129–56.

Boyle P., MacFarlane G.J., Maisonneuve P. et al.. (1990) Epidemiology of mouth cancer in 1989. *J. R. Soc. Med.* **83**, 724–30.

Boyle P., MacFarlane G.J. and Zheng T. Recent advances in the epidemiology of head and neck cancer. *Curr. Opin. Oncol.* **4**, 471–7.

Burke F. J. T. and Frame J. W. (1979) The effect of irradiation on developing teeth. *Oral Surg.* **47**, 11–13.

Carl W. (1980) Dental management and prosthetic rehabilitation of patients with head and neck cancer. *Head Neck Surg.* **3**, 27–42.

Cassileth P.A. (1984) Hematology and hematologic malignancies. *Med. Clin. North Am.* **68**, 531–789.

Cawson R. A. (1969) Leukoplakia and oral cancer. *Proc. R. Soc. Med.* **62**, 6.

Cawson R. A. (1975) Premalignant lesions in the mouth. *Br. Med. Bull.* **31**, 164.

Cawson R.A. and Spector R.G. (1989) *Clinical Pharmacology in Dentistry.* 5th ed. Edinburgh, Churchill Livingstone.

Charak B.S., Parikh P.M., Banavali S.D. et al. (1988) Comparison of clotrimazole with nystatin in preventing oral candidiasis in neutropaenic patients. *Indian J. Med. Res.* **88**, 416–20.

Coleman J. J. (1986) Complications in head and neck surgery. *Surg. Clin. North Am.* **66**, 149–69.

Declerck D. and Vinckier F. (1988) Oral complications of leukemia. *Quintessence* **19**, 575–83.

Degregorio M. W., Lee W. M. F. and Ries C. A. (1982) Candida infections in patients with acute leukaemia: ineffectiveness of nystatin prophylaxis and relationship between oropharyngeal and systemic candidiasis. *Cancer* **50**, 2780–4.

Dreizen S. et al. (1986) Quantitative analysis of the oral complications of anti-leukaemia chemotherapy. *Oral Surg.* **62**, 650–3.

Dunn N.L., Russell E.C. and Maurer H.M. (1990) An update in pediatric oncology. *Pediatr. Dent.* **12**, 10–19.

Editorial (1980) Paraproteinaemia. *Br. Med. J.* **1**, 273–4.

Epstein J.B., Priddy R. W., Sparling T. et al. (1986) Oral manifestations in myelodysplastic syndrome. *Oral Surg.* **61**, 466–70.

Epstein J.B., Schubert M. and Scully C. (1991) Evaluation and treatment of pain in patients with orofacial cancer. *Pain Clinic.* **4**, 3–20.

Fleming P. and Kinirons M. J. (1986) Dental health of children suffering from acute lymphoblastic leukaemia. *J. Paediatr. Dent.* **2**, 15.

Flint S.R., Sugerman P., Scully, C. et al.. (1990) The myelodysplastic syndromes: a predisposing cause of oral ulceration and herpes labialis. *Oral Surg.* **70**, 450–53.

Fortenja S. W., Newman M. G., Lipsey A. I. et al. (1980) Capnocytophaga sepsis: a newly recognised clinical entity in granulocytopenic patients. *Lancet* **i**, 567–8.

Henk J. and Langdon J. (eds) (1985) *Management of Malignant Tumours of the Oral Cavity.* London, Edward Arnold.

Herzon F. S. and Boshier M. (1979) Head and neck cancer–emotional management. *Head Neck Surg.* **2**, 112–18.

Husby G. and Sletten K. (1986) Chemical and clinical classification of amyloidosis 1985. *Scand. J. Immunol.* **23**, 253–65.

Kamp A.A. (1988) Neoplastic diseases in a pediatric population: a survey of the incidence of oral complications. *Paediatr. Dent.* **10**, 25–29.

Kornblut A. D. and de Fries H. O. (ed.) (1979) Symposium on Malignant Disease of the oral Cavity and Related Structures. *Otolaryngol. Clin. North Am.* **12**.

Kuhrer, I. Kuzmits R., Linkesch W. et al. (1986) Topic PGE2 enhances healing of chemotherapy associated mucosal lesions. *Lancet* **i**, 622.

Larson D. L. (1986) Management of complications of radiotherapy of the head and neck. *Surg. Clin. North Am.* **66**, 169–83.

Leading Article (1978) Infection in acute leukaemia. *Lancet* **ii**, 769–70.

Leading Article (1979) Looking at lymphomas. *Lancet* **i**, 306.

Leading Article (1980) Myelofibrosis. *Lancet* **i**, 127–9.

Leading Article (1989) Oral Cancer. *Lancer* **3 ii**, 311–12.

Levendag P.C., Vikram B., Wright R. et al. (1989) Dental problems following surgery and external radiation therapy in patients with advanced carcinomas of the oral cavity and oropharynx. *Acta Oncol.* **28**, 550–5.

Loprinzi C.L., Cianflane S.G., Dose A.M. et al. (1990) A controlled evaluation of an allopurinol mouthwash as prophylaxis against 5-fluorouracil-induced stomatitis. *Cancer* **65**, 1879–82.

Lowe O. (1986) Oral concerns for the pediatric cancer patient. *J. Pedodont.* **11**, 35–46.

McElroy T.N. (1984) Infection in the patient receiving chemotherapy for cancer: oral considerations. *J. Am. Dent. Assoc.* **109**, 454–6.

Murray C. G., Daly T. E. and Zimmerman S. O. (1980) The relationship between dental disease and radiation necrosis of the mandible. *Oral Surg.* **49**, 99–104.

Peterson D. E., Elias E. G. and Sonis S. T. (1986) *Head and Neck Management of the Cancer Patient.* The Hague, Nijhoff.

Peterson D. and Sonis S. (1983) *Oral Complications of Cancer Chemotherapy.* Boston. Nijhoff.

Rand K. H., Kramer B. and Johnson A. C. (1982) Cancer chemotherapy associated symptomatic stomatitis. *Cancers* **50**, 1262–5.

Rodu B., Carpenter J.T. and Jones M.R. (1988) The pathogenesis and clinical significance of cytologically detectable oral candida in acute leukemia. *Cancer* **62**, 2042–6.

Saunders C. M. (1978) *The Management of Terminal Illness.* London, Arnold.

Scully C. (1983) Immunology and oral cancer. *Br. J. Oral Surg.* **21**, 136–46.

Scully C. (1983) An update on mouth ulcers. *Dental Update* **10**, 141–52.

Scully C. (1983) Viruses and cancer: herpes viruses and tumours in the head and neck. *Oral Surg.* **56**, 285–92.

Scully C. (1985) Immunology and virology of oral cancer. In: Henk J. M. and Langdon J. (eds) *Management of Malignant Tumours of the Oral Cavity.* London, Arnold, pp. 14–31.

Scully C., Boyle P. and Tederco B. (1992) The recognition and diagnosis of cancer arriving in the mouth. *Postgrad. Doctor* **15**, 134–41.

Scully C. and Gilmour G. (1986) Neutropenia and dental patients. *Br. Dent. J.* **160**, 436.

Scully C., MacFadyen E. E. and Campbell A. (1982) Orofacial manifestations in cyclic neutropenia. *Br. J. Oral Surg.* **20**, 96–101.

Scully C. and MacFarlane W. H. (1983) Orofacial manifestations in childhood malignancy: clinical and microbiological findings during remission. *J. Dent. Child.* **50**, 121–5.

Scully C., Malamos D., Levers B. G. H. et al. (1986) Sources and patterns of referrals of oral cancer: the role of general practitioners. *Br. Med. J.* **293**, 599–601.

Seto B. G. (1985) Oral mucositis in patients undergoing bone marrow transplantation. *Oral Surg.* **60**, 493–7.

Sinzinger H., Porteder H., Matjka M. et al. (1989) Prostaglandins in irradiation-induced mucositis. *Lancet* **i**, 556.

Stafford R., Sonis S., Lockhart P. et al. (1980) Oral pathoses as diagnostic indicators in leukaemia. *Oral Surg.* **50**, 134–9.

Tsavaris N., Caragiauris P. and Kosmidis P. (1988) Reduction of oral toxicity of 5-fluorouracil by allopurinol mouthwashes. *Eur. J. Surg. Oncol.* **14**, 405–6.

Tweedle D. E. F., Skidmore F. D., Gleave E. N. et al. (1979) Nutritional support for patients undergoing surgery for cancer of the head and neck. *Res. Clin. Forum* **1**, 59–69.

Twycross R. G. (1975) Relief of terminal pain. *Br. Med. J.* **4**, 212–14.

Ueland P. M., Refsum H. and Wesenberg F. (1986) Methotrexate therapy and nitrous oxide anaesthesia. *N. Engl. J. Med.* **300**, 1514.

Wahhin Y.B. and Matsson L. (1988) Oral mucosal lesions in patients with acute leukemia and related disorders during cytotoxic therapy. *Scand. J. Dent. Res.* **96**, 128–36.

Ward–Booth P. and Scully C. (1992) The management of mouth cancer. *Postgrad. Doctor* **15**, 166–75.

Warpeha R. L. (1977) Head and neck surgery. In: Symposium on Complications of General Surgery. *Surg. Clin. North Am.* **57**, 1357–63.

Whittaker J. A. (1980) Advances in the management of adult acute myelogenous leukaemia. *Br. Med. J.* **281**, 960–4.

Williford S.K., Salisbury P.L., Peacock J.E. et al. (1989) The safety of dental extractions in patients with hematologic malignancies. *J. Clin. Oncol.* **7**, 798–802.

Wright W. E. (1985) An oral disease prevention program for patients receiving radiation and chemotherapy. *J. Am. Dent. Assoc.* **110**, 43–7.

Appendix 1 to Chapter 5

Cytotoxic Cancer Chemotherapy Agents

Agent	Used to Treat Mainly	Main Adverse Effects
Actinomycin	Wilms tumour; Rhabdomyo-sarcoma	Nausea
Amsacrine	Acute leukaemias; lymphoma	Cardiotoxic; Hypokalaemia
Bleomycin	Lymphomas; solid neoplasms	Pulmonary fibrosis
Busulphan	Chronic myeloid leukaemia	Pulmonary fibrosis; pigmentation
Carboplatin	Germ cell neoplasms	Nephrotoxic
Carmustine	Lymphoma	—
Chlorambucil	Chronic lymphocytic leukaemia	—
Cisplatin	Germ cell neoplasms	Nephrotoxic; neurotoxic
Crisantaspase		Anaphylaxis
Cyclo-phosphamide	Chronic lymphocytic leukaemia	Cystitis
Cytarabine	Acute leukaemias	—
Dacarbazine	Melanoma	Nausea
Doxorubicin	Wide range of neoplasms	Cardiotoxic
Epirubicin	Wide range of neoplasms	Cardiotoxic
Estramustine	Prostatic carcinoma	—
Ethoglucide	Bladder carcinoma	—
Etoposide	Choriocarcinoma	Nausea
Fluorouracil	Gastrointestinal carcinoma	Nausea
Hydroxyurea	Chronic myeloid leukaemia	Nausea
Ifosfamide	Lymphoma	Cystitis
Lomustine	Lymphoma	Vomiting
Melphalan	Myeloma	—
Mercaptopurine	Acute leukaemias	—
Methotrexate	Acute leukaemias	—
Mitobronitol	Chronic myeloid leukaemia	—
Mitomycin	Lymphoma	Nephrotoxic
Mitozantrone	Breast carcinoma	Cardiotoxic
Mustine	Lymphoma	Nausea and vomiting
Procarbazine	Lymphoma	Disulfiram reaction with alcohol
Razoxane	Sarcoma	—
Thioguanine	Acute leukaemias	—
Thiotepa	Meningeal cancer	—
Treosulfan	Ovarian cancer	—
Vinblastine	Acute leukaemias	Neurotoxic
Vincristine	Acute leukaemias	Neurotoxic
Vindesine	Acute leukaemias	Neurotoxic

Most suppress the bone-marrow. See also Table 5.7.

Appendix 2 to Chapter 5

Support groups in the UK for those with head and neck cancer

Marie Curie Memorial Foundation
28 Belgrave Square, London, SW1X 80Q

Cancer Relief MacMillan Fund,
Anchor House,
15–19 Britten House,
London, SW3 3TZ

BACUP,
121–123 Charterhouse Street,
London, ECIM 6AA

Let's Face It,
c/o Mrs C. Pitt,
Wexham Park Hospital,
Slough,
Berks.

Cancerlink,
17 Britannia Street,
London, WC1X 9JN

Chapter 6

Respiratory Disorders

Respiratory disorders are common, may significantly affect dental treatment and in particular, are often a contraindication to general anaesthesia, opioids, intravenous benzodiazepines and other respiratory depressants.

Cough, the most common symptom, is a reflex which helps defend the respiratory tract but it is abnormal to produce sputum for long periods. Mucoid sputum is often a feature of chronic bronchitis, whereas purulent sputum is produced in acute bronchitis, bronchiectasis or lung abscess. The coughing of blood (haemoptysis) may be a serious event (such as the result of a carcinoma or tuberculosis) but is also common in bronchitis, bronchiectasis and acute infections. Breathlessness (dyspnoea) is particularly ominous if it persists at rest. Wheezing is caused by airways obstruction and is typically a sign of asthma or bronchitis.

Other important signs of respiratory disease include wheezing, cyanosis, finger-clubbing, use of accessory muscles of respiration with indrawing of the intercostal spaces (hyperinflation) and abnormalities in chest shape, movements and breath sounds.

The most useful investigations are chest radiography and spirometric tests. The latter are used to estimate functional capacity of the lungs and overall the most useful, especially for the assessment of obstructive airways disease such as asthma, is the peak expiratory flow rate (PEFR). Spirometry and carbon monoxide perfusion can be used to assess impaired lung ventilation or gaseous exchange. Radionuclide lung scanning, blood gas analysis and sputum cytology or culture are sometimes needed.

RESPIRATORY INFECTIONS

Most respiratory infections begin as viral infections of the upper respiratory tract. The incubation periods are frequently short and rarely exceed 14 days.

Patients with HIV infection and other immunodeficient persons are particularly susceptible to respiratory infections by a great variety of microbes. The otherwise harmless organism *Pneumocystis carinii* is a common cause of fatal pneumonia in such patients.

UPPER RESPIRATORY TRACT INFECTIONS

Upper respiratory tract infections are almost invariably viral, spread readily, are highly infectious in the early stages and have incubation periods of only a few days.
Three main clinical patterns are seen:

1. The common cold syndrome (coryza).
2. Pharyngitis and tonsillitis.
3. Laryngotracheitis.

The common cold syndrome

The common cold syndrome can be caused by many different viruses, but usually a rhinovirus (*Table 6.1*). Nasal discharge and obstruction, with nasopharyngeal soreness, are only too well known. There is only mild systemic upset and serious complications are rare in an otherwise fit patient. However, sinusitis may develop and cause facial pain and tenderness. Tetracyclines, erythromycin or co-trimoxazole appear to be effective for sinusitis due to secondary bacterial invaders; drainage is aided by vasoconstrictors such as ephedrine nasal drops, which improve patency of the maxillary ostium. Earache may result from obstruction of the pharyngotympanic tube by oedema or more seriously by bacterial infection of the middle ear (otitis media).

Illness resembling the common cold can also precede other infections such as measles or influenza.

Table 6.1. Causes of upper respiratory tract infection

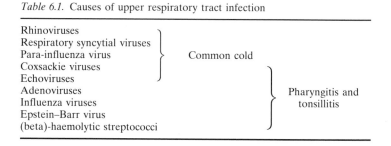

Sinusitis

Infection of the paranasal air sinuses (maxillary, ethmoidal, sphenoidal and frontal) commonly follows an upper respiratory tract infection, and maxillary sinusitis may also follow periapical infection of upper posterior teeth or an oro-antral fistula.

Features of maxillary sinusitis are pain in the cheek and/or upper teeth, worsened by tilting the head or lying down, and nasal obstruction with mucopurulent nasal discharge. There is tenderness over the maxilla, dullness on antral transillumination, and antral radio-opacity or a fluid level on occipitomental radiography.

Sinus opacity is difficult to evaluate. Some studies have shown sinus opacities in up to 50% of children under the age of 6 years. Sinus opacity is sometimes due only to mucosal thickening rather than infection, but a fluid level is highly suggestive of sinusitis. Ultrasonography, CT or MRI may be helpful but the diagnosis can only be confirmed by sinus puncture and aspiration. Nevertheless the history, clinical examination and radiographs are usually suffiently reliable.

Treatment is as described earlier.

Pharyngitis and Tonsillitis

Most cases of pharyngitis and tonsillitis are caused by viruses (*Table 6.1*) but other agents, especially *Streptococcus pyogenes, Mycoplasma pneumoniae* or rarely *Corynebacterium diphtheriae,* may need to be considered in the differential diagnosis.

The throat is sore with pain on swallowing (dysphagia) and sometimes fever and conjunctivitis. Complications, which are rare, include peritonsillar abscess (quinsy). Streptococcal sore throats may be associated with scarlet fever; acute glomerulonephritis or rheumatic fever may occasionally follow but the latter is now a very rare disease. Nevertheless streptococcal throat infections should be treated with penicillin if the patient is not allergic.

Streptococcal sore throat usually responds to penicillin or erythromycin. Ampicillin and amoxycillin should be avoided as they tend to cause rashes, especially in glandular fever.

Herpangina, glandular fever and diphtheria are discussed in Chapter 17.

Laryngotracheitis

Hoarseness, loss of voice and persistent cough are common in laryngotracheitis. In children, partial laryngeal obstruction may cause noisy inspiration (stridor or croup) and is potentially dangerous. Various microbes may be involved, such as respiratory syncytial virus in children particularly.

Dental aspects of upper respiratory tract infections

Most upper respiratory tract infections are innocuous and have no oral manifestations. Oropharyngeal lesions are, however, prominent in herpangina, glandular fever and diphtheria (Chapter 17).

Dental treatment is best deferred until after recovery. General anaesthesia should be avoided since there is often some respiratory obstruction and infection can also be spread down to the lungs. If a general anaesthetic is unavoidable it is best to carry out intubation with a cuffed tube and the patient supine, so that nasal secretions do not enter the larynx. Antimicrobials may be indicated.

Obstructive Sleep Apnoea

Partial upper airways obstruction during sleep can cause snoring and there is an association between obstructive sleep apnoea (OSA), daytime sleepiness and cardiopulmonary complications particularly in obese middle–aged men. Measures devised to overcome these problems include uvulopalatopharyngoplasty (UPPP), nasal continuous airway pressure or even tracheostomy. Only the last two have been shown convincingly to reduce the mortality.

Dental aspects

Recent work suggests that where the obstruction is predominantly hypopharyngeal, surgical advancement of the facial skeleton and hyoid may effectively expand the airway. When there is both oro– and hypopharyngeal obstruction UPPP may need to be combined with mandibulo–maxillary and hyoid advancement. Nasal obstruction may also have to be relieved, but maxillofacial surgery carried out in stages to assess the degree of improvement may relieve nocturnal hypoxia, snoring and daytime sleepiness.

Oronasal obstruction in weak senile patients:
A dangerous degree of dyspnoea and cyanosis has been noted in some weak senile patients, even when awake. The oronasal obstruction resulted from blockage of the nose and lack of teeth or dentures causing the mouth to become tightly closed.

Hypoxia, thus caused, may contribute to the death of these vulnerable patients. Provision of dentures may alleviate this hazard, but a nasal catheter provides a more rapid and simple solution.

LOWER RESPIRATORY TRACT INFECTIONS

Lower respiratory tract infections are frequently viral, although often complicated by bacterial infection, but may be mycoplasmal (atypical pneumonia).

Clinical features vary according to the part of the respiratory tract mainly affected. Bronchitis causes cough, wheezing and sometimes dyspnoea. Bronchiolitis, which is restricted mainly to infants, causes rapid respiration, wheezing, fever and dyspnoea.

Pneumonia is characterized by cough, fever, rapid respiration, breathlessness, chest pain, dyspnoea and shivering. Pneumonia in a previously healthy individual is classed as primary and is usually lobar. Pneumonia may be secondary to some other disorder such as previous viral respiratory infections; aspiration of foreign material; pre-existent lung disease, for example bronchiectasis or carcinoma; or depressed immunity, as a result, for example, of alcoholism or immunosuppression (*Table* 6.2) and is usually bronchopneumonia. *Pneumocystis carinii* pneumonia has been mentioned earlier.

Dental aspects

The majority of lower respiratory tract infections cause substantial incapacity and are contraindications to all but emergency dental treatment. General anaesthesia is hazardous and is absolutely contraindicated. Dental treatment should therefore be deferred until recovery or be limited to relief of pain.

Table 6.2. Factors predisposing to pneumonia

Viral respiratory infections, including colds
Old age
Immobility
Respiratory depression or chest injury
Alcoholism
Immune deficiency (especially HIV infection)
Neurological disorders permitting aspiration of foreign material
Underlying pulmonary disease such as carcinoma or emphysema

Pulmonary Tuberculosis

In the United Kingdom tuberculosis is a problem especially of immigrants; those from the Indian subcontinent and Vietnam have a rate over 50 times that of subjects born in the United Kingdom. Diabetics, alcoholics, severely immunodeficient patients, such as those with HIV infection, vagrants and institutionalized patients are also at risk.

Pulmonary tuberculosis is usually contracted by the inhalation of infected sputum. Inhaled *Mycobacterium tuberculosis* or other mycobacteria, cause lesions subpleurally and in the regional lymph nodes (primary complex). Haematogenous dissemination can lead to genitourinary, bone or joint lesions; the pulmonary lesions may extend and result in a pleural effusion; or lymph node tuberculosis may lead to caseation of the nodes and pressure symptoms, for example on the bronchi. Miliary tuberculosis is characterized by widely disseminated lesions recognized especially in the lungs and in the choroid of the eyes.

Because it frequently passes unrecognized for so long, the mortality from pulmonary tuberculosis is high in native Britons.

Post-primary tuberculosis usually follows the reactivation of an old primary pulmonary lesion and results in lesions ranging from a chronic fibrotic lesion to fulminating tuberculous pneumonIa.

The diagnosis of tuberculosis is suggested by a chronic cough, haemoptysis, loss of weight, night sweats and fever. It is confirmed by physical examination, chest radiography, sputum smears and culture, and tuberculin testing (Mantoux or Heaf test). Erythema nodosum may be seen.

Other (atypical) mycobacteria frequently nowadays cause tuberculosis. *Mycobacterium avium* and *M. intracellulare* can cause pulmonary tuberculosis while *M. scrofulaceum* is a rare cause of tuberculous cervical lymphadenitis, for example.

Patients with HIV infection frequently develop tuberculosis due to atypical mycobacteria as well as *M. tuberculosis;* antimicrobial resistance is increasing.

General management

Chemotherapy is usually effective but must be given for long periods. Alcoholics, vagrants, the mentally handicapped or those with psychiatric disorders frequently default from treatment and, if chemotherapy is less than adequate, bacterial resistance readily develops.

Table 6.3. Anti-tubercular therapy

Drug	Use	Main side-effects
Rifampicin	Initial therapy*	Urine and saliva turn red
		Bullous lesions
	Continuation therapy†	Enhanced liver drug-metabolizing enzymes
		Hepatotoxicity
		Nephrotoxicity
Isoniazid	Initial therapy	Peripheral neuropathy
	Continuation therapy	Hepatotoxicity
Streptomycin	Initial therapy	Vestibular nerve damage
		Circumoral paraesthesiae
Ethambutol	Initial therapy	Ocular damage
Pyrazinamide	Initial therapy	Hepatotoxicity

*Initial therapy = rifampicin + isoniazid + streptomycin or ethambutol for 2 months.
†Continuation therapy = rifampicin + isoniazid for 9 months.

Treatment is started with three drugs in combination in order to avoid the emergence of bacterial resistance, and then continued with two or more antibiotics (*Table 6.3*). Patients are infectious until the sputum is negative to culture but the infectivity is greatly reduced by 2 weeks after the start of chemotherapy.

Dental aspects

Oral manifestations. Oral lesions can develop in pulmonary tuberculosis but are rare. Chronic ulcers, usually of the dorsum of the tongue, are the main oral manifestation. Occasionally the diagnosis of pulmonary tuberculosis is made as the result of biopsy of an oral ulcer. Such cases (usually middle-aged males) may be the result of neglect of symptoms or default from treatment. Unfixed material should also be sent for culture if possible. However the diagnosis is usually confirmed by sputum culture and chest radiographs after granulomas are seen microscopically. Acid–fast bacilli are rarely seen in oral biopsies even with the help of special stains.

Tuberculous cervical lymphadenopathy is the next most common form of the infection to pulmonary disease and is particularly common among those from the Indian subcontinent.

Oral complications of antitubercular therapy are rare (*Table 6.3*).

Dental treatment. Patients with open pulmonary tuberculosis are contagious and should be treated with precautions against cross-infection. The mild symptoms but high infectivity of pulmonary tuberculosis is shown by cases of tuberculous infection of extraction sockets and cervical lymphadenitis in 15 patients treated by an infected member of a dental clinic staff, in Britain. Dental staff are at risk from tuberculosis.

In active tuberculosis, general anaesthesia is contraindicated for dental treatment, because of the risk of contamination of the anaesthetic apparatus or if there is impaired pulmonary function. This could result from pleurocentesis, thoracoplasty or resection which were used before the introduction of effective chemotherapy. Aminoglycosides such as streptomycin enhance the activity of some neuromuscular blocking agents and in large doses may alone cause a myasthenic syndrome during general anaesthesia.

Other factors such as alcoholism (Chapter 19) may also influence dental management.

Legionnaires' Disease (Legionellosis)

The term *Legionnaires' disease* was coined as a result of an outbreak of a previously unrecognized respiratory disease in an American Legion meeting in Philadelphia in 1976. The infection is caused by Gram-negative bacteria of the genus Legionella, usually *L. pneumophila* , which typically causes a lobular type of pneumonia. The latter ranges from discrete patches of inflammmation and consolidation to involvement of whole lobes. A non–pneumonic form of the infection is known as *Pontiac fever.*

The infection spreads mainly through aerosolization of infected water— especially from humidifiers in air–conditioning plants. Those over 45 are predominantly affected and of the 232 cases in England and Wales in 1989, 75 per cent were males. Smokers, the elderly or immunocompromised are particularly susceptible; the overall mortality may be as high as 10 per cent, but over 25 per cent in the elderly and up to 80 per cent in the immunocompromised. By contrast, many younger persons have been exposed to the infections and are seropositive but have remained healthy. However, in an outbreak due to the effluent from the air–conditioning system of Broadcasting House, London, young adults among passers–by in the street developed legionellosis.

Dental aspects

Legionella have been isolated from the stagnant water within dental units and could be disseminated in the dental surgery during aerosolization of water from dental equipment such as air-turbine sprays. Serological studies of dental school personnel have shown a rise in antibodies to Legionella species, that increased with duration of work in the school—suggesting the bacteria could be spread in this way, but it has not been confirmed that the sources were dental equipment.

When dental units have to stand idle for long periods, over holidays or weekends for example, the system should be flushed through, before treating patients.

Lung Abscess

Lung abscess is a localized infection leading to cavitation and necrosis. The clinical features may be very ill-defined and diagnosis rests mainly on the chest radiograph. There is a risk of infection spreading locally or leading to a brain abscess.

Most cases result from pneumonia associated with infection by *Staphylococcus aureus* or *Klebsiella pneumoniae.* Bronchial obstruction by carcinoma or aspiration of foreign bodies are other important causes. A well-known cause of lung abscess is inhalation of a tooth or fragment, or rarely, endodontic instruments, but lung abscesses more often result from aspiration of oral bacteria, particularly anaerobes, even in the absence of dental intervention.

When undertaking endodontics or cementing restorations such as inlays or crowns, a rubber dam or other protective device should *always* be used to avoid the danger of inhalation of these foreign bodies. The main dangers in dentistry are with general anaesthesia, particularly if an inadequate throat pack has been used.

General management

Patients who inhale tooth fragments or dental instruments must have chest radiographs (lateral and postero–anterior) and if necessary, bronchoscopy.

Lung abscesses are usually treated by postural drainage or relief of the obstruction by bronchoscopy and antimicrobial chemotherapy.

Bronchiectasis

Bronchiectasis is dilatation and distortion of bronchi with excess sputum production and poor drainage causing recurrent lower respiratory tract infections. Bronchiectasis is often the result of respiratory damage as a result of measles, whooping cough, bronchiolitis or adenovirus infections in childhood. Some cases follow bronchial obstruction and cystic fibrosis or immunodeficiencies, but in many cases, no cause can be found. The damaged and dilated bronchi lose their ciliated epithelium, and mucus therefore tends to pool. Infection with *S. pneumoniae, H. influenzae* or *P. aeruginosa* is common.

Clinical features of bronchiectasis include overproduction of sputum, which is purulent during exacerbations, a cough (especially during exercise or when lying down) and finger clubbing. There are recurrent episodes of bronchitis, pneumonia and pleurisy. Haemoptysis is not uncommon and, in advanced bronchiectasis, dyspnoea, cyanosis and respiratory failure may develop. Complications include cerebral abscess but amyloid disease is now rare since sepsis can usually be controlled.

General management

Chest radiography and pulmonary function tests are required to establish the severity of bronchiectasis. Postural drainage is important and antimicrobials such as tetracycline, co-trimoxazole or amoxycillin are given for acute exacerbations and for long-term maintenance treatment.

Dental aspects

General anaesthesia is contraindicated in the acute phases and should be avoided in the chronic phase. If a general anaesthetic must be given, safeguards should be taken as for patients with chronic obstructive airways disease and antibiotic cover should be given to prevent dissemination of infection.

OTHER RESPIRATORY DISORDERS

CYSTIC FIBROSIS

Cystic fibrosis (fibrocystic disease: mucoviscidosis) is an inherited disorder of exocrine glands. It is inherited as an autosomal recessive trait and, with an incidence of about 1 in 2000 births, is the most common inherited error of metabolism in the UK and the USA and one of the most common, lethal hereditary disorders.

The essential feature of cystic fibrosis is increased viscosity of mucus. Obstruction of pancreatic ducts by mucus leads to pancreatic insufficiency in childhood with malabsorption and bulky, frequent, foul-smelling fatty stools and growth is frequently stunted (Chapter 7). Diabetes mellitus may be a complication, and some have cirrhosis.

Recurrent respiratory infections may result in bronchiectasis and usually a persistent productive cough. Most patients have recurrent sinusitis and nasal polyps. Viral infections such as measles can have severe sequelae. Cystic fibrosis also affects sweat and salivary glands. Most patients have a sweat sodium concentration in excess of 70 mmol/l (a change also reflected in the saliva) and these changes are used in diagnosis.

General management

Pancreatic replacement therapy (oral pancreatin) is given with each meal: a reduced fat intake and adequate vitamins in the diet are also necessary. Clearance of sputum is helped by regular physiotherapy, water aerosols and bronchodilators (terbutaline or salbutamol). Acetylcysteine may be used as a mucolytic, but its effectiveness is questionable. Vaccination against measles, whooping cough and influenza are important preventive measures while co-trimoxazole or flucloxacillin are effective prophylactic antimicrobials.

Dental aspects

The major salivary glands may become enlarged. Tetracycline staining of the teeth was common, but should rarely be seen now. Enamel hypoplasia may be seen and both dental development and eruption are delayed. Pancreatin may cause oral ulceration if held in the mouth. The low fat, high carbohydrate diet predisposes to caries. General anaesthesia is contraindicated if respiratory function is poor, and liver disease and diabetes may also complicate treatment (Chapter 10).

CHRONIC OBSTRUCTIVE AIRWAYS DISEASE

Chronic obstructive airways disease (COAD: chronic obstructive pulmonary disease, COPD) is most frequently caused by chronic bronchitis and emphysema. Chronic bronchitis is defined as the excessive production of mucus and persistent cough with sputum production for more than 3 months in a year over 3 consecutive years. Emphysema is dilatation of air spaces distal to the terminal bronchioles with destruction of alveoli and a reduction in the alveolar surface area available for respiratory exchange.

Chronic bronchitis and emphysema are usually seen together in Britain, and are exceedingly common especially among cigarette smokers living in cities. Deficiency of the anti-proteolytic enzyme α_1-antitrypsin is a rare cause of emphysema (see Appendix to Chapter 10).

Chronic bronchitis leads to production of excessive, viscous mucus, which is ineffectively cleared from the airway, stagnates and becomes infected with S. pneumoniae and H. influenzae. Patchy areas of alveolar collapse may result. Both chronic bronchitis and emphysema cause cough, sputum and dyspnoea. There is initially an early morning mucoid cough which becomes mucopurulent during exacerbations. Dyspnoea on effort is mild at first, but deteriorates to leave a respiratory cripple ultimately dyspnoeic at rest and especially when recumbent (orthopnoea).

Chronic obstructive airways disease is complicated by chronic hypoxaemia. Eventually the sequence of pulmonary hypertension, right ventricular hypertrophy and cardiac failure (cor pulmonale) develops (Chapter 2). Chronic hypoxaemia leads to central cyanosis which, in association with ankle oedema and raised jugular venous pressure of cor pulmonale, gives rise to a 'blue bloated' appearance. At the other end of the spectrum, chronic obstructive airways disease may produce a 'pink panter' who is severely breathless and pink from vasodilatation caused by CO_2 retention. The reasons for these distinct clinical pictures are unclear.

The diagnosis is made clinically and supported by chest radiography, respiratory function tests and occasionally arterial blood gas estimations.

General management

Patients with chronic bronchitis and emphysema must stop smoking. Exacerbations of bronchitis are managed with co-trimoxazole or amoxycillin. Ipratropium bromide, or other bronchodilators may be beneficial. Respiratory failure and cor pulmonale may also need to be treated.

Dental aspects

The high prevalence of chronic bronchitis and emphysema means that all dental surgeons will have to treat these patients.

Wherever possible, dental treatment should be carried out under local anaesthesia. Patients are best treated in the upright position as they may become increasingly breathless if laid flat. It may also be difficult to use a rubber dam as patients may not tolerate the additional obstruction to breathing.

Patients with COPD should be given a general anaesthetic only if absolutely necessary, and only in hospital after full preoperative assessment. Secretions reduce airway patency and if lightly anaesthetized, the patient may cough and contaminate other areas of the lung. Diazepam and midazolam are also mild respiratory depressants and should not be used for intravenous sedation. Intravenous barbiturates are totally contraindicated.

Patients taking ipratropium may have a dry mouth.

Pre-anaesthetic assessment

Postoperative respiratory complications are more prevalent in patients with pre-existing lung diseases, especially after prolonged operations and if there has been no preoperative preparation. Most patients with pre-existing respiratory disease present no problem if the assessment and anaesthesia have been managed appropriately. Spirometry and carbon monoxide perfusion are essential to assess respiratory function.

The most important single factor in preoperative care is cessation of smoking for at least 1 week preoperatively. Respiratory infections must also be eradicated. Sputum should first be sent for culture and sensitivity, but antimicrobials such as co–trimoxazole or amoxycillin should be started without awaiting results. Treatment can later be altered if necessary. Bronchodilator drugs are useful for bronchospasm. Thorough and frequent chest physiotherapy is important preoperatively and, if there is congestive cardiac failure, diuretics are indicated.

Many anaesthetists suggest that it is safest to avoid premedication. Morphine is certainly contraindicated since it can impair the cough reflex or precipitate bronchospasm. Pethidine can be used if the patient is in pain. Atropine and related antimuscarinics are also best avoided since they dry up the airways and increase the risk of postoperative pulmonary complications.

Postoperative care

Postoperatively there should be close continuous assessment as it is difficult to detect hypoventilation. Arterial blood gases need to be monitored if any problems are anticipated and, rarely, if hypoventilation or excess secretions cannot be controlled by simple means, tracheostomy may be necessary. The 'blue-bloated' type of patient has a high arterial partial pressure of CO_2 ($PaCO_2$) and a low PaO_2. The main stimulus to respiration in these patients is hypoxia and there is little response to raised levels of CO_2. Such patients may hypoventilate postoperatively, especially if the respiratory drive of hypoxia is abolished by giving oxygen.

Bedridden patients with chronic obstructive airways disease may have added complications if given a general anaesthetic. Impaired cardiovascular responses may lead to profound hypotension if agents such as barbiturates are used. Cor pulmonale may be aggravated by the cardiodepressant activity of drugs used in anaesthesia or by the water retention that follows surgery or anaesthesia.

Secondary polycythaemia may predispose to thromboses postoperatively.

ASTHMA

Bronchial asthma is a state of bronchial hyper-reactivity characterized by paroxysmal expiratory wheezing and dyspnoea. Generalized reversible bronchial narrowing is caused by increased bronchial smooth muscle tone, mucosal oedema and congestion, and mucus hypersecretion.

Asthma is common, affects more than 2 per cent of the population and usually begins in childhood or early adult life. Asthma in children is typically allergic (extrinsic asthma) and, although such children are frequently asymptomatic between attacks, they often have had or develop other allergic diseases such as eczema, hay fever and drug sensitivities. This type of asthma, which tends to resolve by adult life, is associated with increased production of IgE on exposure to allergens, and the release of mast cell products which cause bronchospasm and oedema (Chapter 16). Extrinsic asthmatic attacks may be precipitated by allergens in house dust, animal dander, feathers, animal hairs, moulds, milk, eggs, fish, fruit, nuts, nonsteroidal anti-inflammatory agents and some antibiotics. Intrinsic asthma, on the other hand, is not allergic in nature and appears to be related to mast cell instability and hyper-responsive airways. Factors that can initiate an episode of either type of asthma include infections, irritating fumes, exercise, weather changes and emotional stress. Some drugs, particularly beta-blockers such as propranolol, are dangerous in either type of asthma and are absolutely contraindicated.

Children with asthma initially suffer from repeated 'colds' with cough, malaise and fever. Wheeziness with laboured expiration is prominent. The frequency and severity of attacks vary widely between individuals but symptoms are usually worse at night.

Investigations include blood examination for total IgE (usually raised and specific IgE antibody concentrations, skin tests which may help to identify any allergens and chest radiographs. Objective measurement of airways obstruction by a peak flow meter is important and treatment should be based on the amount by which peak flow is reduced.

General management

Management of asthma includes the avoidance of identifiable irritants and allergens, and drug therapy. Sodium cromoglycate is used as an inhalant for prophylaxis particularly in children, but some fail to respond. Selective β_2-adrenoreceptor stimulants (salbutamol, terbutaline, fenoterol or rimiterol) are the safest and most effective bronchodilators for the routine control of asthma. Ipratropium bromide is useful for some patients but particularly those with asthma associated with bronchitis. An alternative is oral sustained release theophylline preparations. These have a prolonged action and are useful for controlling nocturnal asthma. If both of these fail, corticosteroid (beclomethasone or betamethasone valerate) aerosol inhalations may be more effective and taken in conjunction with a bronchodilator, but must be taken regularly. High dose corticosteroid inhalants can cause some degree of adrenal suppression. If these also fail, oral corticosteroid treatment becomes necessary in addition.

Home use of peak flow meters (now available on prescription in Britain) allow patients to monitor progress of their disease and to detect any deterioration, which may require urgent modification of treatment.

Acute asthmatic attacks are usually self-limiting or respond to medication but can occasionally persist despite these measures and continue for hours or days (status asthmaticus). This potentially lethal complication needs emergency hospitalization and treatment.

The patient should be reassured and given nebulized salbutamol, followed by 200 mg of hydrocortisone succinate intravenously. If this fails, intravenous salbutamol or aminophylline (5 mg/kg as a slow intravenous injection over 20 minutes, with cardiac monitoring) may be given. Rapid injection of aminophylline or overdose can cause sudden severe dysrhythmias and death. This risk is increased in patients taking oral theophylline preparations. If severe, unresponsive asthma or status asthmaticus develop, oxygen should be given early and continued during the journey to hospital, if necessary by assisted positive pressure ventilation. Respiratory infections should also be treated.

There are estimated to be at least 2000 deaths from asthma in Britain each year, probably as a result of failure to recognize deterioration, or inadequate treatment.

Dental aspects

Although there are no specific oral complications of asthma, the use of corticosteroid inhalers occasionally causes oral or pharyngeal thrush, while ipratropium bromide (isopropyl atropine, Atrovent) can cause a dry mouth.

Anxiety may occasionally precipitate asthmatic attacks and it is important to attempt to lessen fear of dental treatment by gentle handling and reassurance. Sedation may need to be considered, especially for patients whose asthma is precipitated by anxiety. For this purpose relative analgesia with nitrous oxide and oxygen is preferable to intravenous sedation and give more immediate control of the patient. Sedatives in general are better avoided as, in an acute attack, even benzodiazepines can precipitate respiratory failure.

Asthmatic patients should be asked to bring their usual medication with them when coming for dental treatment. Drugs liable to precipitate an asthmatic attack or anaphylaxis must be avoided: aspirin, mefenamic acid, paracetamol and pentazocine are occasionally responsible. A few patients have *triad asthma* with nasal polyps, asthma and aspirin sensitivity. An asthmatic attack may also be precipitated by drugs causing histamine release directly; morphine and some other opioids, methohexitone, thiopentone, suxamethonium, tubocurarine and pancuronium should also therefore be avoided. Beta-blocker antihypertensive agents such as propranolol can also precipitate severe or life-threatening bronchospasm, and are completely contraindicated.

Allergy to penicillin may be more frequent in asthmatic patients. However, erythromycin is also best avoided, since it may slow the metabolism of theophylline and cause toxicity. Systemic corticosteroid treatment brings with it the risks from steroid complications and operations are dangerous on such patients without adequate preparation.

Dental treatment is best carried out under local anaesthesia. General anaesthesia may be complicated by hypoxia and hypercapnia, which can cause pulmonary oedema even if cardiac function is normal, and cardiac failure if there is cardiac disease. The risk of postoperative collapse of the lung or pneumothorax is also increased. General anaesthesia is therefore best avoided and in any event should only be given by a specialist anaesthetist.

Halothane or better, enflurane or isoflurane are the preferred anaesthetics, but ketamine may be useful in children.

BRONCHOGENIC CARCINOMA

Bronchogenic carcinoma accounts for 95 per cent of all *primary* lung tumours but many other lung tumours are metastases. Bronchogenic carcinoma is the most common cancer in Britain, in males, and is the cause of death in some 10 per cent of them. Bronchogenic carcinoma most frequently affects urban, adult cigarette smokers, and it has become increasingly common in women to the extent that the mortality rate for the two sexes has become equal in the USA where it is the most common type of cancer.

Recurrent cough, haemoptysis, dyspnoea, chest pain and recurrent chest infections are the predominant features. Cerebral metastases are common and can cause headache, epilepsy, hemiplegia or visual disturbances. Hepatic metastases may cause hepatomegaly, jaundice or ascites. Metastases can cause enlargement of the lower cervical lymph nodes. Bone metastases may cause pain, swelling or pathological fracture. Local infiltration may cause pleural effusion, or lesions of the cervical sympathetic chain (Horner's syndrome), brachial neuritis, or recurrent laryngeal nerve palsy. Obstruction of the superior vena cava may cause facial cyanosis and oedema (superior vena cava syndrome).

There are many non-metastatic extrapulmonary effects of bronchogenic or other carcinomas. Loss of weight and anorexia are common. Ectopic hormone production, neuromyopathies, thromboses (thrombophlebitis migrans), finger clubbing, muscle weakness and various skin manifestations may also be seen (Chapter 5) and are sometimes the first manifestations.

The diagnosis of bronchogenic carcinoma is based on history and physical examination supported by radiography, sputum cytology, bronchoscopy and biopsy.

General management

About 25 per cent of patients are suitable for surgery but the 5-year survival after pneumonectomy is only about 25 per cent. Radiotherapy is frequently used but chemotherapy has, in general, given disappointing results. The overall 5-year survival rate is only 8 per cent.

Dental aspects

Metastases in the jaw are only rarely, early or initial manifestations of a carcinoma of the lung. Even more rarely metastases can form epulis-like soft tissue swellings. Pigmentation of the soft palate is another rare early oral manifestation.

Dental treatment under local anaesthesia should be uncomplicated. However, patients with bronchogenic carcinoma often have impaired respiratory function, especially after lobectomy or pneumonectomy and this with any muscle weakness (myasthenic syndrome, Eaton–Lambert syndrome) which may make the patient unduly sensitive to the action of muscle relaxants, make general anaesthesia hazardous. General anaesthesia, if needed, should therefore be carried out by a specialist anaesthetist in hospital.

OCCUPATIONAL LUNG DISEASE

Workers in many industries are exposed to a variety of airborne particles that may cause lung disease. Pulmonary disorders related to the inhalation of dust particles are sometimes grouped as the pneumoconioses.

The clinical significance of these disorders varies widely (Appendix to this chapter). Some, such as siderosis, are benign, while others, such as asbestosis, can cause significant incapacity or cause lethal malignant complications. Berylliosis may be a hazard in some dental technical laboratories. The major complication affecting dental treatment is that of respiratory impairment and for this reason, general anaesthesia may be contraindicated. The physician should be contacted before treatment.

SARCOIDOSIS

Sarcoidosis is a multisystem granulomatous disorder of unknown aetiology. It most commonly affects young adults and typically causes bilateral hilar lymphadenopathy, pulmonary infiltration and skin or eye lesions. It is twice as frequent in females as males.

The aetiology of sarcoidosis is unclear but is associated with limited impairment of cell-mediated immune responses (partial anergy) but no special susceptibility to infection. Sarcoidosis is protean in its manifestations and can involve virtually any tissue (*Table 6.4*). Pulmonary involvement is the most common and important, and causes impaired respiratory efficiency with cough and dyspnoea. Radiological changes may be more severe than suggested by the symptoms. Acute uveitis can progress to blindness. Hypercalcaemia is common and can result in renal damage. There may be an increased susceptibility to malignant lymphoproliferative disease.

General management

Because of its vague and protean manifestations, sarcoidosis appears to be under-diagnosed. In the presence of suggestive clinical features, chest radiography, laboratory investigations (Table 6.4), a Kveim test, a gallium scan of lacrimal and salivary glands, and hilar lymph nodes may be indicated.

Table 6.4. Sarcoidosis—clinical and laboratory findings

1. Systemic symptoms	Fever, weight loss, fatigue
2. Pulmonary	Hilar lymphadenopathy; widespread infiltration
3. Ocular	Acute uveitis, cataracts, glaucoma
4. Lymph nodes	Lymphadenopathy (rarely lymphoma)
5. Dermatological	Erythema nodosum, infiltrates (lupus pernio) around eyes and nose
6. Hepatic	Asymptomatic hepatomegaly, sarcoid liver disease
7. Splenomegaly	
8. Renal	Nephrocalcinosis, renal calculi
9. Joints	Arthralgia, effusion
10. Neurological	Cranial or peripheral neuropathies
11. Skeletal	Cyst-like radiolucent areas
12. Oral/para-oral	Salivary gland swellings, gingival swelling (*see* text)
13. Histological findings	Non-caseating tubercle-like granulomas
14. Immunological findings	1. Anergy (partial)
	Negative response to tuberculin and some other common antigens on skin testing but positive response to Kveim antigen in about 80%
	2. Lymphopenia; reduced numbers of T-cells
	3. Raised serum levels of immunoglobulins
15. Biochemical findings	Hypercalcaemia. Raised serum levels of lysozyme, angiotensin converting enzyme and adenosine deaminase

Mild anaemia, leucopenia and eosinophilia are common. Hypergamma-globulinaemia and a raised ESR are usual; serum albumin levels are reduced. Serum calcium levels are increased because of sensitivity to vitamin D, as are alkaline phosphatase in hepatic sarcoidosis, and lysozyme, adenosine deaminase and serum angiotensin-converting enzyme (SACE).

Histological evidence of non-caseating epithelioid cell granulomas, impaired delayed hypersensitivity reactions to some antigens and a positive Kveim test may be useful. The last is carried out by intracutaneous injection of a heat-sterilized suspension of human spleen or lymph nodes affected with sarcoidosis. After 4–6 weeks the area is biopsied and, if positive, shows well-formed epithelioid granulomas. The test is positive in about 80 per cent of patients.

Patients with only minor symptoms often require no treatment. Cortico-steroids are used especially if there is active ocular disease, progressive lung disease, hypercalcaemia, cerebral involvement or other serious complications.

Dental aspects

Sarcoidosis can involve any of the oral tissues but has a predilection for salivary glands. There is asymptomatic enlargement of the major salivary glands in about 6 per cent of cases (*Fig. 6.1*) and some have xerostomia. Biopsy of minor salivary glands may confirm the diagnosis when other signs of the disease such as a suggestive chest film are present, and avoid the need for more invasive procedures.

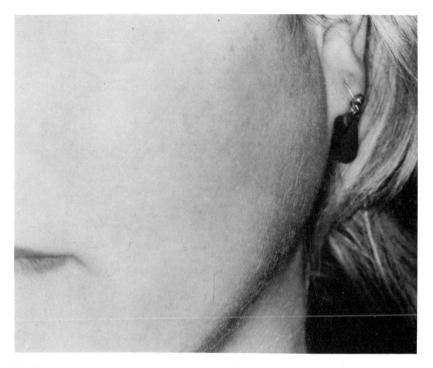

Fig. 6.1. Sarcoidosis presenting with parotid gland swelling.

The association of salivary and lacrimal gland enlargement with fever and uveitis is known as uveoparotid fever (Heerfordt's syndrome). There may be associated cranial neuropathies, especially facial palsy. The salivary gland swellings usually resolve but this may take up to 3 years. Xerostomia is prominent.

Gingival enlargement can be an early or late feature and biopsy shows the typical sarcoid follicles. However, there is a group of patients who have histological features of sarcoid in one or more sites in the mouth, such as the gingivae, but no systemic manifestations and a negative Kveim test. A few of these patients may ultimately develop other more or less systematized disease but probably the majority have isolated lesions. Such cases, where no exogenous cause for the granulomatous reaction can be found, are regarded as having 'sarcoid-like' reactions and treatment is unnecessary. However, patients should be kept under observation for as long as possible.

Management problems of patients with systematic sarcoidosis may include:

1. Respiratory impairment.
2. Uveitis and visual impairment.
3. Renal disease.
4. Jaundice.
5. Corticosteroid treatment.

Other Causes of Granulomatous Reactions

If sarcoid-like follicles are found on biopsy of oral tissues, the differential diagnosis includes sarcoid and the following:

1. Tuberculosis.
2. Crohn's disease and Melkersson–Rosenthal syndrome.
3. As a reaction to some carcinomas.
4. Leprosy.
5. Zirconium.
6. Berylliosis.
7. Brucellosis.
8. Other foreign bodies.

It should be noted that midline granulomas (Chapter 16) are frequently not characterized by epithelioid granulomas histologically.

POSTOPERATIVE RESPIRATORY COMPLICATIONS

Segmental or lobar pulmonary collapse and infection are the most common respiratory complications following surgical operations under general anaesthesia. These complications are more common after abdominal surgery or if there is pre-existent respiratory disease, smoking or occupational respiratory disorders (*see also* Chapter 1).

Postoperative respiratory complications can be significantly reduced by starting physiotherapy preoperatively in patients with respiratory disorders who require prolonged general anaesthesia.

Bronchodilators such as salbutamol may also be of value in preventing complications, especially if there is a strong element of bronchospasm.

If postoperative pulmonary infection develops, physiotherapy and antibiotics should be given and sputum sent for culture. The common microbial causes are *S. pneumoniae* and *H. influenzae;* suitable antibiotics include amoxycillin, erythromycin or co-trimoxazole. Hospital infections may include other micro-organisms such as staphylococci, klebsiella, pseudomonas and other Gram–negative bacteria; microbiological examination of the sputum and antibiotic sensitivities are therefore essential.

ASPIRATION OF GASTRIC CONTENTS (MENDELSON'S SYNDROME)

Inhalation of gastric contents, such as alcoholic vomiting, may cause asphyxia and death. Aspiration of gastric contents into the lower respiratory tract causes pulmonary oedema and can be fatal (Mendelson's syndrome). Aspiration is most likely if a general anaesthetic is given to a patient whose stomach is not empty because, for example, food or drink has been taken or stomach emptying is delayed. Vomiting during anaesthesia, and hence aspiration, is more likely in the last trimester of pregnancy.

The best treatment is prevention, by ensuring that the stomach is empty and by passing an endotracheal tube if not. The endotracheal tube must be passed by a skilled anaesthetist with the patient's head at a lower level than the stomach. Antacids or an H_2 receptor blocker, such as cimetidine may be given by mouth before the anaesthetic to reduce gastric acidity in the event of aspiration.

If gastric contents are aspirated, the pharynx and larynx must be carefully sucked out. Systemic corticosteroids have been recommended, but recent reports have not confirmed any reduction in the mortality.

RESPIRATORY DISTRESS SYNDROMES

Adult respiratory distress syndrome (ARDS) is a sequel to several types of pulmonary injury and discussed in Chapter 13.

Respiratory distress in premature infants may be caused by bronchopulmonary dysplasia and necessitates nasotracheal intubation for many weeks. This may in turn result in midface hypoplasia.

ASPERGILLOMA (ASPERGILLUS FUNGAL BALL)

A large mass of fungal hyphae can form in healthy persons in body cavities and in particular the maxillary antrum, without invasion of the tissues or causing symptoms. Such fungal balls are usually found by chance when a radiograph shows opacity of the antrum when, for example, a root is being removed.

The material from the antrum often appears dry and brownish. Diagnosis is by microscopy, preferably confirmed by culture, for which unfixed material is obviously necessary. Under the microscope the material appears amorphous at low power but the typical branching non-septate hyphae can be seen at high power especially if a stain such as periodic acid Schiff (PAS) is used. Care must be taken, however, to distinguish these harmless fungal balls from invasive rhinocerebral aspergillosis or mucormycosis (*see below*).

Antifungal treatment of aspergilloma in a healthy person is not needed.

RHINOCEREBRAL ASPERGILLOSIS

Invasive aspergillosis is one of the most common opportunistic fungal infections in immunocompromised patients such as those with leukaemia or AIDS, but is far more frequently pulmonary rather than rhinocerebral.

The clinical picture and the microscopy, apart from the morphology of the hyphae, are in essential respects similar to that of a rhinocerebral mucormycosis discussed below, and diagnosis therefore depends on mycological culture, but a distinctive feature of the microscopy is that oxalate crystal formation may be seen.

Though aspergillus is sensitive to amphotericin, treatment is often ineffective because of the underlying disease. The disease is usually fatal once the cranial cavity has become involved. However, there have been a few therapeutic successes as a result of excision of the infected area together with intravenous amphotericin.

A fulminant form of the disease in immunocompromised patients results in gangrenous periostitis and destruction of the nasal cavity and paranasal sinuses within a few days.

RHINOCEREBRAL MUCORMYCOSIS (PHYCOMYCOSIS)

This disease, which has many synonyms as a result of the variety of possible causative fungi, is an infection of the antrum, usually in immunodeficient patients such as those with severe uncontrolled diabetes mellitus, AIDS or leukaemia. Rarely, immunocompetent persons have been affected.

The causative fungi such as Mucor, Rhizopus or Absidia species are ubiquitous saprophytes—growing, for example, on bread or fruit—and for long were thought to be completely harmless. Infection is as a result of inhalation.

Clinical features

Very occasionally the disease appears to follow removal of a root from, or other operative interference with, the antrum, but such treatment is probably more likely to have brought a pre-existing infection to light.

The typical clinical picture is dull sinus pain and congestion, sometimes with a bloodstained nasal discharge associated with a low fever. Deterioration of vision, facial or other cranial nerve palsies and proptosis follow and consciousness is progressively impaired as a result of cranial involvement. Downward spread can cause palatal necrosis and ulceration while laterally the cheek may become inflamed. Blindness, coma and death can follow within 1 or 2 weeks or occasionally even more rapidly.

Diagnosis and Management

In addition to the local clinical picture and any systemic features of the underlying disease there is opacity of the antrum radiographically. Confirmation of the diagnosis is by biopsy showing the ribbon-like non-septate hyphae of irregular width. There is inflammation, sometimes with Langhan's type giant cells and granulation tissue formation, and typically invasion of blood vessels. If possible culture of the fungus should also be carried out.

Treatment is with amphotericin and also, in the case of diabetics, of the underlying ketoacidotic state. This is often successful but in the case of leukaemia and probably also in AIDS the prognosis is likely to be hopeless.

Bibliography

Almeida and Scully C. (1991) Oral lesions in the systemic mycoses. *Curr. Opin Dent.* **1**, 423–8.

Brinker H. (1986) The sarcoidosis-lymphoma syndrome. *Br. J. Cancer* **54**, 467–73.

Brook M.G., Lucas R.E. and Pain A.K. (1988) Clinical features and management of two cases of *Streptococcus milleri* chest infection. Scand. *J. Infect. Dis.* **20**, 345–6.

Cawson R. A. (1960) Tuberculosis of the mouth and throat (with special reference to the incidence and management since the introduction of chemotherapy). *Br. J. Dis. Chest* **54**, 40.

Cawson R.A. and Spector R.G. (1989) *Clinical Pharmacology in Dentistry.* 5th ed. Edinburgh, Churchill Livingstone.

Clarke S. (1976) Respiratory function tests. *Br. J. Hosp. Med.* **15**, 137–53.

Feldman N. T. and McFadden E. R. (1977) Asthma: therapy old and new. *Med. Clin. North Am.* **61**, 1239–51.

Fernald G.W., Roberts M.W. and Boat T.F. (1990) Cystic fibrosis: a current review. *Pediatr. Dent.* **12**, 72–78.

Flenley D. C. (1979) Chronic bronchitis and emphysema. *Medicine (UK)* **22**, 1144–51.

Fotos P. G., Westfall H. N., Synder I. S. et al. (1985) Prevalence of Legionella-specific IgG and IgM antibody in a dental clinic population. *J. Dent. Res.* **64**, 1382–5.

Goldsmith D. and Trieger N. (1980) Pulmonary assessment in the ambulatory patient. *J. Oral Surg.* **38**, 771–3.

Hagan J.L. and Hardy J.D. (1983) Lung abscesses revisited. *Ann. Surg.* **197**, 755–62.

Kaltman S. I. and Sladen A. (1977) Current concepts of the adult respiratory distress syndrome. *Oral Surg.* **35**, 652–9.

Kinirons M.J. (1989) Dental health of patients suffering from cystic fibrosis in Northern Ireland. *Community Dental Health* **6**, 113–20.

Kuhn J.P. (1986) Imaging of the paranasal sinuses: current status. *J. Allergy Clin. Immunol.* **77**, 6–9.

Lindemann R.A., Newman M.G., Kaufman A.K. et al. (1985) Oral colonisation and susceptibility testing of *Pseudomonas aeruginosa* oral isolates from cystic fibrosis patients. *J. Dent. Res.* **64**, 54–57.

McCarthy F. M. (1984) Safe treatment of the emphysema patient. *J. Am. Dent. Assoc.* **106**, 761–6.

Mahaney M. C. (1986) Delayed dental development and pulmonary disease in children with cystic fibrosis. *Arch. Oral Biol.* **31**, 363–7.

Milledge S. and Nunn J. F. (1975) Criteria of fitness for anaesthesia in patients with chronic obstructive lung disease. *Br. Med. J.* **2**, 670 3.

Moser K. M. (1977) Pulmonary embolism. *Am. Rev. Resp. Dis.* **115**, 829–52.

Primosch R. E. (1980) Tetracycline discoloration, enamel defects and dental caries in patients with cystic fibrosis. *Oral Surg.* **50**, 303–8.

Shapiro G.G., Furukawa C.T. and Pierson W.E. (1986) Blinded comparison of maxillary sinus radiography and ultrasound for diagnosis of sinusitis. *J. Allergy Clin. Immunol.* **77**, 59–62.

Smith W. H. R. (1982) Intraoral and pulmonary tuberculosis following dental treatment. *Lancet* **i**, 842–4.

Thompson P. J. et al. (1986) Assessment of oral candidiasis in patients with respiratory disease and efficacy of a new nystatin formulation. *Br. Med. J.* **292**, 699–700.

Thornton J. A. (1969) Problem of anaesthesia and surgery in relation to chronic respiratory disease. MD Thesis, University of London.

Tynan J. J. and Kamiyama K. (1984) Cystic fibrosis and oral health. *J. Canad. Dent. Assoc.* **50**, 833–5.

Appendix to Chapter 6

OCCUPATIONAL LUNG DISEASES

Disorder	Source of causal agent	Group at risk	Clinical significance
Anthracosis	Soot Carbon smoke	Urban dwellers	Benign
Asbestosis	Asbestos (crocidolite or amosite predispose to mesothelioma)	Asbestos workers	Pulmonary fibrosis leading to cor pulmonale Bronchial carcinoma Mesothelioma
Bagassosis	Mouldy sugar cane fibre	Insulation Fertilizers Explosives	Acute pneumonia or bronchiolitis
Barilosis	Barium	Barium miners	Benign
Berylliosis	Beryllium	Fluorescent lamps Various alloys	Chronic respiratory disease leading to cor pulmonale
Byssinosis	Cotton, flax or hemp	Cotton workers	Periodic bronchospasm leading to obstructive airways disease
Coal miner's pneumoconiosis	Coal dust	Coal miners	Largely asymptomatic but may cause fibrosis and emphysema
Kaolin pneumoconiosis	China clay	China clay workers	Resembles silicosis (q.v.)
Siderosis	Iron dust	Welders Grinders	Benign
Silicosis	Silica (quartz) dust	Miners Sandblasting Potters	Pulmonary fibrosis leading to cor pulmonale Tuberculosis
Stannosis	Tin dust	Tin refining	Benign

Chapter 7

Gastrointestinal Disease

ORAL DISEASE

Oral disease is fully discussed in textbooks of oral medicine; this section is restricted to those oral complaints where there may be important medical implications.

ORAL ULCERS

Oral ulcers are very common. Most are traumatic or recurrent aphthae; they are usually of little consequence, but more serious causes of oral ulceration must always be excluded (*Table 7.1*). Particular care must be taken to exclude cancer, blood dyscrasias, mucocutaneous or gastrointestinal disease and HIV infection.

The clinical history is of great value in the differential diagnosis but if there is any doubt investigations, perhaps including biopsy, are essential. The history should establish the time of onset, pattern of recurrence, site, size and duration of the ulcers and may also suggest any systemic disease such as anaemia or other blood dyscrasia, infections, skin, gastrointestinal, eye or genital disease. The typical features of aphthae are summarized in *Table 7.2*. Should the clinical history or examination suggest other causes, specialist advice should be sought.

Recurrent Aphthae (Recurrent aphthous stomatitis, RAS)

Recurrent aphthae are common and, patients' histories suggest that they affect up to 25 per cent of the population at some time. Some groups, for example students, have a higher incidence, but only a minority of patients have ulcers so frequently or severely as to cause them to seek dental or medical advice.

Aphthae typically start in childhood or adolescence and become progressively more troublesome until, when patients reach their twenties or thirties, help is sought. The disease is usually self-limiting and after a variable number of years the ulcers become less frequent or cease altogether. During the course of the disease spontaneous remissions of a month or two are common and this makes evaluation of treatment difficult.

Table 7.1. Causes of oral ulceration

1. Local causes
    Trauma
    Chemical irritation
    Burns
2. Recurrent aphthae, Behçet's and Sweet's syndrome (Chapter 16)
3. Neoplasms
    Squamous cell carcinoma
    Others (Chapter 5)
4. Systemic causes
    (a) *Mucocutaneous diseases* (Chapter 17)
        Lichen planus
        Pemphigus
        Pemphigoid (and localized oral purpura)
        Erythema multiforme
        Epidermolysis bullosa
        Dermatitis herpetiformis and linear IgA disease
    (b) *Connective tissue and other diseases* (Chapter 16)
        Lupus erythematosus
        Reiter's syndrome
    (c) *Blood diseases* (Chapters 3 and 4)
        Leucopenias including HIV disease
        Leukaemias
        Deficiency states or anaemia
    (d) *Gastrointestinal disease* (Chapter 7)
        Coeliac disease
        Crohn's disease
        Ulcerative colitis
    (e) *Drugs*
    (f) *Infections*
        mainly viral (Chapter 17)
        also syphilis and tuberculosis (rarely fungal)

Table 7.2. Features of recurrent aphthae

Minor aphthae
1. Onset usually in childhood or adolescence
2. Often positive family history
3. Recurrences at intervals
4. Usually round or ovoid ulcers
5. Not on attached gingiva or hard palate and rarely on dorsum of tongue
6. Usually form in small crops
7. Most are 2–4 mm in diameter
8. Most heal within 10 days
9. Usually self-limiting. Ulceration typically ceases before middle age

Major aphthae
Uncommon. Ulcers may be one to several centimetres in diameter and persist for months before healing with scarring

Herpetiform aphthae
Uncommon. Ulcers 1–3 mm across and form in crops of 10–100 with widespread erythema

There appears to be a familial basis to the ulceration in some patients. A few show a clear relationship of ulcers with the luteal phase of menstruation, and some with iron, folate or vitamin B_{12} deficiencies. A few patients associate the ulcers with stress, particular foods or trauma and similar ulcers can be a troublesome feature of HIV infection.

Recurrent aphthae are not often medically important—most patients are otherwise healthy. Deficiency states, particularly of iron, folate or vitamin B_{12}, are found in 10–20 per cent of patients. Aphthae may also be associated with some intestinal diseases, notably coeliac or Crohn's disease, or ulcerative colitis, but it is unclear whether the association is always secondary to deficiencies, particularly of iron or folate, or merely coincidental.

A few patients with RAS prove to have Behçet's syndrome (Chapter 16), when there may be genital ulceration, uveitis and other lesions. This diagnosis cannot be made on the basis of oral ulceration alone and management at this stage does not differ from that of RAS. The onset of the different manifestations of Behçet's syndrome may be separated by years and it is always necessary to question the patient specifically about genital ulcers, eye complaints or other lesions. Exceedingly rare causes of ulcers, clinically indistinguishable from RAS, are cyclic neutropenia and other immunodeficiencies. Cyclic neutropenia (the importance of which has been greatly overemphasized in the past) typically causes recurrent infections, fever, malaise and enlarged cervical lymph nodes. Oral ulceration typically appears at 21-day intervals, coincident with the falls in circulating neutrophils, and may be the main manifestation of the disease. In others, severe periodontal disease may develop.

Major aphthae may be the presenting feature of HIV infection. They typically affect the palate and may be associated with pharyngeal or oesophageal ulceration.

In vitro immunological abnormalities have been reported in RAS but there is scant evidence for an autoimmune basis, no association with typical autoimmune diseases and none of the common autoantibodies are found. There is also little evidence for an association with atopic disease.

Management

Patients with aphthae, in addition to a careful history, should be screened haematologically, particularly if the history suggests a systemic disorder or if the ulcers develop or worsen in middle age or later. A full screen includes haemoglobin and blood indices. Serum ferritin (or iron and iron–binding capacity), vitamin B_{12} levels and corrected whole blood or red cell folate levels may sometimes be required (Appendix to Chapter 1).

There is no specific or reliably effective treatment for aphthae. Patients vary widely in their response to various medications and their assessment is complicated by spontaneous remissions or by placebo effects.

A mouthwash of chlorhexidine gluconate (0.2 per cent aqueous solution) is useful to maintain oral hygiene and mitigates ulcers in some patients. Others seem to respond to tetracycline mouthrinses. Topical corticosteroids may sometimes be effective. Hydrocortisone hemisuccinate pellets 2.5 mg (Corlan) dissolved in the mouth up to four times daily should be used continuously, whether ulcers are present or not, unless attacks are infrequent. This regimen should be continued for 2 months then stopped for a month to assess progress and whether the disease has ceased to be troublesome. Triamcinolone acetonide in Orabase paste (Adcortyl in Orabase) can be used, but patients may find it difficult to apply. Betamethasone preparations are sometimes required.

Major aphthae remain a serious problem. Pain may be controlled with the use, topically, of lignocaine gels or viscous solutions. Experimentally, thalidomide and azathioprine may be effective but such treatment is a matter for specialists and no less toxic treatment has been found. In patients with HIV infection major aphthae may respond to zidovudine or thalidomide.

DRY MOUTH

Dry mouth (xerostomia) has many causes (*Table 7.3*). It may be a complaint even when salivary flow is normal but this is psychogenic. Important causes are Sjögren's syndrome, drugs (*see* Appendix to Chapter 19), irradiation of the major salivary glands and HIV infection.

Table 7.3. Causes of dry mouth

1. IATROGENIC
    Drugs (antimuscarinics; sympathominetics)
    Cancer therapy (irradiation of salivary glands, cytotoxic drugs)
    Graft-versus-host disease
2. SALIVARY GLAND DISEASE
    Sjögrens syndrome
    Sarcoidosis
    HIV disease
    Others
3. DEHYDRATION
    Diabetes mellitus
    Diabetes insipidus
    Renal failure
    Haemorrhage
    Other causes of fluid
        loss or deprivation

Drugs

Any drugs with an antimuscarinic or sympathomimetic effect may cause a dry mouth (Appendix to Chapter 19). Tricyclic antidepressants and phenothiazine neuroleptics are some of the most potent causes of xerostomia. However, despite statements to the contrary, neither the commonly used 'tranquillizers', the benzodiazepines nor beta–blockers cause xerostomia. Indeed the latter may be used to relieve dry mouth secondary to anxiety in actors for example, for whom anxiety–induced dry mouth is an occupational hazard. Other antihypertensive agents, such as ganglion blockers, which caused dry mouth are obsolete.

Sjögren's Syndrome

The association of dry mouth (xerostomia) with dry eyes (keratoconjunctivitis sicca) in the absence of rheumatoid arthritis (the features originally observed by Sjögren) is usually now referred to as 'sicca syndrome' (primary Sjögren's syndrome) and the term 'Sjögren's syndrome' (secondary Sjögren's syndrome) is reserved for the association of these features with rheumatoid arthritis, or less frequently with systemic lupus erythematosus, progressive systemic sclerosis, polymyositis, primary biliary cirrhosis or other connective tissue diseases. Indeed the association with Sjögren's syndrome is the single common feature which the connective tissue (collagen vascular) diseases share.

It has been estimated that probably 15 per cent of patients with rheumatoid arthritis develop Sjögren's syndrome and, since the same salivary gland changes can be associated with other connective tissue diseases or can develop in apparent isolation, it is clear that Sjögren's syndrome is relatively common.

Sjögren's syndrome mainly affects middle-aged or older women. The essential changes of Sjögren's syndrome are infiltration of the lacrimal, salivary and other exocrine glands by lymphocytes and plasma cells, with progressive acinar destruction. The parotid glands are chiefly affected but the changes are also detectable in the minor labial glands in most patients. Sicca syndrome shares most of the serological abnormalities of rheumatoid disease, although overt rheumatoid arthritis is not present and there are other differences, as shown in *Table 7.4.* Lymphoma *is* an uncommon but well recognized and lethal complication of Sjögren's and especially, sicca syndrome.

Table 7.4. Sjögren's syndrome—comparison of sub-types

Feature	Primary	Secondary
Connective tissue disease	-	+
Oral involvement	More severe	Less severe
Recurrent sialadenitis	More common	Less common
Ocular involvement	More severe	Less severe
Extraglandular manifestations	More common	Less common
Lymphocyte-aggressive manifestations	More common	Less common
HLA associations	HLA-DR3 HLA-B8	HLA-DR4
Rheumatoid factor	50%	90%
Anti-SS-A (Ro)	5–10%	50–80%
Anti-SS-B (La) antinuclear antigens	54–73%	2–6%
Rheumatoid arthritis precipitin (RAP)*	5%	76%
Salivary duct antibody	10–36%	67–70%

*Also known as SS-C.

Clinically, these syndromes are characterized by oral discomfort caused by the reduced salivary flow, obvious dryness of the mucosa in severe cases and, erythema and lobulation of the tongue. Swelling of the parotids is seen in a minority and, rarely, these glands can also be persistently painful. Late onset of salivary gland swelling may indicate development of a lymphoma.

Table 7.5. Sjögren's syndrome—features and systemic components

1. *Ocular*
   Keratoconjunctivitis sicca
2. *Oral*
   Xerostomia
   Lobulated tongue
   Infections
3. Respiratory tract
   Dryness
4. *Gastrointestinal*
   Dysphagia
5. *Pancreas*
   Subclinical dysfunction
6. *Cutaneous*
   Xeroderma
   Vaginal dryness
   Raynaud's phenomenon
7. *Drug allergies*
8. *Haematological disorders*
   Anaemia
   Leucopenia
9. *Associated autoimmune disorders* (p. 193)

Apart from its dryness, the oral mucosa appears normal but the supervention of candidal infection causes redness and soreness. The main effects of persistent xerostomia are:

1. Discomfort and, in severe cases, difficulty in speaking, swallowing or managing dentures.
2. Disturbed taste sensation.
3. Accelerated caries.
4. Susceptibility to oral candidosis.
5. Susceptibility to ascending (bacterial) sialadenitis.

Surprisingly perhaps, some patients can manage dentures in spite of virtual or complete absence of saliva and many such patients do not complain of dry mouth per se.

In spite of the often troublesome nature of the oral symptoms, the most important effects of Sjögren's syndrome are on the eyes, where drying causes keratoconjunctivitis sicca. This can lead ultimately to impairment or loss of sight. These ocular changes are initially asymptomatic and it is therefore essential for the patient to have an ophthalmological examination.

Bronchial involvement may lead to recurrent respiratory infections and this disease may also involve vaginal glands, pancreas or other organs (*Table 7.5*). Patients with Sjögren's syndrome may develop other autoimmune manifestations such as Raynaud's phenomenon.

HIV Infection

Parotitis is a common feature of HIV infection in children. The infection can also cause salivary gland swellings due to lymphocytic infiltration, and dry mouth. HIV infection should be suspected if a male between the ages of (approximately) 20–40 complains of onset of dry mouth, particularly if associated with parotid swellings.

Though the salivary gland changes in HIV infection are mainly due to lymphocytic infiltration, autoantibody findings typical of Sjögren's syndrome are lacking, and the age and sex distribution are also different.

Management of dry mouth

The history should be directed particularly to discover any drugs likely to cause dry mouth and any symptoms suggestive of connective tissue disease, particularly rheumatoid arthritis, or of diabetes. Dryness of other mucous membranes, particularly of the conjunctivae, should be excluded. Patients with dry eyes may have no symptoms or may complain of grittiness, burning, soreness, itching, or inability to cry. They may wake in the morning with a pustular exudate in the eyes, crusting at the canthuses or have infections of the lids.

Examination should include palpation of the major salivary glands for swelling, and inspection of the eyes. A Schirmer test shows decreased lacrimation. Oral examination may reveal obvious xerostomia with lack of salivary pooling and flow from the duct orifices, frothy saliva, debris on the dorsum of the tongue, or infections (candidosi or sialadenitis) or rampant dental caries. In Sjögren's syndrome the tongue typically becomes lobulated and red.

Since no single investigation will reliably establish the diagnosis of Sjögren's syndrome, a variety of tests *may* have to be carried out. These include the following:

1. Salivary flow rates. Parotid output after stimulation with 10 per cent citric acid can be objectively determined using a suction (Lashley) cup over the parotid duct orifice or by cannulation of the duct. The flow is normally over 1.5 ml/min.

2. Sialography. Hydrostatic instillation of contrast medium typically shows a snow-storm appearance (punctate sialectasis) in well-established cases. Sialography is of course contraindicated if there is acute parotitis.

3. Labial gland biopsy. Biopsy of the parotid is theoretically preferable but labial gland biopsy is easier, safer and reflects the parotid changes in the majority of cases. This is probably the most useful single investigation.

4. Radioactive pertechnetate uptake and concentration in the parotids can be measured by scintigraphy which is sometimes useful, but involves the use of radio–isotopes and depends on the availability of specialized equipment.

5. Haematological examination. The ESR is typically raised and anaemia may be associated with rheumatoid disease.

6. Immunological studies. Typical findings are shown in *Table 7.4,* but the main abnormalities are hypergammaglobulinaemia mainly as a result of the presence of rheumatoid factor, often of antinuclear factors and, frequently, other autoantibodies.

Having said all that, it must be accepted that, since no specific treatment is available, it is arguable whether such intensive investigation is always justifiable. Certainly in a patient with known collagen disease, particularly rheumatoid arthritis, a dry mouth is virtually diagnostic of Sjögren's syndrome. It is, however, essential, as mentioned earlier, to arrange for ophthalmological investigation to exclude or treat early keratoconjunctivitis.

Dry mouth may be helped by frequently sipping water or drinks or using a salivary substitute such as carboxymethyl cellulose preparations such as Hypromellose as frequent, liberal rinses, or Glandosane or Saliva Orthana. Pilocarpine or anticholinesteraseinhibitors such as pyridostigmine may increase salivation if any functional tissue remains, but systemic effects such as diarrhoea may be troublesome.

Preventive dental care is important. Patients have a tendency to consume a cariogenic diet because of the impaired sense of taste–this must be avoided and caries should also be controlled by fluoride applications. Improved oral hygiene and the use of a 0.2 per cent chlorhexidine mouthwash will help to control periodontal disease and other infections.

Denture hygiene is important because of the susceptibility to candidosis and antifungal treatment is often needed (Appendix to Chapter 1).

Generalized soreness and redness of a dry oral mucosa is typically caused by *Candida albicans* and often associated with angular stomatitis. Antifungal treatment is given as rinses of nystatin or amphotericin mixture.

Acute complications such as ascending parotitis should be treated with antibiotics. Pus should be sent for culture and antibiotic sensitivities but, in the interim, a penicillinase-resistant penicillin such as flucloxacillin in combination with metronidazole because of the possible presence of anaerobes, should be started.

Dental treatment. Patients with Sjögren's syndrome who need dental treatment may not be a good risk for general anaesthesia because of the tendency to respiratory infections and complicating factors such as anaemia. There may also be problems in management related to the associated connective tissue disease (Chapter 16).

SIALORRHOEA (HYPERSALIVATION)

A clear distinction should be made between hypersalivation and drooling. Normally, any excess of saliva is swallowed and causes no symptoms. True hypersalivation is very rare, although it may be induced by lesions or foreign bodies in the mouth, by rabies or by drugs such as anticholinesterases (Chapter 19). Often there is no objective evidence for the complaint and it has a psychogenic basis. By contrast, drooling is common in infants, and in patients who have poor neuromuscular coordination or are mentally handicapped, without any increase in production of saliva. If drooling is severe, transplantation of the parotid duct such that it discharges into the pharynx may be effective and the submandibular duct can be moved.

SALIVARY GLAND SWELLINGS

The most common cause of salivary swelling is mumps (Chapter 17), which usually affects children and causes bilateral painful swellings. Other causes

Table 7.6. Causes of salivary gland swelling

1. *Inflammatory*
     Mumps
     Bacterial ascending sialadenitis
     Obstructive sialadenitis
     Sjögren's syndrome
     Sarcoidosis
2. *Neoplastic*
     Pleomorphic adenoma and others
3. *Endocrine and metabolic*
     Alcoholic cirrhosis
     Diabetes mellitus
     Acromegaly
     Malnutrition or bulimia
     Cystic fibrosis
     Chronic renal failure
4. *Drugs (rarely)*
     Isoprenaline
     Phenylbutazone
     Iodides
     Chlorhexidine

include sialadenitis, Sjögren's syndrome, sarcoidosis, some drugs (*Table 7.6*) and HIV infection. Neoplasms (usually pleomorphic adenoma) must also be considered particularly when there is a persistent unilateral swelling in older patients. Painless salivary swelling (sialosis) may also rarely be a feature of alcoholic cirrhosis (Chapter 8), diabetes mellitus, acromegaly (Chapter 10), or bulimia, or may be idiopathic.

FREY'S SYNDROME

Parotidectomy is sometimes followed by sweating and flushing of the preauricular skin on that side, in response to stimulation of salivation (gustatory sweating). Antiperspirants such as 20 per cent aluminium chloride hexahydrate (Driclor) may be effective in controlling sweating.

CERVICAL LYMPH NODE ENLARGEMENT

Causes of cervical lymphadenopathy are shown in *Table 7.7.*

ORAL PIGMENTATION

Most oral pigmentation is racial in origin or are local lesions such as amalgam tattoos. Though they are rare, the most important systemic causes to be excluded are Addison's disease, Nelson's syndrome, melanoma and AIDS. In the last case the pigmentation may be due to treatment with zidovudine,

Table 7.7. Swellings of the cervical lymph nodes

Infections	
Viral:	Viral respiratory infections
	Herpetic stomatitis
	Infectious mononucleosis
	HIV infection
	Others such as rubella
Bacterial:	Dental, tonsil, nose, sinuses, face or scalp
	Tuberculosis and atypical mycobacteria
	Syphilis
	Cat scratch disease
	Staphylococci
	Lyme disease
	Brucellosis
Parasites:	Toxoplasmosis
Unknown:	Mucocutaneous lymph node syndrome (Kawasaki's disease)
Neoplasms	
Primary:	Hodgkin's disease and non-Hodgkin's lymphoma
	Leukaemia, especially lymphocytic
Secondary:	Carcinoma—oral, cutaneous, salivary gland or nasopharyngeal
	Others—malignant melanoma and Ewing's sarcoma
Miscellaneous	
	Sarcoidosis
	Sinus histiocytosis
	Angiolymphoid hyperplasia
	Phenytoin and other drug reactions
	Connective tissue diseases
	Some immunodeficiency diseases

Table 7.8. Oral pigmentation

1. *Racial* (even in some Caucasians)
2. *Congenital*
    Peutz-Jeghers' syndrome (*Table 7.11*)
    Naevi
3. *Acquired*
    Endocrine or metabolic
        Addison's disease
        ACTH therapy
        ACTH-producing tumours (lung cancer)
        Haemochromatosis
        Nelson's syndrome
    Neoplastic
        Melanoma
    Metals
        Amalgam tattoo
        Bismuth, mercury, lead, silver
    Drugs
        Antimalarials
        Cytotoxics (busulphan particularly)
        Oral contraception
        Phenothiazines
        Minocycline
    Others
        AIDS

Table 7.9. Causes of discoloured teeth

	Extrinsic	*Intrinsic*

Most teeth affected	Smoking
	Beverages
	Drugs, e.g. iron,
	    chlorhexidine
	    minocycline
	Poor oral hygiene
		Tetracycline
		Fluorosis
		Amelogenesis imperfecta
		Dentinogenesis imperfecta
		Kernicterus
		Porphyria

One or a few teeth affected	As above	Trauma Caries Internal resorption

occasionally, to Addison's disease secondary to fungal infection or of unknown cause. Pigmentation of the soft palate is a rare manifestation of bronchogenic carcinoma (*Table 7.8*).

DISCOLORATION OF TEETH

Causes are outlined in *Table 7.9*. Most are extrinsic or related to caries or trauma.

TEETHING

Teething is traditionally blamed for a variety of signs and symptoms in infancy. Restlessness, finger-sucking, gum-rubbing and drooling may be associated with the eruption of deciduous teeth. However, teething is not responsible for diarrhoea, fever, convulsions or other systemic disorders; these have systemic causes, usually infections.

BURNING MOUTH

Burning mouth (oral dysaesthesia) is a common complaint in elderly females. It is occasionally a manifestation of deficiency of iron, folic acid or vitamin B_{12}, candidosis, related to denture-wearing or a manifestation of cancer phobia (Chapter 14). The majority of cases have no organic cause. However organic disease must be excluded by appropriate investigation, especially as pernicious anaemia is most common in women in this age group.

HALITOSIS AND DISTURBED TASTE SENSATION

Family and friends are usually more aware of halitosis than the patient. Causes of halitosis are outlined in *Table 7.10*. Similar conditions can cause a bad taste in the mouth (*see also* Chapter 12).

Table 7.10. Causes of halitosis

Oral infections
Dry mouth
Foods
Drugs
Solvent abuse
Alcohol
Chloral hydrate
DMSO (dimethyl sulphoxide)
Smoking
Nasal or antral infections
Systemic disease
Respiratory tract infections
Cirrhosis and liver failure
Renal failure
Diabetic ketosis
Gastrointestinal disease
Psychogenic disorders

One of the most common and manageable causes of halitosis is periodontal disease, in which anaerobes are numerous and frequently produce foul–smelling metabolic products such as sulphides. In such cases also the patient is usually unaware of the displeasure that he causes to others. By contrast, when the patient is concerned about halitosis, there is no organic cause in the majority of cases and the breath does not smell unpleasant. Such patients should be firmly reassured as they may be depressed. In a study of 137 patients troubled by halitosis, 50 were depressed, 36 seemed to be hypochondriacal and most of the remainder had schizophrenia or temporal lobe epilepsy.

CONGENITAL DISORDERS

Some of those which involve the oral cavity and other parts of the gastrointestinal tract are shown in *Table 7.11.*

OESOPHAGEAL DISEASE

DYSPHAGIA

Dysphagia (difficulty in swallowing) is the common symptom of oesophageal disease. It has many possible causes, including disease in the mouth and elsewhere outside the oesophagus (*Table 7.12*), and is sometimes neurotic ('globus hystericus').

Table 7.11. Congenital intestinal disorders

Syndrome	Extra-intestinal features	Gastrointestinal lesions
Familial colonic polyposis	—	Colon polyps, adenocarcinoma
Peutz-Jegher's syndrome	Pigmented macules of mouth lips and digits. Increased risk of neoplasia	Small intestine polyps and carcinoma rarely
Gardner's syndrome (Familial adenomatous polyposis coli)	Osteomas of jaws (especially mandible), epidermal cysts, sebaceous cysts, lipomas, fibroma, dental anomalies	Colon polyps, adenocarcinomas, biliary neoplasia
Juvenile polyposis	—	Inflammatory polyps in small or large intestine
Tylosis (palmar-plantar hyperkeratosis)	Hyperkeratosis of palms and soles	Oral leucoplakia and oesophageal carcinoma
Multiple endocrine adenomatosis, type III	(*see* Chapter 10)	Mucosal neuromas

Table 7.12. Causes of dysphagia

Psychogenic
Organic
1. Xerostomia
2. Inflammatory lesions in mouth or throat
3. Foreign bodies in pharynx
4. Sideropenic dysphagia (Paterson–Kelly syndrome)
5. Pharyngeal pouches
6. Benign stricture
7. Carcinoma
8. Scleroderma
9. External pressure from mediastinal lymph nodes
10. Neurological and neuromuscular causes:
   Achalasia
   Syringobulbia
   Cerebrovascular accidents
   Cerebrovascular disease (pseudobulbar palsy)
   Motor neurone disease
   Guillain-Barré syndrome
   Poliomyelitis
   Diphtheria
   Cerebellar disease
   Myopathies
      Myasthenia gravis
      Muscular dystrophies
      Dermatomyositis

General management

Dysphagia is a symptom that must never be dismissed lightly. The history is often the most important contribution to diagnosis but most patients, unless there are obvious oral causes, should be referred for medical investigation. Chest radiography and a barium swallow examination are usually required unless there are signs of neuromuscular disease. Oesophagoscopy may be needed if there is any suggestion of an organic lesion.

Treatment can be difficult. Surgery is required, particularly for impacted foreign bodies, strictures, pouches, achalasia or carcinoma. The latter has an appallingly poor prognosis (*see Table 5.20*).

Dental aspects

Tonsillitis and pharyngitis are the most common causes of dysphagia, but oral causes include infections or ulcers of the palate, fauces, tongue or floor of the mouth. Almost any infection can cause dysphagia but particularly important are viral infections (herpetic stomatitis, herpangina and glandular fever) and bacterial infections such as pericoronitis. Rarely, pain–dysfunction syndrome by making contraction of the jaw muscles painful causes difficulty in the initiation of the swallowing process.

Infections involving the fascial spaces of the neck, particularly those tracking to the parapharyngeal space, peritonsillar infections and Ludwig's angina (bilateral sublingual and submandibular cellulitis) cause dysphagia which is, nevertheless, a minor feature of these serious diseases.

Oral ulcers can occasionally cause dysphagia. Severe recurrent aphthae are most often responsible, but other causes (*see Table 7.1*), particularly carcinoma, must be excluded. Carcinoma of the posterior lateral border of the tongue is an important cause and can be missed unless examination is thorough.

Dry mouth is an uncommon cause of dysphagia. Dysphagia may be particularly important in disorders of the medulla, since there may be defects of cranial nerves V, VII, IX, X XI or XII (Appendix to Chapter 12).

REFLUX OESOPHAGITIS

Reflux oesophagitis is one of the most common kinds of dyspepsia and, although at one time considered to be a result of hiatus hernia, the relationship between the symptoms and appearances on barium swallow is inconsistent. Oesophageal spasm can complicate the picture.

Symptoms can be effectively relieved by taking frequent small meals, antacids, cimetidine or other H_2 blocker during the day, by reducing obesity and by raising the head of the bed by at least 4 inches.

Some patients are convinced that oral symptoms or disease are caused by 'acid' but, apart from a few genuine cases with persistent regurgitation of gastric contents, which may lead to dental erosion, (*see* Anorexia nervosa and bulimia, Chapter 14), this is no more than a folk myth, probably fostered by advertisements for antacids.

THE STOMACH

NORMAL FUNCTION

Gastric secretions include hydrochloric acid (secreted by parietal cells), pepsin (secreted by chief or peptic cells) and intrinsic factor (secreted by parietal cells).

Gastric mucus contains several glycoproteins which help to protect the mucosa against erosion.

Gastrin stimulates gastric acid secretion and secretion of gastrin is controlled by the inhibitory effects of acid in the antrum or duodenum, decrease in gastric distension and release of the pancreatic hormones, cholecystokinin-pancreozymin and secretin.

Acid secretion is also stimulated by synthetic analogues of gastrin (pentagastrin), by histamine and its analogues, and by hypoglycaemia.

Gastrin acts by inducing local release of histamine which acts on specific (H_2) receptors on the parietal cells which then secrete acid. Drugs such as cimetidine and ranitidine, which block these H_2 receptors, therefore block gastric acid production.

Gastric function tests

Gastric acid secretion in response to various stimuli can be assessed by passing a nasogastric tube and measuring the volume, pH and acid concentration of the aspirate.

PEPTIC ULCER

Peptic ulcer develops in or close to acid-secreting areas, usually in the stomach (gastric ulcer) or proximal duodenum (duodenal ulcer). Acid production is typically normal in those with a gastric ulcer, although zonal gastritis is associated; some, but not all, patients with a duodenal ulcer have acid hypersecretion. Peptic ulcers also complicate conditions characterized by raised gastrin levels. These include Zollinger–Ellison syndrome (a gastrin-producing tumour), hyperparathyroidism (high serum calcium provokes gastrin release) and chronic renal failure (poor gastrin metabolism). Factors that may impair the mucous barrier or otherwise promote peptic ulceration include genetic influences, stress, smoking, diet, environmental factors and drugs, particularly aspirin and other anti-inflammatory analgesics, and corticosteroids. *Helicobacter pylori* appears to play a role in many cases, and its elimination with antimicrobials and bismuth salts may hasten healing.

A characteristic feature of peptic ulcer is epigastric pain which has a variable relationship to meals but is often relieved by antacids. The severity of the pain bears no relationship to the size or severity of the ulceration and many patients with peptic ulcers suffer little more than dyspepsia. Some have no symptoms and the first sign of an ulcer may be one of the complications such as haemorrhage, perforation, or pyloric obstruction with vomiting.

General management

Endoscopy is the most reliable way of confirming the diagnosis but is usually preceded by barium meal radiography. Gastric acid studies or the estimation of serum gastrin levels may also be carried out. Non–drug treatments, particularly bed rest, dietary changes and stopping smoking, and limiting alcohol intake, accelerate the healing of gastric but not duodenal ulcers. Milk, antacids and frequent small meals with no fried foods often relieve symptoms.

Drug treatment is now frequently used. Cimetidine, ranitidine and other analogues are among the most effective drugs and accelerate the healing, particularly of duodenal ulcers. Also effective are pirenzepine, a selective antimuscarinic, sucralfate and bismuth chelate. These may be used in combination with H_2 blockers in intractable cases. Omeprazole, which blocks acid production by inhibiting the parietal cell proton pump mechanism is frequently effective when H_2 blockers fail. Drug treatment may have to be maintained as relapses may follow.

Partial gastrectomy is usually reserved for those with complications but is effective and also has the advantage that it eliminates the need for long term drug treatment, Gastric ulcers are managed by antrectomy with gastroduodenal anastomosis; duodenal ulcers are managed usually with vagotomy and pyloroplasty or antrectomy.

Dental aspects

There are no oral manifestations of peptic ulcer unless there is anaemia from gastrointestinal bleeding, or surgical procedures. Anaemia may also complicate treatment, particularly general anaesthesia. Persistent regurgitation of gastric acid as a result of pyloric stenosis can cause severe dental erosion, typically of the palatal aspects of the upper anterior teeth and premolars. Drugs that cause gastric ulceration, or increase bleeding from such ulcers, should not be given to patients with peptic ulcers. Such drugs include aspirin, other non-steroidal anti-inflammatory analgesics and corticosteroids. Cimetidine may delay benzodiazepine clearance but the effect is not clinically significant. Complications of surgery, relevant to dentistry mainly follow total resections. They include deficiencies of vitamin B_{12}, folate or iron, and attacks of hypoglycaemia, but should not be seen now.

CANCER OF THE STOMACH

The stomach is one of the most frequent sites of cancer, which typically causes no symptoms until late. The prognosis is poor, with about a 7 per cent 5-year survival rate (see Table 5.20). Men are affected nearly twice as often as women. The aetiology of gastric cancer is unclear but may include genetic influences, atrophic gastritis, achlorhydria and possibly, ingestion of carcinogens. Patients with pernicious anaemia have an increased incidence of gastric cancer.

The symptoms of gastric cancer may closely mimic peptic ulcer, a common complaint being indigestion or vague upper abdominal pain. Later, anorexia, loss of weight, nausea, vomiting or melaena (stools black and tarry with blood) and anaemia may develop. The tumour spreads locally to cause pain, and may obstruct the intestine to cause vomiting, or bile duct to cause jaundice. Jaundice may also be caused by liver metastases and deposits may form in the peritoneum (causing ascites), lungs, bones or brain.

The diagnosis of gastric cancer is usually suggested by radiography but confirmed by gastroscopy and biopsy. Most patients are treated by surgery, but unfortunately, it is frequently only palliative.

Dental aspects

Metastases to the jaw from gastric carcinomas are probably more frequent than from many other cancers but are still rare. They are usually in the body of the mandible and may cause swelling, pain, paraesthesia, loosening of teeth or sockets that fail to heal, or be found as ragged radiolucent areas, sometimes with resorption of roots. Other rare manifestations are shown in *Table 5.19*. Occasionally metastases from a gastric carcinoma may be first detected in a lower cervical lymph node, usually on the left side (Troisier's sign).

Oral signs of anaemia can be an initial feature and it is worth emphasizing that iron deficiency in a male should always be regarded with suspicion, since it usually results from chronic haemorrhage, often from the gastrointestinal tract and then not infrequently due to an ulcer or neoplasm.

Anaemia or obstructive jaundice may complicate dental treatment. Pernicious anaemia (*see* Chapter 4) may precede development of gastric cancer.

THE SMALL INTESTINE

Normal function

The small intestine is the main area of digestion and absorption of food. Digestion depends on intestinal and pancreatic enzymes acting on food previously exposed to salivary amylase and gastric acid and pepsin. Bile salts facilitate the absorption of fats and the fat-soluble vitamins (A, D, E and K); gastric intrinsic factor is needed for the absorption of vitamin B_{12} in the terminal part of the ileum. Iron and folate are absorbed in the duodenum, most other substances in the jejunum.

General aspects of small intestine disease

Malabsorption is the main feature of most of these disorders. Lassitude, weakness, loss of weight or failure to thrive, vitamin deficiencies and anaemia are common. Diarrhoea or steatorrhoea, and sometimes abdominal discomfort are the main complaints, but in the later stages there are manifestations of chronic deficiencies.

Diseases of the small intestine of most significance include coeliac disease and Crohn's disease, but other causes of malabsorption include surgery, infestations and drugs.

COELIAC DISEASE (GLUTEN-SENSITIVE ENTEROPATHY)

Coeliac disease affects about 1 in 1800 of the population. There is hypersensitivity or toxic reaction of the small intestine mucosa to the gliadin component of gluten—a group of proteins present in wheat, rye, barley and possibly oats. Destruction of villi (villous atrophy) and inflammation follow ingestion of gluten and can result in malabsorption, abdominal pain and steatorrhoea or more subtle symptoms—coeliac disease is one of the great mimics in medicine.

Stunting of growth is sometimes conspicuous but, at the opposite extreme, symptoms can be minimal or absent and the diagnosis is made only after some complication develops; indeed, the diagnosis is not uncommonly missed. Recurrent aphthae, anaemia or infertility are examples of non–specific effects that may ultimately lead to the diagnosis at almost any age.

General management

The diagnosis of coeliac disease depends on the clinical features, particularly those of malabsorption and its complications, such as low blood folate and carotene levels (the screening method of choice) and findings of antibodies of gliadin and to endomysium. Jejunal biopsy should show villous atrophy. The biopsy, if positive, is repeated after a gluten-free diet has been maintained for about 3 months. In children the same procedure is used, except that an additional biopsy is carried out after a test challenge of gluten, as it is essential to establish the diagnosis with certainty from the outset and to eliminate such conditions as self–limiting but prolonged postinfectious gastroenteritis which can cause a histologically similar lesion.

Nutritional deficiencies should be rectified and a gluten-free diet adhered to. Patients require continued supervision, as there is often difficulty in keeping to the diet. Coeliac disease may also occasionally be complicated by gastrointestinal malignancy, especially lymphoma of the small intestine.

Dental aspects

Coeliac disease may be found in up to 5 per cent of patients with recurrent aphthae and should be suspected if there are any other symptoms suggestive of small intestine disease. Other oral complaints include glossitis, burning mouth or angular stomatitis. Short stature associated with diarrhoea and enamel defects are particularly suggestive of early onset coeliac disease. A surprisingly wide range of foods and beverages contain gluten and care must be taken not to interfere with the gluten-free diet. Anaemia may complicate treatment.

Dermatitis herpetiformis

Dermatitis herpetiformis is an uncommon chronic skin disease related to coeliac disease. It usually affects males past middle age, and causes an itchy papulovesicular eruption, usually on the extensor surfaces of the upper limbs and trunk. It leaves pigmented areas on healing. Diagnosis is established by demonstrating deposits of IgA at the papillae at the epithelial basement membrane zone (BMZ), with papillary tip microabscesses and a sub-epithelial split. Anti-endomysial antibodies may be detectable.

Serum immune complexes are often found, but decline if the patient is put on a gluten-free diet which, if strictly adhered to, may be of considerable benefit.

Dental aspects

Oral lesions in dermatitis herpetiformis are usually innocuous but may be erythematous, vesicular, purpuric or sometimes erosive. Patients are usually managed with dapsone, which rarely causes a lichenoid eruption, or sulphapyridine, which may cause erythema multiforme. Rarely, dermatitis herpetiformis is a complication of internal cancer (*see Table 5.19*). Linear IgA disease is a rare variant in which the IgA deposits are linear at the BMZ. Similar oral manifestations to dermatitis herpetiformis may be seen.

CROHN'S DISEASE (REGIONAL ENTERITIS OR ILEITIS)

Crohn's disease is an inflammatory disease of unknown cause that, with ulcerative colitis is one of a spectrum of diseases which have many features in common and are termed *chronic inflammatory bowel disease.* Crohn's disease can affect any part of the gastrointestinal tract but especially the ileocaecal region, typically with ulceration, fissuring and fibrosis of the wall. Microscopically, a submucosal chronic inflammatory infiltrate with non-caseating granulomas is found.

The manifestations of Crohn's disease depend on its severity and the site affected. Small intestinal involvement may cause abdominal pain that often mimics appendicitis, with malabsorption or abnormal bowel habits. Colonic Crohn's disease may mimic ulcerative colitis and is frequently associated with chronic perianal disease. ·

Complications include gastrointestinal obstruction, internal or external fistulas, perianal fissures, abscesses, troublesome arthralgia and sometimes renal damage (renal stones or infections). There is also a slightly increased predisposition to small bowel carcinoma.

General management

The diagnosis of Crohn's disease is confirmed by sigmoidoscopy, rectal mucosal biopsy and radiography. Barium enemas of large and small bowel, or barium meal and follow-through, are required. Rectal biopsies often show typical granulomas when Crohn's disease affects either the large or small intestine. Haematological examination may show deficiencies of iron, folate or vitamin B_{12}. The ESR and acute phase proteins such as C-reactive protein and seromucoid are usually raised but the serum potassium, zinc and albumin are depressed.

The major differential diagnoses include ulcerative colitis, tuberculosis, ischaemic colitis, infections, infestations such as giardiasis, and lymphoma. Management includes correction of nutritional deficiencies, but there is no specific treatment. Sulphasalazine or corticosteroids may be useful in acute disease; olsalazine and mesalazine are newer alternatives which lack sulphonamide side effects. Any of these may be supplemented with metronidazole, and azathioprine may be used in unresponsive patients. Surgery (usually resection) becomes necessary at some stage in most patients with intestinal Crohn's disease, but nearly 50 per cent relapse within 10 years of operation and, overall, treatment is unsatisfactory.

Dental aspects

Oral lesions may be caused by Crohn's disease itself, by associated nutritional defects, or may be coincidental. Oral lesions of Crohn's disease include ulcers, facial or labial swelling (*Fig.* 7.1), mucosal tags or 'cobblestone' proliferation of the mucosa. Some of these patients may have asymptomatic intestinal disease, or develop intestinal disease later. Melkersson–Rosenthal syndrome (facial swelling, facial palsy and fissured tongue) and cheilitis granulomatosa may possibly also be

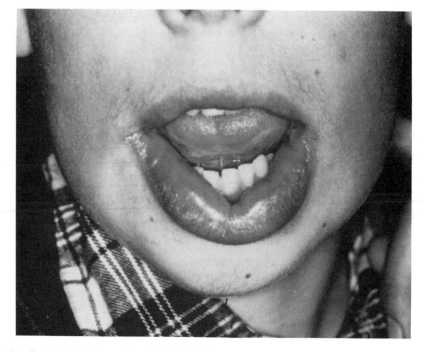

Fig. 7.1. Facial and labial swelling in Crohn's disease.

incomplete manifestations of Crohn's disease. Patients with atypical ulcers, especially when they are large,linear and ragged, or those with recurrent facial swellings should have biopsy of the mucosa in addition to other investigations. Biopsies in oral Crohn's disease typically show granulomas and lymphoedema and in their absence diagnosis is somewhat speculative. Sarcoidosis and tuberculosis are the main differential diagnoses. Microscopically similar granulomatous lesions may also be seen in the absence of systemic disease and may possibly result from reactions to some foods or medicaments. This condition has been termed 'orofacial granulomatosis' but this should not be confused with midfacial (midline) granuloma syndrome (Chapter 16).

Oral effects of malabsorption may also be seen. Dental management may be complicated by any of the problems associated with malabsorption or by corticosteroid or other immunosuppressive treatment.

An increased prevalence of caries in Crohn's disease has been reported. There is also continued investigation of the possibility that (as suggested in the 1930s when the disease was first described) the fine particulate matter in toothpastes may an aetiological factor, as a result of the relative impermeability of the intestinal mucosa to insoluble material.

PEUTZ–JEGHERS SYNDROME (*see* Table 7.11)

THE PANCREAS

ACUTE PANCREATITIS

Acute pancreatitis may be precipitated by gallstone disease, alcoholism, hypercalcaemia, hyperlipidaemia, viral infections such as mumps, drugs such as corticosteroids or phenothiazines, or various other factors.

Acute pancreatitis causes acinar damage and activation of enzymes leading to local fat necrosis and systemic effects such as severe abdominal pain, nausea, vomiting and shock. Mild pancreatitis usually resolves in a few days, but in fulminating pancreatitis the patient is severely ill with retroperitoneal haemorrhage, pleural effusion and paralytic ileus. Metabolic complications include hypocalcaemia, hyperbilirubinaemia, hyperglycaemia and raised serum levels of alkaline phosphatase, the transaminases, amylase and lipase. Radiology and ultrasonography aid the diagnosis.

The mortality in acute pancreatitis is 15–25 per cent. Treatment of shock and metabolic complications and relief of pain are essential.

CHRONIC PANCREATITIS

Chronic pancreatitis is of similar aetiology to acute pancreatitis; gallstone disease and alcoholism are frequently aetiological factors but malnutrition, hyperparathyroidism, haemochromatosis, hyperlipidaemia, carcinoma, cystic fibrosis and other factors may be implicated.

Chronic pancreatitis results in acinar atrophy and deterioration in both endocrine and exocrine function. Abdominal pain is severe. Chronic dull pain is punctuated by episodes of acute pancreatitis. Many patients have abnormal glucose tolerance or frank diabetes mellitus, and weight loss is common.

Exocrine dysfunction is confirmed by a decrease in the volume, bicarbonate content and enzyme content of pancreatic secretions. Serum levels of amylase and lipase are often raised; faecal levels of chymotrypsin are depressed. Pancreatic steatorrhoea is suggested by high faecal fat and undigested faecal meat fibres.

Radiography demonstrates pancreatic calcification, especially in alcoholic pancreatitis, and the diagnosis may be supported by barium meal, duodenography, cholangiographic findings and endoscopy.

Management includes analgesics, treatment of diabetes and the oral administration of pancreatic enzymes to aid digestion.

Dental aspects

Factors, predisposing to or resulting from pancreatitis, that might influence dental management include:

1. Bleeding due to vitamin K malabsorption (Chapter 3).
2. Alcoholism (Chapter 19).
3. Hyperparathyroidism (Chapter 10).
4. Diabetes mellitus (Chapter 10).
5. Cystic fibrosis (Chapter 6).
6. Narcotic abuse because of severe pain (Chapter 19).

PANCREATIC TUMOURS

Pancreatic carcinoma appears to be increasing in incidence and is now about one-tenth as common as bronchogenic carcinoma. Carcinomas frequently involve the head of the pancreas and invade locally to cause biliary obstruction, pancreatitis and diabetes mellitus. Extra-pancreatic complications such as peripheral vein thrombosis (thrombophlebitis migrans) are also common. Radiography or percutaneous transhepatic cholangiography may be of diagnostic help.

Pancreatic carcinoma has the worst prognosis of any cancer (*see Table 5.20*). It is usually treated surgically, often with a bypass to relieve obstructive jaundice for as long as possible.

Dental aspects

In many cases the poor prognosis of pancreatic cancer may significantly influence the dental treatment plan (Chapter 5). Biliary obstruction may lead to bleeding tendencies, especially if there are hepatic metastases, and diabetes mellitus may be an added complication.

THE LARGE INTESTINE

ULCERATIVE COLITIS

Ulcerative colitis is an inflammatory disease of part or the whole of the large intestine and frequently of the rectum. The aetiology is unknown but psychosomatic symptoms are often associated. Women are slightly more frequently affected, particularly young adults.

Typical features are painless bloody diarrhoea with stools containing intermixed mucus. In severe cases there is abdominal pain, fever, anorexia and weight loss. Extra-abdominal signs of ulcerative colitis may be minimal unless there are complications such as iron deficiency anaemia caused by blood loss. However, arthralgia, uveitis, finger clubbing, erythema nodosum and other skin lesions such as pyoderma gangrenosum may be seen. An increase in platelets and some clotting factors may lead to thromboembolism. Various types of liver disease may complicate ulcerative colitis. The most serious complication is, however, carcinoma of the colon, which is up to 30 times more frequent than in the general population.

General management

Apart from routine examinations, all patients must have sigmoidoscopy and rectal biopsy to establish the diagnosis. Colonoscopy is also necessary if any polyps are seen radiographically. Patients with early onset colitis or with disease persisting for more than 10 years are most likely to develop colonic carcinoma and regular colonoscopy is needed.

Treatment includes sulphasalazine and local corticosteroids, often by enema. Systemic steroids may be required in acute exacerbations. A high fibre diet is indicated and any anaemia needs treatment. If symptoms are severe, the response to medical treatment is poor, or complications such as pyoderma gangrenosum or haemorrhage develop, colectomy should be carried out. This also eliminates the risk of malignant change and is curative.

Dental aspects

Oral manifestations in ulcerative colitis are rare but include pyostomatitis gangrenosum (chronic ulceration), pyostomatitis vegetans (multiple intraepithelial microabscesses) and discrete haemorrhagic ulcers or lesions related to anaemia. Since uveitis, skin lesions and mouth ulcers can be found in ulcerative colitis it is important to differentiate it from Behçet's syndrome (Chapter 16). Management complications may include anaemia and those associated with corticosteroid therapy.

DIVERTICULAR DISEASE

Diverticular disease includes both diverticulosis (diverticula of the large intestine) and diverticulitis (inflammation of the diverticula), but these can rarely be reliably distinguished. The disorder is common, affecting up to 25 per cent of adults over middle age, and involves particularly the descending and pelvic colon. Diverticular disease may result from a low fibre diet.

Diverticular disease may be asymptomatic but is often accompanied by dyspepsia, abdominal pain, constipation and flatulence. Complications include pericolic abscess, perforation or fistula formation.

Management includes a high fibre diet and reassurance. There are no management problems in dentistry, although codeine should be avoided.

IRRITABLE BOWEL SYNDROME (SPASTIC COLON)

This is a common cause of recurrent abdominal pain in which there is increased tone and activity of the colon, abnormal bowel habits and other symptoms. It may affect up to 30 per cent of the population and is the most common cause of referral to gastroenterologists. There is frequently a positive family history and patients frequently have anxious personalities. Many also have migraine or psychogenic oral symptoms such as pain-dysfunction syndrome, sore tongue or atypical facial pain (Chapter 14).

A high fibre diet is said frequently to be effective in controlling the bowel symptoms.

FAMILIAL POLYPOSIS COLI

This is an autosomal dominant condition in which multiple adenomatous polyps affect the rectum and colon. Carcinomatous change usually supervenes. Familial polyposis coli is a feature of Gardner's syndrome (Chapter 17; *Table 7.11*) with multiple exostoses of the jaws which also appear to be more common in patients with non-familial colorectal cancer than in the general population.

CARCINOMA OF THE COLON

Carcinoma of the colon is common. The peak incidence is in the sixth or seventh decades and the carcinoma usually arises in the rectum or pelvic (sigmoid) colon.

Carcinoma of the colon may cause abdominal pain, change in bowel habit, weight loss or complications such as anaemia, intestinal obstruction or perforation.

Abdominal examination may reveal a mass. Sigmoidoscopy and barium enema are needed and colonoscopy may be required. Surgical resection is the usual treatment, while radiotherapy may be useful for dealing with pain from recurrences. Spread is frequently to the liver. The 5-year survival rate is overall about 30 per cent (*see Table 5.20*).

Dental aspects

Anaemia resulting from chronic intestinal haemorrhage can cause oral signs or symptoms or complicate dental management. Mandibular osteomas may, as mentioned earlier, be markers of an increased risk of colorectal cancer.

ANTIBIOTIC-ASSOCIATED (PSEUDOMEMBRANOUS) COLITIS

Most of the orally administered antimicrobials can cause diarrhoea, but clinically significant colitis is rare. The most severe type was staphylococcal enterocolitis, usually caused by prolonged heavy doses of tetracyclines, particularly after bowel surgery. Now that the cause is recognized this type of colitis has become rare.

Lincomycin and clindamycin cause pseudomembranous colitis more frequently than other antibiotics, as a result of proliferation of toxigenic strains of clostridia, particularly *Clostridium difficile,* which are resistant to low concentrations of these antibiotics. However pseudomembranous colitis is not known to follow clindamycin in a single dose, which is now recommended for the prophylaxis of infective endocarditis as an alternative to penicillin. Other antibiotics usually allow the survival of more competitors to *Clostridium difficile* which cannot so readily proliferate as a consequence. Even so, other antimicrobials including the penicillins can cause colitis occasionally.

Clinically, antibiotic colitis is characterized by painful diarrhoea and passage of mucus. In some cases, in elderly debilitated patients especially, there is passage of blood and pseudomembranous material (necrotic mucosa), occasionally resulting in death.

Pseudomembranous colitis usually responds to oral vancomycin or metronidazole.

Bibliography

Beutner, E.H., Kumar, V., Chorzelski, T.P. (1989) Screening for celiac disease. *N. Engl. J. Med.* 320, 1087–8.

Black, M.J.M., Gunn, A. (1990) The management of Frey's syndrome with aluminium chloride hexahydrate antiperspirant. *Ann. R. Coll. Surg. Eng.* 72, 49–52.

Carpenter I. V. (1978) The relationship between teething and systemic disturbances. *J. Dent. Child.* 45, 37–40.

Cataldo E., Covino M. C. and Tesone P. E. (1981) Pyostomatitis vegetans. *Oral Surg.* 52, 172.

Cawson R. A. and Kerr G. A. (1964) Syndrome of jaw cysts, basal cell tumours and skeletal anomalies. *Proc. R. Soc. Med.* 57, 799.

Cawson R.A. and Spector R.G. (1989) *Clinical Pharmacology in Dentistry.* 5th ed. Edinburgh, Churchill Livingstone.

Challacombe S. I., Scully C., Keevil B. et al. (1983) Serum ferritin in recurrent oral ulceration. *J. Oral. Pathol.* 12, 290–99.

Chan S., Scully C., Prime S.S. et al. (1991) Pyostomatitis vegetans: oral manifestations of ulcerative colitis. *Oral Surg.* 72, 689–92.

Cooke W.T. and Holmes G.K.T. (1984) *Coeliac Disease.* Edinburgh, Churchill Livingstone.

Daniels T. E. and Cawson R. A. (1976) Disorders of the salivary glands. *Med. Int.* 2, 1146–8.

Epstein J.B. and Scully C. (1992) The role of saliva in oral health and the causes and effects of xerostomia. *J. Can. Dent. Assoc.* 58, 217–21.

Epstein J.B. Stevenson–Moore P. and Scully C. (1992) Management of xerostomia. *J. Can. Dent. Assoc.* 58, 140–3.

Grattan C.E.H. and Scully C. (1986) Oral ulceration: a diagnostic problem. *Br. Med. J.* **292**, 1093–4.

Gray R. L. M. (1978) Pigmented lesions of the oral cavity. *J. Oral Surg.* **36**, 950–5.

Jarvinen V., Meurman J.H., Hyvarinen H. et al. (1988) Dental erosion and upper gastrointestinal disorders. *Oral Surg.* **65**, 298–303.

Jones I.H. and Mason D.K. (1990) *Oral Manifestations of Systemic Disease.* 2nd ed. London, Balliere Tindall.

Kinsner J.B. and Shorter R.G. (1982) Recent developments in 'non-specific' inflammatory bowel disease. *N. Engl. J. Med.* **306**, 775–837.

Lamey P.I., Carmichael F. and Scully C. (1985) Oral pigmentation, Addison's disease and results of screening. *Br. Dent. J.* **158**, 297–305.

Leading Article (1984) An irritable mind or an irritable bowel? *Lancet* **ii**, 1249–50.

Leading Article (1989) A lump in the throat. *Lancet* **i**, 534.

Leading Article (1989) xerostomia and its management. *Lancet* **i**, 884.

Leading Article (1991) Oral granulomatosis. *Lancet* **38**, 20–1

Lu D.P. (1982) Halitosis: an etiologic classification, a treatment approach, and prevention. *Oral Surg.* **54**, 521–6.

Porter S.R. and Scully C. (1991) Aphthous stomatitis: overview of aetiopathogenesis and management. *Clin. Exp. Dermatol.* **16**, 235–43.

Porter S.R., Scully C. and Flint S.R. (1988) Haematological status in recurrent aphthous stomatitis compared with other oral disease. *Oral Surg.* **66**, 41–44.

Rasmussen P. and Espelid I. (1980) Coeliac disease and dental malformation. *J. Dent. Child.* **47**, 424.

Rooney T. P. (1984) Dental caries prevalence in patients with Crohn's disease. *Oral Surg.* **57**, 623–4.

Scully C. (1978) Mouth ulcers. *Update* **17**, 1431–50.

Scully C. (1982) The mouth in general practice. *Dermatol. Practice* **1**, 19–29.

Scully C. (1982) Serum B microglobulin in recurrent aphthous stomatitis and Behçet's syndrome. *Clin. Exp. Dermatol.* **7**, 61–64.

Scully C. (1983) An update on mouth ulcers. *Dent. Update* **10**, 141–52.

Scully C. (1986) Sjögren's syndrome: review of immunopathogenesis: clinical and laboratory features and management in relation to dentistry. *Oral Surg.* **62**, 510–23.

Scully C. (1987) *The Mouth in Health and Disease.* London, Heinemann.

Scully C. (1989) Oral parameters in the diagnosis of Sjögren's syndrome. *Clin. Exp. Rheumatol.* **7**, 113–18.

Scully C. (1992) Non-neoplastic diseases of the major and minor salivary glands: a summary update. *Br. J. Oral Maxillofac. Surg.* **30**, 244–7.

Scully C. and Cawson R. A. (1986) Common dental disorders. *Med. Int.* **2**, 1129–33.

Scully C. and Cawson R. A. (1986) White, red and pigmented patches. *Med. Int.* **2**, 113–842.

Scully C. and Matthews R.W. (1983) Mouth ulcers. *Update* **26**, 693–700.

Scully C. and Porter S.R. (1989) Recurrent aphthous stomatitis: current concepts of aetiological pathogenesis and management. *J. Oral Pathol. Med.* **18**, 21–27.

Scully C., Russell R. I., Cochran K. M. et al. (1982) Crohn's disease of the mouth; an early indicator of intestinal involvement. *Gut* **23**, 198–201.

Scully C. and Shepherd J. (1986) *Slide Interpretation in Oral Diseases and Oral Manifestations of Systemic Diseases.* Oxford, Oxford University Press.

Shanahan F. and Weinstein W.M. (1988) Extending the scope of celiac disease. *N. Engl. J. Med.* **319**, 782–3.

Snyder M. B. and Cawson R. A. (1976) Oral changes in Crohn's disease. *J. Oral Surg.* **34**, 594–9.

Strober W. and James S. P. (1986) The immunologic basis of inflammatory bowel disease. *J. Clin. Immunol.* **6**, 415–33.

Swann J. L. (1979) Teething complications, a persisting misconception. *Postgrad. Med.* **55**, 24–5.

Thompson W.G. (1984) The irritable bowel. *Gut* **25**, 305–20.

Trau H. (1982) Peutz–Jegher's syndrome and bilateral breast carcinoma. *Cancer* **50**, 788–92.

Wiesenfeld D., Ferguson M. M., Mitchell D. N. et al. (1985) Orofacial granulomatosis: clinical and pathological analysis. *Q. J. Med.* **213**, 101–13.

Worsae N., Christensen K. C. and Schiodt M. (1982) Melkersson–Rosenthal syndrome and cheilitis granulomatosa. *Oral Surg.* **54**, 404–13.

Wray D. and Scully C. (1986) The sore mouth. Med. Int. 2,1134–7.

Chapter 8

Hepatic Disease

The main problems in the management of patients with liver disease are:

1. Impaired drug detoxification.
2. Bleeding tendencies.
3. Transmission of viral hepatitis.

Liver diseases fall into three broad groups but there is some overlap. The main groups are shown in *Table 8.1*.

Liver diseases can have many effects (*Table 8.2*). Impaired degradative and excretory activity in parenchymal liver disease often results in the accumulation of drugs and metabolites in the body. Bilirubin, the breakdown product of haemoglobin, is normally conjugated in the liver to produce a water-soluble form for excretion. This bilirubin ester is excreted in bile and colours the faeces. If bilirubin is not conjugated (enzyme defect or parenchymal liver disease) or excreted (biliary obstruction) it accumulates in the body and colours the skin and mucous membranes (jaundice). Failure of the bilirubin to reach the intestine (obstructive diseases) results in pale faeces but dammed-back bilirubin spills over into, and darkens, the urine. Bile salts, which are needed for the

Table 8.1. Causes of liver disease

1. *Congenital hyperbilirubinaemia*
     Rhesus incompatibility
     Prematurity
     Gilbert's syndrome
     Crigler–Najjar syndrome
     Biliary atresia
     Others
2. *Parenchymal liver disease* (hepatocellular disease)
     Viral hepatitis
     Chronic hepatitis
     Cirrhosis
     Primary biliary cirrhosis
     Drug-induced hepatitis
     Others
3. *Extrahepatic biliary obstruction*
     Gallstones
     Carcinoma of pancreas
     Others

Table 8.2 Manifestations of liver diseases

Disorder	Main diseases	Consequences	Clinical features
Impaired bilirubin metabolism	Congenital hyperbilirubinaemia Hepatocellular disease	Hyperbilirubinaemia	Jaundice
Impaired bilirubin excretion	Extrahepatic obstructions Hepatocellular disease	Hyperbilirubinaemia Bilirubinuria	Jaundice Dark urine Pale stools
Impaired excretion of bile salts	Extrahepatic obstruction Hepatocellular disease	Rise in serum alkaline phosphatase +5′ nucleotidase Fat malabsorption → malabsorption of fat-soluble vitamins (especially vitamin K) → prolonged prothrombin time	Pruritus Fatty stools Bleeding tendencies
Impaired liver cell metabolism	Hepatocellular disease	Impaired clotting factor synthesis → prolonged prothrombin time Impaired albumin synthesis Impaired drug metabolism Rise in serum transaminases	Bleeding tendencies Oedema Coma or neurological disorders
Disorganized liver structure	Cirrhosis	Portal venous hypertension	Splenomegaly Bleeding from oesophageal varices

absorption of fats, are also held back and the faeces therefore become fatty. Malabsorption of fats also causes impaired absorption of fat-soluble vitamins such as vitamin K. Accumulation of bile salts is thought to be responsible for the itching, nausea, anorexia and vomiting seen in some forms of liver disease.

Impaired drug metabolism means that CNS depressants such as sedatives, analgesics and general anaesthetics may be potentiated and can even cause coma. Glucose metabolism is also disturbed and there may be disorders of calcium and sex steroid metabolism.

The synthesis of plasma proteins including most clotting factors is depressed in severe liver disease. Impaired absorption of vitamin K also leads to decreased synthesis of clotting factors. Patients with liver disease may therefore have hypoalbuminaemia and also bleeding tendencies that may be difficult to control. Other factors such as excess fibrinolysins, aggravate the bleeding tendency and both the prothrombin and activated partial thromboplastin times are prolonged (Chapter 3).

Chronic liver disease is also associated with obstruction to the portal circulation leading to portal hypertension, varices in the oesophagus and the risk of fatal haemorrhage and hepatic encephalopathy. Portal obstruction can lead to hepatic encephalopathy and chronic bleeding may cause anaemia.

Liver damage is reflected in a rise in various enzymes released into serum. Serum levels of aspartate transaminase (AST, sometimes called serum glutamine-oxaloacetate transaminase or SGOT), alanine transaminase (ALT, sometimes called serum glutamic pyruvate transaminase or SGPT) and γ-glutamyl transpeptidase (GGT) are often raised in parenchymal liver disease and GGT is particularly raised in alcoholic liver disease. Rises in the levels of these enzymes may, however, also be seen if there is tissue damage elsewhere. Biliary canalicular enzymes such as 5'-nucleotidase and alkaline phosphatase may be increased in the serum in obstructive jaundice, but again the enzymes are not totally specific.

1. CONGENITAL DISORDERS ASSOCIATED WITH JAUNDICE (HYPERBILIRUBINAEMIA)

Transient jaundice is common in neonates but usually of little consequence. More severe neonatal jaundice can be caused by prematurity or rhesus incompatibility and can lead to kernicterus (damage to the basal ganglia of the brain). This can be fatal or cause epilepsy or choreoathetosis (with or without mental defect) and deafness in survivors. Rare familial hepatic disorders characterized by jaundice are summarized in *Table 8.3*. The most common of this group is Gilbert's syndrome in which the serum level of total (but not conjugated) bilirubin is raised; bilirubin does not enter the urine and other liver functions are quite normal. Gilbert's syndrome is benign. However if the patient starves, takes alcohol or has a general anaesthetic, he may become jaundiced. After an anaesthetic the jaundice may be confused with the many other, more serious causes of postoperative jaundice (*see Table 8.16*). Severe congenital jaundice can result from biliary atresia or be intrahepatic. It rarely causes kernicterus but may lead to portal hypertension, hepatic coma or respiratory infection.

Table 8.3. Features of congenital hyperbilirubinaemias

	Gilbert's syndrome	*Crigler–Najjar syndrome*	*Dubin–Johnson syndrome*	*Rotor syndrome*
Prognosis	Usually benign	Usually lethal	Benign	Benign
Bilirubinaemia	Unconjugated	Unconjugated	Conjugated	Conjugated
Pigment in urine	—	—	+	+
Associated problems	—	Kernicterus	—	—

Other benign congenital disorders are rare, but include the Dubin–Johnson and Rotor syndromes. The Crigler–Najjar syndrome is more serious and can cause kernicterus as the bilirubin levels rise, and the condition is usually fatal in early childhood.

Dental aspects of congenital jaundice

Disorders associated with an early rise in serum levels of conjugated bilirubin (mainly rhesus disease) can cause dental hypoplasia and a greenish discoloration of the teeth. The familial disorders cause little problem except for the need to differentiate them from more serious liver disease. The more serious disorders may lead to a bleeding tendency and impaired drug metabolism (*see below*).

2. PARENCHYMAL LIVER DISEASE

The most common causes of parenchymal liver disease are summarized in *Table 8.1*. Many of the disorders may significantly affect dental management but only general aspects are considered here. Further details are given under the specific disorders.

Dental aspects

Impaired drug detoxification and excretion.   The effects of drugs in parenchymal liver disease are not entirely predictable. Factors determining the response include the type and severity of the liver disease, as well as induction of hepatic drug-metabolizing enzymes by previous medication. Drugs, particularly the barbiturates, liable to cause respiratory depression are especially dangerous.

Brain metabolism is abnormal and the brain becomes more sensitive to a variety of drugs. Encephalopathy or coma can thus be precipitated by sedatives, hypnotics, tranquillizers or narcotics. The effects may also be enhanced by reduced protein-binding of the drug resulting from hypoalbuminaemia.

Anticoagulants can cause uncontrollable haemorrhage since clotting factor synthesis is depressed and broad-spectrum antibiotics (at least in theory) may further reduce vitamin K availability by destroying the gut flora. Aspirin and most other non-steroidal anti-inflammatory analgesics such as indomethacin should be avoided because they aggravate the haemorrhagic tendency and because of the risk of gastric haemorrhage in those with portal hypertension or those with peptic ulcers, which are not uncommon in liver disease (*Table 8.4*).

Tetracyclines, erythromycin estolate, chlorpromazine, monoamine oxidase inhibitors and phenylbutazone which, in varying degrees, are hepatotoxic should be avoided where possible or used in lower doses.

Table 8.4. Drug use in patients with liver disease

	Contraindicated	*Use instead*
Central nervous system depressants	Barbiturates Opioids Phenothiazines	Pethidine* Benzodiazepines*
General anaesthetics	Methohexitone Thiopentone Halothane	Isoflurane Nitrous oxide Local anaesthetics
Muscle relaxants	Suxamethonium	Curare
Analgesics	Aspirin Codeine Mefenamic acid Phenylbutazone Indomethacin	Paracetamol*
Antidepressants	Monoamine oxidase inhibitors	Tricyclics*
Antimicrobials	Tetracyclines Erythromycin estolate Talampicillin	Penicillin Erythromycin stearate Amoxycillin
Others	Prednisone Diuretics Oral contraceptives Methyldopa Biguanides Lomotil Liquid paraffin Anticoagulants Anticonvulsants	Prednisolone

*Give reduced dose.

Local anaesthesia is safe and relative analgesia is preferable to intravenous sedation with a benzodiazepine. General anaesthesia, if unavoidable, must be given by a specialist anaesthetist. Premedication with opioids must be avoided; pethidine and phenoperidine appear to be fairly well tolerated but benzodiazepines are preferred. Benzodiazepines are preferable to thiopentone for induction; isoflurane is preferable to halothane (*see* Halothane hepatitis, p. 237).

Suxamethonium (Scoline) is best avoided since the reduction in cholinesterase activity in liver disease causes increased sensitivity to this neuromuscular blocker. Nitrous oxide with pethidine or phenoperidine appears to be suitable for anaesthesia but it is essential to avoid hypoxia.

Impaired haemostasis.   Impaired haemostasis leads to haemorrhage, especially into the gastrointestinal tract from oesophageal, gastric or duodenal erosions. In addition to the clotting defects, portal venous hypertension in cirrhosis leads to the formation of oesophageal varices which may rupture causing severe haemorrhage. Patients with parenchymal liver disease can therefore present serious problems if surgery is carried out. If the prothrombin time is increased vitamin K_1 10 mg parenterally (phytomenadione) should be given daily for several days preoperatively in an attempt to improve haemostatic function. If there is an inadequate response as shown by the prothrombin time, a transfusion of fresh blood may be required. Repeated gastrointestinal bleeding may cause anaemia (Chapter 4) or be fatal.

Underlying disease.   There may be underlying disease such as alcoholism (Chapter 19), autoimmune disease, hepatitis B, C or D antigen carriage or diabetes (Chapter 10).

Other complications.   Acute renal failure may complicate hepatic failure (hepatorenal syndrome) but the precise mechanism is obscure.

VIRAL HEPATITIS

The term 'viral hepatitis' usually refers to liver infection by hepatitis A, hepatitis B with or without delta agent, or non-A non-B hepatitis (particularly hepatitis C) viruses. Most, except hepatitis A, constitute a cross–infection risk in dentistry as they are transmitted parenterally. Other viruses are occasionally responsible (*Table 8.5*). Hepatitis B is discussed first because of its importance in dentistry but in the absence of a vaccine as yet, hepatitis C may become a more significant problem.

Hepatitis B (Serum Hepatitis, Homologous Serum Jaundice)

In the general population of the UK only 20 per cent of cases of viral hepatitis are hepatitis B. This infection is endemic throughout the world, especially in institutions, in cities and in poor socioeconomic conditions. Spread of

Table 8.5. Causes of viral hepatitis

Hepatitis A virus
Hepatitis B virus
Non-A non-B viruses (hepatitis C and E particularly)
Delta agent (hepatitis D)
Epstein–Barr virus (infectious mononucleosis)
Herpes simplex
Cytomegalovirus
Coxsackie B virus
Yellow fever

hepatitis B is mainly parenterally (via blood or blood products), particularly by intravenous drug abuse, sexually (especially among male homosexuals) and perinatally. The incidence of hepatitis B has been increasing but now seems to be declining in Britain.

The disease has an incubation period of 2–6 months, and has an acute mortality of less than 2 per cent. In a very few outbreaks the death rate has been as high as 30 per cent, particularly where there is also infection with the delta agent (*see also* p. 227).

Clinical aspects

The effects of hepatitis B virus (HBV) infection range from subclinical infections without jaundice (anicteric hepatitis) in the vast majority of cases, to fulminating hepatitis, acute hepatic failure and death. Most patients recover completely and suffer no untoward effect apart perhaps from some persistent malaise.

The prodromal period of 1–2 weeks is characterized by anorexia, malaise and nausea. Muscle pains, arthralgia and rashes are more common in hepatitis B than hepatitis A and there is often fever. As jaundice becomes clinically evident the stools become pale and the urine dark due to bilirubinuria. The liver is enlarged and tender, and pruritus may be troublesome (*Table 8.6*). Serum enzyme estimations are useful in diagnosis: aspartate transaminase (AST) and alanine transaminase (ALT) are raised in proportion to the severity of the illness and alkaline phosphatase, α-fetoprotein and serum bilirubin levels are also raised.

In the absence of complications, infection with hepatitis B appears to confer immunity. A high proportion of staff working in developing countries or in institutions for the mentally handicapped develop antibody to hepatitis B surface antigen in spite of a low incidence of overt hepatitis. This suggests that active immunity can be acquired naturally.

Table 8.6. Viral hepatitis: clinical features and biochemical changes

Stage	Clinical features	Serum bilirubin	Aspartate transaminase	Alanine transaminase	Alkaline phosphatase
Prodrome	Anorexia Lassitude Nausea Abdominal pain	N or ↑	↑	↑↑	N or ↑
Clinical hepatitis	As above plus Jaundice Pale stools Dark urine Pruritus Fever Hepatomegaly	↑	↑	↑↑↑	N or ↑

Arrows indicate a value above normal (N).

Complications of hepatitis B

Carrier state. Hepatitis B progresses to a carrier state, in which virus persists within the body, in 5–10 per cent of cases, more frequently in anicteric infections or those contracted early in life. In most patients who contract hepatitis B, viraemia precedes the clinical illness by weeks or months and lasts for some weeks thereafter before clearing completely. Carriers, however, may remain positive for up to 20 years, although some 5–10 per cent of carriers lose the hepatitis antigen each year. The carrier state appears to complicate anicteric hepatitis mainly, and may not therefore be suspected clinically. However, certain groups of patients, especially those who have received blood products and those who have immune defects, are predisposed to the carrier state. These 'high risk' groups are shown in *Table 8.7*. Most carriers are healthy but others, especially those with persistently abnormal liver function tests, develop chronic liver disease.

The prevalence of carriers in the normal population varies considerably, being low (about 0.2 per cent) in Western Europe and North America, rising to 5 per cent in the Middle East, up to 40 per cent in some parts of West Africa and even higher in Indo-China. Over 75 per cent of some populations such as Australian aboriginees (hence the term 'Australia antigen') are carriers.

Chronic hepatitis. Chronic liver disease appears especially to complicate insidious hepatitis B with mild or absent jaundice but continued malaise. The very young and old are particularly at risk, as are those who have persistent serum markers (HBsAg, HBeAg, and anti-HBc and DNA polymerase, *see Table 8.8* for details).

Cirrhosis (see p. 234).

Hepatocellular carcinoma. Epidemiological evidence has implicated hepatitis B virus (HBV) in the aetiology of hepatoma as a consequence of the cirrhosis. HBV nucleic acid acid has also been detected in this tumour.

Table 8.7. Viral hepatitis—high-risk groups for HBsAg carriage

1. Patients receiving blood products or multiple plasma or blood transfusions (e.g. haemophilia, thalassaemia) (especially in the Far East or Africa)
2. Immunosuppressed or immunodeficient patients (e.g. post-transplantation or due to malignant disease)
3. Residents and staff of long-stay institutions (especially for the mentally handicapped)
4. Health care and laboratory personnel (especially surgeons)
5. Intravenous drug abusers
6. Sexually active individuals (especially male homosexuals)
7. Patients from the Third World (especially Africa and Asia)
8. Tattooing and acupuncture (especially in the Far East)
9. Certain other disorders (e.g. Down's syndrome, polyarteritis nodosa)
10. Consorts of patients with hepatitis or any of the above groups
11. Some chronic liver diseases

Table 8.8. Serum markers of Hepatitis B infection in relation to progress of disease

	HBsAg	Anti-HBs	HBeAg*	Anti-HBe	HBcAg	Anti-HBc	DNA polymerase*
Late incubation	+	−	+	−	Liver only	−	++
Acute hepatitis	++	−	±	−	Liver only	++	+
Recovery (immunity)	−	++	−	+	−	+	−
Asymptomatic carrier state	++	−	−	±	−	++	±
Chronic active hepatitis	++	−	+	−	−	+	±

+ = Serum level elevated.
*Presence implies high infectivity.

Polyarteritis nodosa (see Chapter 16).

Serological markers of hepatitis B

Electron microscopy shows three types of particle in serum from patients with hepatitis B. The Dane particle probably represents intact hepatitis virus, and consists of an inner core containing DNA and core antigens (HBcAg), and an outer envelope of surface antigen (HBsAg). The smaller spherical forms and the tubular forms probably represent excess HBsAg. The other antigen from hepatitis B is the e antigen (HBeAg). Serological markers are useful in diagnosis and are of prognostic value in hepatitis B (*Table 8.8*).

Hepatitis B surface antigen and antibody. HBsAg (Australia antigen, hepatitis associated antigen, hepatitis B antigen) is a non–infectious protein found transiently in those with acute hepatitis B, and persists in those chronically infected with the virus (carriers) and in some who are non-infectious.

In a typical case of hepatitis B, HBsAg develops 20–100 days after exposure, is detectable in the serum for 1–120 days and then disappears. The serum becomes negative for HBsAg about 6 weeks after the onset of clinical jaundice and in most instances antibody (anti-HBs) develops and is detectable in the serum for many years thereafter. Persistence of HBsAg beyond 13 weeks of the clinical illness often implies a carrier state. The presence of anti-HBs in the absence of HBsAg implies recovery and immunity. Vaccination with hepatitis B vaccine, which consists of HBsAg, elicits an anti-HBs response.

Hepatitis B e antigen and antibody. The e antigen (HBeAg) is a soluble protein found only in serum that is also HBsAg-positive. However, only about 25 per cent of those who are HBsAg-positive are also HBeAg-positive and infectious. HBeAg is indicative of active disease and high infectivity. If HBeAg persists beyond about 4 weeks of the onset of symptoms the patient will probably remain infectious and develop chronic liver disease.

Development of antibody to HBeAg (anti-HBe) and loss of HBeAg usually indicates complete recovery and loss of infectivity. Asymptomatic HBsAg carriers often possess anti-HBe, and are usually a lower infective risk than those with HBeAg and DNA polymerase (super-carriers).

Hepatitis B core antibody. The core antigen of the Dane particle is found in liver biopsies in acute hepatitis B but not in serum.

Serum antibody to HBcAg (anti-HBc) is a sensitive marker of viral replication indicating current or recent infection. Anti-HBc associated with anti-HBs appears to indicate recovery and immunity to hepatitis. However, if anti-HBs is absent, anti-HBc suggests the carrier state or chronic hepatitis.

DNA polymerase. The core of the Dane particle contains the enzyme DNA polymerase which appears transiently in the serum early in the course of viral B hepatitis: if demonstrable in HBsAg carriers it, like HBeAg, appears to imply high infectivity.

General management of hepatitis B

Patients with hepatitis may benefit from bed rest and a high carbohydrate diet and should avoid hepatotoxins such as alcohol. Normal human immunoglobulin may confer some protection against hepatitis B but the evidence is dubious. Any such protection presumably depends on the titre of antibody to hepatitis B (anti-HBs), which varies between batches of sera.

Passive immunity may be temporarily conferred by high titre hepatitis B immunoglobulins (HBIG) but is only indicated for groups at risk or following accidental exposure when it should be given with active immunization (hepatitis B vaccine). Hepatitis B immunoglobulins should be given to non-immune subjects after acute exposure to infected material. The degree and duration of protection are, however, uncertain and it is not known whether immunoglobulin affects the sequelae of hepatitis B infection.

Active immunity as conferred by the hepatitis B vaccine is the most effective prophylaxis (p. 225).

Adenine arabinoside or acyclovir, and interferon are under trial for the treatment of *chronic* hepatitis B and may be of value.

Sources of infection by hepatitis B in the dental surgery

Although pure parotid saliva does not contain HBsAg, saliva collected from the oral cavity may contain hepatitis B antigens and nucleic acid (presumably derived from serum) and may be a source for non-parenteral transmission. However, the risk of transmission by this route appears to be low except where there is very close contact, as in families or children's nurseries or sexual contact, or possibly needlestick injuries. Hepatitis B can also be transmitted by human bites.

Blood, plasma or serum can be infectious: indeed, as little as 0.0000001 ml of HBsAg-positive serum can transmit hepatitis B. The main danger is from needlestick injuries and some 25 per cent of these may transmit HBV infection if the instrument has been used on HBV-infected patients.

Risk of infection in dental personnel

About 1 in 1000 of the UK population are HBsAg carriers. Even among *high-risk* patients attending dental hospitals (*Table 8.7*) less than 10 per cent are HBsAg carriers and 75 per cent of these are probably non-infectious (HBeAg-negative). There is clear evidence of unvaccinated dentists and other dental personnel contracting hepatitis, but several reports indicate that the risk is fairly low, especially if precautions are taken. Surveys in Scandinavia and Israel have failed to show a risk to general dental practitioners significantly greater than that to the population at large, but there is a greater risk for oral surgeons and periodontologists, and for those working with high-risk patients.

Vaccination against hepatitis B substantially reduces this risk and since use of this vaccine has become widespread, there are now few cases of hepatitis B among British dental staff. Good cross–infection control also reduces the risk.

Risk of transmission of infection to patients. Dental procedures can transmit hepatitis B to patients, although recent studies suggest that the dental surgery is no longer a significant source of transmission, if adequate precautions are taken.

In earlier studies, HBsAg carriage has been found in about 1 per cent of dental practitioners, who have occasionally transmitted the infection to their patients and in the USA in particular, oral surgeons appear to have been responsible for minor outbreaks in which there have been a few fatalities. Carriers of HBV can reduce, but not eliminate the risk of transmission of HBV by wearing surgical gloves.

Practitioners ill with hepatitis should stop dental practice until fully recovered. HBsAg-positive personnel should follow the precautions outlined below, and must wear protective clothing, gloves and mask. Testing for HBeAg may prove useful in identifying those individuals likely to spread hepatitis B, and HBeAg–positive dental surgeons may be advised to discontinue practice. HBeAg-positive personnel should certainly not treat immunologically compromised patients.

Hepatitis B vaccination

The current vaccine against HBV infection is Engerix B a recombinant vaccine of HBsAg. After vaccination anti-HBs develops, and confers protection against HBV infection. Vaccination also protects indirectly, against delta hepatitis. Immediate side-effects from the vaccine are minimal and no long-term reactions have been reported. Vaccination is recommended for all clinical dental staff, especially those working with high-risk groups. Protection probably persists for 3–5 years, but thereafter, booster immunization may be needed.

Dental management of the patient with jaundice, hepatitis, or a history of either

Jaundice is not a disease *per se* but the manifestation of several diseases. Although jaundice usually signifies liver disease the possibility that jaundice is a result of haemolytic anaemia should be considered.

In the presence of clinical jaundice or where, in the absence of jaundice, there are abnormal liver function tests, operative intervention should be avoided unless imperative. The responsible physician should be consulted for the diagnosis and for advice on management of dental treatment. The main problems in management (bleeding tendency and drug sensitivity) have been outlined above.

A more frequent problem for the dental surgeon is the patient with a past history of jaundice who requires dental treatment. It is wise in this event to try to establish the probable diagnosis. Jaundice just after birth is common, usually physiological and rarely of consequence. Jaundice during childhood is often caused by hepatitis A—also of little consequence. Jaundice in the teenager or young adult may be due to viral hepatitis (B, delta agent or non-A non-B). Jaundice in middle age or later is more likely to be obstructive.

It is not practical to screen all patients with a history of jaundice for viral carriage and even if it were possible, most carrier states follow anicteric hepatitis and would therefore not be suspected. Further, failure to detect HBsAg does not confirm absence of infectivity for hepatitis B, unless there is other evidence suggesting past infection and immunity (the presence of anti-HBs, and anti-HBe or anti-HBc). Testing will not exclude non-A non-B hepatitis carriage nor other infections.

The groups *most* likely to be carrying HBV are those with a recent history of hepatitis (often male homosexuals or intravenous drug abusers or both), or patients from Africa or South-east Asia. Such patients may also be carrying other infections. Venepuncture, where necessary, should be carried out in conformity with the current code of practice for cross–infection control. The bottle should be clearly labelled and the necessary laboratory request forms completed before venepuncture. Equipment necessary for venepuncture should be laid out on a plastic or metal tray, so that there is no contamination of working surfaces, and glutaraldehyde 2 per cent (Cidex) or sodium isocyanurate should be readily available for disinfection in the event of spillage of blood.

The operator should be experienced in venepuncture and should wear a gown and disposable rubber gloves. Ten millilitres of blood are withdrawn into a plastic 20 ml syringe or into a vacuum syringe. The needle must not be resheathed but removed with a needle removal device and immediately discarded into a suitable impermeable disposal container. The blood is gently introduced into the glass bottle with care not to contaminate the outer surface of the bottle. The bottle is closed and sealed securely in a plastic bag (coloured red or yellow) labelled as infected or biohazard. The syringe, mask and gloves are disposed of into a plastic bag and similarly labelled.

Management of patients positive for HBsAg and HBeAg. It is important to avoid penalizing HBsAg-positive patients by refusing them treatment since such actions may lead the patient to conceal the fact that he may be positive or is at risk. Furthermore, since most positive patients are unidentified, refusal to treat known carriers would not significantly reduce the risk to the operator.

Asymptomatic carriers of HBsAg: Although asymptomatic carriers of HBsAg may be infective, those whose serum is anti-HBe-positive/DNA-polymerase–

negative are a *very* low risk and can be treated in general dental practice provided that accepted precautions are taken.

Asymptomatic carriers whose serum is HBeAg-positive/DNA-polymerase–positive are the highest risk and may need to be managed in hospital dental departments that have appropriate facilities. Many carriers have other problems that influence their management (for example, HIV infection or drug abuse). Only staff who are immune (anti–HBs positive) should carry out dental treatment on very high risk patients.

Patients with acute hepatitis B: If patients are known to be incubating hepatitis B or are in the acute or convalescent stages of hepatitis, dental treatment should be deferred where possible until after recovery is complete. Virus is usually cleared by about 3 months after symptomatic recovery and then serological examination should be carried out to detect HBsAg and HBeAg carriage.

Essential emergency dental care during incubation or acute hepatitis should be carried out in a hospital department with appropriate precautions against transmission of infection. Due regard must be taken for the fact that the liver damage may influence dental treatment.

Symptomatic carriage of HBsAg: Patients with HBsAg carriage who also have liver or other disease should be treated in a hospital department as indicated above.

The Delta Agent (Hepatitis D Virus)

Delta agent (Δ agent) is an incomplete RNA virus carried within the hepatitis B particle and will only replicate in the presence of HBsAg. Delta agent is found worldwide and is endemic especially in the Mediterranean littoral and among intravenous drug abusers. It is not endemic in Northern Europe or the US but some haemophiliacs have acquired the infection and the prevalence is increasing. The incubation period is unknown. Delta agent spreads parenterally, mainly by shared hypodermic needles. Risk groups are as for HBV (*Table 8.7*). Delta infection may coincide with hepatitis B or superinfects patients with chronic hepatitis B. Infection may produce a biphasic pattern with double rises in liver enzymes, and bilirubin. Delta infection does not necessarily differ clinically from hepatitis B but it can cause fulminant hepatitis with a high mortality rate. Delta agent antigen and antibody can now be assayed: Δ antigen indicates recent infection; Δ antibody indicates chronic hepatitis or recovery. Vaccination against HBV protects against Δ agent.

Non-A Non-B Hepatitis (NANBH) and Hepatitis C

Hepatitis C accounts for at least 90 per cent of cases of post-transfusion NANB hepatitis and is responsible for much sporadic viral hepatitis, particularly in intravenous drug abusers, among whom its prevalence is increasing. By contrast, transfusion–associated hepatitis C is declining and will presumably decline rapidly once blood is routinely tested for it. Hepatitis C has a similar incubation period to hepatitis B (usually less than 60 but up to 150 days). The illness is usually less severe and shorter than hepatitis B, but 25–80 per cent have abnormal liver function tests after one year and many go on to chronic liver disease and liver cancer. Hepatitis C is responsible for a substantial proportion

Table 8.9. Comparative features of more common forms of viral hepatitis relevant to dentistry

	Hepatitis A (infectious hepatitis)	Hepatitis B (serum hepatitis)	Non-A non-B-hepatitis* (hepatitis C)	Delta agent (hepatitis D)
Incubation	2–6 weeks	2–6 months	2–22 weeks	?
Main route of transmission	Faecal-oral	Parenteral	Parenteral	Parenteral
Severity	Mild	May be severe	Moderate	Severe
Complications	Rare	Relatively few → chronic liver disease hepatoma polyarteritis nodosa chronic glomerulonephritis	Many → chronic liver disease ? other complications	Can cause fulminant hepatitis
Carrier state possible	No	Yes	Yes	Yes
Acute mortality	0.1 per cent	1–2 per cent	?	?

*Several forms.

of patients with chronic liver disease and may account for a significant number of those who were thought to have autoimmune hepatitis.

Serological tests (ELISA) are available to detect the C100–3 polypeptide of the hepatitis C virus, but anti–HCV IgG is usually not detectable until 1–3 months after the acute infection and may take up to a year to appear. A more sensitive method using the polymerase chain reaction (PCR) to detect viral sequences has also been developed but is not suitable for mass screening. The timing of its application is also critical as viraemia in HCV fluctuates. Testing for hepatitis C antigen by PCR suggests that most of those who are seropositive by immune assay are viraemic and (despite the presence of antibody) are infective, but radio–immune assay underestimates the prevalence of HCV.

Table 8.10. Precautions to prevent transmission of blood-borne viral infections in the dental surgery

1. The patient should be regarded as potentially infectious.
2. All dental staff should wear gloves, protective eye-wear, mask and gown. Staff with any exposed skin wounds must ensure those are covered.
3. All working surfaces should be covered with plastic sheeting or cling film.
4. Wherever possible, disposable instruments should be used.
5. To avoid any possible aerosol spread of HBV, HIV, other viruses and opportunistic organisms, ultrasonic scalers should not be used. Air-rotors should be used with a rubber dam.
6. To avoid needle-stick injuries, needles should not be bent, broken or removed from disposable syringes.
7. Intraoral radiographs can be taken provided each film pack is wrapped in a sealable plastic envelope before use. The cone of the X-ray machine should be wrapped in plastic sheeting or cling film.
8. A portable suction system should be used and a metal container used as a spitoon.
9. Dental impressions can be taken using a silicone-based material. The dental laboratory should have prior notice of the patient's high-risk status. Before pouring up, the impressions should be soaked in 2 per cent glutaraldehyde for 1 h, rinsed and then immersed in 2 per cent glutaraldehyde for a further 3 h. The dimensional stability of impressions is not affected by this process.
10. All disposable instruments and waste should be placed in puncture-resistant sharps containers (e.g. burn-bins) and double wrapped in plastic bags. The outer bag should be labelled as a biohazard containing contaminated waste. These should then be incinerated by the local health authority.
11. All non-disposable instruments that can be sterilized should first be physically cleaned in detergent and warm water and then sterilized. This can either be by saturated steam or by hot air. Boiling water is not sufficient.
    All non-disposable instruments that cannot be autoclaved should be soaked in 2 per cent glutaraldehyde for 1 h, washed in detergent and warm water to remove all debris, and then left to soak in 2 per cent glutaraldehyde; this should be left for 3 h at least.
12. All external surfaces of equipment and contaminated working surfaces should be cleaned with freshly prepared sodium hypochlorite at a concentration of 10 parts/10^6 available chlorine (1 in 10 dilution of household bleach). This should be left on the surfaces for 30 min before rinsing off. Metallic surfaces can be sterilized with 2 per cent glutaraldehyde solution; this should be left on for 3 h. Non-exposed surfaces can be simply washed down with hypochlorite or glutaraldehyde.
13. All non-disposable garments can be washed in a conventional automatic washing machine provided the washing cycle includes a 10 min period of 90°C water temperature.

Carriers of hepatitis C and any other form of non-A non-B hepatitis should be managed with the precautions recommended for HBV or HIV carriers (*see below*). The hepatitis C virus has been found in saliva and infection has been reported after a human bite. There is as yet no vaccine available against hepatitis C.

Precautions aginst cross–infection in the dental surgery (Table 8.10)

Organizations such as the British and the American Dental Associations have produced useful guidelines for cross–infection control but the essentials are summarized here.

Equipment: All working surfaces should be covered with disposable material. Disposable instruments should be used wherever possible and local anaesthetic cartridges and needles must *never* be re-used for any other patient.

Used equipment, should be clearly identified as infected and always handled with gloves before disposal into an impervious container, or washing and autoclaving.

Sterilization: Instruments, needles etc. must be placed in an impervious container before sterilization or incineration, and must be labelled as infective. Disposable instruments, dressings etc. should be incinerated. Non-disposable instruments should be rinsed in an effective disinfectant (*Table 8.11*) and sterilized immediately by autoclaving (134°C for 3 min) or hot air (160°C for 1 h). In hospital practice, ethylene oxide gas (10 per cent concentration in carbon dioxide) at 55–69°C for 8–10 h can be used. It should be emphasized that solutions of ethyl or isopropyl alcohol, quaternary ammonium compounds or chlorhexidine cannot be guaranteed to inactivate viruses. *Boiling instruments in a dental boiling water bath for 30 min is also unreliable.*

Non-disposable instruments and dental impressions that cannot be sterilized by heat should be disinfected by immersion for at least 1 h (preferably overnight) in a suitable disinfectant such as 2 per cent glutaraldehyde (*Table 8.11*).

Working areas are disinfected with 2 per cent glutaraldehyde, or hypochlorite (1 per cent available chlorine). Since HBsAg remains stable in blood stains for up to 6 months at room temperature and the survival of the other viruses is uncertain, spillage of blood should be disinfected by dropping a napkin on the area and flooding it with 2 per cent glutaraldehyde.

Protection of dental staff: All staff must be educated in the possible dangers of hepatitis, HIV and other infections, their modes of transmission and the precautions necessary to prevent cross-infection, particularly vaccination against

Table 8.11. Disinfectants active against Hepatitis B viruses and HIV

Disinfectant	Concentration	Trade name	Shelf life	Comments
Hypochlorite	10% of stock solution	Chloros, Domestos, Milton	Prepare fresh	Corrosive to metals
Glutaraldehyde	2%	Cidex	14 days	Care: may burn skin or mucosa

HBV. Immunocompromised staff should probably be absolved from the responsibility of treating infected patients.

The most effective measure in avoiding infection is extreme precaution against accidental cuts and pricks from instruments or needles. Protective clothing, namely surgical gown, gloves, mask and eye protection should be worn at *all* times during the treatment of all patients and also during the disinfection and cleaning of instruments and dental surgery. Surgical gloves alone, do not provide adequate protection against hepatitis; they are readily perforated, often microscopically, and should be changed between patients. Gloves, masks and other protective clothing must not be worn or taken elsewhere, unless in an impervious container clearly labelled as infective. Clothing should be autoclaved before laundering. These precautions are summarized in *Table 8.10*.

Should the skin be punctured by an instrument that has been used on a patient, the area of skin should be liberally rinsed in water and the advice of the nearest public health laboratory or hospital microbiologist sought. Where appropriate, blood from the patient on whom the instrument was used, and from the wounded person should be tested for HBeAg, delta and HIV antibodies to determine the possible risks.

Note: The use of surgical gloves during treatment of all patients has been advised in the preceding sections. Heavy domestic rubber gloves should be worn during instrument cleaning.

Chronic Hepatitis

Chronic hepatitis is a term applied to two inflammatory diseases of quite different prognoses *chronic persistent hepatitis* and *chronic active hepatitis*.

Chronic persistent hepatitis

Chronic persistent hepatitis is a benign condition, often of unknown aetiology but sometimes complicating viral hepatitis or other diseases (*Table 8.12*).

The main features are persistent lassitude and fatigue, intolerance of fats and alcohol, and an enlarged tender liver. Laboratory investigations show raised serum transaminases but normal levels of bilirubin, alkaline phosphatase, albumin and immunoglobulins. The diagnosis is confirmed by liver biopsy.

The prognosis is good and no specific treatment is required, but complete recovery may take some years and is aided by abstention from hepatotoxic agents.

Chronic active hepatitis

Chronic active hepatitis, by contrast, is a serious condition that frequently leads to cirrhosis. Chronic active hepatitis may be immunologically mediated (so-called lupoid hepatitis) or caused by various other factors (*Table 8.12*).

Lupoid hepatitis mainly affects women and is asymptomatic or causes mild fatigue. It may, however, be associated with arthralgia, diabetes, thyroiditis,

Table 8.12. Causes of chronic active and chronic persistent hepatitis

Causes	Chronic active hepatitis	Chronic persistent hepatitis*
Hepatitis B, or non-A non-B	+	+
Autoimmune	+	−
Alcoholism	+	+
Inflammatory bowel disease	−	+
Wilson's disease	+	−
α_1-Antitrypsin deficiency	+	−
Aspirin	+	+
Cytotoxic agents	−	+
Halothane	+	−
Isoniazid	+	+
Methyldopa	+	+
Paracetamol	+	+

Adapted from: Sherlock S. (1979) *Medicine (UK)* **18**, 908.
*Chronic persistent hepatitis may follow chronic active hepatitis.

haemolytic anaemia, ulcerative colitis, renal tubular acidosis, pulmonary infiltration or amenorrhoea. There is often a Cushingoid appearance, hepatosplenomegaly and recurrent episodes of acute hepatitis with jaundice. Lupoid hepatitis is characterized by negative HBsAg, hyperimmunoglobulinaemia G, smooth muscle autoantibodies, antinuclear antibodies, lupus erythematosus (LE) cells and HLA B8/DR3.

Chronic active hepatitis caused by hepatitis B virus mainly affects males, especially those who have been frequently exposed to hepatitis B (eg some homosexuals), some immigrants and the immunologically compromised. The condition may be asymptomatic or have features of chronic liver disease but only moderate rises in serum bilirubin, transaminases and immunoglobulins. In contrast to lupoid hepatitis, smooth muscle autoantibodies are not a prominent feature. Serological findings include positive HBsAg, HBeAg and anti-HBc. This type of hepatitis may progress to cirrhosis or hepatoma.

General management of chronic active hepatitis

Prednisolone is effective mainly for lupoid hepatitis. Corticosteroids may be used alone or with azathioprine in chronic active hepatitis and hepatotoxic agents should be avoided. Interferon is indicated for HBeAg positive patients.

Dental aspects of chronic active hepatitis

There are no common oral problems in chronic active hepatitis but Sjögren's syndrome is relatively common in lupoid hepatitis and oral lichen planus may develop. Hepatotoxic agents, aspirin and paracetamol should be avoided.

Other management problems include:

1. Chronic liver disease.
2. HBsAg carriage.
3. Corticosteroids.
4. Complicating disorders such as other autoimmune disorders, diabetes, Wilson's disease or α_1-antitrypsin deficiency.

Hepatitis A (Infectious Hepatitis)

Hepatitis A is endemic throughout the world. Spread is mainly by the faecal–oral route and by the consumption of contaminated food particularly raw shellfish, or water. The incubation period is 2–6 weeks but the disease is frequently subclinical or anicteric and has a mortality of less than 0.1 per cent. Infectious hepatitis usually affects children and gives long-lasting immunity and, since many adults have had the infection, there is little risk of a further attack if subsequently exposed to the virus.

The clinical features of hepatitis A are similar to those of hepatitis B but muscle pains, rashes and arthralgia are rare (*Table 8.9*). Recovery is usually uneventful, the blood and faeces become non-infective during or shortly after the acute illness and there is no evidence either of a carrier state or of the progression of hepatitis A to chronic liver disease.

The diagnosis can be confirmed by demonstrating serum antibodies to the virus (HAAb). No treatment is usually needed. Normal human immunoglobulin may prevent or attenuate the clinical illness, but does not necessarily prevent infection. It is used mainly in sporadic outbreaks. A vaccine is available prophylaxis in travellers to Asia and Africa where there is a high endemic rate.

Hepatitis A and dentistry

Hepatitis A is communicable for only about 2–3 weeks—or the latter half of the incubation period until a few days after the onset of jaundice.There appears to be no evidence to transmission of hepatitis A in dentistry.

Hepatitis E

A NANB virus transmitted enterically and causing a disease similar to hepatitis A has recently been identified as the hepatitis E virus, which is an unenveloped single–stranded RNA virus.

Enterically transmitted NANB hepatitis is epidemic in India, South East Asia, parts of the CIS and Africa. It has a high mortality (up to 40 per cent) in pregnant women.

Hepatitis E is not known to be transmitted during dentistry but is a hazard to travellers particularly to the countries mentioned earlier.

CIRRHOSIS

Cirrhosis is a late result of parenchymal liver damage, leading to fibrosis, nodular regeneration and vascular derangement. Cirrhosis is a non–specific reaction to a wide variety of factors (*Table 8.13*). The aetiology is, however, known in only relatively few cases: most are idiopathic (cryptogenic cirrhosis) or, increasingly frequently, alcoholic, but cirrhosis can also be a sequel to hepatitis B and NANB.

Table 8.13. Causes of cirrhosis

Adults
Idiopathic (cryptogenic)
Alcoholism
Hepatitis B
Hepatitis non-A non-B
Chronic active hepatitis
Primary biliary cirrhosis
Wilson's disease
α_1-Antitrypsin deficiency
Haemochromatosis
Congestive cardiac failure
Children
Cystic fibrosis
Chronic active hepatitis
Wilson's disease
α_1-Antitrypsin deficiency
Galactosaemia

Cirrhosis chiefly affects the middle-aged or elderly. The main features result from hepatocellular damage or portal venous hypertension (*Table 8.14*) but cirrhosis is frequently asymptomatic in the earlier stages. Anorexia, malaise and

Table 8.14. Cirrhosis—clinical features

Jaundice
Ascites
Swollen ankles
Gastrointestinal haemorrhage
Mental confusion
Hepatomegaly
Splenomegaly
Finger clubbing
Skin manifestations
    Spider naevi
    Palmar erythema
    Opaque nails
    Sparse hair
Other occasional manifestations
    Parotid swelling
    Gynaecomastia
    Bleeding (liver failure)
    Portal hypertension and varices

weight loss are common. Jaundice, hepatosplenomegaly, ascites, gastrointestinal haemorrhage, palmar erythema, spider naevi, finger clubbing, opaque nails, pigmentation, fluid retention, bruising and other features may be present. Alcoholic cirrhosis may have associated parotid swelling (sialosis), Dupuytren's contracture, gastric ulceration or pancreatitis.

Laboratory tests are non-specific with no consistent pattern of abnormalities. Serum bilirubin levels, immunoglobulins, transaminases and alkaline phosphatase may be raised. Serum albumin is often low. Haematological abnormalities include a prolonged prothrombin time, anaemia, macrocytosis, thrombocytopenia and sometimes leucocytosis.

Cirrhosis is a serious disorder with complications which include:

1. Portal–systemic encephalopathy, which can be precipitated by drugs, gastrointestinal haemorrhage or a high protein diet and lead to coma.

2. Haemorrhage from oesophageal varices causing anaemia or death. (Blood may be vomited—haematemesis.)

3. Ascites.

4. Diabetes mellitus.

5. Hepatoma.

6. Peptic ulceration.

General management

Where a specific cause has been identified it should be treated if possible, and in those with chronic active hepatitis, interferon, corticosteroids or immunosuppressives may be indicated. Adequate nutrition is maintained and the management is mainly directed towards the prevention and treatment of complications.

Dental aspects

Routine dental treatment can usually be carried out without any particular problem. The physician should be contacted if surgery or general anaesthesia is needed. Surgery is hazardous in view of bleeding tendencies, diabetes, anaemia, drug therapy, possible HBV or NANB virus carriage or infection, and poor wound healing. In advanced cirrhosis, surgery, and particularly general anaesthesia, are so hazardous that the patient should be referred to hospital for treatment. Alcoholism may be a problem.

PRIMARY BILIARY CIRRHOSIS

Primary biliary cirrhosis (PBC) is a rare, progressive, inflammatory disorder of intrahepatic bile ducts. It begins with non-suppurative destructive cholangitis and culminates in cirrhosis. The vast majority of patients with PBC are middle-aged women. Patients may be asymptomatic for many years but eventually complain of weakness, lethargy, weight loss, pale stools and dark urine, jaundice and pruritus. The biochemical features also resemble those of obstructive jaundice. Complications include skin pigmentation and xanthomas, osteomalacia, or the complications of any chronic liver disease. PBC may be complicated by other connective tissue diseases particularly systemic sclerosis (scleroderma) or Sjögren's syndrome. Most patients have serum autoantibodies to mitochondria, and hyperimmunoglobulinaemia.

General management

Cholestyramine is often needed to relieve pruritus. Vitamins A, D and K are required (intramuscularly) and oral medium-chain triglycerides improve nutrition. Penicillamine may be of benefit.

Dental management

Sjögren's syndrome complicates 70 per cent or more cases of PBC (Chapter 16); oral lichen planus is an occasional complication. Penicillamine occasionally causes polymyositis (Chapter 11), pemphigus or myasthenia. Penicillamine may also cause lichenoid lesions, oral ulceration and loss of taste; zinc supplements may then help.

Patients with PBC may present similar management problems to those with other parenchymal liver diseases.

DRUG-INDUCED LIVER DISEASE

Many drugs, especially alcohol, may induce liver damage. In some cases this is a predictable dose-related effect, while in others the damage is unpredictable and may be related to an immunological reaction.

Dose-related damage may be induced especially by alcohol, tetracyclines, carbon tetrachloride or paracetamol, but many other drugs may be responsible (Table 8.15).

Damage that is unpredictable and may be immunologically mediated is induced by many other drugs (Table 8.15), especially halothane, the phenothiazines and sulphonamides.

Table 8.15. Drug and chemically-related liver disease

Dose-related liver damage	Non-dose-related liver damage
Alcohol	Halothane
Tetracyclines	Sulphonamides
Ketoconazole	Erythromycin estolate
Paracetamol	Anti-thyroid drugs
Methyldopa	Phenytoin
Isoniazid	Nitrofurantoin
Methyltestosterone and anabolic steroids	Phenylbutazone
Vinyl chloride and carbon tetrachloride	Phenothiazines

Dental aspects

The major problems in dentistry are those created by the tetracyclines, erythromycin estolate, halothane and, possibly, aspirin.

Tetracyclines.   The extent of liver damage is related to the blood levels and the danger of hepatotoxicity is therefore increased if there is impaired urinary excretion. However, there is a risk of liver damage only if massive doses of tetracyclines are administered.

Erythromycin estolate.   Erythromycin estolate, is potentially hepatotoxic but the effect is reversible when the drug is stopped. Erythromycin stearate is not hepatotoxic.

Halothane.   Abnormal liver function tests and occasionally jaundice or liver failure may follow any general anaesthetic and may result from such factors as contaminated infusions or the stress of surgery (*see Table 8.16*), so that it is difficult to establish the relationship of hepatic reactions to the anaesthetic agent itself. The frequency of reactions to halothane is at a level low enough to have very little impact on postoperative mortality and morbidity. However, halothane can undoubtedly cause hepatitis which may follow a single exposure in 1 in 35000 cases.

Transient impairment of liver function appears after halothane as after other anaesthetics, but there is evidence that liver damage is more common in middle-aged females, the obese and especially when anaesthetics are given repeatedly at intervals of less than a month. There also appears to be a genetic susceptibility.

The reaction may be some form of hypersensitivity but the precise mechanism is uncertain and pre-existing liver disease does *not* appear to be a contributory factor.

Clinically, halothane hepatitis causes pyrexia developing after a week postoperatively. Malaise, anorexia and jaundice may then appear, and if the jaundice is severe, the prognosis is very poor.

Unfortunately there are no dependable criteria or laboratory tests to indicate when halothane is truly contraindicated. Serum antibodies reacting with halothane–altered liver membrane determinants have been reported in about 75 per cent of patients, but as with antibodies to penicillin, few patients have a reaction on a further exposure. Nevertheless it is now advised, that halothane should not be given repeatedly, or within a period of 6 months, and never to any patient who has had malaise, pyrexia or jaundice after halothane anaesthesia.

Enflurane and isoflurane.   Enflurane and particularly, isoflurane do not induce hepatitis in those who have had an episode of halothane hepatitis. In many hospitals isoflurane has, despite its cost, replaced halothane, particularly to carry out several operations on the same patient at short intervals

Aspirin and Reye's sydrome.   There is some evidence that the use of aspirin in children who have an upper respiratory tract infection, chickenpox, influenza or other viral infections, may rarely precipitate liver damage with encephalopathy (Reye's syndrome). Aspirin is therefore contraindicated for children under 12, except for certain specific diseases. Paracetamol in moderate dosage only is now the preferred analgesic and antipyretic in most circumstances.

Since this precaution seems to have been widely implemented the mortality from Reye's syndrome has declined significantly and the disease has become rare. In the period 1989/1990 there were only 7 confirmed cases in the UK and Ireland.

3. EXTRAHEPATIC BILIARY OBSTRUCTION

The main causes of obstructive jaundice are gallstones and carcinoma of the pancreas (see Table 8.1).

Dental aspects of obstructive jaundice

The main danger in surgery on the patient with obstructive jaundice is excessive bleeding resulting from vitamin K malabsorption. Surgical intervention should be deferred wherever possible in the presence of jaundice until haemostatic function returns to normal. If surgery is essential, vitamin K_1 should be given parenterally at a dose of 10 mg daily for several days in an attempt to correct the bleeding tendency (Chapter 3).

General anaesthesia in a severely jaundiced patient can lead to renal failure (hepatorenal syndrome). If general anaesthesia is unavoidable it must be given by a specialist anaesthetist; hypotension must be avoided and the anaesthetist will usually give an intravenous infusion of mannitol to cause osmotic diuresis and help prevent renal complications.

Gallstones

Gallstones are a frequent problem, especially with advancing age. Cholesterol-containing stones are the most common and the aetiology is usually unclear. Some patients on clofibrate, oral contraceptives or oestrogens appear to be predisposed to develop gallstones. Pigment gallstones may be a problem in chronic haemolytic anaemias (hereditary spherocytosis, thalassaemia or sickle cell anaemia).

Gallstones are often asymptomatic. Passage of the stones into the bile ducts, however, may precipitate acute cholecystitis, biliary colic, obstructive jaundice or acute pancreatitis.

Obstructive jaundice is characterized by pruritus, dark urine and pale stools. There is a rise in serum bilirubin esters, alkaline phosphatase, 5'-nucleotidase, a-glutamyl transpeptidase and transaminases. Radiology is a useful diagnostic adjunct.

General management of obstructive jaundice due to gallstone disease

Cholecystectomy is usually indicated in obstructive jaundice due to gallstones, but lithotripsy and medical treatment with chenodeoxycholic acid have a place in the treatment of asymptomatic stones.

Dental aspects of obstructive jaundice due to gallstone disease

Oral surgical intervention should be deferred wherever possible in the jaundiced patient in view of the risk of haemorrhage. Other potential problems such as the hepatorenal syndrome, have been discussed above.

POSTOPERATIVE JAUNDICE

Postoperative jaundice was mentioned in Chapter 1. It is a problem of some importance and may be caused by several factors (*Table 8.16*).

Table 8.16. Causes of postoperative jaundice

1. Increased bilirubin load
    Haemolysis due to haemolytic anaemia or incompatible transfusions
    Resorption of blood from large haematoma
2. Hepatocellular disease
    Halothane and other drug-induced hepatitis
    Gilbert's syndrome
    Viral hepatitis
    Shock
    Sepsis
3. Obstructive jaundice
    Bile duct damage
    Gallstone disease
    Pancreatitis

Bibliography

Blogg C. E. (1986) Halothane and the liver: the problem revisited and made obsolete. *Br. Med. J.* **292**, 1691–2.
Bouchier A. D. (1981) Diagnosis of jaundice. *Br. Med. J.* **283**, 1282.
Brown B. R. (1985) Halothane hepatitis revisited. *N. Engl. J. Med.* **313**, 1347–8.
Cawson R.A. and Spector R.G. (1989) *Clinical Pharmacology in Dentistry.* 5th ed. Edinburgh, Churchill Livingstone.
Centers for Disease Control (1982) Hepatitis B vaccine safety: report of an inter-agency group. *Morbidity and Mortality Weekly Report* **31**, 465–7.
Dinsdale R. C. W. (1985) *Viral Hepatitis, AIDS and Dental Treatment.* London, British Dental Journal.
Editorial (1980) The liver and halothane again. *Br. Med. J.* **1**, 1197–8.
Editorial (1980) Hepatitis B vaccines. *Br. Med. J.* **1**, 203.
Editorial (1980) Halothane and hepatitis. *Lancet* **i**, 203.
Editorial (1980) Hepatitis B virus infections among surgeons. *Lancet* **ii**, 300.

Editorial (1986) Halothane-associated liver damage. *Lancet* **i**, 1251–2.

Farrell G., Prendergast D. and Murray M. (1985) Halothane hepatitis. *N. Engl. J. Med.* **313**, 1310–14.

Gelman S. (1986) Halothane hepatotoxicity again? *Anesth. Analg.* **65**, 831–4.

Matthews R. W., Dowell T. B. and Scully C. (1987) Acceptance of hepatitis vaccination by auxillary dental personnel. *Health Trends* **19**, 22–7.

Matthews R. W., Hislop S. and Scully C. (1986) The prevalence of hepatitis B markers in high risk dental patients. *Br. Dent. J.* **161**, 294–96.

Matthews R.W., Scully C. and Dowell T. B. (1986) Acceptance of hepatitis B vaccine by general dental practitioners in the United Kingdom. *Br. Dent. J.* **161**, 371–73.

Matthews R.W., Scully C. and Dowell T.B. (1989) Attitudes and practices regarding control of cross-infection in general dental practice. *Health Trends* **21**, 10–12.

Morisaki I., Abe K., Tong L.S.M. et al. (1990) Dental findings of children with biliary atresia: report of seven cases. *J. Dent. Child.* May, 220–3.

Porter S.R. and Scully C. (1990) Non-A, Non-B hepatitis and dentistry. *Br. Dent. J.* **168**, 257–61.

Samaranyake L. P., Scully C., Dowell T. B.et al. (1988) New data on the acceptance of the hepatitis B vaccine by dental personnel in the United Kingdom. *Br. Dent. J.* **164**, 74–7.

Schiff E. R., de Medina M.D., Kline S. N.et al. (1986) Veterans Administration cooperative study on hepatitis and dentistry. *J. Am. Dent. Assoc.* **113**, 390–6.

Scully C. (1985) Hepatitis B: an update in relation to dentistry. *Br. Dent. J.* **159**, 321–8.

Scully C. et al. (1986) Use of the airotor in hepatitis B surface antigen carriers. *Br. Dent. J.* **161**, 355–56.

Scully C., Panthin L., Samaranyake L.P. et al. (1990) Increasing acceptance of hepatitis B vaccine by dental personnel but reluctance to accept hepatitis B carrier patients. *Oral Surg.* **69**, 45–7.

Scully C. and Porter S. R. (1987) Acquired immune deficiency syndrome and viral hepatitis. In: *Infection Control in General Practice*, Martin M. (ed.) ICI.

Scully C. and Samaranyake L.P (1992) *Clinical Virology in Dentistry and Oral Medicine*. Cambridge, Cambridge University Press.

Scully C. et al. (1985) Lichen planus and liver diseases: how strong is the association? *J. Oral. Pathol.* **14**, 224–226.

Shovelton D. S. (1982) The prevention of cross-infection in dentistry. *Br. Dent. J.* **153**, 2601.

Sims W. (1980) The problem of cross-infection in dental surgery with particular reference to serum hepatitis. *J. Dent.* **8**, 20–6.

Taylor, T.W.S. (1986) Halothane and the liver. *Br. Med. J.* **293**, 335.

Workshop Report (1986) *Br. Dent. J.* **160**, 131–4.

Zuckerman A. J. (1982) Priorities for immunization against hepatitis B. *Br. Med. J.* **284**, 686–8.

Chapter 9

Genitourinary and Renal Disorders

The common diseases of the genitourinary tract are infections, usually of the bladder or urethra. These usually have little relevance for dental care, although the symptoms may cause the patient to defer treatment for a few days. However, such infections may suggest that the patient is at risk from sexually transmitted diseases. Furthermore, several of the less common renal disorders pose special problems of dental management. Some previously fatal chronic renal diseases can also now be managed successfully, so that the number of patients with chronic renal disease and those treated with renal transplants who may require dental care is increasing. The dental management of these patients may be complicated by the underlying renal disorder and by many aspects of the medical or surgical treatment. Problems associated with the impaired excretion of drugs, hypertension, immunosuppression, anaemia and hepatitis virus carriage are common.

CHRONIC RENAL FAILURE AND RENAL TRANSPLANTATION

Chronic renal failure (CRF) results from progressive and irreversible renal damage as indicated by a reduced glomerular filtration rate (GFR) persisting for more than 3 months.

The causes of chronic renal failure include chronic glomerulonephritis, chronic pyelonephritis, congenital renal anomalies, hypertension and diabetes.

CRF is asymptomatic at first, but later there is significant impairment of all renal functions with effects on virtually all body systems. The symptoms and signs of CRF depend on the degree of renal malfunction. Early features are nocturia and anorexia. Advanced CRF is complicated by many problems (*Table 9.1*), especially hypertension and anaemia. 'Uraemia' is the term applied to the clinical and biochemical syndrome caused by advanced renal failure.

General management

Renal function may remain relatively adequate for long periods if the progress of the renal lesion is slow, but any stress, infection or urinary tract obstruction may precipitate symptoms. Initial management aims to reduce the level of blood

Table 9.1. Chronic renal failure: clinical features

1. *Metabolic*
   Nocturia and polyuria
   Thirst
   Glycosuria
   Increased serum urea, creatinine, lipids and uric acid
   Electrolyte disturbances
   Secondary hyperparathyroidism
2. *Cardiovascular*
   Hypertension
   Congestive cardiac failure
   Pericarditis
   Cardiomyopathy
   Atheroma
3. *Gastrointestinal*
   Anorexia
   Nausea and vomiting
   Hiccoughs
   Peptic ulcer and gastrointestinal bleeding
4. *Neuromuscular*
   Weakness and lassitude
   Drowsiness leading to coma
   Headaches
   Disturbances of vision
   Sensory disturbances
   Tremor
5. *Dermatological*
   Pruritus
   Bruising
   Hyperpigmentaton
6. *Haematological*
   Bleeding
   Anaemia
   Lymphopenia
7. *Immunological*
   Liability to infections

urea, electrolytes etc. by dietary control, but dialysis or transplantation becomes essential if function deteriorates. Despite the tendency to inexorable deterioration, acute complications such as uncontrolled hypertension, congestive cardiac failure, infections, urinary tract obstruction and biochemical disturbances should be controlled or promptly treated where possible.

General management therefore includes:

1. Low protein diet.
2. Potassium restriction.
3. Salt or water control.
4. Dialysis, peritoneal or renal, followed when appropriate and possible by renal transplantation.
5. Treatment of symptoms and complications such as hiccough, vomiting, fits and calcium loss.
6. Prevention of further renal damage (antibiotics or antihypertensives).

Intermittent peritoneal or renal dialysis is valuable but inevitably regular renal transplantation is needed. Haemodialysis is carried out, often at home or as an outpatient, for two to three 6–hourly sessions per week. An arteriovenous fistula is created surgically at the wrist to facilitate the introduction of infusion lines. The patient is heparinized during dialysis in order to keep both the infusion lines and the dialysis machine tubing patent. Control of infection is of paramount importance during haemodialysis as infection with hepatitis viruses or HIV is possible. Over 70 per cent of patients on haemodialysis survive 5 years.

Renal transplantation is now commonplace. Patients need to be immuno-suppressed, usually with a corticosteroid plus a steroid-sparing drug such as azathioprine or cyclosporin, to prevent graft rejection. They are therefore liable to infection (Chapter 16).

Dental aspects

In children with CRF, growth is usually retarded and tooth eruption is delayed. There may be malocclusion and enamel hypoplasia with brownish discoloration but tetracycline staining of the teeth should no longer be seen.

The oral mucosa may be pale because of anaemia, and there may be oral ulceration, a dry mouth, halitosis and a metallic taste. Insidious oral bleeding and purpura can also be a manifestation. The salivary glands may swell, salivary flow is reduced, there are protein and electrolyte changes and there is calculus accumulation. Recent studies indicate a *lower* caries rate and less periodontal disease in children with CRF.

A variety of white lesions may be seen. Oral candidosis may be persistent, especially in the immunosuppressed patient, or mixed bacterial plaques may develop on the oral mucosa. In other patients a form of keratosis resembling white sponge naevus, or hairy leukoplakia may develop in the absence of HIV infection. Rarely dental infections may spread with serious complications such as cavernous sinus thrombosis or metastatic infections, and oral bacteria are an important source of bacteraemias. Cyclosporin may cause gingival hyperplasia as may nifedipine which is frequently used to control hypertension.

Osseous lesions include loss of the lamina dura, osteoporosis and osteolytic areas (renal osteodystrophy). Secondary hyperparathyroidism may lead to giant cell lesions. There may be abnormal bone repair after extractions, with socket sclerosis.

The main management problems are with patients in CRF and with the immunosuppressed post-transplant patient who has had severe CRF and has been dialysed. Treatment may be complicated by:

1. Impaired drug excretion.
2. Corticosteroid or other immunosuppressive therapy (Chapter 10).
3. Hypertension (Chapter 2).
4. Infections at arteriovenous shunts.
5. Bleeding tendencies and anticoagulant therapy (Chapter 3).
6. Infections with hepatitis B, or other viruses (Chapters 8 and 16).

7. Anaemia (Chapter 4).
8. Renal osteodystrophy.
9. The underlying disease.
10. Dysrhythmias predisposed to by hyperkalaemia.

Drugs. Many drugs are excreted mainly by the kidney and may therefore have undesirably enhanced or prolonged activity if doses are not reduced in renal failure. Some drugs such as tetracycline, cephaloridine, phenacetin, phenylbutazone and aminoglycosides are directly nephrotoxic. Tetracyclines can also cause nitrogen retention and worsen renal function.

Few of the drugs likely to cause complications in CRF are used in dentistry. However, antimicrobials, hypnotics and anaesthetics may need to be given in reduced doses (*Table 9.2*) and, except in emergency, should be prescribed only after consultation with the renal physician.

Fluoride supplements can usually safely be given for caries prophylaxis.

Antimicrobials: Erythromycin, cloxacillin, doxycycline, fucidin and cephalothin can be given in standard dosage. The doses of some, such as penicillins other than cloxacillin, metronidazole and cephaloridine, should be reduced, since very high serum levels may be toxic to the central nervous system. Benzylpenicillin has a significant potassium content and may be neurotoxic and may therefore be contraindicated. The anti-anabolic effect of most tetracyclines can cause increasing nitrogen retention and acidosis in CRF: they should be avoïded, but doxycycline and minocycline can be safely given.

Analgesics: Excretion of aspirin and other non-steroidal anti-inflammatory analgesics is delayed and in any event, gastrointestinal irritation and bleeding

Table 9.2. Modifications to drug usage in chronic renal failure*

Type of drug	Best avoided	Dosage reduction needed	No dosage change usually required
Antimicrobials	Tetracycline	Benzylpenicillin	Cloxacillin
	Oxytetracycline	Ampicillin	Erythromycin
	Streptomycin	Amoxycillin	Cefsulodin
	Sulphonamides†	Methicillin	Fucidin
	Talampicillin	Cephaloridine	Doxycycline
	Inosine pranobex	Metronidazole	Minocycline
		Co-trimoxazole	Cephalothin
		Vancomycin	
		Acyclovir‡	
Analgesics	Aspirin	Opoids	Codeine
	Phenacetin	Pentazocine	
	Phenylbutazone	Pethadine	
		Propoxyphene	
		Paracetamol	
Hypnotics and	Phenobarbitone	Chlorpromazine	Diazepam
sedatives	Antihistamines	Promethazine	Chloral hydrate
		Chlordiazepoxide	Sodium amytal

See also current British National Formulary: for anaesthetics *see* text. Non-depolarizing muscle relaxants should be avoided. All drug doses should be kept to a minimum.
†Suphadimidine appears to be safe.
‡Systemic.

may be associated with CRF. Aspirin should therefore be avoided. Phenacetin is nephrotoxic and is in any case obsolete. Analgesics that can be safely used in renal disease include codeine and dihydrocodeine.

Hypnotics and sedatives: Diazepam or chloral hydrate can be used. Long-acting barbiturates (phenobarbitone) are contraindicated since their excretion is delayed. Chlordiazepoxide may produce depression and lethargy in patients with CRF and is best avoided. Antihistamines or drugs with antimuscarinic side-effects may cause dry mouth or urinary retention.

Anaesthetics: Local anaesthesia is safe unless there is a severe tendency. General anaesthesia should only be carried out in hospital by a specialist anaesthetist. Some of the difficulties with general anaesthesia are that patients with CRF are highly sensitive to the myocardial depressant effects of halothane or cyclopropane, and may develop hypotension at moderate levels of anaesthesia. Myocardial depression and cardiac dysrhythmias are especially likely in those with poorly controlled metabolic acidosis and hyperkalaemia. Enflurane is metabolized to potentially nephrotoxic organic fluoride ions and therefore should only be used with caution if other nephrotoxic agents are used concurrently. Isoflurane is probably safer. Induction with methohexitone followed by very light general anaesthesia with nitrous oxide is generally the technique of choice. In dental practice local anaesthesia should be used—with relative analgesia if necessary.

Other drugs: Antacids containing magnesium salts should not be given as there may be magnesium retention. Antacids containing calcium or aluminium bases may impair the absorption particularly of tetracyclines, but also of penicillin-V and sulphonamides. Cholestyramine, sometimes used in CRF, may also interfere with the absorption of penicillins. Many are on antihypertensive therapy, digoxin and diuretics (Chapter 2), which may also complicate management. Some have peptic ulceration which is a further contraindication to aspirin.

Immunosuppressive therapy: Patients with renal transplants are immunosuppressed, usually with corticosteroids and azathioprine, and may need steroid supplementation or antimicrobial cover during dental treatment (Chapter 10).

Postoperative complications.   Major surgical procedures may be complicated by hyperkalaemia as a result of tissue damage, acidaemia and blood transfusion. Hyperkalaemia predisposes to dysrhythmias and may cause cardiac arrest. Dialysis is avoided postoperatively if possible since heparinization is required.

Hypertension.   Hypertension is common in CRF and may affect dental treatment, and these patients are also liable to atherosclerosis.

Infections at arteriovenous shunts and transplants.   Dental surgery should be covered by antibiotic prophylaxis in view of the susceptibility of immunosuppressed patients to infections, especially at the arteriovenous fistulas or of the transplant. These patients may therefore need to be managed with precautions similar to those at risk from infective endocarditis (Chapter 2). An alternative is to give 500 mg vancomycin i.v. during dialysis, which gives cover for at least a day.

The veins of the forearms and the saphenous veins are lifelines for patients on regular haemodialysis. If, therefore, the dentist has to give (for example) intravenous diazepam or midazolam, or take blood, other veins such as those at or above the elbow should be used in case there is consequent thrombophlebitis.

Bleeding tendencies. Haemostasis is poor in CRF as a result of impaired platelet function. There may be defective platelet aggregation, decreased platelet Factor III and increased prostacyclin (prostaglandin I,) leading to poor platelet aggregation, and vasodilatation. The bleeding time is often prolonged and there is also an ill-defined clotting defect. Patients on haemodialysis are also heparinized during dialysis. Careful haemostasis should therefore be ensured if oral surgical procedures are necessary (Chapter 3). Dental treatment is best carried out on the day after dialysis, when there has been maximal benefit from the dialysis and the effect of the heparin has worn off, but the haematologist should first be consulted. Should bleeding be prolonged, cryoprecipitate and DDAVP may achieve haemostasis.

Infections. Infections are not only poorly controlled by the patient with CRF, especially if he is immunosuppressed, and may spread locally as well as giving rise to septicaemia or distant contiguous spread, but also increase tissue catabolism causing clinical deterioration. Infections can be difficult to recognize as signs of inflammation are masked. Odontogenic infections should therefore be treated vigorously and surgical procedures covered with antimicrobials (*Table 9.2*). Oral candidosis can usually be managed with topical nystatin, amphotericin or miconazole (*Fig. 9.1*). Aspergillosis and other fungal infections occasionally develop. Mixed bacterial oral mucosal plaques may respond to the appropriate antibiotic, trypsinization and possibly to an aqueous chlorhexidine (0.2 per cent) mouthwash. Some patients carry enterococci in plaque. Carriage of hepatitis viruses is common in haemodialysed or immunosuppressed patients, and patients with CRF should be kept away from sources of hepatitis (Chapter 8). Other infections such as herpes simplex or zoster, cytomegalovirus, toxoplasmosis and *Pneumocystis carinii,* to which the immunosuppressed patient is prone, are discussed in Chapter 16. Oral herpes simplex and zoster infections can be prevented, deferred or ameliorated by prophylactic low dose oral acyclovir.

Anaemia. CRF is invariably complicated by anaemia which is a contraindication to general anaesthesia if the haemoglobin is below 10 g/dl. Blood transfusions are best avoided in view of the risk of transmitting hepatitis and other viruses.

Other complications. Patients on immunosuppressive treatment after renal transplantation have a greatly increased incidence of malignant disease, particularly lymphomas and, to a lesser extent, skin and lip cancer. Cases have also been reported of oral keratosis, squamous cancer and of Kaposi's sarcoma in these patients.

Renal osteodystrophy. Renal osteodystrophy appears to cause increasing symptoms after the start of regular haemodialysis. Phosphate retention in CRF leads to depression of plasma calcium levels and subsequently increased

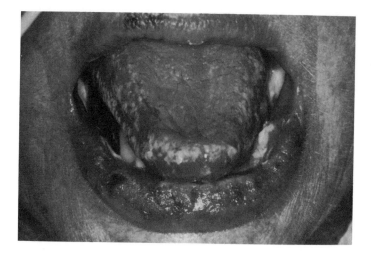

Fig. 9.1. Thrush (acute pseudomembranous candidosis) frequently implies underlying disease, in this instance immunosuppression with corticosteroids and azathioprine in a patient who has a renal transplant for chronic renal failure caused by diabetes mellitus.

parathyroid activity (secondary hyperparathyroidism). Parathyroid hyperplasia may eventually become adenomatous and irreversible (tertiary hyperparathyroidism) Phosphate retention may also interfere with vitamin D metabolism, and calcium absorption is thereby reduced, further contributing to the osteodystrophy. Vitamin D metabolism is also impaired by the renal disease. Patients may therefore be treated with calcium carbonate, aluminium hydroxide (to reduce phosphate levels) or the active vitamin D metabolite 1,25-dihydrocholecalciferol (1, 25-DHCC or its synthetic analogue DHCC). Parathyroidectomy may be necessary (Chapter 10).

Underlying diseases and complications. Consideration must be given to the effect on dental management of underlying diseases, such as diabetes (Chapter 10), systemic lupus erythematosus, polyarteritis nodosa (Chapter 16), myelomatosis and amyloidosis (Chapter 5), or complications such as peptic ulceration (Chapter 7).

THE NEPHROTIC SYNDROME

The nephrotic syndrome is characterized by massive proteinuria with hypoalbuminaemia, oedema and hyperlipidaemia. Oedema, especially of the face, genitals and lower limbs, and transudates in serous cavities (especially the peritoneal cavity) may result. Loss of immunoglobulins (especially IgG) in the urine predisposes to infections, often pneumococcal. Initially there is neither hypertension nor increased blood urea, but the serum cholesterol is raised. Loss of cholecalciferol-binding protein may lead to vitamin D deficiency, secondary hyperparathyroidism and bone disease. Loss of antithrombin III and increased Factor VIII may cause increased blood coagulability and result in thromboses.

The main causes of nephrotic syndrome are minimal change disease, diabetic nephropathy and systemic lupus erythematosus.

Treatment is aimed at reducing proteinuria, controlling infections, preventing thromboembolic complications and removing or treating the basic cause of the nephrotic syndrome. Treatment may include corticosteroids together with a low salt but high protein diet. Prophylactic antimicrobials may also be given.

Dental aspects

Many of the considerations in the management of the patient in chronic renal failure are also applicable to the nephrotic patient.

Drugs.   Long-term corticosteroid therapy is the main problem (Chapter 10).

Infections.   Treatment with corticosteroids and other factors such as electrolyte imbalance, hypoproteinaemia and hypoimmunoglobulinaemia predispose to infections.

Cardiovascular and haematological disorders.   Patients with the nephrotic syndrome are susceptible to cardiovascular disease (atheroma) because of hypercholesterolaemia. The blood concentrations of Factor VIII, fibrinogen and other clotting factors are also raised, leading to a hypercoagulable state. This may lead to spontaneous thromboses, especially in patients treated with corticosteroids. Immobilized patients are often, therefore, treated with heparin.

RENAL STONES

Renal stones are not uncommon. They may be seen on radiography or cause symptoms of renal colic or secondary renal damage. Although no underlying systemic disease is usually identified, stones may complicate gout, hyperparathyroidism, hyperoxaluria, cystinosis or renal tubular acidosis. There is no known predisposition to salivary calculi or dental calculus formation.

SEXUALLY TRANSMITTED DISEASES

See Chapters 16 and 17.

Bibliography

Brenner B. M. and Rector F. C. (1981) *The Kidney*, 2nd ed. Philadelphia. Saunders.
Buckley D. J. et al. (1986) Control of bleeding in severely uraemic patients undergoing oral surgery. *Oral Surg.* **61**, 546–9.

Burton J. R. (1972) Aspergillosis in four renal transplant recipients: diagnosis and effective treatment with amphotericin. *Ann. Intern. Med.* **77**, 383–8.

Cawson R. A. (1964) Defects of enamel structure in renal osteodystrophy. *Br. Dent. J.* **117**, 141.

Cawson R.A. and Spector R.G. (1989) *Clinical Pharmacology in Dentistry.* 5th ed. Edinburgh, Churchill Livingstone.

Chow M. H. and Peterson D. S. (1979) Dental management for children with chronic renal failure undergoing hemodialysis therapy. *Oral Surg.* **48**, 34–8.

Ciechanover M. (1980) Malrecognition of taste in uraemia. *Nephron* **26**, 20–2.

Cross A. S. and Steigbigel R. T. (1976) Infective endocarditis and access site infections in patients on hemodialysis. *Medicine* **55**, 453–66.

Eigner T. L., Jastak J. T. and Bennett W. M. (1986) Achieving oral health in patients with renal failure and renal transplants. *J. Am. Dent. Assoc.* **113**, 612–6.

Epstein S. R., Mandel I. and Scopp I. W. (1980) Salivary composition and calculus formation in patients undergoing hemodialysis. *J. Periodontol.* **51**, 336–9.

Fillastre J. P. and Godin M. (1980) Prescribing for patients with renal failure. *Medicine (UK)* **25**, 1299–303.

Fraser C.G. (1985) Urine analysis: current performance and strategies for improvement. *Br. Med. J.* **291**, 321–5.

Greenberg M. S. and Cohen G. (1977) Oral infection in immunosuppressed renal transplant patients. *Oral Surg.* **43**, 879–85.

Heard E., Staples A. F. and Czerwinski A. W. (1978) The dental patient with renal disease: precautions and guidelines. *J. Am. Dent. Assoc.* **96**, 792–6.

Hovinga J., Roodvoets A.R. and Guillard J. (1975) Some findings in patients with uraemic stomatitis. *Maxillofac. Surg.* **3**, 125–7.

Janson R. A. (1980) Treatment of the bleeding tendency in uraemia with cryoprecipitate. *N. Engl. Med.* **303**, 318–22.

Kellett M. (1983) Oral white plaques in uraemic patients. *Br. Dent. J.* **154**, 366–8.

Krekeler G., Whilms H.and Akuamoa-Boateng E. (1980) Inflammatory pathology in the dental system in renal transplantation. *Int. J. Oral Surg.* **9**, 383–6.

Leading Article (1988) Is routine urinalysis worthwhile? *Lancet* **i**, 747.

Milam S. B. and Cooper R. L. (1983) Extensive bleeding following extractions in a patient undergoing chronic hemodialysis. *Oral Surg.* **55**, 14–16.

Remuzzi G. (1977) Prostacyclin-like activity and bleeding in renal failure. *Lancet* **ii**, 1195–7.

Scully C. (1979) Orofacial manifestations of disease. *Hospital Update* **5**, 923.

Seale L., Jones C. J. and Kathpalia S., (1985) Prevention of herpes virus infections in renal allograft recipients by low dose oral acyclovir. *JAMA* **254**, 3435–8.

Shasha S. M. (1983) Salivary content in hemodialysed patients. *J. Oral Med.* **38**, 67–70.

Sheil A. G. R. (1977) Cancer in renal allograft recipients in Australia and New Zealand. *Transplant. Proc.* **9**, 1133.

Smyth C. J., Halpenry M. K. and Ballagh S. J. (1987) Carriage rates of enterococci in the dental plaque of haemodialysis patients in Dublin. *Br. J. Oral Maxillofac. Surg.* **25**, 21–33.

Stoufi E. D., Sonis S. T. and Shklar G. (1986) Significance of the head and neck in late infection in renal transplant recipients. *Oral Surg.* **62**, 524–8.

Stuart F. P., Simonian S. J. and Hill J. L. (1976) Special considerations in surgical management of patients on hemodialysis and after successful kidney transplantation. *Surg. Clin. North Am.* **56**, 15–19.

Tyldesley W. R., Rotter E. and Sells R. A. (1979) Oral lesions in renal transplant patients. *J. Oral Pathol.* **8**, 53–9.

Uthman A. A. (1975) Viral hepatitis and the dental treatment of renal dialysis and kidney transplant patients. *J. Oral Med.* **30**, 70–2.

Westbrook S. D. (1978) Dental management of patients receiving hemodialysis and kidney transplants. *J. Am. Dent. Assoc.* **96**, 464–8.

Zazgornik J., Schmidt P., Thurner J. et al. (1975) Klinik und therapie der pilzinfektionen nach nieren-transplantation. *Dtsch. Med. Wochenschr.* **100**, 2082–6.

Chapter 10

Endocrine and Metabolic Diseases

THE HYPOTHALAMUS AND PITUITARY

The hypothalamus controls pituitary function but is itself under the control of higher centres. The posterior pituitary is a downgrowth from the base of the brain and is connected by neurones with the hypothalamus. The posterior pituitary (neurohypophysis) stores two hormones produced by the hypothalamus—vasopressin (antidiuretic hormone, ADH) and oxytocin; and neurophysin. The anterior pituitary (adenohypophysis) originates as an outgrowth from the stomatodeum (Rathke's pouch). It produces seven hormones (*Table 10.1*) and controls many metabolic activities.

Although anatomically distinct from the hypothalamus, the anterior pituitary falls under its influence by factors passing through a portal venous system. Feedback control influences both the amount of hypothalamic hormone secreted and the response of the pituitary to a particular hypothalamic hormone.

POSTERIOR PITUITARY HYPOFUNCTION

Diabetes Insipidus

Diabetes insipidus is a rare disease characterized by production of an excessive volume of dilute urine. Diabetes insipidus is caused either by lack of antidiuretic hormone (ADH) secretion (cranial diabetes insipidus) or renal insensitivity to ADH action (nephrogenic diabetes insipidus).

Cranial diabetes insipidus is more common and can be caused by trauma, a tumour or vascular disease in the region of the hypothalamus or pituitary, or it may be idiopathic. The disorder may be temporary—especially after head injuries. Polyuria and persistent thirst are the main features, but a lesion in the hypothalamic area may also cause pressure on the optic chiasma leading to visual defects, or raised intracranial pressure and headaches.

The diagnosis of diabetes insipidus is established by demonstrating inability to concentrate the urine during a water-deprivation test. Skull radiographs, visual field charting and also tests of anterior pituitary function are used to assess the local extent of disease.

Table 10.1. Pituitary hormones

Hormone	Effects
Anterior pituitary	
Growth hormone (GH)	Growth (diabetogenic)
Thyroid-stimulating hormone (TSH)	Stimulates thyroid hormone synthesis and release
Adrenocorticotrophin (ACTH)	Stimulates glucocorticoid synthesis and release
Prolactin	Lactation
Luteinizing hormone (LH)	Gonadotrophin
Follicle-stimulating hormone (FSH)	Gonodotrophin
Melanocyte-stimulating hormone (MSH)	Pigmentation
Posterior pituitary	
Antidiuretic hormone (ADH)	Water reabsorption in renal distal tubules and collecting ducts
Oxytocin	Lactation
	Uterine contraction

Diabetes insipidus is treated with the ADH-like peptide desmopressin or other drugs having an antidiuretic action such as chlorpropamide.

Dental aspects of diabetes insipidus

Dentistry is usually uncomplicated by this disorder except for dryness of the mouth. Transient diabetes insipidus can be a complication of head injury.

Syndrome of Inappropriate Antidiuretic Hormone Secretion (SIADH)

Excessive ADH levels may be caused by some tumours (especially some lung cancers), drugs (carbamazepine and chlorpropamide). They occasionally follow maxillofacial or head injuries, anaesthesia, or even elective maxillofacial surgery, possibly because of trigeminal stimulation. The SIADH is characterized by water retention, overhydration causing confusion, behavioural disturbances, ataxia and dysphagia. Patients with SIADH are treated with fluid restriction, corticosteroids or demeclocycline.

ANTERIOR PITUITARY HYPOFUNCTION

The usual causes of hypopituitarism are local hypothalamic or pituitary lesions. There may be individual or more frequently multiple hormone deficiencies. The results of hypopituitarism (*Table 10.2*) are essentially hypofunction of the target glands.

Surgery may be needed if there are tumours, cranial nerve defects or hydrocephalus. Substitution therapy is needed for deficiency states.

Table 10.2. Hypopituitarism—clinical effects

Sequence of development of hormone defects	Effects
1. LH	Impotence
FSH	Amenorrhoea
	Infertility
	Loss of pubic hair
2. GH	Impaired growth in child
3. Prolactin	Failure of lactation if post-partum (Sheehan's syndrome)
4. ACTH	Hypoadrenocorticism
5. TSH	Hypothyroidism

For abbreviations *see Table 10.1*

Dental aspects of hypopituitarism

General anaesthesia is usually contraindicated since there may be no TSH (leading to hypothyroidism) nor ACTH (leading to hypoadrenocorticism). Patients are at risk from adrenal crisis and hypopituitary coma.

Hypopituitary coma may be precipitated by stress (trauma, surgery, general anaesthesia or infection) much in the way that an adrenal crisis may be caused. Hypopituitary coma may also be precipitated by sedatives or hypnotics.

Hypopituitary coma should be treated with an immediate intravenous injection of 200 mg hydrocortisone sodium succinate. Blood should be taken for assay of glucose, thyroid hormones and cortisol, and 25–50 g dextrose should be given intravenously if there is hypoglycaemia. Oxygen should be given by face mask, medical assistance summoned and emergency admission to hospital arranged.

ANTERIOR PITUITARY HYPERFUNCTION

Growth Hormone Excess: Gigantism and Acromegaly

Overproduction of growth hormone causes gigantism before the epiphyses have fused, and acromegaly thereafter. All the organs, soft tissues and skeleton enlarge and the disorder may be complicated by diabetes mellitus, hypertension, cardiomyopathy, hypercalcaemia and osteoarthrosis. Local pressure effects from the pituitary tumour may cause hypopituitarism, compression of the optic chiasma (leading to visual field defects) and raised intracranial pressure. Acromegaly is one of the few endocrine diseases that can be instantly recognized—even in a passer-by in the street—by the appearance of the face and hands (*Fig.* 10.1). However, many cases go unrecognized for long periods.

Diagnosis and management

Skull radiography (to demonstrate pituitary enlargement), CT and MRI scans, visual field assessment (to detect optic chiasma involvement), glucose tolerance

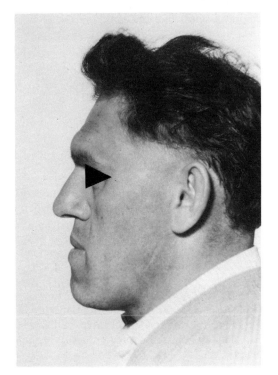

Fig. 10.1. Acromegaly.

tests (to exclude diabetes and to assess the plasma growth hormone response), growth hormone levels and assessment of remaining pituitary function are required.

The pituitary adenoma may be resected or the whole gland may have to be irradiated. Hypopituitarism or diabetes insipidus follow such treatment. Bromocriptine may be used but is rarely effective alone.

Dental aspects of growth hormone excess

Mandibular enlargement leads to class III malocclusion with spacing of the teeth and thickening of all soft tissues (*Fig* 10.1). Orthognathic surgery may therefore be needed and fatalities have followed such surgery in the past, because of airways obstruction. Otherwise, dental management may be complicated by:

1. Diabetes mellitus.
2. Hypertension.
3. Cardiomyopathy and dysrhythmias.
4. Hypopituitarism.
5. Kyphosis and other deformities affecting respiration may make general anaesthesia hazardous. The glottic opening may be narrowed and the cords' mobility reduced. A goitre may further embarrass the airway.
6. Thromboembolic phenomena.

Rarely, acromegalics have Cushing's syndrome or hyperparathyroidism due to associated multiple endocrine adenoma syndrome (p. 284).

ACTH Excess (*see* Cushing's syndrome, p. 262)

ADRENAL CORTEX

The adrenal cortex produces a series of corticosteroids, mainly the glucocorticoids, cortisol (hydrocortisone) and corticosterone, and the mineralocorticoid, aldosterone.

ADRENOCORTICAL HYPOFUNCTION

Adrenocortical hypofunction may be due to a congenital defect in the biosynthesis of corticosteroids (congenital adrenal hyperplasia), acquired adrenal disease (primary hypoadrenocorticism) or ACTH deficiency (secondary hypoadrenocorticism).

Primary Hypoadrenocorticism (Addison's Disease)

Hypoadrenocorticism is a rare disease characterized by atrophy of the adrenal cortices and failure of secretion of cortisol and aldosterone. In most cases there are circulating autoantibodies to the adrenal cortex. Patients with autoimmune Addison's disease also have a higher incidence of other endocrine deficiencies (Chapter 16) and occasionally, chronic mucocutaneous candidosis is associated. Other causes such as adrenal tuberculosis, histoplasmosis (occasionally secondary to HIV infection), malignancy, haemorrhage, sarcoidosis, amyloidosis or adrenalectomy for metastatic breast cancer are rare.

Lack of cortisol predisposes to hypotension and hypoglycaemia. The hypothalamopituitary axis is stimulated by the low serum cortisol and there is therefore increased release of pro-opiomelanocortin which has ACTH and melanocyte stimulating hormone (MSH) activity. Lack of aldosterone leads to sodium depletion, reduced extracellular fluid volume and hypotension. Patients with hypoadrenocorticism therefore suffer from fatigue, lethargy, anorexia, nausea, vomiting, diarrhoea, hyperpigmentation, weight loss, dizziness and postural hypotension (*Table 10.3*).

More important, the lack of adrenocortical reserve makes patients vulnerable to any stress such as infection, injury, surgery or anaesthesia, though they may be asymptomatic otherwise.

Table 10.3. Hyper- and hypoadrenocorticism—clinical features

Hyperadrenocorticism	*Hypoadrencocorticism*
Weight gain	Weight loss
Truncal obesity	Skin pigmentation
Weakness	Weakness
Hypertension	Hypotension
Hirsutism	Anorexia, nausea and vomiting
Amenorrhoea	Mucosal pigmentation
Cutaneous striae	
Personality changes	

Secondary Adrenocortical Insufficiency

Secondary adrenocortical insufficiency is caused by steroid therapy (p. 257) or ACTH deficiency as a result of hypothalamic or pituitary disease. Secondary adrenocortical insufficiency may therefore be associated with other endocrine defects, but there is no hyperpigmentation (ACTH levels are low) and blood pressure is virtually normal (aldosterone secretion is normal).

Congenital Adrenal Hyperplasia

Congenital adrenal hyperplasia is the term given to a group of rare autosomal recessive inborn errors of corticosteroid metabolism characterized by lack of cortisol (adrenal insufficiency) and androgen excess. Aldosterone secretion is also lacking in some of these disorders.

Nelson's Syndrome

This rare syndrome may affect up to 40 per cent of persons who have had bilateral adrenalectomy, usually to control breast cancer metastases or Cushing's syndrome. This results in increasing pituitary activity and sometimes adenoma formation. Large amounts of ACTH are released and there is cutaneous pigmentation. Some 10 per cent develop oral pigmentation.

Diagnosis and management of hypoadrenocorticism

The blood pressure should be measured, as hypotension is frequent. Blood should be taken for plasma cortisol estimation (10 ml in lithium heparin orange tube, or plain tube) at 8.00 or 9.00 am. In hypoadrenocorticism the basal cortisol level is usually lower than 100 nmol/l, but in early disease the cortisol levels may still be in the low normal range and therefore a short tetracosactrin (Synacthen) test (ACTH stimulation) is indicated as described below. Plasma electrolytes are normal in many cases, unless a crisis is imminent, but the plasma sodium level may be low and the potassium raised. There is often also hypoglycaemia.

Estimation of serum ACTH levels differentiates primary (ACTH raised, usually above 200 ng/l) from secondary (ACTH low or normal) hypoadrenocorticism.

Other investigations that may be helpful include radiography or CT scans of the skull (for pituitary abnormalities), chest (for tuberculosis) or abdomen (for adrenal calcification suggestive of tuberculosis or a mycosis). Serum should be tested for autoantibodies to various tissues—specially endocrine glands. Most patients are treated with oral hydrocortisone and fludro-cortisone.

The main complication of hypoadrenocorticism is an acute adrenal crisis (Addisonian crisis or shock). Acute adrenal crisis is characterized by collapse, bradycardia, hypotension, profound weakness, hypoglycaemia, vomiting and dehydration. This may be the first manifestation of the disease and results from failure of the adrenocortical response to stress.

The Synacthen test. Plasma is collected before and 30 minutes after 250 μg of tetracosactrin (synthetic ACTH: Synacthen) is injected intramuscularly. In health the plasma cortisol level normally doubles from at least 200 nmol/l to more than 500 nmol/l after tetracosactrin. In hypoadrenocorticism the basal cortisol level is low and does not rise after tetracosactrin is given.

Dental aspects. Pigmentation of the mucosa of a brown or black colour is seen in over 75 per cent of patients with Addison's disease, but is not a feature of corticosteroid-induced hypoadrenocorticism or of hypoadrenocorticism secondary to hypothalamopituitary disease. Hyperpigmentation is related to high levels of MSH and affects particularly areas normally pigmented or exposed to trauma (for example in the buccal mucosa at the occlusal line, or the tongue, but also the gingivae). Other causes of oral pigmentation (Chapter 7) (especially racial pigmentation) need to be differentiated but, though it is a rare cause, Addison's disease must be considered particularly if there is hypotension, weakness, weight loss, anorexia, nausea, vomiting or abdominal pain.

The diagnosis is established by (*a*) assay of plasma fluorogenic corticosteroids (cortisol) which in hypoadrenocorticism are lower than 6 μg/100 ml (170 nmol/l) at 8.00 to 9.00 a.m. and (*b*) failure of synthesis of cortisol in response to ACTH stimulation (Synacthen test).

The danger of dental treatment in the patient with hypoadrenocorticism is of precipitating hypotensive collapse, and therefore corticosteroids must be given preoperatively. This is discussed more fully below under the section on systemic corticosteroid therapy, the most frequent cause of hypoadrenocorticism.

SYSTEMIC CORTICOSTEROID THERAPY

Corticosteroids are used either to replace missing hormones (in Addison's disease or after adrenalectomy) or for immunosuppression (*Table 10.4*). Corticosteroids can therefore mask the presence of many serious diseases that may influence dental care as well as causing suppression of the adrenocortical response to stress.

Table 10.4. Some uses of systemic corticosteroids

Allergic disorders	Asthma
Connective tissue disorders	Rheumatoid arthritis (rarely)
	Systemic lupus erythematosus
Renal disorders	Nephrotic syndrome
	Renal transplants
Gastrointestinal disorders	Ulcerative colitis
	Crohn's disease
Blood dyscrasias	Idiopathic thrombocytopenia
	Lymphocytic leukaemia
	Lymphoma
Adrenal insufficiency	Addison's disease
	Adrenalectomy
	Hypopituitarism
Mucocutaneous diseases	Pemphigus

COMPLICATIONS OF CORTICOSTEROID THERAPY

The long-term use of corticosteroids can cause many side-effects (*Fig.* 10.2), often beginning soon after the start of treatment (*Table 10.5*). The most significant effect is suppression of ACTH secretion, leading to adrenal atrophy and failure to respond to stress. Corticosteroids in high doses also cause a significant morbidity or mortality, particularly from infection, perforated or bleeding peptic ulcers, diabetes and hypertension and their complications. In children

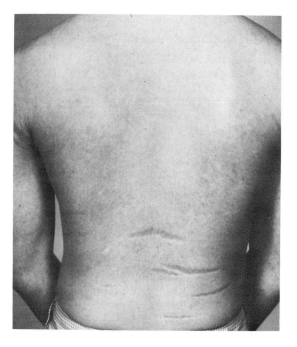

Fig. 10.2. Systemic corticosteroid therapy causes several complications, including cutaneous striae, as here.

Table 10.5. Systemic corticosteroid therapy—complications

Immunosuppressive	Increased susceptibility to infections
Cardiovascular	Hypertension
	Myocardial infarction
	Cerebrovascular accidents
	Hypotensive crises
Metabolic	Hypothalamic–pituitary–adrenal suppression
	Impaired glucose tolerance or diabetes mellitus
	Growth retardation
	Loss of sodium and potassium
	Osteoporosis
	Fat redistribution (moon face and buffalo hump)
Gastrointestinal	Peptic ulcer
Neurological	Mood changes
	Psychosis
	Cataracts
Dermatological	Acne
	Striae
	Bruising

there may be growth retardation. These complications may be reduced but not abolished if steroids are given on alternate days, or by substituting ACTH therapy where practical.

Corticosteroids and Suppression of Adrenal Function

Adrenal corticosteroids are an essential part of the body's response to stresses such as trauma, infection, general anaesthesia or operation. At times of stress there is normally an increase of corticosteroid production and the size of the response is related to the degree of stress. In the absence of such a response there is rapidly developing hypotension, collapse and death.

The hypothalamus is in overall control of adrenocortical function by producing releasing factors that stimulate the pituitary to release adrenocorticotrophic hormone (ACTH or corticotropin). ACTH stimulates the production of adrenal corticosteroids. Circulating steroids control hypothalamic activity by a negative feedback mechanism.

The function of the hypothalamic–pituitary–adrenocortical axis (HPA) is disrupted if the pituitary or adrenal cortex ceases to function as a result of trauma, surgery or disease, or if exogenous corticosteroids are given. Administration of corticosteroids results in negative feedback to the hypothalamus, reduced ACTH secretion and consequent adrenocortical atrophy. The adrenal cortex is then unable to produce the necessary steroid response to stress, and acute adrenal insufficiency (adrenal crisis) is precipitated.

Suppression of the HPA axis becomes more severe as the dose of steroids exceeds physiological levels (more than about 7.5 mg/day of prednisolone), especially if treatment is prolonged. However, adrenal function may even be suppressed for up to a week after cessation of steroid treatment lasting only 5 days. If steroid treatment is for longer periods, adrenal function may be suppressed for 2–12 months after the cessation of treatment. Adrenal suppression is less when the exogenous steroid is given on alternate days or as a single morning dose (rather than as divided doses through the day). Corticotrophin (ACTH) was formerly used in the hope of reducing adrenal suppression, but the response is variable and unpredictable, and wanes with time.

Patients on, or who have been on, corticosteroid therapy within the past year are therefore at risk from adrenal crisis if they are not given supplementary corticosteroids before and during periods of stress. Patients should be warned of this danger and should carry a steroid card indicating the dosage and responsible physician (*Fig.* 10.3). Metal bracelets or necklets with the diagnosis engraved are available, for example, from Medic Alert Foundation, 9 Hanover Street, London W1R 9HF (*see Figs* 1.3, 1.4).

Dental aspects

Susceptibility to infection is increased and there is a predisposition to oral candidosis. Bacterial infections tend to be more frequent and severe. Wound healing is impaired in systemic corticosteroid therapy and wound infections are more frequent. In addition to careful aseptic surgery, prophylactic antimicrobials may, therefore, be indicated.

I am a patient on–

STEROID

TREATMENT

which must not be

stopped abruptly

and in the case of intercurrent illness

may have to be increased

full details are available

from the hospital or general→

practitioners shown overleaf

STC1

INSTRUCTIONS

1 DO NOT STOP taking the steroid drug except on medical advice. Always have a supply in reserve.

2 In case of feverish illness, accident, operation (emergency or otherwise), diarrhoea or vomiting the steroid treatment MUST be continued. Your doctor may wish you to have a LARGER DOSE or an INJECTION at such times.

3 If the tablets cause indigestion consult your doctor AT ONCE.

4 Always carry this card while receiving steroid treatment and show it to any doctor, dentist, nurse or midwife whom you may consult.

5 After your treatment has finished you must still tell any new doctor, dentist, nurse or midwife that you have had steroid treatment.

Fig. 10.3. Steroid Warning Card: this is a blue card that should be carried at all times by patients on systemic corticosteroids in view of the danger of an adrenocortical crisis and collapse if the patient is subjected to trauma, stress or anaesthesia. (With the kind permission of the Controller of Her Majesty's Stationery Office).

Adrenocortical function is likely to be suppressed if:

1. The patient is currently on corticosteroids.
2. Corticosteroids have been taken regularly for more than 1 month during the past year.

Systemic corticosteroids cause the greatest risk but there can also be adrenocortical suppression from extensive application of steroid skin preparations, particularly if occlusive dressings are used. During intercurrent illness or infection, after trauma, or before operation or anaesthesia, these patients require a considerable increase in steroid dosage. Minor operations under local anaesthesia may be covered by giving oral steroids 2–4 hours pre- and postoperatively (100 mg hydrocortisone or 20 mg prednisolone or 4 mg dexamethasone) or, better, by giving intravenous hydrocortisone immediately before operation (*see below*). Intravenous hydrocortisone must be immediately available for use if the patient collapses or the blood pressure falls. General anesthesia must be given only in hospital by a specialist anaesthetist. Cover should be provided, by giving at least 100–200 mg hydrocortisone sodium succinate intramuscularly or intravenously (with the premedication) and then 6-hourly for a further 24–72 hours (*Table 10.6*). The blood pressure must also be carefully watched during surgery and especially during recovery, and steroid supplementation given immediately if the blood pressure starts to fall. Corticosteroids given by intramuscular injection are more slowly absorbed and reach lower plasma levels than when given intravenously or orally.

Drugs, especially sedatives and general anaesthetics, are a hazard and it is extremely important to avoid hypoxia, hypotension or haemorrhage. Patients may also require special management as a result of diabetes, hypertension, poor wound healing, or infections.

Aspirin and other non-steroidal anti-inflammatory agents should be avoided as they may increase the risk of peptic ulceration in those on corticosteroids. Osteoporosis introduces the danger of fractures when handling the patient.

Topical corticosteroids for use in the mouth are unlikely to have any systemic effect but predispose to oral candidosis.

ACUTE ADRENAL INSUFFICIENCY

Acute adrenal insufficiency has several causes (*Table 10.7*) and is managed as follows:

1. Lay the patient flat with the legs raised.
2. Give 200 mg hydrocortisone intravenously.
3. Summon medical assistance.
4. Take blood for glucose (Dextrostix) and electrolyte estimation.
5. Give glucose if there is hypoglycaemia (25 g orally or intravenously).
6. Put up an intravenous infusion of normal saline or glucose-saline. Give 1 litre over 2 hours together with 200 mg hydrocortisone sodium succinate, repeating this at 4–6-hourly intervals as required and monitor the blood pressure.

Table 10.6. Suggested management of patients with a history of systemic corticosteroid therapy

	No steroids for previous 12 mth	Steroids taken during previous 12 mth	Steroids currently taken
Conservative dentistry or minor surgery (e.g. single extraction) under LA	No cover required	Give hydrocortisone 200 mg orally,* or i.v. preop.†	Give hydrocortisone 200 mg orally* or i.v. preop.† Continue normal steroid medication postop.
Intermediate surgery (e.g. multiple extractions, or surgery under GA)	Consider cover if large doses of steroid were given. Test adrenocortical function (ACTH stimulation test)	Give hydrocortisone† 200 mg i.v. preop. and i.m. 6-hourly for 24 hours	Give hydrocortisone† 200 mg i.v. preop. and i.m. 6-hourly for 24 hours. Then continue normal medication
Major surgery or trauma (e.g. maxillofacial surgery)	Consider cover if large doses of steroid were given. Test adrenocortical function (ACTH stimulation test)	Give hydrocortisone† 200 mg i.v. preop. and i.m. 6-hourly for 72 hours	Give hydrocortisone† 200 mg i.v. preop. and i.m. 6-hourly for 72 hours. Then continue normal medication

*Hydrocortisone given orally 2 hours preoperatively
†Hydrocortisone sodium succinate (e.g. Ef-Cortelan soluble) or phosphate given immediately preoperatively and monitor blood pressure.

Table 10.7. Causes of hypotensive adrenal crisis

1. In a patient on systemic corticosteroids
    Trauma
    Operation
    Anaesthesia
    Infection
2. Addison's disease (causes of stress as above)
3. Post-adrenalectomy
4. Waterhouse-Friderichsen syndrome (adrenal haemorrhage caused by septicaemia, anti-coagulants or epilepsy)
5. Congenital adrenal hyperplasia
6. Hypopituitarism

7. Determine and deal with the underlying cause (*Table 10.7*) when the blood pressure has been stabilized. Control of pain and infection are particularly important and steroid supplementation must be continued for at least 3 days after the blood pressure has returned to normal.

Subacute adrenal insufficiency (corticosteroid withdrawal syndrome). Subacute adrenal insufficiency develops if corticosteroid dosage is reduced too quickly after replacement therapy in postsurgical patients with Cushing's syndrome. Features include lethargy, abdominal pain, hypotension and psychological disturbances. Scaly desquamation of the facial skin, particularly of the forehead, is a characteristic sign. Hydrocortisone replacement needs to be increased if there are signs of adrenal insufficiency.

ADRENOCORTICAL HYPERFUNCTION

Adrenocortical hyperfunction may lead to release of excessive glucocorticoids (Cushing's disease), mineralocorticoids (Conn's syndrome or hyperaldosteronism) or androgens (congenital adrenal hyperplasia).

Cushing's Syndrome and Disease

Cushing's disease is caused by excess glucocorticoid production by adrenal hyperplasia secondary to excess ACTH production by pituitary adenomas, or occasionally by adrenal or other tumours which produce ectopic ACTH. Cushing's syndrome is clinically similar but caused by primary adrenal disease (adenoma or rarely carcinoma). The two terms are often used interchangeably. A similar syndrome is produced by systemic corticosteroid therapy (*see Table 10.5*) and, rarely, by the multiple endocrine adenoma syndromes (*see Table 10.19*).

The most obvious features are obesity affecting particularly the face (moon face) (*Fig. 10.4*), interscapular region (buffalo hump) and trunk, but with relative sparing of the limbs. Hypertension has more serious effects and the breakdown of proteins with conversion to glucose leads to hyperglycaemia and diabetes

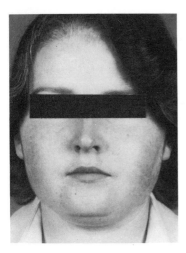

Fig. 10.4. Moon face in a patient with Cushing's syndrome.

mellitus, osteoporosis, muscle weakness, thinning of the skin, purpura and striae. Acne is common and many patients become hirsute. Hyperpigmentation is uncommon and usually suggests that excess ACTH production is the cause.

Diagnosis and management

The plasma cortisol levels may be informative but are not always raised in Cushing's syndrome and it is better to look for absence of diurnal variation in cortisol levels, which are normally highest early in the morning and lowest at midnight. A corticotrophin–releasing hormone stimulation test should be used and 24 hour urine should be assayed for free cortisol. Another useful screening test is to measure plasma cortisol at 8.00–9.00 a.m. after giving 1 mg dexamethasone orally at midnight to suppress the adrenals temporarily (low dose overnight dexamethasone suppression test). Normally, the latter reduces cortisol levels below 5 µg/1100 ml, but in Cushing's syndrome there is no such reduction. Other special dexamethasone tests or sampling from the inferior petrosal sinus are needed to distinguish pituitary from adrenal causes of Cushing's syndrome. However MRI may demonstrate a pituitary tumour. ACTH levels and other investigations are also required.

Corticotrophin–releasing hormone (CRH) stimulation test: This test depends on the fact that the pituitary is responsive to CRH, whereas adrenal tumours and other tumours producing ectopic ACTH, are not.

Baseline ACTH and cortisol levels are first obtained, CRH is then given. An exaggerated increase in plasma ACTH and cortisol levels is given by patients with pituitary Cushing's syndrome but not by patients with other types of Cushing's syndrome.

The responsible glands are irradiated or excised. About 10 per cent of patients subjected to bilateral adrenalectomy develop pituitary ACTH-producing adenomas with hyperpigmentation and symptoms related to the pituitary tumour (Nelson's syndrome).

Dental aspects of Cushing's syndrome

There are no specific oral manifestations of Cushing's syndrome or disease, but, though it may be hard to believe, patients have been referred for a suspected dental cause of the swollen face.

Patients once treated are maintained on replacement therapy and then are at risk from an adrenal crisis if subjected to operation, anaesthesia or trauma.

Management complications may therefore include:

1. Need for corticosteroid cover.
2. Hypertension.
3. Cardiovascular disease.
4. Diabetes mellitus.
5. Psychosis.
6. Vertebral collapse or myopathy causing limited mobility.
7. Multiple endocrine adenomatosis (MEA I, *see Table 10.19*).

HYPERALDOSTERONISM

A rare tumour or hyperplasia of the adrenal cortex results in primary hyperaldosteronism (Conn's syndrome). Secondary hyperaldosteronism may complicate cirrhosis, nephrotic syndrome, severe cardiac failure or renal artery stenosis.

High aldosterone secretion leads to potassium loss and sodium retention. Loss of potassium often results in muscle weakness, polyuria and polydipsia, and, since it is associated with a metabolic alkalosis, may lead to tetany. Sodium retention leads to hypertension but rarely to oedema.

The aldosterone antagonist, spironolactone, is given until the affected glands can be excised.

Dental aspects

In the untreated patient, hypertension and muscle weakness are the main complications. Competitive muscle relaxants should be used with restraint if a general anaesthetic is needed, as they can cause profound paralysis.

If bilateral adrenalectomy has been carried out, the patient is at risk from collapse during dental treatment and therefore requires corticosteroid cover.

THE ADRENAL MEDULLA

The adrenal medulla secretes noradrenaline and adrenaline, which are normally released in response to hypotension, hypoglycaemia and other stress, their release being regulated by the central nervous system.

PHAEOCHROMOCYTOMA

Phaeochromocytomas are rare, usually benign tumours, producing excessive catecholamines. The tumours most commonly form in the adrenal medulla but may arise in other neuroectodermal tissues such as paraganglia or the sympathetic chain. Phaeochromocytomas may occasionally be associated with neurofibromatosis, or with endocrine tumours particularly medullary carcinoma of the thyroid and hyperparathyroidism (multiple endocrine adenomatosis: MEA II or III, *see Table 10.19*). There is often then a familial incidence.

The typical features of phaeochromocytoma are episodes of anxiety, palpitations, sweating, pyrexia, flushing, hypertension, headache and epigastric discomfort. Attacks may be accompanied by tachycardia, dysrhythmias, hypertension and glycosuria.

Diagnosis and management

Diagnosis of a phaeochromocytoma is supported by finding excessive urinary catecholamine metabolites such as vanillylmandelic acid (VMA) or metanephrines. Plasma catecholamines (collected at rest in the supine position) may also be increased. The site of the tumour is localized by such techniques as venous catheterization, arteriography, computerized axial tomography and radionuclide scanning.

The tumour is excised after the blood pressure has been controlled with an alpha-blocking agent, such as phenoxybenzamine, and a beta-blocker.

Dental aspects

Phaeochromocytoma is occasionally associated with oral mucosal neuromas (MEA III syndrome, *see Table 10.19*). Factors likely to complicate treatment include acute hypertension and dysrhythmias. Dental treatment should therefore be deferred until after surgical treatment of the phaeochromocytoma. A general anaesthetic must not be given to the untreated patient.

Patients who have had adrenal surgery for phaeochromocytoma may suffer from hypoadrenocorticism, since the adrenal cortex is inevitably damaged at operation. These patients therefore require steroid cover at operation.

THE THYROID

The normal thyroid produces two main hormones, thyroxine (T4) and triiodothyronine (T3). These hormones are stored as iodide-rich 'thyroid colloid' and released under the influence of thyroid stimulating hormone (TSH) from the pituitary.

The diagnosis of thyroid disease is mainly made on clinical grounds, from the history and examination, and laboratory tests. There are many such tests but they may give conflicting results and no one alone is sufficiently reliable or comprehensive (*Table 10.8*).

T4 and T3 are bound to plasma proteins and only a small amount is free in plasma. It is, however, the free hormones that are biologically important. The free thyroxine index is useful since measurement of free T4 is difficult. The index is the ratio of T4 to binding protein (binding protein is equivalent to T3 uptake).

Table 10.8. Tests of thyroid function

Test	Hyperthyroidism	Hypothyroidism
1. Hypothalmic–pituitary–thyroid axis		
Serum TSH	↓	↑*
TRH test (release of TSH by TRH)	ND	↓*
2. Thyroid function		
Radio-iodine uptake	↑†	ND
3. Concentration of serum thyroid hormones		
Serum T4	↑	↓
Serum T3	↑	↓
Free thyroxine index	↑	↓
T3 resin uptake	↑	↓
4. Other tests		
Thyroid autoantibodies	LATS	Thyroglobulin autoantibodies

*Depressed in pituitary hypofunction.
†Not suppressed by administration of T3.
Note: Basal metabolic rate not now used as a test.
LATS, Long acting thyroid stimulator; ND, not done.
Arrows indicate raised or lowered values.

Goitre

A goitre is an enlarged thyroid gland. A goitre is usually a consequence of thyroid hyperplasia secondary to excessive TSH levels caused by decreased circulating thyroid hormone. Thyroid cancer and hyperthyroidism may also cause goitre (*Table 10. 9*)

Diagnosis and management of goitre

Thyroid function is assessed to determine whether it is normal (euthyroid), hyperactive (hyperthyroid) or hypoactive (hypothyroid), and the cause of the goitre is sought.

Most goitres do not require surgery but it is indicated if there is a danger of airways obstruction as shown by cough, voice changes, dyspnoea, tracheal deviation or dysphagia. A large goitre may also need to be reduced for cosmetic reasons.

Table 10.9. Causes of goitre

1. Graves' disease (toxic goitre)
2. Low iodine intake or natural goitrogens (endemic goitre)
3. Drugs
   Thiouracil
   Carbimazole
   Potassium perchlorate
   Lithium
   Phenylbutazone
4. Dyshormonogenesis
5. Carcinoma
6. Hashimoto's thyroiditis
7. Physiological (puberty; pregnancy)

Dental aspects of goitre

A rare cause of goitre is a medullary carcinoma of the thyroid which can be part of a multiple endocrine adenomatosis syndrome (MEA II and MEA III, *see Table 10.19*). In the latter, numerous small plexiform neuromas are found in the oral mucosa, lips, eyelids and skin. The patient may also have a Marfanoid habitus and diarrhoea.

Dental management in other types of goitre may be influenced by changes in thyroid function, by the underlying cause of the goitre, or by complications such as respiratory obstruction.

Lingual Thyroid

The thyroid develops as a downgrowth from the foramen caecum at the junction of the posterior third with the anterior two-thirds of the tongue. Rarely thyroid tissue remains in this area and may be seen as a lump. It is often asymptomatic but may cause dysphagia; hypothyroidism may be associated. A lingual thyroid may not be suspected until the lump in the tongue has been excised and examined histologically, but if possible, should not be excised unless normal functioning thyroid tissue is identified in the neck.

The diagnosis can be confirmed by iodine 123 or 131, or technetium 99 uptake in the tongue or by biopsy. The lesion can also be demonstrated by CT scanning *without* contrast.

Treatment depends on the size of the lingual thyroid but thyroxine may be needed and the lingual thyroid ablated by surgery or iodine 131.

HYPOTHYROIDISM

Hypothyroidism may be primary (thyroid disease) or secondary (hypothalamic or pituitary dysfunction). Most cases of hypothyroidism are associated with autoantibodies to thyroglobulin or thyroid microsomes. Surgical removal of too much thyroid tissue, or destruction by irradiation, are important causes of hypothyroidism in a previously hyperthyroid patient. Congenital thyroid disorders are rare.

Hypothyroidism is often unrecognized and subclinical hypothyroidism, with raised TSH but normal T4 levels, may be found in up to 10 per cent of postmenopausal females. Hypothyroidism may cause weight gain, lassitude, dry skin, loss of hair, cardiac failure or ischaemic heart disease, anaemia, neurological or psychiatric changes, hoarseness, bradycardia or hypothermia (*Table 10.10*), and may be complicated by coma. The respiratory centre is hypersensitive to drugs such as opioids or sedatives. Congenital hypothyroidism (cretinism) has similar features, together with an enlarged tongue and mental handicap.

Table 10.10. Hypo- and hyperthyroidism—typical clinical features

Hypothyroidism	Hyperthyroidism
Cold intolerance	Heat intolerance
Decreased sweating	Excess sweating
Dry cold skin	Warm moist skin
Loss of hair	
Decreased appetite	Increased appetite
Weight gain	Weight loss
Bradycardia	Tachycardia (atrial fibrillation)
Angina	Heart failure
Hoarseness	
Slow reactions	Tremor
Constipation	Diarrhoea
Slow cerebration, poor memory	Irritability
Psychosis	Psychosis

Diagnosis and management

The diagnosis is confirmed by demonstrating a reduced free thyroxine index (p. 266). The serum TSH is raised in primary hypothyroidism but depressed in secondary hypothyroidism.

Symptomatic patients are managed with daily oral thyroxine sodium. Treatment is always started slowly, but especially so if there is evidence of ischaemic heart disease, as angina, myocardial infarction or sudden death may be precipitated.

Dental aspects

The main danger is of precipitating myxoedema coma by the use of sedatives (including diazepam), opioid analgesics (including codeine), other tranquillizers and general anaesthetics. These drugs should therefore either be avoided or the dose reduced. Hypotension and hypoadrenocorticism may be associated with hypothyroidism and diminished cardiac output and bradycardia are common.

Anaemia or ischaemic heart disease (Chapter 2) are often complications Local anaesthesia is therefore preferable to general anaesthesia.

General anaesthesia, if unavoidable, should be delayed if possible until thyroxine has been started and in any event must be given in hospital by a specialist anaesthetist since it can precipitate circulatory failure.

Occasional additional problems are associated hypopituitarism and other autoimmune disorders such as Sjögren's syndrome.

HYPERTHYROIDISM

Most cases of hyperthyroidism are associated with a diffuse goitre (Graves' disease, primary hyperthyroidism) and thyroid-stimulating autoantibodies. Secondary hyperthyroidism is associated with thyroid nodules or nodular goitre.

Hyperthyroidism causes weight loss, anorexia, vomiting or diarrhoea, anxiety, tremor, sweating, tachycardia and heat intolerance. Eye signs such as lid lag, lid retraction and exophthalmos are also characteristic (*Table 10.10, Fig.* 10.5). Cardiac disturbances such as dysrhythmias (especially atrial fibrillation) or cardiac failure may complicate it, particularly in the older patient.

Diagnosis and management

The diagnosis of hyperthyroidism should be confirmed by determination of the plasma levels of T3 and T4. The free thyroxine index is also raised in hyperthyroidism. The TRH test is negative since raised thyroid hormone levels suppress the response.

Treatment may be medical, with antithyroid drugs or ^{131}I, or surgical. Carbimazole is the usual antithyroid drug. Beta-blockers achieve rapid control

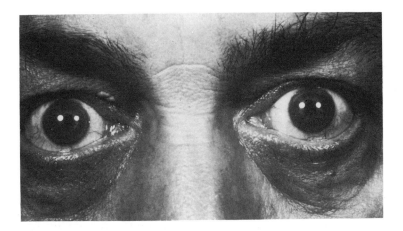

Fig. 10.5. Exophthalmos in hyperthyroidism.

of many of the signs and symptoms of hyperthyroidism (since the latter causes sympathetic overactivity) and are useful preoperatively. Care must be taken if beta-blocker treatment is stopped, since a thyroid crisis can be precipitated within 4 hours. Antithyroid drugs very rarely have side-effects such as rashes and agranulocytosis but nearly 50 per cent of patients have a relapse. [131]I is effective, but not infrequently results in hypothyroidism. Surgery is effective, but leads eventually to hypothyroidism in about 30 per cent of cases, but hypoparathyroidism or recurrent laryngeal nerve palsy are now rare complications.

Dental aspects

The hyperthyroid patient is at risk from general anaesthesia because of the risk of precipitating dangerous dysrhythmias. General anaesthesia must not therefore be given in the dental surgery until the disease is treated. If needed urgently, general anaesthesia should be given by a specialist anaesthetist in hospital. Patients with untreated hyperthyroidism may be also difficult to deal with as a result of heightened anxiety and irritability. The sympathetic overactivity may lead to fainting but the risks of giving adrenaline-containing local anaesthetics in moderate amounts are more theoretical than real. If there is anxiety on this score, prilocaine with felypressin can be given but is not known to be safer.

Benzodiazepines may potentiate antithyroid drugs, and nitrous oxide, which is more rapidly controllable, is probably safer for dental sedation. Sedation is desirable since anxiety may precipitate a thyroid crisis.

Thyroid (thyrotoxic) crisis is dangerous and characterized by anxiety, tremor and dyspnoea and can go on to ventricular fibrillation. It may be precipitated by infection or surgery, or by premature cessation of antithyroid treatment. Medical assistance is essential as treatment of a crisis requires the use of potassium iodide and propylthiouracil, and propranolol or chlorpromazine.

After treatment of hyperthyroidism the patient is at risk from hypothyroidism which may pass unrecognized. This point must especially be borne in mind if a general anaesthetic is required.

Medical treatment of hyperthyroidism with carbimazole occasionally leads to agranulocytosis which may cause oral or oropharyngeal ulceration. Otherwise the treated thyrotoxic patient presents no special problems in dental treatment.

THE PARATHYROIDS

The parathyroid glands produce parathyroid hormone (PTH) which regulates a normal plasma calcium level by acting on the kidneys, gastrointestinal tract and bone. PTH secretion is stimulated by a fall in the level of the plasma ionized calcium. PTH increases the renal reabsorption of calcium and decreases phosphate reabsorption. PTH also increases bone resorption: both mineral and matrix are degraded and imino acids such as hydroxyproline thus released are

Table 10.11. Parathyroid function tests

	Calcium*	Phosphate*	Alkaline phosphatase	Urea*
Primary hyperparathyroidism				
without bone lesions	↑	↓	N	N
with bone lesions	↑	N or ↓	↑	N or ↑
Secondary hyperparathyroidism				
due to renal failure	N or ↓	N or ↑	N or ↑	↓
due to malabsorption	N or ↓	↓	↑	N
Tertiary hyperparathyroidism				
with bone lesions	↑	N or ↓	↑	N or ↑
without bone lesions	↑	↓	N	N or ↑
Hypoparathyroidism	↓	↑	N	N
Pseudo-hypoparathyroidism	↓	↑	N	N
Pseudo-pseudohypoparathyroidism	N	N	N	N
Vitamin D deficiency	↓	N or ↓	↑	N

*Serum concentrations.
Arrows indicate values above or below normal (N).

not re-used but excreted in the urine. The excess bone turnover is reflected in a rise in the plasma level of calcium and of the osteoblastic enzyme alkaline phosphatase (*Table 10.11*).

HYPOPARATHYROIDISM

Thyroidectomy is still the most frequent cause of hypoparathyroidism. The idiopathic form of the disease is rare. Tetany is the classic feature of hypoparathyroidism, with numbness and tingling of arms and legs, facial twitching (Chvostek's sign), carpopedal spasms (Trousseau's sign) and even laryngeal stridor. Plasma calcium is low and phosphate often raised (*Tables 10.11, 10.12*). Some cases of idiopathic hypoparathyroidism may be associated with other endocrine defects, particularly hypoadrenalism (polyendocrinopathy syndrome) and sometimes chronic mucocutaneous candidosis (Chapter 16).

Postsurgical hypoparathyroidism is relatively transient and resolves when the remaining parathyroid tissue undergoes compensatory hyperplasia.

Idiopathic hypoparathyroidism has as its typical features tetany and stridor, cataracts, calcification of the basal ganglia, defects of the teeth and, occasionally, chronic mucocutaneous candidosis and other endocrinopathies—especially hypoadrenocorticism—associated with multiple autoantibodies (Chapter 16).

Pseudohypoparathyroidism is characterized by normal or raised PTH secretion but the tissue receptors do not respond. The clinical features are similar to idiopathic hypoparathyroidism but the patients are short in stature and have small fingers but no defects of the teeth. Patients of similar appearance but with normal biochemistry are termed pseudo-pseudohypoparathyroidism.

Table 10.12. Clinical features of hypo- and hyperparathyroidism

Hypoparathyroidism	Hyperparathyroidism
Tetany	Renal stones
Epilepsy	Nephrocalcinosis
Candidosis*	Bone resorption
Cataracts*	Peptic ulcer: pain
Psychiatric disorders	Psychiatric disorders
	Polyuria
	Constipation
	Hypertension
	Weakness
	Acute pancreatitis

*Only in some types of congenital hypoparathyroidism.

Dental aspects

Oral manifestations of idiopathic hypoparathyroidism may include enamel hypoplasia, shortened roots with osteodentine formation, delayed eruption and sometimes chronic mucocutaneous candidosis which can be resistant to antimycotic treatment. There may be facial paraesthesia and facial twitching caused by tetany (Chvostek's sign). Dental management may be complicated by:

1. Tetany.
2. Epilepsy.
3. Psychiatric problems or mental handicap.
4. Hypoadrenocorticism or other endocrinopathies such as diabetes mellitus.
5. Dysrhythmias.

HYPERPARATHYROIDISM

Hyperparathyroidism may be primary, secondary or tertiary.

Primary hyperparathyroidism is usually caused by an adenoma. Rare causes are carcinoma of the parathyroids or the genetic disorder, familial hypocalciuric hypercalcaemia, in which there is impaired sensing of plasma calcium by the parathyroids and kidneys. Hyperparathyroidism is most commonly a disease of postmenopausal women. The main features are hypercalcaemia, renal disease and, less commonly, skeletal disease. Most patients have renal calcifications and often hypertension, dysrhythmias and peptic ulceration (*see Table 10.12*). Bone pain, pathological fractures, giant cell tumours, bone rarefaction or pancreatitis are now rare.

Hyperparathyroidism may occasionally be familial and associated with tumours of other endocrine glands (MEA I, II and III).

Measurements of serum calcium require attention to detail since: (*a*) the level must be interpreted in relation to the serum albumin level, and (*b*) changes may only be intermittent.

Ten millilitres of blood should be collected into a plain container, the venepuncture being performed (*a*) in the fasting patient, and (*b*) without venous stasis (take the tourniquet off before aspirating).

Estimation of serum calcium levels should be repeated several times at intervals of a few days to exclude hypercalcaemia.

In hyperparathyroidism there is hypercalcaemia, the plasma phosphate level is low or normal, the plasma alkaline phosphatase level is normal (unless there is bone involvement when the level is raised) and urinary calcium excretion is increased (*see Table 10.11*).

Parathyroidectomy is usually needed. Medical treatment such as vitamin D (1,25-dihydroxycholecalciferol) is useful in those with severe bone disease.

Secondary hyperparathyroidism is a response to low plasma calcium caused by chronic renal failure or prolonged dialysis, or severe malabsorption and is increasing in frequency. In contrast to primary hyperparathyroidism renal stones are uncommon; the main manifestation is bone disease (usually renal osteodystrophy) which often responds to active vitamin D hormone (1,25-DHCC) but not to dietary vitamin D (cholecalciferol). Parathyroidectomy may, however, be needed.

Tertiary hyperparathyroidism follows prolonged secondary hyperparathyroidism which has become autonomous. Parathyroidectomy is then required.

Dental aspects

Dental changes in hyperparathyroidism, which include loss of the lamina dura, generalized bone rarefaction and giant cell lesions, are late and uncommon. Giant cell lesions of hyperparathyroidism (brown tumours) are rare but histologically indistinguishable from central giant cell granulomas of the jaws. If, therefore, a giant cell lesion is found, particularly in a middle-aged patient or in a patient with renal failure, parathyroid function should be investigated.

Dental treatment in hyperparathyroidism may be complicated by:

1. Hypertension.
2. Cardiac dysrhythmias.
3. Renal disease.
4. Peptic ulcer.
5. Sensitivity to muscle relaxants.
6. Bone fragility.
7. Pluriglandular disease (*see Table 10.19*); MEA I (diabetes or Cushing's syndrome); MEA II or III (phaeochromocytoma).
8. Hepatitis B in secondary or tertiary hyperparathyroidism, resulting from renal dialysis.

THE PANCREAS

Insulin, produced by the β-cells of the islets of Langerhans, is the main pancreatic hormone but several other hormones such as glucagon, gastrin and vasoactive peptides are produced.

DIABETES MELLITUS

Diabetes mellitus is one of the most common endocrine disorders and is characterized by persistently raised blood glucose levels (hyperglycaemia). Diabetes affects at least 2 per cent of the population but is recognized in only about 50 per cent of those affected and its prevalence appears to be increasing. Diabetes is the result of an absolute or relative deficiency of insulin from a variety of causes.

Diabetes is usually a primary disorder and only a few cases are secondary to diseases such as haemochromatosis or other endocrinopathies (*Table 10.13*).

Table 10.13. Diabetes melitus—causes

1. *Primary*
    (a) Juvenile onset (insulin-dependent; IDDM)
          Genetic Type IA
          Autoimmune Type IB
          (viral?)
    (b) Maturity onset (non-insulin dependent; NIDDM)
          Genetic Type II non-obese
          Obesity Type II obese
2. *Secondary to:*
    (a) Pancreatic damage
          Chronic pancreatitis
          Haemochromatosis
    (b) Endocrine abnormalities
          Cushing's syndrome
          Corticosteroid therapy
          Acromegaly
          Phaeochromocytoma
          Glucagonoma
          Somatostatinoma
          Insulin resistance
    (c) Many rare genetic syndromes

The two main types of primary (idiopathic) diabetes are the maturity-onset (Type II) non-insulin dependent (NIDDM) and the less common insulin-dependent juvenile (Type I or IDDM) forms.

Non-insulin-dependent diabetes mainly affects obese, middle-aged patients. The onset is gradual. Most patients with this type of diabetes can be managed on diet and oral hypoglycaemic drugs but they are often resistant to insulin effects.

Insulin-dependent diabetes generally develops before the age of 25. There may be a genetic basis to this type of diabetes and possibly a viral aetiology; some cases appear to follow an attack of mumps or a Coxsackie virus infection. The onset is relatively acute, typically with thirst, polyuria (especially at night), hunger and loss of weight. Lipolysis with increased production of fatty acids leads to over-production of acetoacetate which is converted to the other ketone bodies, hydroxybutyrate and acetone. These cause acidosis and thus hyperventilation. Ketone bodies also appear in the urine (ketonuria).

Diagnosis of diabetes mellitus

Glycosuria, conveniently detected by means of Clinistix or B–M Stix, is usually indicative of diabetes mellitus but should be confirmed by blood glucose levels. Fasting blood glucose levels higher than 8 mmol/l or random blood glucose higher than 11 mmol/l confirm the diagnosis. Fasting blood glucose levels less than 6 mmol/l and random blood glucose less than 8 mmol/l exclude the diagnosis. A glucose tolerance test is only justified when blood glucose levels are borderline (about 7 mmol/l, fasting) and the clinical picture is not completely convincing. The absence of glycosuria does not completely exclude diabetes.

Acute Complications of Diabetes

The course of diabetes is variable. Some patients, particularly non-insulin-dependent diabetics, are readily controlled, while others are difficult to control (brittle diabetes) and prone to ketosis, severe acidosis and hyperglycaemia (diabetic coma). Many insulin-treated patients are liable to hypoglycaemia, due to an imbalance between food intake and insulin therapy.

Hyperglycaemic (diabetic ketoacidotic) coma. Hyperglycaemic coma is the result of a relative or absolute deficiency of insulin and, in patients under treatment, may be precipitated by several factors (*Table 10.14*). Diabetic coma usually has a slow onset over many hours, with increasing drowsiness and signs of:

Table 10.14. Comparative features of hypo- and hyper-glycaemic comas and their treatment

Hypoglycaemic coma	Hyperglycaemic coma
1. Known diabetic	1. Diabetes may be unrecognized
2. Too much insulin or too little food or too much exercise or alcohol	2. Too little insulin or Infection, myocardial infarct, acute abdominal infection
3. Adrenaline release causes: Sweaty warm skin Rapid bounding pulse Dilated (reacting) pupils Anxiety, tremor Tingling around mouth	3. Acidosis causes: Vomiting Hyperventilation Ketonuria
4. Cerebral hypoglycaemia causes: Confusion, disorientation Headache Dysarthria Unconsciousness Focal neurological signs, e.g. fits	4. Osmotic diuresis and polyuria; Dehydration Hypotension Tachycardia Dry tongue and skin Abdominal pain, acetone breath
5. Take blood for sugar estimation If conscious give 25 g glucose orally If comatose give 20 mg 20% dextrose i.v. and on arousal 25 mg orally If unrestrainable for i.v. injection give glucagon 1 mg i.m.	5. Put up infusion to rehydrate Take blood for baseline sugar, electrolytes, urea, Hb and PCV Call ambulance

1. Dehydration (dry skin, weak pulse, hypotension).
2. Acidosis (deep breathing).
3. Ketosis (acetone smell on breath, vomiting).

Hypoglycaemic coma. Hypoglycaemic coma is usually the result of failure to take food, or overdosage of insulin, hypoglycaemic drugs or alcohol. Hypoglycaemic coma is of rapid onset and may resemble fainting. There is adrenaline release often with anxiety, irritability and disorientation before consciousness is lost. The pulse is strong and bounding, and the skin sweaty. By contrast, in diabetic coma the pulse is weak and skin dry (*Table 10.14*).

Coma in a diabetic patient is usually due to hyper- or hypoglycaemia but other possible causes of loss of consciousness should always be considered (Chapter 18). Furthermore, coma in a diabetic may be due to hyperglycaemia in the absence of significant ketosis (hyperosmolar non-ketotic coma) or, rarely, to lactic acidosis.

Less common causes of hypoglycaemia are shown in *Table 10.15*.

Table 10.15. Causes of hypoglycaemia

Common (Diabetics)
1. Excess insulin or oral hypoglycaemic drug
2. Missed meal
3. Exercise
Rare (Non-diabetics)
4. Insulinoma
5. Hepatic disease
6. Hypoadenocorticism
7. Hypopituitarism
8. Functional hypoglycaemia
9. Beta blockers

Management of coma in the diabetic patient

The cause should be established as soon as possible, but hypoglycaemia needs urgent treatment.

Cause of collapse not immediately apparent. If possible take blood for glucose measurement with Dextrostix (Ames) and if there is any doubt about the cause never give insulin but immediately give glucose as a diagnostic test. This will cause little harm in hyperglycaemic coma but will improve hypoglycaemic coma. Insulin, by contrast, can cause severe brain damage or kill a hypoglycaemic patient.

If the patient is conscious, immediately give 10 g sugar or equivalent glucose solution by mouth (*Table 10.16*). If the patient is comatose, take a blood sample for glucose estimation (2 ml blood in a yellow cap bottle containing fluoride) and give 10–20 ml of 20–50 per cent sterile dextrose intravenously.

Table 10.16. Treatment of hypoglycaemia

Patient conscious	Patient unconscious
2 teaspoons sugar *or* 3 lumps sugar *or* 3 Dextrosol tablets *or* 60 ml Lucozade *or* 15 ml Ribena *or* 90 ml Cola drink* *or* 1/3 pt milk	20 ml 20% or 50% dextrose i.v. *or* 1 mg glucagon i.m.

Not Diet-Cola or Diet Pepsi

Hypoglycaemic coma. Hypoglycaemia must be quickly corrected or brain damage can result. Glucose should be given as described above. If a vein cannot be found, glucagon 1 mg can be given intramuscularly. On arousal the patient should be given glucose orally.

Hyperglycaemic coma. If it is certain that collapse is due to hyperglycaemic ketoacidotic coma, the first priority is to establish an intravenous infusion line and start rapid rehydration. Blood should be taken for baseline measurements of glucose, electrolytes and pH. Raised plasma ketone body levels can be demonstrated with Ketostix (Ames). Insulin is then started—either 20 units i.m. stat. then 6 units hourly, or 6 u/h as an i.v. infusion. The intravenous infusion is required to correct dehydration, and electrolyte (especially potassium) losses, and to facilitate the administration of insulin. Medical help should be obtained as soon as possible (*see Table 10.14*).

Chronic Complications of Diabetes

Diabetes mellitus causes serious chronic complications; microangiopathy, macroangiopathy and neuropathy involve the eyes, kidneys and cardiovascular system (*Table 10.17*). Ischaemic heart disease or renal failure may significantly affect management and occasionally there are associations with autoimmune disorders, especially Addison's disease.

Management of Diabetes

The objectives of treatment are to control the blood glucose at near normal levels and to avoid acute or chronic complications, especially hypoglycaemic attacks. All diabetics should carry a card indicating the diagnosis, treatment schedule and physician in charge. Some diabetics wear a Medic-Alert device (*see Figs 1.3, 1.4*), and all should be advised to do so.

Diet. Diabetics should have meals at regular intervals, with a high fibre and relatively high carbohydrate contents but avoiding sugars. The caloric intake

Table 10.17. Chronic complication of diabetes

Circulatory	Atherosclerosis leading to ischaemic heart disease, cerebrovascular disease and peripheral gangrene
	Diabetic microangiospathy
Ocular	Retinopathy
	Cataracts
Renal	Renal failure
Neuropathies	Peripheral polyneuropathy
	Mononeuropathies
	Autonomic neuropathy, causing postural hypotension and cardio-respiratory arrest
Infections	Candidosis
	Staphylococcal infections

should be strictly related to physical activity. The efficacy of the diet is controlled by checking the weight and glucose levels, either by urinalysis, or by home glucose monitoring. Non-insulin-dependent diabetics test their urine for glucose at intervals from daily to once a week (Clinistix Ames) and adjust drugs or diet to keep the urine free of glucose. Insulin-dependent diabetics should test their urine 2–4 times daily and/or measure their own blood glucose levels (Dextrostix, Ames).

Elderly, obese diabetics often manage with diet control alone or with diet and oral hypoglycaemic agents. The young generally require insulin as well.

Oral hypoglycaemic agents. Sulphonylureas act mainly by stimulating the release of insulin from the pancreas. Chlorpropamide is potent, has a long action (up to 24 hours), ismildly antidiuretic and may predispose to cardiovascular complications by causing fluid retention. Chlorpropamide, therefore, is best avoided in the elderly, especially those with cardiovascular disease, as it may worsen congestive cardiac failure. Glibenclamide is short-acting and potent, but is a mild diuretic. Tolbutamide is short-acting and of lower potency, and since it is less likely to cause unwanted hypoglycaemia in the early hours of the morning following a breakfast dose the previous day, it is preferred for the elderly. Several other sulphonylureas are available: all may enhance, or be enhanced by, aspirin, anticoagulants, monoamine oxidase inhibitors, beta-blockers or clofibrate.

Biguanides (metformin) affect the absorption and metabolism of glucose and reduce appetite.

Guar gum and other fibres retard glucose absorption slightly.

Insulin. Insulin is given by injection. The dose varies widely between patients and also depends on the type of preparation, diet and exercise. Infection or trauma also increase insulin requirements.

Insulin may be given as soluble insulin which has a rapid onset and short action, or as long-acting preparations (insulin zinc suspension). Neutral insulins purified to be virtually non-antigenic (monocomponent insulins) and human (recombinant) insulins have been introduced. In younger insulin-dependent diabetics, the best regimen is a mixture of short- and intermediate-acting insulin given twice-daily—before breakfast and before the evening meal. Older insulin-treated diabetics often manage on one injection a day.

Long-term assessment of control can now be achieved by estimation of the blood level of Fructosamine, or glycosylated haemoglobin (HbA_1c). This is normal adult haemoglobin that binds glucose, remains in circulation for the life of the erythrocyte and therefore acts as a cumulative index of diabetic control.

Dental aspects of diabetes mellitus

There are no specific oral manifestations of diabetes mellitus but even well-controlled diabetics have a slightly more severe periodontal disease than controls. Initially tooth development appears to be accelerated but, after the age of 10 years, is retarded. If control is poor, severe periodontitis or oral candidosis may develop. Severe diabetes with ketoacidosis predisposes to and is the main cause of mucormycosis originating in the paranasal sinuses and nose (Chapter 16). A dry mouth may result from dehydration and occasionally there is swelling of the salivary glands (sialosis), possibly due to autonomic neuropathy. The tongue may show glossitis and alterations in filiform papillae or (it is said) there may be burning sensations in the absence of physical changes. Oral mucosal lichenoid reactions may result from the use of chlorpropamide and some other antidiabetic agents (Appendix to Chapter 19) but the 'Grinspan syndrome' (diabetes, lichen planus and hypertension) may be purely coincidental associations of common disorders probably related to drug use. Chlorpropamide may cause facial flushing.

Dental disease and treatment may disrupt the normal pattern of food intake and can interfere with diabetic control. A little forethought will prevent diabetics from collapsing in the waiting room at lunchtime from hypoglycaemia caused by missing a meal.

Special management considerations apply to the diabetic who is to undergo anything more than very minor procedures (*Table 10.18*) since the effects of stress and trauma may raise insulin requirements and precipitate ketosis. Orofacial infections should be vigorously treated as they also may precipitate ketosis.

General anaesthesia may be complicated especially by:

1. Chronic renal failure.
2. Ischaemic heart disease.
3. Autonomic neuropathy.

Autonomic neuropathy can lead to postural hypotension and impaired ability to respond to hypoglycaemia. Severe autonomic neuropathy carries a risk of cardiorespiratory arrest if a general anaesthetic is given.

However, the main danger to diabetics during operation is that of hypoglycaemia. General anaesthesia for the diabetic is therefore a matter for the specialist anaesthetist.

Table 10.18. Management of diabetics requiring general anaesthesia*

	Non insulin-dependent diabetics†		Insulin-dependent diabetics
	Minor operations e.g. few extractions	Major operations e.g. maxillofacial surgery	Any operation
Before operation		Stop biguanides. If on chlorpropamide, change to tolbutamide 1 week preop.	Stabilize on at least b.d. insulin for 2–3 days preop. One day preop. use only short-acting insulin (Actrapid soluble or neutral)
During operation	Omit oral hypoglycaemic. Estimate blood glucose level		Do not give sulphonylurea or subcutaneous insulin on day of operation. Estimate blood glucose level. Set up intravenous infusion of 10 per cent glucose 500 ml containing Actrapid or Leo neutral insulin 10 units plus KCl 1 g at 8.00 a.m. Infuse over 4 h. Estimate blood glucose and potassium levels 2-hourly. Adjust insulin and potassium to keep glucose at 5–10 mmol/l and normokalaemic
After operation	Estimate blood glucose 4 h postop.		Continue infusion 4-hourly. Estimate blood glucose 4-hourly. Estimate potassium 8-hourly
When resuming normal diet	Start sulphonylurea or other usual regimen	Start sulphonylurea	Stop infusion. Start Actrapid or Leo neutral insulin and over the next 2 days: Start normal insulin regimen

*Adapted, with permission, from Alberti and Thomas (1979).
†If well controlled, otherwise treat as insulin-dependent.

Routine non-surgical procedures. Routine dental treatment or short minor surgical procedures under localanaesthesia can be carried out with no special precautions apart from ensuring that treatment does not interfere with eating. The dose of adrenaline used in dental local anaesthetic solution is unlikely to increase blood glucose levels significantly. Treatment is best carried out just after breakfast and routine antidiabetic medication, to allow the diabetic to have lunch.

Surgical procedures. The essential requirement is to avoid hypoglycaemia but to keep hyperglycaemia below levels which may be harmful because of delayed wound healing or phagocyte dysfunction. The desired whole blood glucose levels are therefore 120–180 mg/dl (3 to 5 mmol/l).

Precautions required during oral surgery in diabetics depend mainly on:

1. The type and severity of the diabetes and complications such as autonomic neuropathy that may predispose to hypotension or cardiac arrest.
2. The type of anaesthetic.
3. The extent of surgery.
4. The extent of interference with normal feeding postoperatively.

Many different management regimens have been suggested and each patient requires individual handling: the following therefore provides only general guidelines and the diabetician should always decide the regimen.

Diabetics controlled by diet alone. These diabetics are often obese or elderly with little liability to ketosis and if they are well controlled many can tolerate minor surgical procedures, such as single extractions under local anaesthetic, without problems. A brief general anaesthetic can be given without special precautions apart from monitoring the urine sugar before the operation and on recovery, at 2-hourly intervals. However, such patients must have the anaesthetic in hospital, so that if ketonuria develops, blood sugar levels can be rapidly estimated.

Not all such patients are necessarily well controlled. In this case, or if more major surgery is planned, the patient should be admitted to hospital preoperatively for assessment and possible stabilization with insulin. The blood sugar should be monitored during and after operation.

Diabetics controlled by diet and oral hypoglycaemics. Patients controlled by oral hypoglycaemic drugs may tolerate minor oral surgical procedures under local anaesthesia, providing that normal meals are not interrupted. Well-controlled patients can safely have short simple procedures carried out under general anaesthesia in hospital without insulin, but the blood glucose should be monitored 2-hourly.

If diabetic control is poor, if the patient is on large doses of drugs or if more major surgery is planned, a suggested regimen is as follows:

1. Admit to hospital 2 days preoperatively for assessment and stabilization.
2. Metformin must be stopped at least 2 days preoperatively as it tends to cause lactic acidosis.

3. Chlorpropamide must be stopped at least 3 days, or preferably a week preoperatively because of its prolonged action and changed to tolbutamide or glibenclamide or, better, to soluble insulin 3 times daily.

4. At 8.00 to 9.00 a.m. on the day of operation, blood is taken for glucose estimation and an intravenous infusion line is put up.

5. Infusion of 10 per cent glucose (500 ml) containing 10 mmol potassium chloride and insulin 5 units (if the blood glucose is less than 6 mmol/l) or insulin 10 units (if the blood glucose is higher than 6 mmol/l) appears to be satisfactory. The blood glucose is monitored regularly and this regimen is continued at 100 ml/h until normal food can be taken orally.

6. The infusion is then stopped and the oral hypoglycaemic restarted.

Diabetics on insulin. Minor surgical procedures under local anaesthetic can be carried out in well-controlled diabetics with no change in the insulin regimen, providing that normal diet has, and can, be taken and that the procedure is carried out within 2 hours of breakfast and the morning insulin injection. In a well-controlled diabetic, minor operations under general anaesthesia, such as simple single extractions, can often be carried out safely by operating early in the morning and withholding both food and insulin until after the procedure.

More protracted procedures such as multiple extractions must only be carried out in hospital, with the following precautions:

1. Patients should be admitted preoperatively for assessment.

2. Before the operation, the patient should be put on soluble insulin and stabilized. Insulin may need to be given twice or three times daily, and control is confirmed by estimation of blood sugar (fasting, midday and before the evening meal).

3. The operation should be carried out early in the morning and booked first in the list, so that any delays in the operation schedule will not impair diabetic control.

4. At 8.00 to 9.00 a.m. blood should be taken for glucose estimation and an intravenous infusion set up giving glucose 10 g, soluble insulin 2 units and potassium 2 mmol/hour (GIK infusion), until normal oral feeding is resumed—at which time the patient can be returned to the preoperative insulin regimen.

5. Blood glucose should be monitored at 2–4-hourly intervals until the patient is feeding normally.

Blood glucose levels can be estimated in the laboratory or by using Dextrostix (Ames) with the aid of a Reflectance meter or Glucocheck machine.

PANCREATIC TUMOURS

Carcinoma of the head of the pancreas is the most common pancreatic tumour and the carcinoma with the shortest survival time. Hormone–secreting pancreatic tumours are as follows:

Glucagonoma. These pancreatic tumours are frequently malignant and release large amounts of glucagon, a hormone that causes hyperglycaemia and abnormal glucose tolerance. Estimation of plasma glucagon levels differentiates glucagonomas from diabetes mellitus—the main cause of hyperglycaemia. Glucagon levels may also be increased in patients taking danazol.

A major clinical feature of glucagonoma is a distinctive bullous or pustular skin lesion (necrotic migratory erythema), but there is often also weight loss, anaemia and hypercholesterolaemia.

Severe oral lesions have been reported in many patients and include bullae, erosions and angular stomatitis

Other hormone-secreting pancreatic tumours have been reported but are rare. Insulinomas are the most common cause of hypoglycaemia in those not taking insulin. The Zollinger–Ellison syndrome of diarrhoea and duodenal ulceration, due to a gastrin-secreting tumour, may be part of the multiple endocrine adenoma syndrome (MEA I), whilst vasoactive peptides seem to be responsible for the watery diarrhoea, hypokalaemia and achlorhydria (WDHA) syndrome, which often includes hyperglycaemia.

Multiple endocrine adenoma (MEA). MEA syndromes, also known as the multiple endocrine neoplasia (MEN) syndromes, are rare autosomal dominant diseases affecting several endocrine glands (*Table 10.19*). Their main relevance to dentistry is the presence in Type III of oral mucosal neurofibromas, particularly along the margins of the tongue. These tumours may lead to the diagnosis of this potentially lethal disease. All types,however, can cause difficulties in dental management as a result of the endocrine overactivity.

ENDOCRINE AND METABOLIC MANIFESTATIONS OF CANCER

Tumours of various kinds, especially bronchial carcinoma, can be the site of ectopic production of polypeptide hormones or other biologically active substances (Appendix to this chapter).

Carcinoid syndrome where there is overproduction of 5–hydroxytryptamine, facial flushing is characteristic; it is sometimes also seen in phaeochromocytoma, where there is release of sympathomimetic enzymes. Other causes are shown on p. 303.

INBORN ERRORS OF METABOLISM

A vast number of rare metabolic disorders result from inherited enzyme defects. Most are recessive traits which do not appear unless both parents are heterozygous carriers. The disease appears in one in four (in statistical terms) of the offspring of heterozygous parents often as a result of marriage of first cousins.

All but a few of the inborn errors of metabolism are rare and unlikely to be encountered in dental practice. Many are quite innocuous (for example hereditary pentosuria) but others, especially suxamethonium sensitivity, malignant

Table 10.19. Multiple endocrine adenoma syndromes—tissues affected

MEA type	Pituitary	Parathyroid	Thyroid	Adrenals	Pancreas	Others
MEAI (Wermer's syndrome)	+++	+++	++	+++ Cushing's	+++ Zollinger–Ellison Insulinoma Others	Carcinoid Lipomas Gastrinoma
MEAII (IIa) (Sipple syndrome)	–	++	+++ Medullary cell Ca. in 100%*	+++ Phaeochromo-cytoma in 33%	–	Dermal neuroma
MEAIII (IIb)	–	–	+++ Medullary cell Ca in up to 80–100%	+ Phaeochromo-cytoma in 70%	–	Oral mucosal neuromas Marfanoid skeletal anomalies Visual disturbances

*Causes raised serum calcitonin levels and reduced serum calcium levels.

hyperpyrexia and porphyria, although rare, can seriously complicate dental management and especially general anaesthesia.

Many of these disorders are associated with mental handicap or neurological disease. Some inborn errors of metabolism have a particularly high prevalence in certain racial groups. This section includes the inborn errors of metabolism of most significance in dentistry. Other inborn errors of metabolism are tabulated in the Appendix to this chapter.

It must be repeated that most of these disorders will be encountered rarely in general practice, although in certain situations—especially in paediatric clinics or institutions for the handicapped—they are more common.

SUXAMETHONIUM SENSITIVITY

Suxamethonium (Scoline) is a depolarizing neuromuscular blocker acting similarly to acetylcholine. This agent has a brief action due to its rapid destruction by the plasma cholinesterase, and is therefore widely used for muscle relaxation during the induction of general anaesthesia.

About 1 in 3000 patients are abnormally sensitive to the action of suxamethonium because of a defect in plasma cholinesterase. This is an autosomal recessive trait. If given suxamethonium, patients with this defect remain paralysed for several hours and unable to breathe. They therefore die unless artificially ventilated until the drug action abates.

Abnormal sensitivity to suxamethonium may also result from some other diseases (*Table 10.20*, Appendix to Chapter 19) or may be some sort of hypersensivity reaction (*see* Chapter 16).

Patients with suspected suxamethonium sensitivity must not be given it with a general anaesthetic in the dental surgery but should be referred to hospital for specialist attention.

Table 10.20. Conditions in which the action of suxamethonium may be prolonged

Suxamethonium sensitivity
Myopathies; dystrophia myotonica and myotonia congenita
Myasthenia gravis
Liver disease
Renal disease
Burns
Malignant hyperpyrexia
Drugs
    Trasylol
    Cyclophosphamide
    Procaine
    Phenothiazines
    Pancuronium
    Cytotoxic drugs

MALIGNANT HYPERTHERMIA (MALIGNANT HYPERPYREXIA)

Malignant hyperthermia is a rare inherited condition affecting about 1 in 12 000 children, and 1 in 40 000 adults. It is characterized by a rapid rise in temperature when the patient has a general anaesthetic or another drug which can trigger an attack. The mortality rate, in the absence of treatment, may approach 80 per cent.

Males are predominantly affected and 40 per cent of reported cases have been in children under 14 years of age. Two forms of malignant hyperthermia are recognized—an autosomal dominant type where the individuals are normal between attacks, and a recessive type affecting young boys who have various congenital abnormalities including short stature. Patients with myotonia congenita, myotonic dystrophy, central core disease and Evan syndrome (proximal wasting; short stature; kyphoscoliosis) are particularly susceptible.

Local anaesthesia is safe and the main drugs liable to precipitate malignant hyperthermia are the potent inhalational anaesthetic agents such as halothane, and muscle relaxants including suxamethonium and curare–like (non–depolarizing) agents. Intravenous anaesthetic agents are usually safe (*Table 10.21*). The syndrome may develop after a single anaesthetic exposure or after several uneventful anaesthetics.

Malignant hyperpyrexia has been reported after administration of nitrous oxide but this is extremely rare. The brevity of most dental anaesthetics is possibly a factor that makes hyperpyrexial reactions rare in dentistry.

Amide local anaesthetic agents including lignocaine and prilocaine were thought to be weak triggering agents but this has been dismissed.

Inquiry into the family history is essential before giving a general anaesthetic as there are no absolutely reliable predictive tests. Unfortunately, absence of reaction to a previous anaesthetic does not exclude the possibility of a reaction on the next occasion.

The importance of the family history is emphasized by the fact that a dental patient reported to the writers had had 14 relatives die under general anaesthesia. Understandably, this patient was less than enthusiastic about the idea of a general anaesthetic for dental purposes.

In a member of an affected family raised serum creatine kinase and pyrophosphate levels are indicative of susceptibility, but nearly one-third of patients have

Table 10.21. Drug use in malignant hyperpyrexia in susceptible subjects

	Contraindicated	Use
Muscle relaxants	Suxamethonium	Pancuronium
	Curare	
Premedication	Atropinics	Diazepam
General anaesthetics	Halothane	Methohexitone
	Ether	Thiopentone
	Cyclopropane	Nitrous oxide
	Ketamine	
	Enflurane	
Antidepressants	Tricyclic antidepressants	
	Monoamine oxidase inhibitors	

normal levels of creatine kinase. Excessive *in vitro* response of muscle to halothane, suxamethonium or caffeine, and raised myophosphorylase A levels, may be detected in patients but muscle biopsy is necessary for these tests.

The onset of malignant hyperthermia may be detected by poor muscular relaxation after induction of anaesthesia or complete failure of the jaw to relax after suxamethonium has been given. However, it is controversial whether masseter spasm is a reliable early sign of the onset of malignant hyperthermia. Suxamethonium, unlike pancuronium or vecuronium, causes jaw stiffness in many normal children, but intense muscle spasm may be significant.

There is a rise in temperature with tachycardia or dysrhythmias and hypotension. Late complications include pulmonary oedema, acute renal failure and disseminated intravascular coagulation. Malignant hyperthermia is a medical emergency with a high mortality rate.

Dental aspects of malignant hyperthermia

If a positive family history is obtained, dentistry can usually be safely carried out under local anaesthesia or relative analgesia. For major oral surgery, specialist anaesthetic care is needed and thiopentone or methohexitone is used. In the event of hyperthermia, surgery must be stopped and the patient cooled. Oxygen and a bicarbonate intravenous infusion (2 mEq/kg) to counteract the metabolic acidosis, should also be given. Dantrolene sodium (1–2 mg/kg i.v. every 5–10 min to a total dose of 10 mg/kg) or procainamide are effective in controlling the disease. Dantrolene given preoperatively and postoperatively for about 3 days (4–7 mg/kg/ day) may prevent hyperthermia.

Dental infections should be quickly and effectively treated since they also may precipitate attacks.

NEUROLEPTIC MALIGNANT SYNDROME

A rare but potentially lethal complication of the use of certain non-anaesthetic drugs such as phenothiazines and other neuroleptics, and tricyclic or monoamine oxidase inhibitor antidepressives, is known as *neuroleptic malignant syndrome.* The salient features are hyperthermia, muscle rigidity, fluctuating consciousness and autonomic dysfunction (pallor, tachycardia, labile blood pressure and sweating). The relationship to malignant hyperthermia is unknown. The causative drug should be stopped and dantrolene or bromocriptine should be given but the syndrome may persist for several days.

HYPERLIPOPROTEINAEMIA (HYPERLIPIDAEMIA)

The main plasma lipids are triglycerides, cholesterol ester and phospholipids (lecithin, sphingomyelin etc). Non-esterified fatty acids and cholesterol are also present. Plasma lipoproteins are responsible for the transport of lipids and

Table 10.22. Primary hyperlipoproteinaemias

Type		Main manifestations
I	Hypertriglyceridaemia (hyperchylomicronaemia)	Xanthomas Acute pancreatitis (Rare)
II	Hyperbetalipoproteinaemia (hypercholesterolaemia)	Atherosclerosis Ischaemic heart disease Xanthomas and xanthelasmas (Common)
III	Dysbetalipoproteinaemia (broad-beta disease)	Atherosclerosis Peripheral vascular disease Xanthomas Hyperglycaemia (Rare)
IV	Endogenous	Mild glucose intolerance Hyperuricaemia Atherosclerosis Xanthomas (Common)
V	Mixed hyperlipidaemia	Acute pancreatitis Xanthomas (Rare)

cholesterol within the body. The lipoproteins are divided into four groups based on their density and electrophoretic mobility.

Hyperlipoproteinaemia can be primary or secondary. Primary hyperlipoproteinaemias are often genetically determined (*Table 10.22*). Their importance is that several of them are characterized by accelerated atherosclerosis and premature death from ischaemic heart disease. Secondary hyperlipoproteinaemias may be caused by diabetes, hypothyroidism, nephrotic syndrome, liver disease, alcoholism and use of oral contraceptives.

Dental aspects of the hyperlipoproteinaemias

Premature coronary heart disease may result from hyperlipoproteinaemias, especially type II. Other factors such as hypertension, diabetes or smoking further increase the risk of coronary heart disease. Occasionally patients with hyperlipoproteinaemias may be recognized by the presence of cutaneous xanthomas (xanthelasmas) on the eyelids (*Fig.* 10.6). Xanthomas consist of slightly raised yellowish plaques. Although seen in familial dysbetalipoproteinaemia and then associated with accelerated atherosclerosis and heart disease, xanthelasmas are not specific to type II hyperlipoproteinaemia. A unique feature of this disorder, however, is the association of prominent xanthomas on the elbows and knees, especially with yellow to orange discoloration of the palmar creases.

Type IV and V hyperlipoproteinaemias may be complicated by sicca syndrome.

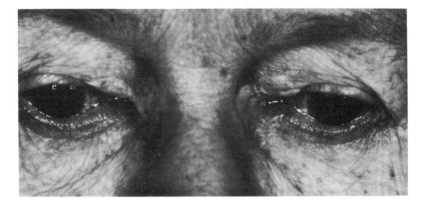

Fig. 10.6. Xanthelasma in familial hyperlipidaemia: such lesions may suggest a high risk of ischaemic heart disease.

Hypolipoproteinaemias

Pulpal calcifications and unusual odontomes may be found in high density lipoprotein deficiency (Tangier disease).

THE PORPHYRIAS

Porphyrias are inborn errors of haem metabolism. Porphyrias are divided into two main groups according to the principal site of the enzyme defect, namely in the liver or the red blood cells. The latter group (the erythropoietic porphyrias) are exceedingly rare and only the hepatic porphyrias, particularly variegate and acute intermittent porphyria, are important in dentistry (*Table 10.23*).

Variegate porphyria is estimated to affect 1 in 400 South Africans of Afrikaner descent. The main features are attacks of acute, severe abdominal pain accompanied by neuropsychiatric and cardiovascular disturbances. The neurological disturbance is typically a peripheral sensory and motor neuropathy but respiratory embarrassment or major convulsions can develop. Tachycardia and hypertension develop in the majority and may be followed by postural hypotension. Barbiturates, some other drugs, fasting, acute infections and pregnancy can precipitate attacks, but between attacks patients may appear normal apart from severe photosensitivity rashes which affect about 80 per cent of Afrikaner patients. These rashes typically cause hyperpigmentation of the face and hands (exposed areas).

Acute intermittent porphyria shows essentially the same features but the attacks may be even more severe and end in fatal respiratory failure. Rashes are not, however, a feature.

The diagnosis of the acute hepatic porphyrias is confirmed by demonstrating aminolaevulinic acid and porphobilinogen in the urine.

Table 10.23. The porphyrias

Hepatic porphyrias
    Acute intermittent porphyria (AIP)
    Hereditary coproporphyria
    Variegate porphyria
    Cutaneous porphyria
Erythropoietic porphyrias
    Erythropoietic protoporphyria
    Congenital porphyria

The essentials of treatment of attacks are, if possible, to stop the administration of the triggering drug and to give fluids, electrolytes and glucose by intravenous infusion.

Dental aspects

Barbiturates (including the intravenous barbiturates) and other drugs (*Table 10.24*) liable to precipitate attacks are absolutely contraindicated. Prevention of attacks by the avoidance of these drugs is the essential precaution, but local anaesthetics are safe.

Erythropoietic porphyria is characterized by red discoloration of the teeth, hypertrichosis, severe mutilating photosensitivity rashes and haemolytic anaemia. Fewer than 100 cases have probably ever been reported, but it has

Table 10.24. Drug use in porphyria

	Drugs not to be used	*Drugs safe to use*
1. Intravenous anaesthetics	Barbiturates Althesin†	
2. Analgesics	Pentazocine	Aspirin Paracetamol Codeine Opicids
3. Antimicrobials	Sulphonamides*	Penicillins Tetracyclines Erythromycin
4. Antidepressants and sedatives	Chlordiazepoxide Barbiturates Imipramine Meprobamate	Diazepam Chlorpromazine Promazine Metoclopramide
5. Others	Dichloralphenazone Carbamazepine Corticosteroids Oral contraceptives Phenytoin Chlorpropamide	Sodium valproate

*Co-trimoxazole contains a sulphonamide.
†Not now available

been suggested that this disease might have been the source of the werewolf legend because of the red teeth (thought to be dripping with blood), the hairy distorted facial features and the avoidance of daylight.

HAEMOCHROMATOSIS

Haemochromatosis is an uncommon disorder of iron metabolism characterized by high serum ferritin levels and deposition of iron, as haemosiderin, in many tissues particularly the liver, abdominal lymph nodes, skin, adrenals, pancreas, salivary glands and heart. A sicca syndrome may be a complication. A fibrotic reaction to these deposits can result in cirrhosis, skin pigmentation, adrenocortical insufficiency, diabetes (bronze diabetes) or cardiomyopathy, any of which can affect dental management. Treatment is by venesection.

HOMOCYSTINURIA

Homocystinuria is an inborn error of methionine metabolism with an autosomal recessive inheritance. Affected patients are tall with a Marfanoid appearance, joint hypermobility, ectopia lentis and visual and mental deterioration. Blood vessel abnormalities together with increased platelet adhesiveness predispose to thromboembolism, both spontaneously and postoperatively. Dextran 40 or 70 infusion intravenously perioperatively may reduce the thromboembolic risk.

ORAL CONTRACEPTIVES

Oral contraceptives are usually mixtures of synthetic oestrogens and progestogens which may act in several ways, especially by inhibiting ovulation by an action on the hypothalamic–pituitary axis, by altering the composition of uterine cervical mucus and by impeding implantation of the ovum.

The major risk in taking oral contraceptives is the increased incidence of thromboembolic disease (thrombosis of deep veins and coronary or cerebral thrombosis). However, the incidence of cardiovascular or cerebrovascular disease is normally so low in young women that these diseases are still uncommon even with a four- or fivefold increase in incidence in this group.

Hypertension, diabetes, jaundice and liver tumours, usually benign, are amongst the many other disorders increased in incidence in those taking oral contraceptives (*Table 10.25*). Most side-effects are thought to be caused by the oestrogen component, which is now only 50 µg or less.

Table 10.25. Side-effects of oral contraceptives

1. Mild
     Nausea
     Depression
     Loss of libido
     Breast pain
     Fluid retention
     Weight gain
2. Moderate
     Intermenstrual bleeding
3. Serious
     Thromboembolic disease* and hypertension*
     Myocardial infarction*
     Gallstones
     Liver tumours

Note: Side-effects are low compared with the risks associated with pregnancy.
*More frequent in smokers and older women.

Dental management of patients taking oral contraceptives

Worsening gingivitis and possibly a slight increase in severity of periodontitis may result from oral contraceptive use. There may also be an increased risk of dry sockets after third molar extractions and, on radiography, there may be jaw radiopacities or altered trabecular patterns.

The predisposition to myocardial infarction, thromboembolic disease and hypertension theoretically necessitates precautions if operation under general anaesthesia is required. However, if the patient is otherwise well, general anaesthesia in the dental chair is not contraindicated.

In spite of the risk of thromboembolism, the disadvantages of discontinuing oral contraceptives before dental general anaesthesia outweigh the advantages.

The main drugs that may interfere with the action of contraceptive pills and as a result may increase the risk of pregnancy are shown in *Table 10.26.*

Oral contraceptives may interact with anticoagulants to disturb anticoagulant control and they can impair the effect of tricyclic antidepressants.

Table 10.26. Some drugs interacting with oral contraceptives to produce risk of pregnancy

Significantly
  Barbiturates
  Anticonvulsants (phenytoin, carbamazepine, primidone)
  Dichloralphenazone (Welldorm)
  Rifampicin
Slightly (not necessarily significant)
  Oral antibiotics (particularly ampicillin, amoxycillin, metronidazole and tetracyclines)

PREGNANCY

Routine dental treatment of pregnant women under local anaesthesia is safe but general anaesthesia, some drugs and possibly radiography may endanger either fetus or mother. Infection control is particularly important in this group.

THE FETUS

Any woman of childbearing age is a potential candidate for pregnancy but may not be aware of pregnancy for 2 or more months, when, unfortunately, the fetus is most vulnerable. Fetal development during the first 3 months (trimester) of pregnancy is a complex process of organogenesis and the fetus is then especially at risk from developmental defects. Ten to twenty per cent of all pregnancies abort at this time, often because of fetal defects. Most developmental defects are of unknown aetiology but, in addition to hereditary influences, infections and drugs, such as alcohol and smoking, can be implicated in some cases. The only safe course of action is therefore to protect the patient as far as possible from infections and to avoid the use of drugs, particularly general anaesthetics, and radiography during the first trimester.

In the second and third trimesters the fetus is growing and maturing but can still be affected by drugs, such as tetracyclines, infections and possibly other factors.

Despite the existence of a few disastrous exceptions, notably thalidomide and some retinoids, very few drugs have been *proved* to be teratogenic for humans.

Mercury. Concern has been expressed, particularly in Sweden, about the risk of placental transfer of mercury as a result of exposure to the metal during pregnancy. However, measurements taken at the Department of Odontological Toxicology at the Karolinska Institute, on female dental personnel and their newborn babies and non–exposed controls have shown no significant differences in the plasma mercury levels nor in the fetal/maternal ratios of mercury levels.

Experimental and clinical data do not suggest that there should be any restriction on use of amalgams or work restriction of dental personnel, provided that work practices are up to accepted standards.

THE MOTHER

Pregnancy is a major event in any woman's life and is associated with physiological changes affecting especially the endocrine and cardiovascular systems, and often with changes in attitude, mood or behaviour. Endocrine changes cause nausea and vomiting and increased pigmentation, particularly of the nipples and sometimes the face (chloasma).

Diabetic control can be difficult, since insulin requirements increase, and pregnant diabetics need specialist attention. Pregnancy is a diabetogenic stress; glycosuria is not uncommon and glucose tolerance is reduced. However, these disturbances of carbohydrate metabolism usually resolve after pregnancy.

Cardiovascular changes in pregnancy include an increase in both blood volume and cardiac output. Initially there may be a slight decrease in blood pressure with the possibility of syncope or postural hypotension. In later pregnancy 10 per cent of patients may become hypotensive if laid supine, when the gravid uterus compresses the inferior vena cava and impedes venous return to the heart (supine hypotension syndrome: *see below*).

The increased cardiac output is associated with tachycardia. Expansion of the blood volume may cause an apparent anaemia but in about 20 per cent of pregnant females true anaemia also develops, mainly because of fetal demands for iron and folate. Most patients are given both of these haematinics. Pregnancy may worsen pre-existing anaemias, especially sickle cell anaemia.

An important complication of pregnancy is hypertension, which leads to increased morbidity and mortality in both fetus and mother. Hypertension may be asymptomatic but, when associated with oedema and proteinuria (pre-eclampsia), may culminate in eclampsia (hypertension, oedema, proteinuria and convulsions) which may be fatal. The fetus is at risk because of possible placental separation or damage leading to prematurity, fetal lung damage or intrauterine death. Hypertensive pregnant patients should therefore rest as much as possible and have antihypertensive treatment.

A further complication of pregnancy is increased blood coagulability which can lead to venous thrombosis, particularly postoperatively (Chapter 2) or occasionally disseminated intravascular coagulopathy (Chapter 3).

Dental aspects of pregnancy

Oral complications of pregnancy include aggravation of pre-existent gingivitis (pregnancy gingivitis), sometimes with localized swelling (pregnancy epulis). Pregnancy gingivitis begins at about the second month and persists until parturition. Improved oral hygiene and scaling reduce gingivitis and both conditions may resolve after parturition. Occasionally epulides need removal.

The teeth do not of course lose calcium as a result of fetal demands and there is no reason to expect caries to become more active unless the mother develops a capricious desire for sweets.

Pregnancy is the ideal opportunity to begin a preventive dental education programme and to advise on fluoride administration to the infant. Prenatal fluorides are not indicated as there is little evidence of benefit to the fetus.

In a few women subject to recurrent aphthae, ulcers may stop (or occasionally become more severe) during pregnancy.

Radiography should be avoided, especially in the first trimester even though dental radiography is unlikely to be a significant risk. Nevertheless, if essential, patients must wear a lead apron and exposure must be minimal.

Drug treatment should be avoided where possible, especially in the first trimester (*Table 10.27*). Any drug may endanger the fetus and though in many cases the risk is largely theoretical, administration of drugs should be avoided as far as possible.

Tetracyclines may cause tooth discoloration but other drugs may be teratogenic (*Table 10.27*). Unfortunately many women are unaware of being pregnant in the early part of the first trimester and therefore it is preferable to avoid giving any drugs to women of childbearing age, unless absolutely essential.

When drug treatment is unavoidable, penicillin, cephalosporins and erythromycin (stearate or ethyl succinate) are probably safe antimicrobials while paracetamol and codeine or dihydrocodeine are probably safe analgesics.

Dental treatment is best carried out during the second trimester, but the same precautions still apply. Advanced restorative procedures are probably best postponed until the periodontal state improves after parturition and prolonged sessions of treatment are better tolerated.

Table 10.27. Drug use in pregnancy

	To be avoided	Preferable
Analgesics	Aspirin Mefenamic acid Dextropropoxyphene Pentazocine Diamorphine	Paracetamol
Antimicrobials	Tetracyclines Metronidazole Aminoglycosides Co-trimoxazole Sulphonamides Rifampicin	Penicillin Erythromycin Cephalosporins Sulphisoxazole
Premedication	Long-acting benzodiazepines (e.g. diazepam) Opioids	Temazepam
Anaesthesia	Barbiturates	Nitrous oxide
Others	Etretinate Antidepressants Carbamazepine Corticosteroids Danazol Thalidomide Colchicine	Halothane

In the third trimester the supine hypotension syndrome may result if the patient is laid flat. The patient should therefore be put on one side to allow venous return to recover. Elective dental care should be avoided in the last month of pregnancy, as it is uncomfortable for the patient. Moreover, premature labour or even abortion may also be ascribed to dental treatment without justification. Because of the risk of such coincidental mishaps it is wise to avoid giving any drugs, possibly even local anaesthetics, and postponing as much treatment as possible until after parturition particularly in those with a history of abortions and those who have at last achieved pregnancy after years of failure.

General anaesthesia and sedation

General anaesthesia and possibly sedation with diazepam or midazolam are particular hazards and must be avoided in the first trimester and in the last month of pregnancy. In addition, when a general anaesthetic is unavoidable but there is a mishap to the fetus, the mother is likely to blame the anaesthetist, even though this may be quite unjustifiable. Yet another hazard is an increased tendency to vomiting during induction, in the third trimester.

Despite such considerations and the results of animal experiments, there is scanty evidence of teratogenic effects in humans from exposure to general anaesthetic agents. It is possible that barbiturates and benzodiazepines are teratogenic but the greater risk is late in pregnancy when they may induce respiratory depression in the fetus. Nitrous oxide, though able to interfere with vitamin B_{12} and folate metabolism does not appear to be teratogenic though it is advisable to limit the duration of exposure.

HAZARDS TO PREGNANT DENTAL STAFF

Chronic exposure to inhalational anaesthetic agents or mercury vapour, and exposure to infections by some viruses, such as cytomegalovirus or rubella may pose occupational risks to pregnant dental staff.

LACTATION

Since drugs may pass from mother to fetus, care should be taken in their use (*Table 10.28*). Cephalexin is a useful antimicrobial as it is not secreted in the milk. Fluoride passes into breast milk and if the local water supply contains more than 1 mg/l fluoride, supplements are not indicated for the breast-fed infant.

Table 10.28. Drug use in lactating mothers

	May be contraindicated	*Use instead*
Analgesics	Aspirin (high dose)	Aspirin (low dose)
	Dextropropoxyphene	Paracetamol
		Codeine
		Mefenamic acid
Antimicrobials	Tetracyclines	Penicillins
	Co-trimoxazole	Erythromycin
	Metronidazole	Rifampicin
	Sulphonamides	Cephalosporins
	Aminoglycosides	
Premedication	Atropine	Benzodiazepines (low dose)
	Chloral hydrate	Phenothiazines (low dose)
	Beta blockers	
Others	Antidepressants	
	Etretinate	
	Carbamazepine	
	Corticosteroids (high dose)	Corticosteroids (low dose)

PREMATURITY

Increasing survival rates of premature infants has revealed several long-term sequelae, including orofacial defects. Some 20–55 per cent of affected children have enamel hypoplasia, compared with 2 per cent of controls. Factors involved range from birth trauma to infections or metabolic and nutritional disorders. Calcium disturbances are also common.

Laryngoscopy can damage the unerupted maxillary anterior teeth and intubation with an oropharyngeal tube can cause grooving of the anterior maxillary ridge. Fortunately, the latter has few serious consequences.

THE MENOPAUSE

The menopause is the termination of a woman's productive life and is marked by cessation of menstrual periods. The menopause can start at any age between 40 and 55 years.

In most women the menopause is not associated with serious physical or emotional complications. Some gain weight, lose some muscle tone and may develop a few hairs on the chin or upper lip. Hot flushes, when the patient feels a wave of heat passing over the body, are, however, common. Flushes may be momentary or last several minutes and their frequency is very variable. Hot flushes appear to be caused by vasomotor instability and may sometimes be controlled by oestrogens.

Psychological disorders are not uncommon in the menopause. They are usually mild and include dizziness and insomnia, but depression or paranoia may develop.

Dental aspects

The menopause has been blamed for many problems, although age itself is usually responsible. This period of life is, however, associated with emotional disturbances and stresses, particularly, no doubt, partly as a result of the changing pattern of family life. Depression is relatively common at this time.

Atypical facial pain and oral dysaesthesias are most common but there is little evidence of benefit from steroid sex hormones (Chapter 14). Dryness of the mouth and so-called desquamative gingivitis are not hormonal in origin; Sjögren's syndrome, lichen planus and mucous membrane pemphigoid are all more common in the middle-aged or older, and particularly in females.

DIETARY DISORDERS

OBESITY

Obesity rather than malnutrition is the main nutritional problem in the Western World. Although many fat people believe that they have a glandular cause for their obesity, this is hardly ever the case and obesity simply results from eating more than the body needs. Obesity can however *occasionally* be the result of hypothalamic disease (Fröhlich's Laurence–Moon–Biedl, or Prader–Willi syndromes *see* Appendix to Chapter 20) and can also be caused by endocrinopathies (hypothyroidism, Cushing's disease or insulinoma).

Obesity predisposes to or aggravates several disorders (*Table 10.29*).

There is about a threefold increase in premature deaths in obese patients. Management includes calorie restriction, more exercise and possibly appetite suppressants such as fenfluramine for a limited period.

Table 10.29. Complications of obesity

Cardiovascular
    Hypertension
    Ischaemic heart disease
    Varicose veins
Respiratory
    Cor pulmonade
Metabolic and endocrine
    Diabetes mellitus
    Hyperlipoproteinaemias (type II, III and IV)
Gynaecological
    Uterine prolapse
    Polycystic ovaries
    Amenorrhoea
Orthopaedic
    Accidents
    Painful osteoarthritis
Psychological
    Depression
Gastrointestinal
    Hiatus hernia (and other hernias)
    Gallstones
    Colonic disease (diverticulitis/carcinoma)

Dental aspects of obesity

Jaw wiring of obese patients appears to be an effective and safe way of substantially reducing weight in those in whom simpler methods fail, but relapse frequently follows this extreme measure.

Dental treatment in the obese patient may be complicated by diabetes or cardiovascular disease, or, rarely, by an organic cause of the obesity. Cardiac dysrhythmias may be produced by the interaction of halogenated anaesthetics and large doses of amphetamines or amphetamine–like appetite suppressants (all Controlled Drugs) which should be discontinued a week before general anaesthesia.

The total work of breathing is increased in obese patients and even at rest obese patients need to ventilate more than normal. Respiration is further impaired in the supine position.

Some 10 per cent of grossly obese persons have hypoventilation, cor pulmonale and episodic somnolence (Pickwickian syndrome).

Lactovegetarianism

Frequent intake of a lactovegetarian diet may result in dental erosion. Citrus fruits, vinegar and acidic berries are especially responsible, particularly if ingested just before retiring to sleep.

Vegetarians and Vegans

Complete absence of meat products can lead to vitamin B_{12} deficiency (Chapter 4) though the latter is surprisingly rare in vegans. Vegetarians may have less caries than others.

Malnutrition

Certain types of latent malnutrition may predispose to mouth ulcers, glossitis and angular stomatitis (Chapter 4). Severe malnutrition can result from anorexia nervosa or bulimia (Chapter 14). Secondary immunodeficiencies with a predisposition to oral ulceration and necrotizing gingivitis may result from severe malnutrition. Sialosis is a rare effect.

Bibliography

Alberti K. G. M. M. and Thomas D. J. B. (1979) The management of diabetes during surgery. *Br. J. Anaesth.* **51,** 693–710.
Bainton R. (1986) Interaction between antibiotic therapy and contraceptive medications. *Oral Surg.* **61,** 453–5.
Barba M. W., Post A. C. and Duncan W. K. (1985) Dental treatment of a malignant hyperthermia susceptible child. *Pediatr. Dent.* **7,** 61–5.
Blinkhorn A. S. (1981) Dental preventive advice for pregnant and nursing mothers—sociological implications. *Int. Dent. J.* **31,** 14–22.
Brownell A. K. W. and Paaruke R. T. (1986) Use of local anaesthetics in malignant hyperthermia. *CMAJ* **134,** 992–4.
Brunt L. M. and Wells S. A. (1985) The multiple endocrine neoplasia syndromes. *Invest. Radiol.* **20,** 916–7.
Cantin R. Y., Poole A. and Ryan J. F. (1986) Malignant hyperthermia. *Oral Surg.* **62,** 389–92.
Carson J. M. and van Sickels J. E. (1982) Preoperative determination of susceptibility to malignant hyperthermia. *J. Maxillofac. Surg.* 432–5.
Catellani J. E., Harvey S., Erickson S. T. et al. (1980) Effect of oral contraceptive cycle on dry socket (localized alveolar osteitis). *J. Am. Dent. Assoc.* **101,** 777–80.
Cawson R. A. and James J. (1973) Adrenal crisis in a dental patient having systemic steroids. *Br. J. Oral Surg.* **10,** 305.
Chiodo G. T. and Rosenstein D. I. (1985) Dental treatment during pregnancy: a preventive approach. *J. Am. Dent. Assoc.* **110,** 365–8.
Chow A. W. and Jewesson P. J. (1985) Pharmacokinetics and safety of antimicrobial drugs during pregnancy. *Rev. Infect. Dis.* **7,** 287–313.
Cook D. M. and Kendall J. W. (1980) Cushing syndrome: current concepts of diagnosis and therapy (Medical Progress). *West. J. Med.* **132,** 111–22.
Desmonts J. M., Lehouelleur J., Redmond P. et al. (1977) Anaesthetic management of patients with a phaeochromocytoma review of 102 cases. *Br.J. Anaesth.* **49,** 991.
Douglas M. J. and McMorland G. H. (1986) The anaesthetic management of the malignant hyperthermia susceptible patient. *Can. Anaesth. Soc. J.* **33,** 371–8.
Editorial (1980) Corticosteroids and hypothalamic–pituitary–adrenocortical function. *Br. Med. J.* **280,** 813–14.
Editorial (1985) Measuring serum calcium. *Br. Med. J.* **290,** 728–9.
Ellis F. R. and Halsall P. J. (1980) Malignant hyperpyrexia. *Br. J. Hosp. Med.* **24,** 318–27.
Fuks A. B., Kaufman E. and Galiti D. (1980) Comprehensive dental treatment under general anaesthesia for patients with homocystinuria. *J. Dent. Child.* **102,** 340–2.
Garrow J. S. and Gardiner G. T. (1981) Maintenance of weight loss in obese patients after jaw wiring. *Br. Med. J.* **282,** 858–60.
Gislen G. Nilsson K. O. and Matsson L. (1980) Gingival inflammation in diabetic children related to degree of metabolic control. *Acta Odontol. Scand.* **38,** 241–6.
Goss A. N. (1980) Treatment of massive obesity by prolonged jawimmobilization for edentulous patients. *Int. J. Oral Surg.* **9,** 253–8.
Jashi J. V. (1980) A study of interaction of low dose combination oral contraceptive with ampicillin and metronidazole. *Contraception* **22,** 643–52.
Keith O., Flint S. and Scully C. (1989) Lingual abscess in a patient with anorexia nervosa. *Br. Dent. J.* **167,** 71–2.
Kennon S., Tasch E. G. and Arm R. N. (1978) Considerations in the management of patients taking oral contraceptives. *J. Am. Dent. Assoc.* **97,** 641–3.

Kinirons M. J. and Glasgow J. F. T. (1985) The chronology of dentinal defects related to medical findings in hypoparathyroidism. *J. Dent.* **13,** 346–9.

Lamey P. J.,Carmichael F. and Scully C. (1985) Oral pigmentation, Addison's disease and the results of screening for adrenocortical insufficiency. *Br. Dent. J.* **158,** 297–8.

Lessof M. H. (1977) Reducing the problems of corticosteroid therapy. *Br. J. Hosp. Med.* **17,** 380–5.

Linkosalo E. and Markkanen H. (1985) Dental erosions in relation to lactovegetarian diet. *Scand. J. Dent. Res.* **93,** 436–41.

Luyk N. H., Anderson J. and Ward-Booth R. P. (1985) Corticosteroid therapy and the dental patient. *Br. Dent. J.* **159,** 12–17.

McAndrew P. G., Nicholl A. D. J. and Beck P. R. (1982) The syndrome of inappropriate antidiuretic hormone secretion. *Br. J. Oral Surg.* **20,** 256–9.

Mazze R I. (1986) Nitrous oxide during pregnancy. *Anaesthesia* **41,** 897–9.

Montgomery D. A. D. and Welbourn R. B. (1975) *Medical and Surgical Endocrinology.* London, Arnold.

Murrah V. A. (1985) Diabetes mellitus and associated oral manifestations: a review. *J. Oral Pathol.* **14,** 271–81.

Newrick P.G., Bowman C., Green D. et al. (1991) Parotid secretion in diabetic autonomic neuropathy. *J. Diabetic Complications* **5,** 35–7.

Page M. M. B. and Watkins B. J. (1978) Cardio-respiratory arrest and diabetic autonomic neuropathy. *Lancet* **i,** 14.

Pandit S. K., Kothary S. P. and Cohen P. J. (1979) Orally administered Dantrolene for prophylaxis of malignant hyperthermia. *Anesthesiology* **50,** 156–8.

Porter S. R., Malamos D. and Scully C. (1986) Mouth–skin interface, 2: Connective tissue and metabolic disorders. *Update* **33,** 94–96.

Rehorst E. D. and de Groot G W. (1976) Preoperative management of glucocorticoid-dependent pedodontic patients. *J. Am. Dent. Assoc.* **93,** 809–12.

Scully C. (1979/80) Orofacial manifestations of disease. 5: Endocrine and metabolic disorders and iatrogenic disease. *Dent. Update* **7,** 175; *Hosp. Update* **6,** 9.

Seow W K. (1986) Oral complications of premature birth. *Aust. Dent. J.* **31,** 23–9.

Sessler D. I. (1986) Malignant hyperthermia. *J. Pediatr.* **109,** 9–14.

Smith N. J. D. (1982) Dental radiography during pregnancy. *Br. Dent. J.* **152,** 346.

Spiegel R. J., Vigersky R. A., Oliff A. I. et al (1979) Adrenal suppression after short-term corticosteroid therapy. *Lancet* **i,** 630–3.

Whelan J., Redpath T. and Buckle R. (1982) The medical and anaesthetic management of acromegalic patients undergoing maxillofacial surgery. *Br. J. Oral Surg.* **20,** 77–83.

Williamson L. W., Lorson E. L and Osbon D. B. (1980) Hypothalamic–pituitary–adrenal suppression after short-term dezamethasone therapy for oral surgical procedures. *J. Oral Surg.* **38,** 20–8.

Appendix to Chapter 10

INBORN ERRORS OF METABOLISM

Disease	*Management problems*
Abetalipoproteinaemia	Ataxia: haemorrhage
Acatalasaemia	Gingival ulceration
Acid lipase deficiency	Mental handicap: anaemia
Acrodermatitis enteropathica	Severe oral ulceration: neuropathies
Adenosine deaminase deficiency	Immunodeficiency
α_1-antitrypsin deficiency	Hepatic disease: emphysema
Argininaemia	Spasticity: mental handicap: epilepsy
Aspartylglucosaminuria	Mental handicap
Cerebrotendinous xanthomatosis	Dementia: ataxia: paresis: cataracts
Cholinesterase deficiency	Suxamethonium sensitivity
Chronic granulomatous disease	Lymph node abscesses (cervical etc.)
	Liability to severe bacterial infections
Combined hyperlipidaemia	Atherosclerosis
Congenital adrenal hyperplasia	Hypoadrenocorticism
Crigler-Najjar syndrome	Jaundice
Cystinosis	Renal disease
Cystinuria	Renal disease
Diphosphoglycerate mutase deficiency	Anaemia
Dubin-Johnson syndrome	Jaundice
Dysbetalipoproteinaemia	Atherosclerosis
Fabry's disease	Neuropathy: thromboses: renal failure: pulmonary failure
Familial dysautonomia (Riley–Day syndrome)	Sensitive to barbiturates: dysphagia: sialorrhoea: insensitive to pain: mental handicap: epilepsy: blood pressure labile
Familial goitre	Hypothyroidism
Fanconi syndrome	Aminoaciduria: osteomalacia
Fucosidosis	Mental handicap
Galactosaema	Mental handicap: hepatic disease: cataracts: hypoglycaemia
Gilbert's disease	Jaundice
GM_1 gangliosidosis	Mental handicap: epilepsy: blindness
GM_2 gangliosidosis	„ „ „ „
(a) Tay-Sachs disease	„ „ „ „
(b) Sandhoff disease	„ „ „ „
Gaucher's disease	Mental handicap: spasticity: thrombocytopenia: leucopenia
Glucose 6-phosphate dehydrogenase deficiency	Haemolytic anaemia
Glutaric aciduria	Hypoglycaemia
Glycogen storage disease:	
I	Hypoglycaemia: caries: bleeding tendency
II	Cardiomyopathy: respiratory infection: neurological abnormalities
III	Hypoglycaemia
IV	Hepatic disease: cardiac failure
VI	Mild hypoglycaemia
VIa	„ „ „ „
O	„ „ „ „
Gout	Renal disease: hypertension: atherosclerosis
Haemochromatosis	Diabetes: hepatic disease: cardiomyopathy

Disease	*Management problems*
Hereditary angio-oedema	Airways obstruction
Hereditary fructose intolerance	Hepatic disease: hypoglycaemia
Hereditary oroticaciduria	Severe anaemia: leucopenia
Hereditary spherocytosis	Haemolytic anaemia
Hexokinase deficiency	Anaemia
Histidinaemia	Hearing deficit: speech deficit: infections: mental handicap
Homocystinuria	Mental handicap: epilepsy: blindness: hepatic disease: chest deformities: thrombotic disease
Hypercalcaemia	Renal disease: cardiac subaortic stenosis: mental handicap
Hypercholesterolaemia	Atherosclerosis
Hypercystinuria	Renal disease
Hyperornithinaemia	Mental handicap
Hyperoxaluria .	Renal disease
Hypertriglyceridaemia	Atherosclerosis: pancreatitis
Hypophosphatasia	Skeletal abnormalities: dental hypoplasia
Krabbe disease	Mental handicap: blindness
Lecithin/cholesterol,acetyltransferase deficiency	Haemolytic anaemia : atherosclerosis: renal disease
Lesch-Nyhan syndrome	Mutilation of tongue or lips: mental handicap: epilepsy: athetosis
Lipoprotein lipase deficiency	Pancreatitis
Lysinuria	Epilepsy
Mannosidosis	Mental handicap
Metachromatic leucodystrophy	Mental handicap: blindness: psychoses
Methionine malabsorption	Epilepsy
Mucolipidosis (I cell disease)	Mental handicap: blindness: valvular heart disease
Mucopolysaccharidoses (MPS):	
I Hurler syndrome	Mental handicap:blindness:cardiac disease: temporomandibular joint trismus
II Hunter syndrome	As in MPS I
III Sanfilippo syndrome	Mental handicap
IV Morquio syndrome	Blindness: chest deformity: aortic valve disease: enamel hypoplasia
V Ullrich Scheie syndrome	Blindness: valvular heart disease
VI Maroteaux–Lamy syndrome	Mental handicap: blindness
VII	Mental handicap
Myeloperoxidase deficiency	Candidosis
Niemann Pick disease	Mental handicap: epilepsy: pancytopenia
Neuronal ceroid lipofuscinoses	Mental handicap: epilepsy: blindness
Orotic aciduria	Megaloblastic anaemia
Oxalosis	Renal disease
Phenylketonuria	Mental handicap: epilepsy
Porphyrias	Drug sensitivities: neuropathies: hypertension
Primary hypophosphataemia (vitamin D-resistant rickets)	Dwarfism: rickets: dental abscesses
Prolinaemia	Epilepsy: deafness
Purine nucleoside phosphorylase deficiency	Immunodeficiency
Pyruvate kinase deficiency	Anaemia
Renal glycosuria	Glycosuria (confusion with diabetes)
Refsum's disease	Blindness: deafness
Rotor syndrome	Jaundice
Transcobalamin II deficiency	Macrocytic anaemia: pancytopenia
Triosephosphate isomerase deficiency	Anaemia

Disease	Managementproblems
Tyrosinaemia	Hepatic disease
Tyrosinosis	Myaesthenia: epilepsy
Wilson's disease (hepatolenticular degeneration)	Hepatic disease: renal disease: spasticity: tremor
Wolman's disease	Mental handicap
Xeroderma pigmentosum	Skin cancers

ENDOCRINE AND METABOLIC EFFECTS OF SOME CANCERS

Substance released	Most common tumours responsile	Disease caused	Features
ACTH	Bronchial carcinoma Bronchial carcinoid Phaeochromocytoma Pancreatic carcinoma Parotid carcinoma	Cushing's syndrome	See p. 262
Antidiuretic hormone (ADH)	Bronchial carcinoma Hodgkin's disease Pancreatic carcinoma	SIADH	See p. 251
Parathormone (PTH) and prostaglandins	Almost any squamous cell carcinoma Renal carcinoma Breast cancer	Hypercalcaemia	Vomiting, constipation, polyuria, polydipsia, psychosis, abdominal pain
Thyroid stimulating hormone (TSH)	Trophoblastic tumours	Hyperthyroidism	See p. 268
Human chorionic gonadotrophin (HCG)	Pancreatic carcinoma Hepatoblastoma Breast cancer	Precocious puberty	
Erythropoietin	Fibroids Breast cancer Adrenal tumours Bronchial carcinoma Hepatoma Phaeochromocytoma	Polycythaemia	
Gastrin	Pancreatic carcinoma	Zollinger–Ellison syndrome	Multiple small-intestinal ulcers Diarrhoea
5-Hydroxytryptamine and other vaso-active substances	Ileocaecal carcinoma Bronchial carcinoma	Carcinoid syndrome	Symptoms mainly if there are hepatic metastases Flushing, broncho-spasm, diarrhoea Right-sided valvular heart lesions (especially pulmonary stenosis)

Chapter 11

Diseases of the Musculoskeletal System

Of the two components of the skeletal system, the joints are considerably more frequently affected by disease than the bones. The jaws and temporomandibular joints are part of this system but they are rarely involved by systemic disease and few skeletal diseases affect the management of the dental patient directly. However, access to the surgery or getting into or out of the chair may be difficult.

DISEASES OF BONE

GENETIC SKELETAL DISEASES

Many genetic disorders of the skeleton are rare and of little clinical importance in dentistry. Their main features are summarized in the Appendix to this chapter and only the more relevant disorders are discussed here.

Osteogenesis Imperfecta (Fragilitas Ossium)

Osteogenesis imperfecta (brittle bone disease) is a rare inherited autosomal dominant disorder with a frequency of 1 in 20 000 births. The gene for dentinogenesis imperfecta, one of the more common heritable defects of the teeth, is closely related. There are several variants (*Table 11.1*).

The basic defect in osteogenesis imperfecta, as in Marfan's and Ehlers Danlos syndromes, appears to be in Type I collagen formation, and although osteoblasts are active the total amount of bone formed is small and is mostly woven in type. The long bones are typically normal in length with epiphyses of normal width but slender shafts, frequently giving a trumpet-shaped appearance.

The bones are fragile and multiple fractures follow minimal trauma. Healing is rapid but usually with distortion and the ultimate effect in severe cases is gross deformity causing dwarfism. The frequency of fractures usually tends to diminish after puberty. The parietal regions of the skull may bulge outwards causing eversion of the upper part of the ear. Other defects are blue sclerae, deafness, easy bruising and weakness of tendons and ligaments causing loose-jointedness

Table 11.1. Osteogenesis imperfecta—subtypes

Type	Inheritance	Bone disease	Stature	Extraskeletal involvement
I*	AD	Mild: fractures in childhood	Almost normal	Common. Blue sclerae: otosclerosis: thin aortic valves: hypermobile joints: ‡Dentinogenesis imperfecta ±
II	AR	Severe: skull virtually unossified: multiple fractures: lethal	—	—
III	AR some sporadic	Progressive: few can walk unaided	Reduced	Blue sclerae. No dentinogenesis imperfecta
IV	AD	Severe	Reduced	Sclerae not blue. Dentinogenesis imperfecta common
V	Varied	Mild	Almost normal	Loose-jointedness a prominent feature

AD. Autosomal dominant.
*Constitutes 80 per cent of all cases.

and often hernias. The severity and extent of the disease is very variable but occasionally clinical difficulties may be caused by chest deformities or cardio-vascular disease such as mitral valve prolapse or aortic incompetence.

Dental aspects

In those with associated dentinogenesis imperfecta, the teeth may have the characteristic abnormal translucency and brown or purplish colour. The enamel may therefore adhere poorly to the dentine and be progressively shed under the stress of mastication. By adolescence the teeth may be worn down to the gum margins but obliteration of the pulp chamber by dentine usually prevents exposure of the pulp. The softness of the dentine, however, makes the fitting of post crowns impractical so that extraction and replacement by dentures is the usual form of treatment in severe cases. In spite of the brittleness of most of the skeleton the jaws rarely fracture. Dental extractions can usually there-fore be safely carried out in most patients but care should obviously be taken to support the jaws and to use minimal force.

Apart from the obvious management problems related to bone fragility, there may be a risk from general anaesthesia if there are chest deformities or cardiac complications with a risk of infective endocarditis.

Care should be taken not to confuse children with brittle bone syndrome from those who have been subjected to physical abuse (Chapter 14)

Achondroplasia

Achondroplasia is a defect in cartilaginous bone formation, often inherited as an autosomal dominant trait. Defective long bone growth leads to dwarfism with short limbs, a normal spine length with lumbar lordosis and an apparently large head (circus dwarf). Nasal septal and base of skull growth is impaired so that the bridge is depressed and skull bossed. Many patients are otherwise completely normal, but spinal deformity can be severe and occasionally cause spinal cord compression.

Dental aspects

The only significant dental aspects are orthodontic in nature as a result of malocclusion but diabetes and kyphosis may cause management problems.

Cleidocranial Dysplasia (Cleidocranial Dysostosis)

Cleidocranial dysplasia is a defect mainly of membrane bone formation often inherited as an autosomal dominant. The defects mainly involve the skull and clavicle. The head is large with bulging frontal bones and a persistent metopic (frontal) suture. The fontanelles persist and there are numerous wormian bones. The middle facial third is hypoplastic leading to a relative mandibular protrusion, and the nasal bridge is depressed.

The clavicles are either absent or defective thus conferring the unusual ability to approximate the shoulders anteriorly (*Fig.* 11.1). Other skeletal defects such as kyphoscoliosis or pelvic anomalies may be associated.

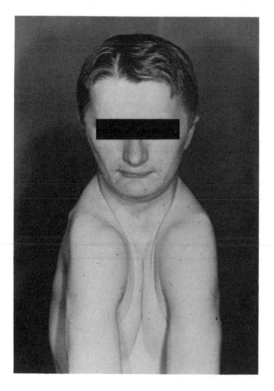

Fig. 11.1. Cleidocranial dysostosis.

Dental aspects

Apart from the facial anomalies there may be persistence of the deciduous dentition, unerupted permanent teeth and multiple supernumeraries, twisted roots, malformed crowns and dentigerous cysts. The associated problems are dealt with in textbooks of oral surgery.

Osteopetrosis (Albers–Schönberg Disease)

Osteopetrosis (marble-bone disease) is a rare disorder of variable severity characterized by a general increase in bone density probably as a result of a defect in osteoclastic activity and hence of the bone remodelling mechanism. The bones, though abnormally dense are weak.

In mild osteopetrosis there may be no symptoms and the diagnosis is made incidentally by radiography. Other patients suffer bone pain, fractures or osteomyelitis. Fractures, though common, usually heal normally.

In more severe disease (malignant infantile osteopetrosis) added complications can be cranial neuropathies leading, for example, to optic atrophy. Hydrocephalus, epilepsy and mental handicap are less frequent.

The medullary cavities are filled with bone, and anaemia is common in spite of extramedullary haemopoiesis in the liver, spleen and lymph nodes. Macrophages and neutrophils are defective. Serum levels of acid phosphatase are raised but calcium and phosphate levels are normal. Treatment is unsatisfactory. Corticosteroid therapy may be of some help but marrow transplantation may be the only hope.

Dental aspects

The face may be broad with hypertelorism, snub nose and frontal bossing. There may be retarded tooth eruption. Radiography shows increased bone density and thickness, especially obvious in the skull.

Trigeminal or facial neuropathies may complicate the disease and fracture of the jaw or osteomyelitis may complicate extractions. Once established, infection is difficult to eradicate, so that surgery should be minimally traumatic, mucoperiosteal flaps preferably not raised and antibiotic cover should be used. Eruption of posterior teeth may be complicated by osteomyelitis. Other management problems may include anaemia (Chapter 4) and corticosteroid therapy (Chapter 10).

Marfan's Syndrome

Marfan's syndrome is an autosomal dominant disorder of connective tissue with skeletal, ocular and cardiovascular manifestations. The disease has a prevalence of about 1 in 10 000 and is of such variable expression that diagnosis may be difficult and there can be confusion with other, rare disorders (*Table 11.2,* Appendix to this chapter).

Table 11.2. Marfan's Syndrome

Autosomal dominant	TMJ subluxation
Disproportionately long limbs	Cardiovascular defects
Arachnodactyly	Dilatation of ascending aorta
Loose joints	Dissecting aneurysm
Pectus excavatum	Aortic regurgitation
Ectopia lentis	Mitral valve prolapse
Mental handicap (sometimes)	Blue sclerae in some

Note: Marfan's syndrome shares the features of loose-jointedness, cardiac valvular defects and ocular lesions with various of the subtypes of Ehlers–Danlos syndrome. However, the most obvious distinguishing feature of Marfan's syndrome is the long, thin body habitus and long slender fingers.

Skeletal manifestations are increased length of tubular bones so that patients are tall with wide arm span and excessively long spider-like fingers (arachnodactyly). Ligaments are so lax that hyperextensibility, subluxation or dislocation of joints and hernias are common. Lung cysts may lead to spontaneous pneumothorax and respiratory function can also be impaired by kyphoscoliosis.

The eyes are affected in most patients and the lens subluxes or dislocates in 80 per cent—often causing visual impairment.

Cardiovascular abnormalities affect 90 per cent of patients with Marfan's syndrome. Aortic dissection can be life-threatening. There is often severe aortic and mild mitral incompetence. Death in the fifth decade is common.

It has been suggested that Abraham Lincoln may have had Marfan's syndrome. His facial appearance and build possibly indicate the appearance of a mild case. However, casts of his hands, which were broad and strong, disprove this idea.

Dental aspects

The palatal vault is high in Marfan's syndrome and temporomandibular joint dysfunction or recurrent subluxation may be a prominent symptom.

Management may be complicated by chest deformities and cardiovascular abnormalities, which may be contraindications to general anaesthesia, and there is a risk of infective endocarditis (Chapter 2).

A Marfanoid body build may also be a feature of the multiple endocrine adenoma syndrome (MEA III) (Chapter 10).

Ehlers–Danlos Syndrome

Ehlers–Danlos syndrome is a group of disorders of collagen formation (*Table 11.3*) characterized by hyperextensible skin, propensity to bruising and loose-jointedness. The most common forms are inherited as autosomal dominant traits while the remainder are recessive. There have been recent advances in the understanding of some of the molecular abnormalities of collagen in

Table 11.3. Ehlers—Danlos syndrome—subtypes

Subtypes	Inheritance	Skin		Joints	Special features
		Hyperextensibility	Fragility and bruising	Hypermobility	
I (gravis)	AD	++	++	++	Parrot face. Frequent musculoskeletal disorders. Mitral valve prolapse
II (mitis)	AD	+	+	+	Mitral valve prolapse. Bruising common
III (benign hypermobile)	AD	±	+	++	Dislocations, haemarthrosis, early onset arthritis. Mitral valve prolapse
IV (ecchymotic)	AR	±	+++	± Digits only	Bleeding from major arteries. Cerebrovascular accidents, severe purpura from minimal trauma, spontaneous rupture of bowel, skull defects
V (sex-linked)	X-linked	++	+	±	Frequent musculoskeletal disorders. Males only
VI (ocular or hydroxylysine deficient)	AR	++	±	++	Fragile cornea and sclera. Multiple ocular defects, deafness, often early loss of sight
VII (multiple congenital dislocation or arthrochalasis multiplex congenita)	AR	+	±	++	Early onset of multiple dislocations. Some laxity of ligaments, short stature
VII (periodontal)	AD	±	±	±	Severe early onset periodontitis and loss of teeth. Blue sclerae
IX (skeletal and urinary tract dysplasia)	AR	−	±	±	—
X (fibronectin deficiency)	AR	±	±	±	Bleeding tendency

AD, Autosomal dominant; AR, autosomal recessive.

Ehlers–Danlos syndrome so that the nature of the subtypes in earlier reports of oral manifestations in this group of diseases may be uncertain.

There is wide variation in the clinical features of the different types of Ehlers–Danlos syndrome but hypermobility of the joints is the best known manifestation. Typical features, seen in varying degrees in the whole group, are as follows.

The skin is typically soft, abnormally extensible, feels fine and thin and may appear lax in some sites. Even when it appears normal, it may be possible to pull the skin of the cheek out for one or two inches. Fragility of the skin and oral mucosa may cause wounds to gape or to split after slight trauma. Slow healing may leave fragile scars with a tissue-paper texture while easy ('spontaneous') bruising may mimic purpura caused by haematological disease.

Hypermobility of the joints may be extreme (India-rubber man) but the severity varies in the different subtypes. It may be possible to hyperextend the fingers until they are at right angles to the back of the hand and to pull the thumb back until it touches the forearm. Recurrent, semi-spontaneous dislocation may result.

Internal complications affecting the cardiovascular system (especially mitral valve prolapse or conduction defects), gastrointestinal tract, urinary tract and respiratory system also result from weakness of their connective tissue component. Mitral valve prolapse (floppy valve syndrome), which is associated especially with Type III Ehlers–Danlos syndrome, may confer susceptibility to infective endocarditis or lead to rapid development of mitral insufficiency and heart failure with resulting anaesthetic hazards. Spontaneous rupture of major arteries can cause fatal haemorrhage. Internal bleeding can cause abdominal emergencies while widespread purpura can readily be mistaken for haematological disease with haemorrhagic tendencies but is unlike any of the latter because of the combination of subcutaneous, submucosal and deep bleeding which, though of vascular origin, may mimic a coagulation defect such as haemophilia, clinically.

Haemostatic function is usually normal but platelet defects have occasionally been reported. The latter may be caused by the same defect that underlies the connective tissue disorder.

Dental aspects

The most severe vascular abnormalities are seen in Type IV (ecchymotic type) in which there is severe semi-spontaneous purpura with extensive ecchymoses and also weakness of arterial walls.

Severe bleeding from the gingivae, especially after toothbrushing, or from extraction sockets, may sometimes be the main complaint. Post-extraction bleeding is likely to be most severe in Type IV.

Type VIII Ehlers–Danlos syndrome is of special interest to periodontists in view of the early onset of periodontal disease, which is widespread and severe with early loss of teeth.

Other, incidental oddities that may be seen in Ehlers–Danlos syndrome may include the ability to touch the nose with the tip of the tongue and dental abnormalities. The teeth may be small with short or abnormally shaped roots, and large numbers of pulp stones. Hypermobility of joints is severe in Types I, VI and VII and in all of these, dislocation of the temporomandibular joint is a possibility.

Patients with mitral valve prolapse may develop heart failure with attendant risks during anaesthesia and there is also a risk of infective endocarditis (Chapter 2).

Pseudoxanthoma Elasticum

Pseudoxanthoma elasticum is a rare autosomal recessive disorder of connective tissue characterized by yellow papular or reticular skin lesions, visual impairment and cardiovascular abnormalities.

The skin is hyperextensible, as in the Ehlers–Danlos syndrome, and there may be blue sclerae and loose-jointedness. Abnormalities in the eye include streaks beneath the retina (angioid streaks) and often haemorrhages and scarring.

Cardiovascular involvement includes calcification of elastic tissue in vessel walls leading to poor peripheral blood flow, causing intermittent claudication, and ischaemic heart disease. Hypertension is common. Some patients develop hypothyroidism; others bleed from the upper gastrointestinal tract, uterus, renal or respiratory tracts.

Some patients have a normal lifespan but others succumb to haemorrhage, cardiac disease or cerebrovascular accidents.

Dental aspects

Skin lesions may be seen around the face and mouth and there may be nodules in the lips, or sometimes in the mouth. Dental management may be complicated particularly by cardiovascular disease.

Diseases of Calcium Metabolism and Bone

Localized bone diseases such as osteomyelitis or tumours are not within the remit of this text and reference should be made to oral pathology texts. Hyperparathyroidism is discussed in Chapter 10.

The main factors controlling bone metabolism and blood calcium levels include the following:

1. Vitamin D is taken in the diet and absorbed from the upper small intestine with other fat–soluble vitamins. Precursors are also synthesized in the skin under the influence of sunlight. The most active metabolite is produced by hepatic and then renal conversion of precursors to 1,25-dihydroxycholecalciferol (DHCC), a process enhanced by parathyroid hormone and low phosphate levels. The active metabolite controls bone metabolism, enhances calcium absorption and incidentally, affects the proliferation of various cells other than those of bone.

2. Active vitamin D and parathyroid hormone promote intestinal transport of calcium and phosphate to maintain their normal extracellular fluid levels.

3. Parathormone (PTH) secretion is regulated by blood calcium levels: when these fall, PTH is secreted, accelerates the removal of calcium from bones to raise the blood calcium level and enhances the formation of active vitamin D.

4. Calcitonin opposes the action of parathormone and lowers the blood calcium level, mainly by increasing the deposition of calcium in the bones.

5. Several other hormones, including corticosteroids, oestrogens and thyroxine, affect bone formation and metabolism to varying degrees.

Bone is a dynamic tissue which is being constantly remodelled throughout life. It is a reservoir of calcium, magnesium, phosphate and other ions necessary for many homeostatic functions.

Osteoblasts secrete osteoid which becomes mineralized during bone development by the deposition of calcium phosphate, both as hydroxyapatite and amorphous calcium phosphate, in this matrix. The resorption of bone is carried out by multinucleated osteoclasts, and mononuclear cells. During the growth period, bone develops by the remodelling and replacement of cartilage to form the long bones, or in the case of the flat membrane bones, by mineralization of osteoid matrix. Increase in the length of bones is dependent on epiphyseal growth whilst increase in the width and thickness is the result of periosteal deposition.

When bone is resorbed, calcium and phosphate are removed and released into the extracellular fluid. Osteoclasts are rich in acid phosphatase which may be released into the serum in significant amounts where there is widespread osteolysis. Osteoblasts, on the other hand, contain alkaline phosphatase, the level of which rises in the serum when osteoblastic activity increases. Mineralization depends on the extracellular fluid calcium and phosphate levels.

Rickets and Osteomalacia

Rickets is a disease of childhood characterized by defective skeletal mineralization. Osteomalacia is a disease with the same pathogenesis but affects adults in whom there is failure of mineralization of replacement bone in the normal process of bone turnover. Causes include one or more of the following:

1. Nutritional deficiency of vitamin D.
2. Failure of vitamin D synthesis in the skin because of lack of sunlight.
3. Vitamin D malabsorption.
4. Renal disease: loss of calcium, loss of phosphate, acidosis and impaired vitamin D metabolism.
5. Vitamin-D-resistant rickets: an X-linked defect of renal reabsorption of phosphate (familial hypophosphataemia).
6. Prolonged treatment with drugs such as phenytoin or occasionally phenobarbitone, rifampicin or others, leading to accelerated metabolism of vitamin D.
7. Excessive calcium demands in pregnancy and lactation.
8. Liver disease can lead to impaired absorption of vitamin D.
9. Isoniazid interferes with vitamin D metabolism.
10. Vitamin D–dependent rickets—a defect of the enzyme required to form 1,25–dihydroxycholecalciferol.

Vitamin D is abundant in fish liver oil and animal livers, and is synthesized in the skin under the influence of sunlight. Rickets and osteomalacia can, therefore, be a result of a dietary deficiency in poorly nourished communities, especially among Indian and Pakistani immigrants living in northern Britain. In this group, a contributory factor may be the eating of chapatties of wholemeal flour containing phytates which bind calcium and impair its absorption.

Osteomalacia is most prone to develop in adult women as a result of the demands of pregnancy and lactation, in malabsorption states, or in the presence of any cause of impairment of absorption of vitamin D.

Chronic renal failure can also cause osteomalacia, because of excess calcium loss and inability of the diseased kidneys to synthesize the active metabolite of vitamin D. Similar problems may complicate vitamin-D-resistant rickets, renal tubular acidosis or the Fanconi syndrome (see Appendix to Chapter 10).

In rickets, the bones are weak and readily deformed. The bones also fracture easily but incompletely (pseudo-fractures). In addition, affected infants and young children are often listless and irritable, the muscles are weak and hypotonic and they suffer bone pains.

In osteomalacia the inadequate mineralization and excess formation of osteoid matrix (rachitic rosary), unsupported by calcium salts weakens the bones. Deformity of weight-bearing bones is, therefore, the most obvious consequence. The plasma calcium level tends to be low with normal or low phosphate levels (see Table 10.11). Alkaline phosphatase levels are raised.

Management

The management of rickets and osteomalacia is to ensure an adequate intake of vitamin D and calcium. Complications, such as bone deformity, must also be treated.

Dental aspects

The teeth escape surprisingly well from the effects of rickets. Dental defects are seen only in unusually severe cases, but eruption of the teeth may be retarded. Vitamin D deficiency is not a contributory cause of dental caries. The jaws may show abnormal radiolucency.

In malabsorption syndromes there may be secondary hyperparathyroidism (Chapter 10) or vitamin K deficiency (Chapter 3), with endocrine or bleeding disorders respectively and oral manifestations of malabsorption (Chapter 4).

In vitamin D-resistant rickets (familial hypophosphataemia), the skull sutures are wide and there may be frontal bossing, but dental complaints frequently bring notice to the disease. The teeth have large pulp chambers, abnormal dentine calcification and are therefore liable to pulpitis and multiple, apparently spontaneous dental abscesses. Since even minimal caries or attrition can lead to pulpitis, preventive care and prophylactic occlusal coverage are needed.

Osteoporosis

Osteoporosis is a deficiency of both bone matrix and calcium salts. The bone is structurally normal but there is too little of it (osteopenia). Overall it is probably the most common disease of bone and contributes to approximately 1 500 000 fractures a year in the USA and in Britain, is estimated to cost the National Health Service £750 000 000 a year.

Diminishing bone mass is a normal concomitant of ageing, but there are several other causes (*Table 11.4*). Women after the menopause are mainly affected and the chief complications are fractures, particularly of the neck of the femur or of the vertebral bodies causing gradual collapse of the spine. Low back pain is common. There are often no biochemical abnormalities but there may be increased urinary loss of calcium and hydroxyproline, and in a group of women who lose bone particularly fast, urinary tests can be informative.

Table 11.4. Causes of osteoporosis

Senile	Corticosteroid therapy
Post-menopausal	Hyperthyroidism
Hypogonadism	Alcoholism
Cushing's syndrome	Immobilization

Until recently there have been no simple methods of quantifying bone mass and of recognizing osteoporosis before bones start to fracture. Dual X–ray absorptiometers (Dexa equipment) now allow rapid assessment but are currently available only at a limited number of specialist centres.

Management

The control of osteoporosis is often only partially successful and depends on the underlying cause, if it can be identified. Hormone replacement therapy (oestrogen plus progesterone) may be effective in postmenopausal women and may also help to relieve other postmenopausal symptoms such as flushing. However oestrogens can cause vaginal bleeding and there is a slightly increased risk of breast cancer. Alternative treatments are diphosphonates and in particular etidronate, and calcitonin. The latter, however, has to be given by injection. Additional calcium and 1 α-hydroxy vitamin D may also be helpful.

Dental aspects

There are no specific oral manifestations of osteoporosis and the association of osteoporosis with excessive alveolar bone loss in the elderly has been difficult to confirm because of the lack, until recently, of objective methods of quantifying bone mass. Patients with osteoporosis may have any of the problems of the elderly (Chapter 15) and may be at risk during general anaesthesia if there has been vertebral collapse and chest deformities.

Hypercalcaemia of Neoplasia and Sarcoidosis

In these conditions hypercalcaemia results from excessive calcium absorption from the intestine, probably as a result of overproduction of 1,25–dihydroxyc-holecalciferol.

Hypercalcaemia–Supravalvular Aortic Stenosis Syndrome

This syndrome, sometimes termed Williams' syndrome, comprises in its rare complete form, infantile hypercalcaemia, characteristic so–called elfin facies, supravalvular subaortic stenosis or other cardiovascular abnormalities and mental deficiency. Most such cases appear to be sporadic. Hypercalcaemia typically remits in infancy but leaves growth deficiency, osteosclerosis and craniostenosis. Despite the mental defect, these children may be sociable and talkative ('cocktail party manner').

Dental aspects

Dental defects are varied but may include hypodontia, microdontia and hypoplastic, bud–shaped teeth. The upper arch may be disproportionately wide and overlap the lower.

Masseter spasm has been reported in a child with William's syndrome during general anaesthesia with halothane and suxamethonium. However, malignant hyperthermia did not develop and it is not clear whether these children are particularly prone to this complication.

Tumoral Calcinosis

Tumoral calcinosis is a rare disease characterized by ectopic, soft tissue calcifi-cations but normocalcaemia. Dental and periodontal changes are typical features and serve as markers of the severity of the disorder: early onset periodontitis has been reported.

Fibrous Dysplasia

Fibrous dysplasia may affect a single bone (monostotic) or is less commonly multiple (polyostotic) and occasionally then can be part of Albright's syndrome. The aetiology is unknown. The natural history of cherubism also has some features in common with fibrous dysplasia but may cause bilateral lesions of the maxilla causing the eyes to 'upturn towards heaven'.

The essential feature of the osseous lesions of fibrous dysplasia is replace-ment of an area of bone by fibrous tissue and production of a localized swelling. The process typically starts in childhood and, as the skeleton matures, the lesions ossify progressively and ultimately, when skeletal growth ceases, usually become stabilized.

Monostotic fibrous dysplasia is more common in females, and frequently involves the mandible or maxilla.

Polyostotic fibrous dysplasia may affect either sex and may involve over 50 per cent of the skeleton, but is uncommon. The lesions may be unilateral and 50 per cent of patients have abnormal skin hyperpigmentation of a *café-au-lait* type, especially over the dorsum of the trunk and limbs usually on the same side as the bone lesions (*Fig.* 11.2). Precocious puberty is seen mainly in females but occasionally other endocrine disturbances are present.

Albright's syndrome comprises polyostotic fibrous dysplasia with pigmentation of the skin and precocious puberty in females. There are episodic rises in serum oestrogen and falls in gonadotropin levels.

Radiography shows a cystic or ground-glass appearance according to the stage. Serum calcium and phosphate levels are normal but, in many, the serum alkaline phosphatase level is high and urinary hydroxyproline raised.

Management

Patients are usually managed by surgery and sometimes calcitonin. Testolactone is effective treatment for the precocious puberty of Albright's syndrome.

Dental aspects

The facial bones are frequently involved in monostotic fibrous dysplasia and in 25 per cent of cases of polyostotic disease facial deformity is the presenting feature.

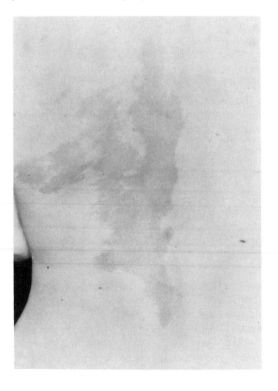

Fig. 11.2. Albright's syndrome: *café-au-lait* pigmentation on the back.

Fibrous dysplasia is typically a self-limiting condition that ceases to progress after adolescence in most cases. Surgery can then be used to correct any cosmetic defect. Radiotherapy should be avoided, as osteosarcomas have been reported after such treatment.

Monostotic fibrous dysplasia is not a medical problem but it is possible for the polyostotic type of the disease to be unrecognized when the facial lesions are the most obvious feature. Hyperthyroidism or diabetes mellitus may occasionally be associated with polyostotic fibrous dysplasia and therefore may, rarely, complicate treatment.

Mucosal pigmentation has been reported in Albright's syndrome but is rare. In the differential diagnosis, it may be confused with that of Addison's disease while the skin pigmentation may simulate that of neurofibromatosis. From the histological viewpoint the lesions of fibrous dysplasia may show foci of giant cells and differentiation from hyperparathyroidism or giant cell granuloma may have to be considered.

Paget's Disease of Bone (Osteitis Deformans)

Paget's disease is a common disorder characterized by progressive deformity and enlargement of bones. Radiographic evidence of its presence can be found in more than 5 per cent of those over 55 years of age in the UK. There appears to be considerable geographic variation in the prevalence of Paget's disease but there is always a male predominance.

The aetiology of Paget's disease is unknown but a slow virus may be involved. Its essential features are total disorganization of the normal orderly replacement of bone and an anarchic alternation of bone resorption and apposition. In the earlier stages resorption predominates (osteolytic phase) but later apposition takes over and, as disease activity declines, the affected bones become enlarged and dense (sclerotic stage).

Clinically, symptoms are absent in the early stages which can only be detected radiologically. The effects are most apparent in the elderly. One or many bones may be affected, and in the polyostotic type the axial skeleton is mainly involved. The hands and feet are usually spared. Other possible complications of Paget's disease are bone pain, deformities or pathological fractures, and sometimes compression of cranial nerves with such effects as deafness or impairment of vision. In some cases bone pain is intense and responds poorly to analgesics. Rarely there is brain-stem compression. If the disease is widespread, hypervascularity of the bones can produce, in effect, an arteriovenous fistula and high-output cardiac failure. Development of osteosarcoma is a recognized, but uncommon, complication and possibly affects fewer than 0.1 per cent of cases overall.

General management of Paget's disease

Diagnosis is made on the clinical and radiographic features, and chemical changes. The serum alkaline phosphatase level is grossly raised when many bones are affected and osteocalcin levels increased. There is then also increased urinary hydroxyproline excretion but, in general, little or no change in calcium or phosphate levels. Radionuclide scanning shows increased uptake of technetium diphosphonate. Currently the most effective treatment is with disodium etidronate, a diphosphonate. Less commonly, calcitonin is used; it is given by injection and may effectively relieve bone pain and deafness but is immunogenic.

Dental aspects

When the skull is affected a typical early feature is a large irregular area of relative radiolucency (osteoporosis circumscripta). Later basilar invagination may be seen with also a 'cotton wool' appearance of the vault of the skull on radiography.

The jaws are relatively rarely affected; the maxilla more often than the mandible. Typically, enlargement of the maxilla causes symmetrical bulging in the malar region (leontiasis ossea, *Fig.* 11.3). There is increased radio-opacity with the loss of the normal landmarks and an irregular cotton–wool appearance. The intraoral features are gross symmetrical widening of the alveolar ridges, sometimes loss of lamina dura, root resorption and hypercementosis often forming enormous craggy masses which may become fused to the surrounding bone. Pulpal calcification may be seen.

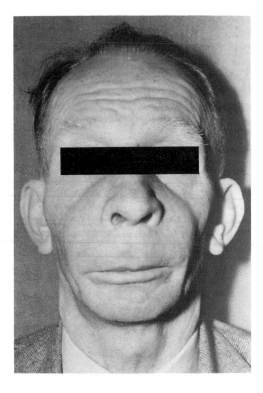

Fig. 11.3. Leontiasis ossea in Paget's disease.

Serious complications follow efforts to extract severely hypercementosed teeth. Attempts using forceps may fail to move the tooth, or cause fracture of the alveolar bone. Alternatively, the tooth may be mobilized but retained as if in a ball-and-socket joint. In the early stages of the disease, the highly vascular bone may bleed freely; later, the poor blood supply to the bone makes it susceptible to chronic suppurative osteomyelitis as a result of such trauma.

If hypercementosis is severe, a surgical approach with adequate exposure should be used for extractions, and prophylactic administration of an antibiotic such as penicillin (immediately before and for 3 or 4 days after the operation) may help to prevent postoperative infection.

In the edentulous patient, dentures have to be replaced as the alveolar ridge enlarges.

If the patient is in heart failure, the usual precautions (Chapter 2) have to be taken but, since general anaesthesia may be needed for extractions, this aspect of the disease needs to be kept in mind. Chest deformity may also complicate general anaesthesia.

Localized, but rapidly growing and often painful swelling is suggestive of osteosarcoma. However, this is particularly rare in the jaws where no fully authenticated case appears to have been reported. Benign giant cell tumours of the jaws may, however, be seen.

DISEASES OF JOINTS

OSTEOARTHRITIS

Osteoarthritis is a common disease, and is especially painful in the weight-bearing or traumatized joints in the elderly. Osteoarthritis has been traditionally regarded essentially as a wear-and-tear phenomenon, but excessive stress on the joints, as a result of occupation for example, does not, of itself, necessarily predispose to it. The disease has a significant systemic component which leads to disordered regulation of chondrocyte activity and failure of repair of articular cartilage. However, this may be aggravated by other kinds of disturbance of joint function or abnormal internal stresses, caused for example by operations such as meniscectomy.

The essential change in osteoarthritis is degeneration of articular cartilage with compensatory thickening of the underlying bone which becomes exposed. The bone is at first smooth and shiny but later the surface becomes roughened, cystic spaces form beneath and bone proliferates at the joint margins. Exposure and collapse of the cystic cavities, together with continued peripheral proliferation, cause progressive deformity.

The main clinical feature is usually pain with stiffness, progressively reduced function and deformity of one or more of the larger joints, such as the hips or knees, which are heavily stressed.

In contrast to rheumatoid arthritis, there are no systemic symptoms, clinically obvious inflammation of affected joints or serological changes. Osteophytes formed at the margins of the distal interphalangeal joints of the fingers produce Heberden's nodes, which are a hallmark of the disease.

The characteristic radiographic features of osteoarthritis include:

1. Narrowing of the joint space.
2. Marginal osteophyte formation (lipping).
3. Subchondral bone sclerosis.
4. Bone 'cysts' (rounded areas of radiolucency just beneath the joint surface).
5. Deformity.

General management

Weight reduction, physiotherapy, heat treatment and the use of various appliances are helpful. Anti-inflammatory analgesics are usually needed and arthroplasty may prevent disablement in advanced disease.

Dental aspects

Osteoarthritis has been described in temporomandibular joints in some elderly patients. However, patients with osteoarthritis of other joints do not appear to have significantly more involvement of the temporomandibular joints than controls. The radiographic severity of temporomandibular joint osteoarthritis does not correlate with symptoms, although palpable crepitus may be common.

Patients should not therefore be made anxious by being told of such findings, since osteoarthritis of this joint is rarely of clinical significance.

Dental management may otherwise be complicated by age (Chapter 15) or a bleeding tendency if the patient takes high doses of aspirin. There is no evidence of a need for antibiotic prophylaxis before dental treatment in most patients with prosthetic joints. In the largest published study, a single case out of 1855 joint infections followed dental intervention and it is questionable whether any of the rare, late infections of prosthetic hip joints that have been reported to follow dental treatment, have been due to oral bacteria. Infections of prosthetic joints are typically by non-oral micro-organisms such as staphylococci which are frequently penicillin–resistant. A syndrome of dry mouth and osteoarthritis (sialo-adenitis, osteoarthritis, xerostomia: SOX) has been described but needs confirmation.

Following joint replacement, patients may be anticoagulated for a few weeks (Chapter 3).

Rheumatoid Arthritis

Rheumatoid arthritis is a multisystem disease, but joint pain and damage are the most prominent features (*Table 11.5*). The disease appears to be immunologically mediated. An abnormal immunoglobulin is formed in the joint tissues and an auto-antibody to the abnormal immunoglobulin (rheumatoid factor, RF), is produced in response. It is postulated that immune complex (antigen–antibody complex) formation may then lead to the activation of complement, inflammation and synovial damage.

Table 11.5 Rheumatoid arthritis—features and complications

Joints	Arthritis
	Tenosynovitis
	Laxity of ligaments
	Subluxation
	Spinal nerve root compression
Non-specific features	Fever
	Malaise
	Fatigue
Dermal, oral and para-oral	Palmar erythema
	Various rashes
	Subcutaneous nodules
	Sjögren's syndrome (dry mouth)
	Temporomandibular arthritis
	Oral drug lesions
Muscle	Weakness
	Wasting
Bone	Osteoporosis
Eyes	Sjögren's syndrome (dry eyes)
	Episcleritis, scleritis or scleromalacia
Cardiovascular	Pericarditis
	Myocarditis
	Valvulitis
	Vasculitis
Haematological	Anaemia
	Leucopenia
	Thrombocytopenia
Respiratory	Pleurisy and pleural effusion
	Nodules in lung
	Fibrosis
	Bronchiolitis
Neurological	Various neuropathies
Renal	Various nephropathies
	Amyloidosis
Hepatic	Abnormal liver function tests

Rheumatoid arthritis is a widespread disease which probably affects about 2 per cent of the population in Britain and the USA. Women are affected approximately three times as frequently as men.

The onset is typically between the ages of 30 and 40 and is often insidious, with increasing stiffness of the hands or feet which is worse in the morning. In the acute stage there is aching, swelling, redness, tenderness and limitation of movement of the joints.

The disease usually first affects the small joints of the hands and feet symmetrically—later the wrists, elbows, ankles and knees are commonly involved. The interphalangeal joints typically become spindle-shaped as a result of joint swelling with muscle wasting on either side (*Fig.* 11.4). In some cases the onset is acute with fever and malaise in addition to the joint pain. Other common manifestations are tenosynovitis, subcutaneous nodules, leucocytosis and anaemia. Clinically apparent effects on other systems are less common. The anaemia is typically normochromic (anaemia of chronic disease) and can be severe. Other laboratory findings are shown in *Table 11.6*.

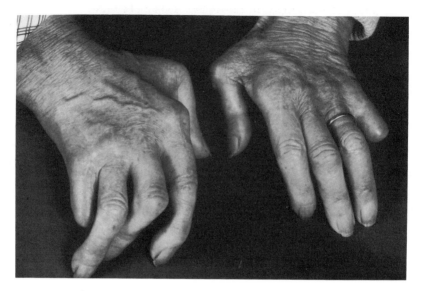

Fig. 11.4. Rheumatoid arthritis showing the characteristic deformities affecting the hands, particularly the deviation of the fingers (ulnar deviation).

General management

The serological marker of rheumatoid arthritis is rheumatoid factor, which is present in 60–70 per cent. It is detected by the sensitive latex agglutination test in which IgG-coated latex particles are agglutinated if the patient's serum contains IgM autoantibody to IgG. The Rose–Waaler test, using agglutination of sensitized sheep erythrocytes, is less sensitive but more specific for rheumatoid arthritis. In so-called seronegative cases, rheumatoid factor may be IgG rather than the typical IgM and is therefore not detected by these routine methods. Antinuclear antibodies are also often found but are usually in low titre (*Table 11.6*).

Radiographic features are soft tissue swelling and widening of the joint space due to accumulation of fluid in the early stages. Later there is increasing osteoporosis of the adjacent bone, cyst-like spaces and narrowing of the joint space. Ultimately there may be severe bone destruction and deformity, but ankylosis does not follow.

Table 11.6. Laboratory findings in rheumatoid arthritis

Test	Typical findings
Full blood count	Normocytic hypochromic anaemia
	Mild leucocytosis (or leucopenia)
	Mild thrombocytopenia
Erythrocyte sedimentation rate	Raised
Protein electrophoresis	Hypergammaglobulinaemia
Rheumatoid factor—latex agglutination	Positive
Antinuclear antibodies	Positive in 20–60 per cent

The main aspects of management are:

1. Rest in acute phases, but between these episodes maintenance of mobility of the affected joints.
2. Non-steroidal anti–inflammatory drugs
3. Other drugs such as gold, penicillamine or, if all else fails, corticosteroids. The last has the disadvantage that the disease is worsened when it is withdrawn.
4. Haematinics in an attempt to treat anaemia.
5. Physiotherapy.

Non-steroidal antinflammatory agents are the safest and most effective drugs and should be given in increasing doses until the side-effects become disproportionately great in relation to the benefits.

Among other problems of severe rheumatoid arthritis is depression associated with persistent pain and restriction of activity, so that antidepressant treatment may sometimes be needed.

Dental aspects

The main oral complication of rheumatoid arthritis is Sjögren's syndrome (Chapter 7). Patients may also have severely restricted manual dexterity and consequent difficulty maintaining adequate oral hygiene. In spite of the predilection of rheumatoid arthritis for small joints, the temporomandibular joints are often painless but there may be limitation of opening or stiffness. Radiographic changes, however, are common and consist of erosions, flattening of the joint surfaces and marginal proliferation. Pain felt in the joint itself and tenderness on palpation is not significantly more common than in control subjects but there may be referred pain. The temporomandibular joint, therefore, shows radiographic changes of rheumatoid arthritis more frequently than is often suspected but symptoms are usually slight. Even when the disease is severe, pain from the temporomandibular joint appears to trouble only a minority. (*Table 11.7*).

The drugs used in rheumatoid arthritis are a cause of oral side-effects (*Table 11.8*) and high dose aspirin may cause a bleeding tendency. Iron deficiency anaemia secondary to ·gastrointestinal blood loss caused by aspirin can also produce oral manifestations (Chapter 4) or, with the anaemia of rheumatoid disease, may be severe enough to affect management. A few patients are treated with corticosteroids. In some patients, as a result of weakness of the ligaments of the neck, dislocation of the atlanto-axial joint or fracture of the odontoid peg can readily follow sudden jerking of the head. Disastrous accidents of this sort have been known to follow adjustment of the head-rest of older types of dental chair, or sudden extension of the neck during the induction of general anaesthesia. Patients with joint prostheses may require antibiotic cover before surgical procedures.

Felty's Syndrome

Felty's syndrome comprises rheumatoid arthritis, splenomegaly and lymphadenopathy. These patients are at risk from infections because of

Table 11.7. Rheumatoid arthritis of the temporomandibular joint

Type*	TMJ disease	TMJ symptoms	TMJ radiographic findings	Occlusal and facial features
I	Early adult	Continuous dull pain; limitation of movement; crepitus	Erosive changes	Normal
II	Advanced	Variable pain; crepitus; loss of mobility	Gross erosive changes and loss of condylar height	Open bite Decreased ramus height Increased anterior facial height
III	Arrested	Often none	Loss of condylar shape	Open bite Decreased ramus height Increased anterior facial height
IV	Idiopathic condylar resorption	Variable symptoms including subluxation or dislocation	Flattened, shortened condylar stump	Open bite Decreased ramus height Increased anterior facial height

*After Kent et al. (1986).

leucopenia and may suffer severe oral ulceration or oropharyngeal infections, including chronic sinusitis. Management can also be complicated by anaemia and mild thrombocytopenia.

Juvenile Rheumatoid Arthritis (Childhood Polyarthritis)

Although uncommon compared with adult rheumatoid arthritis, it is estimated that at least 10 000 children suffer from this distressing and often crippling group of diseases. One important form of this disease predominantly affects girls in late childhood, affects virtually any joint and is associated with rheumatoid nodules, mild fever, anaemia and malaise. Rheumatoid factor is positive in all cases and antinuclear antibodies are present in 75 per cent. Over 50 per cent develop severe arthritis and deformity. There are, however, several subtypes of juvenile chronic arthritis of which Still's disease is one.

Table 11.8. Drugs in rheumatoid arthritis: oral side-effects

Corticosteroids	Candidosis
Gold	Lichenoid reactions
Pencillamine	Loss of taste Lichenoid reactions Severe ulceration
Antimalarials	Lichenoid reactions
Non-steroid anti-inflammatory agent	Lichenoid reactions (rarely) Ulceration

At its worst, juvenile arthritis is considerably more severe than the adult disease and can lead to gross deformity.

Damage to the temporomandibular joint of various types has occasionally been described. Complete bony ankylosis has been reported and it has been suggested that micrognathia may develop in 4–25 per cent.

Psoriatic Arthritis

Joint disease closely resembling rheumatoid arthritis is sometimes a feature of psoriasis. However, psoriatic arthritis is usually milder, can affect the lower spine and sacro-iliac joints and there are no characteristic serological abnormalities.

When psoriatic arthritis affects the temporomandibular joint, the clinical effects are slight. In spite of the high prevalence of psoriasis (which may affect 2–3 per cent of the population), oral mucosal lesions are exceedingly rare and histologically verified oral psoriasis has been reported on few occasions. The oral lesions are not conspicuous and typically consist of pale, somewhat translucent plaques that are usually associated with pustular psoriasis. Psoriasis may occasionally be treated with methotrexate which may cause oral ulcers.

Note: Severe damage to the temporomandibular joint, including bony ankylosis, has been reported in the past in rheumatoid, psoriatic and other non-infective arthritides. However, in view of recent surveys doubt must be expressed about whether these earlier reports were of uncomplicated disease or whether the diagnoses would fulfil current strict criteria. However, even if these reports are valid, the effects they describe are quite exceptional.

Infective Arthritides of the Temporomandibular Joint

Infective arthritides of the temporomandibular joint are very rare but may follow penetrating wounds, extension from adjacent septic areas or haematogenous dissemination. Possible causes are *Neisseria gonorrhoeae, Haemophilus influenzae, Staphylococcus aureus,* or *Mycobacterium tuberculosis.* Ankylosis can be a complication.

Lyme Disease

Lyme disease is caused by a spirochaete *Borrelia burgdorferi* which is mainly transmitted by ixodes ticks from deer. It is considerbly more common in the USA than in Great Britain but cases are seen in most parts of the world.

The first sign is usually a rash (erythema marginatum chronicum) which spreads outwards from the site of the insect bite. Arthritis may develop in the acute phase and be transient, or later be persistent. The knees are typically most severely affected.

Other effects include neurological involvement which may result in facial palsy, and lymphadenitis. Lyme disease of the temporomandibular joint has been reported but is rare even in endemic areas in the USA.

Gout

Primary gout is an inborn error of metabolism which causes raised serum levels of uric acid and deposition of urates, especially in the joints. Secondary gout, which is considerably more common, is usually caused by the effects of drugs or radiotherapy of myeloproliferative diseases releasing large amounts of purines into the blood.

Primary gout is partly genetically determined and mainly affects adult men. Contrary to popular belief, over-eating and drinking do not *cause* gout, but food rich in purines (such as fish roe), or an alcoholic 'binge', can precipitate an attack in those with the underlying metabolic disorder.

In gout, phagocytosis of urate crystals by polymorphs results in release of lysosomal enzymes and acute inflammation.

Gouty tophi are masses of urate crystals which, in joints, interfere mechanically with function and also destroy bone and cartilage to cause a severe, deforming arthritis. Chronic tophaceous gout is often associated with renal disease.

Extra-articular tophi typically form in the helix of the ear and are conspicuous as almost white, hard, subcutaneous nodules. The overlying skin may become necrotic and allow extrusion of semi-solid masses of urates.

Clinically, an acute attack of gout (typically in a man in his forties) causes sudden and intensely severe joint pain, usually in the big toe, associated with fever, leucocytosis and raised serum uric acid levels.

Gout leads to renal disease which, unless treated, leads to fatal renal failure in up to 25 per cent of patients. Many gouty patients are obese, middle-aged males and there is a high incidence of hyperlipidaemia, hypertension, diabetes mellitus and atherosclerosis with their attendant complications.

General management

Serum should be taken for estimation of uric acid and possibly for renal function tests, especially in chronic tophaceous gout. Secondary gout should be investigated for the underlying disorder.

Colchicine and indomethacin relieve an acute attack. Colchicine, however, can cause severe side-effects so that anti-inflammatory analgesics, but not aspirin, which interferes with uricosuric agents, may be more suitable.

Allopurinol can be used to decrease uric acid production. In severe cases uric acid levels can be lowered by the use of uricosuric agents such as probenecid or sulphinpyrazone.

Dental aspects

Gout can affect the temporomandibular joint but only rarely. The chief importance of this disease is its important associations with hypertension, ischaemic heart disease, cerebrovascular disease, diabetes mellitus and renal disease. Aspirin is contraindicated as it interferes with the action of uricosuric agents.

Drugs used for the treatment of gout, particularly allopurinol, can also occasionally cause severe oral ulceration (*see* Appendix to Chapter 19).

In a rare inborn error of metabolism (Lesch–Nyhan syndrome), hyperuricaemia is associated with mental handicap, choreoathetosis and compulsive self-mutilation, as a result of the lips being chewed away and of self-inflicted injuries especially to the face and head, despite the pain it obviously causes.

Ankylosing Spondylitis

Ankylosing spondylitis is a chronic inflammatory arthritis predominantly affecting the spine, mainly in young males. Up to 1 in 250 males are affected. Ankylosing spondylitis is partly genetically determined and a positive family history is sometimes obtained. The aetiology is unknown but over 90 per cent of patients are HLA-B27.

The synovial changes resemble those of rheumatoid arthritis, but inflammation involves the insertions of ligaments and tendons and is followed by ossification, forming bony bridges which fuse adjacent vertebral bodies or cause ankylosis of other joints.

The onset is usually insidious, with low back pain and stiffness followed by increasing pain and tenderness in the sacro-iliac region. The hip joints may also be involved. Over the course of years the back becomes fixed in extreme flexion with the result that chest expansion is limited and respiration impaired. About 25 per cent of patients develop ocular lesions (uveitis or iridocyclitis) and about 10 per cent develop cardiac disease—usually aortic insufficiency or conduction defects.

On radiography, the spine shows progressive squaring-off of the vertebrae which become rectangular, and then, as intervertebral ossification develops, a bamboo spine appearance is produced. The sacro-iliac joints typically become obliterated.

General management

Apart from a raised ESR, mild anaemia and the association with HLA-B27 there are no significant laboratory findings. Autoantibodies are not found.

Treatment consists of anti-inflammatory analgesics to control pain and allow the back to be kept as mobile as possible. Phenylbutazone and its analogues, or indomethacin, may be used but all can cause side-effects which are sometimes severe. Physiotherapy and exercises are also essential. Occasionally, radiotherapy to the spine is needed but this carries with it the risk of leukaemia.

Dental aspects

Ankylosing spondylitis can affect the temporomandibular joints in about 10 per cent of patients, especially those over 40 years of age with widespread disease. However, temporomandibular joint symptoms are usually mild with little pain but usually some trismus. Very occasionally the disability is severe enough to require condylectomy.

General anaesthesia can be hazardous because of severely restricted opening of the mouth, impaired respiratory exchange associated with severe spinal deformity, or cardiac disease with aortic insufficiency.

Reiter's Disease

Reiter's syndrome comprises arthritis, urethritis and conjunctivitis, but there are numerous other effects and it is commoner now to speak of Reiter's disease. The pathogenesis is unknown but it appears to be a post-infective response, particularly after gut infections such as *Shigella flexneri* or *Salmonella typhimurium*. The disease may also follow sexually transmitted infection but urethritis is a feature of the disease itself. Reiter's disease almost exclusively affects males between 20 and 40 years of age, about 80 per cent of whom are HLA–B27 positive. The arthritis is chronic or recurrent and migratory and affects the small joints of the hands and feet and also the weight-bearing joints in asymmetrical fashion. Fever, malaise and loss of weight may accompany the acute symptoms. The conjunctivitis is usually bilateral and iritis may sometimes develop.

Characteristic skin lesions of hyperkeratotic thickening, which can be gross, affect the palms and soles (keratoderma blenorrhagica). The penis may have circinate lesions (circinate balanitis) resembling those seen in the mouth.

Leucocytosis is common and the ESR is often raised. The urethritis is purulent but sterile on culture. Like ankylosing spondylitis there is the strong association with HLA-B27, but no findings confirming an immunological mechanism for this disease have yet been described.

Anti-inflammatory analgesics are used to control the acute phase of the disease, which usually subsides within a few months but may recur.

Dental aspects

The possibility of sexually transmitted disease should be considered in the differential diagnosis.

Oral lesions are said to be very frequent but are transient and painless and often, therefore, unnoticed. The most characteristic lesion is a pattern of scalloped white lines surrounding reddish areas and closely resembling one variant of migratory glossitis (geographic tongue), but affecting any part of the mouth.

DISEASES OF MUSCLES

Muscle diseases (myopathies) are uncommon and rarely either cause oral manifestations or affect dental management.

Genetic Myopathies

The genetic myopathies comprise the muscular dystrophies and the myotonic disorders.

Muscular Dystrophies

Muscular dystrophies are a group of uncommon genetically determined diseases but nevertheless are now the main crippling diseases of childhood in the West. They are characterized by degeneration of muscle, leading to progressive weakness and often death or other complications (*Table 11.9*).

Duchenne muscular dystrophy is the most common form and is a recessive sex-linked disorder with an incidence of about 1 in 5000 live male births. The pelvic girdle is affected first and the disease appears as the infant begins to walk: there is a waddling gait and severe lumbar lordosis. The child has difficulty in standing and, after lying down, typically has to climb up his legs in order to stand (Gower's sign). The shoulder girdle is also weak, and winging of the scapulae is characteristic. Weakness spreads to all other muscles but tends to spare those of the head, neck and hands. The affected muscles enlarge (pseudo-hypertrophy) but the child is crippled and, before puberty, becomes confined to a wheelchair.

Cardiac disease (cardiomyopathy), respiratory impairment and intellectual deterioration complicate this disease at an early stage, and patients usually die in their twenties.

Dental aspects

In those muscular dystrophies where there is facial myopathy (classical in the facioscapulohumeral type) there is lack of facial expression and, often, inability to whistle. Malocclusions, especially expansion of the arches, may be seen, but there is no abnormal susceptibility to dental disease.

Cardiomyopathies and respiratory disease are the usual causes of death in Duchenne dystrophy and are contraindications to general anaesthesia.

Myotonic Disorders

Myotonic disorders are a group of conditions characterized by abnormally slow relaxation after muscle contraction. There are four main myotonic disorders:

Myotonia congenita (Thomsen's disease) is a generalized myotonia without weakness that appears in infancy but there are no other problems.

Myotonia congenita (Becker type) appears later in childhood and is characterized by muscle hypertrophy. Patients may have dental management problems resulting from treatment with corticosteroids or phenytoin, or from susceptibility to malignant hyperthermia (Chapter 10).

Paramyotonia congenita causes myotonia and weakness after exposure to cold.

Dystrophia myotonica (Steinert's myotonic dystrophy) is the most disabling form of myotonia and can lead to ptosis, progressive facial weakness, cataracts, testicular atrophy and frontal baldness. The onset typically becomes apparent in the third decade.

There is atrophy of the temporalis, masseter and sternomastoid muscles, (producing a swan neck appearance) and sometimes, distal limb weakness and

Table 11.9. Muscular dystrophies

Type	Inheritance	Muscles affected	Pseudo-hypertrophy	Onset	Progress	Other features
Duchenne (pseudohypertrophic)	X-linked	All	Usual	Early childhood	Rapid	Cardiomyopathy Death in early adulthood
Becker	X-linked	All	Usual	Late childhood	Variable	More benign than Duchenne type
Childhood muscular	AR	All	Usual	Late childhood	Variable	More benign than Duchenne type
Limb girdle (Erb)	AR	Pelvic and shoulder girdles	Occasional	Adolescence	Variable	Severely disabling May be cardiomyopathy
Facioscapulohumeral	AD	Starts in face and shoulder	Rare	Adolescence	Slow	Most benign type Normal life expectancy Pouting of lips with facial weakness
Scapuloperoneal	AD or X-linked	Scapular Peroneal	Occasional	Adolescence	Slow	Cardiac conduction defects
Congenital muscular	AR	All	Rare	Birth	Variable	Relatively benign
Distal myopathy	AD	Distal	Rare	Any age	Slow	—
Oculopharyngeal	AD	Facial and sterno-mastoid	Rare	Adult	Slow	Dysphagia may be prominent Weakness of masticatory muscles and tongue

AD, Autosomal dominant; AR, autosomal recessive.
Adapted from: Hewer R.L. (1979) In: Read A. E., Barritt D. W. and Hewer R.L. (ed.) *Modern Medicine.* Tunbridge Wells, Pitman Medical.

wasting. Myotonia in the tongue causes difficulty in speaking (dysarthria) and there may also be difficulty in masticating food.

Other complications include cardiac conduction defects, respiratory impairment, mild endocrinopathies, intellectual deterioration and personality changes.

Dental aspects of myotonic dystrophy

Atrophy of the masticatory muscles leads to an open mouth posture. There may also be dysphagia, dysarthria and increased caries. General anaesthesia may be a risk because of:

1. Cardiac conduction defects.
2. Suxamethonium sensitivity (Chapter 10).
3. Respiratory impairment.
4. Behavioural problems.
5. Malignant hyperthermia (Chapter 10).

The Dystonias (see Chapter 12)

Other Genetic Myopathies (*see Table 11.10*)

Table 11.10. Metabolic myopathies

1. Endocrine
    Acromegaly
    Hyperthyroidism
    Hypothyroidism
    Cushings syndrome and steroid therapy
    Hyperaldosteronism
    Diabetes mellitus
2. Bone disease
    Hyperparathyroidism
    Osteomalacia
    Chronic renal failure
3. Drugs
    Alcohol
    Diuretics
    Carbenoxolone
    Vincristine
    Cimetidine
    Tryptophan
4. Malignant hyperthermia
5. Neuromuscular disorders
    Peroneal muscular atrophy (Charcot–Marie–Tooth disease)
    Hypertrophic polyneuritis (Dejerine–Sottas disease)
    Glycogen storage diseases
    Mitochondrial myopathies

ACQUIRED MYOPATHIES

Polymyositis and Dermatomyositis

Polymyositis and dermatomyositis are rare inflammatory myopathies which are immunologically mediated. Muscle weakness and pain are the main features. Polymyositis is usually associated with a variety of systemic abnormalities and if there are associated skin lesions is known as dermatomyositis. Circulating autoantibodies of various types are frequently present: in a few cases, other connective tissue diseases or distant neoplasms are associated.

Polymyositis and dermatomyositis usually develop between the fifth and sixth decades. Women are affected twice as often as men. The onset is characteristically insidious but is occasionally acute, with weakness usually of the pelvic girdle and the proximal limb muscles, especially those of the legs. Speaking and swallowing may become difficult. In severe cases, weakness may make patients bedridden and ultimately, atrophy, contracture and calcinosis of muscles can develop.

A characteristic rash affects about 30 per cent of patients with polymyositis. It is dusky and violaceous (heliotrope) with a butterfly distribution across the bridge of the nose and adjacent cheeks but may spread to the upper part of the body. Small ulcerated skin lesions may develop over bony prominences.

Raynaud's phenomenon and features of the other connective tissue diseases, particularly scleroderma, may be associated in about 20 per cent of cases, especially those with dermatomyositis, and other complications include myocarditis and fibrosing alveolitis. Underlying malignant disease is found in up to 10 per cent and is the main cause of death.

General management of polymyositis

Raised serum levels of the enzymes creatinine phosphokinase (CPK), aldolase and aspartate transaminase (AST) may be found and the diagnosis is confirmed by electromyography and muscle biopsy.

The most effective drugs are corticosteroids or other immunosuppressants, but these are much less effective when there is underlying malignant disease.

Dental aspects of polymyositis

A minority of patients have pharyngeal weakness. Oral lesions have rarely been reported in polymyositis/dermatomyositis but it has been suggested that they may be found in 10–20 per cent of patients. These oral lesions appear to be variable in character and comprise dark or purplish erythema and oedema of the oral mucosa and possibly also of the gingival margins. Small whitish patches occasionally with shallow ulceration may also develop and bear some resemblance to the oral lesions of lichen planus or lupus erythematosus.

Dental management may be complicated by corticosteroid therapy or associated disorders such as other connective tissue diseases, including Sjögren's syndrome (Chapter 7).

CRANIAL ARTERITIS AND POLYMYALGIA RHEUMATICA

These disorders are vasculitides, not myopathies, but are relatively common causes of muscle pain and headache in the middle-aged and elderly.

The basic lesion, which may be immunologically mediated, is inflammation of the walls of medium-size arteries with prominent giant cells. There is obliteration of the vessel lumen and ischaemia of the part supplied.

Clinically, giant cell arteritis usually either affects the craniofacial region, and is then called cranial or temporal arteritis, or alternatively it can be more widespread, affecting particularly the shoulder and pelvic regions and is then known as polymyalgia rheumatica. The common feature of these diseases is muscle pain caused by ischaemia, but the eyes and other structures can also be affected leading to blindness.

Cranial Arteritis

The most common complaint is severe unilateral throbbing headache. Women are predominantly affected, usually after the age of 55. The headache is acute and can be mainly in the temporal region or more widespread. The temporal artery is typically prominent, tortuous and tender. Biopsy of an affected part of the vessel confirms the diagnosis. Associated features are malaise, fever and usually a greatly raised ESR.

The most severe complication of cranial arteritis is ischaemia of the optic nerve causing blindness, which in the absence of treatment may develop in up to 30 per cent of patients and it is obligatory to give systemic corticosteroids (60 mg prednisone daily reducing as the ESR returns to normal) as soon as the diagnosis is made to prevent this complication. The clinical response to these drugs is rapid.

Dental aspects

Ischaemic pain in the muscles of mastication can cause severe pain when eating and has been reported in 20 per cent of these patients. This is sometimes called 'claudication' of the masticatory muscles but, though they share the feature of ischaemic muscle pain, it seems unreasonable to suggest that the masticatory muscles are limping—the literal meaning of claudication.

A rare manifestation of cranial arteritis is ischaemic necrosis and gangrene of the tongue and it is probably the only cause of this unusual and unpleasant phenomenon.

The most important aspect is to differentiate the masticatory pain of cranial arteritis from temporomandibular-pain-dysfunction syndrome by the later onset, greater severity of pain, the high ESR and, often, local signs of inflammation of the temporal artery. There is no diagnostic serological test. Artery biopsy is the one confirmatory diagnostic measure and even this may be negative as the lesions are patchily distributed. Accurate diagnosis is, however, essential because of the danger of blindness.

Temporal arteritis may occasionally have to be differentiated from trigeminal neuralgia where the pain can also be triggered by mastication. The pain of trigeminal neuralgia is, however, different in character and distribution, systemic symptoms are absent, the ESR is normal and there is usually a good initial response to carbamazepine.

Systemic corticosteroids may complicate dental management.

Polymyalgia Rheumatica

Polymyalgia rheumatica can co-exist with cranial arteritis, or develop as a separate entity. The age and sex distribution, and associated systemic disturbances, are the same and the typical arterial changes may be found. In polymyalgia rheumatica there is pain, stiffness and weakness across the shoulders, in the upper arms and in the pelvic region radiating into the thighs. In most cases the disease is ultimately self-limiting though it frequently persists for 1–2 years. In the absence of cranial symptoms relatively small doses of corticosteroids usually give rapid relief. The dose should be adjusted to bring the ESR to and maintained to keep it at the normal level.

Dental aspects

The main oral and perioral features have been mentioned earlier. Patients may be on treatment with systemic corticosteroids.

Eosinophilia Myalgia Syndrome

Tryptophan may be used as an antidepressant or for the treatment of insomnia. This syndrome, first described in 1989 in patients taking tryptophan, has an abrupt onset of myalgia with oedema of the extremities, rashes of various types and peripheral eosinophilia. About a third of patients have had to be hospitalized and some have died from an ascending polyneuropathy and respiratory failure.

The disease has mainly been seen in the US and appears to be caused by a contaminant of trytophan. It is a rare cause of facial pain but tryptophan has now been withdrawn in Britain and can only be given under exceptional circumstances to individual, named patients.

MYASTHENIA GRAVIS (*see* Chapter 12)

Bibliography

Audran M. and Kumar R. (1985) The physiology and pathophysiology of vitamin D. *Mayo Clin. Proc.* **60**, 851–66.
Avioli L. V. and Krane S. M. (1978) *Metabolic Bone Disease.* New York, Academic Press.

Beard C. J. et al. (1986) Neutrophil defect associated with malignant infantile osteopetrosis. *J. Lab. Clin. Med.* **108**, 498–505.

Bjorvatn K., Gilhuus-Moe O. and Aarskog D. (1979) Oral aspects of osteopetrosis. *Scand. J. Dent. Res.* **87**, 245–52.

Carlsson G. E., Koop S. and Oberg T. (1979) Arthritis and allied disease of the temporomandibular joint. In: Zarb G. A. and Carlsson G. E. (ed.) *Temporomandibular Joint Function and Dysfunction*. Copenhagen, Munksgaard, pp. 269–320.

Cartells S. et al. (1986) Plasma osteocalcin levels in patients with osteogenesis imperfecta. *J. Pediatr.* **109**, 81–91.

Cawson R. A. and Scully, C. (1986) Temporomandibular joint disorders. *Medicine Int.* **2**, 140–41.

Cawson R.A. and Spector R.G. (1989) *Clinical Pharmacology in Dentistry*. 5th ed. Edinburgh, Churchill Livingstone.

Chesley L.D. and Van Gilder J.W. (1990) Eosinophilic myalgia syndrome masquerading as facial pain. *J. Oral Maxillofac. Surg.* **48**, 980–1.

Culver J. and Robinson K. (1978) Exodontics in a patient with Felty syndrome. *J. Oral Surg.* **36**, 135–7.

Dubovitz V. (1978) *Muscle Disorders in Childhood*. Philadelphia, Saunders.

Editorial (1977) Planning treatment for rheumatoid arthritis. *Br. Med. J.* **1**, 1120.

Editorial (1984) Osteogenesis imperfecta 1984. *Br. Med. J.* **289**, 394–5.

Eskinazi D. (1989) Is systematic antimicrobial prophylaxis justified in dental patients with prosthetic joints? *Oral Surg.* **66**, 430–1.

Fadavi S. and Rowold E. (1990) Familial hypophosphatemic vitamin D resistant *J. Dent. Child.* 212–5.

Feuillan P. P. et al. (1986) Treatment of precocious puberty in the McCune–Albright syndrome with the aromatase inhibitor testolactone. *N. Engl. J. Med.* **315**, 1115–19.

Frame B. (1978) Osteomalacia: current concepts. *Ann. Intern. Med.* **89**, 966.

Freedus M. S., Schaaf N. G. and Ziter W. D. (1976) Orthognathic surgery in osteogenesis imperfecta. *J. Oral Surg.* **34**, 830–4.

Friedman R. D., Joe J. and Bodak G. L. Z. (1980) Myotonic dystrophy. *Oral Surg.* **50**, 229–32.

Guralnick W., Kaban L. B. and Merrill R. G. (1978) Temporomandibular joint afflictions *N. Engl. J. Med.* **229**, 123–9.

Hill C. M. (1980) Death following dental clearance in a patient suffering from ankylosing spondylitis—a case report with discussion on management of such problems. *Br. J. Oral Surg.* **18**, 73–6.

Holbrook W. P., Turner E. P. and MacIver J. E. (1979) Felty's syndrome. *Br. J. Oral Surg.* **17**, 157–60.

Horton W.A. and Schinke R.N. (1980) Osteopetrosis: further heterogeneity. *J. Pediatr.* **97**, 580–8.

Hosking D. J. (1982) *Paget's Disease of Bone*. London, Update Publications.

Jacobson J. J., Millard H. D. and Plezia R. (1986) Dental treatment and late prosthetic joint infections. *Oral Surg.* **61**, 413–17.

Jacobsen P. L. and Murray W. (1980) Prophylactic coverage of dental patients with artificial joints: a retrospective analysis of thirty-three infections in hip prostheses. *Oral Surg.* **50**, 130–3.

Jaspers M. T. and Little J. W. (1985) Prophylactic antibiotic coverage in patients with total arthroplasty: current practice. *J. Am. Dent. Assoc.* **111**, 943–8.

Jowsey J. (1977) *Metabolic Diseases of Bone*. Philadelphia, Saunders.

Kent J. N., Carlton D. M. and Zide M. F. (1986) Rheumatoid disease and related arthropathies. *Oral. Surg.* **61**, 432–9.

Leading Article (1979) Reiter's syndrome. *Lancet* **ii**, 567.

Leading Article (1980) Learning from Ehlers–Danlos. *Lancet* **ii**, 1062–3.

Leading Article (1987) Vitamin D: new perspectives. *Lancet* **i**, 1122–3.

McCarty D. J. (1979) *Arthritis and Allied Conditions*, 9th ed. Philadelphia, Lea & Febiger.

McGowan D. A. and Hendrey M. L. (1985) Is antibiotic prophylaxis required for dental patients with joint replacements? *Br. Dent. J.* **158**, 336–8.

Medsger T.A. (1990) Tryptophan-induced eosinophilia-myalgia syndrome. *N. Engl. J. Med.* **322**, 926–8.

Migliorisi J. A. and Blenkinsopp P. T. (1980) Oral surgical management of cleidocranial dysostosis. *Br. J. Oral Surg.* **18**, 212–20.

Morgan-Hughes J. (1980) Diseases of muscle. *Medicine (UK)* **34**, 171–31.

Mulligan R. (1980) Late infections in patients with prostheses for total replacement of joints: implications for the dental practitioner. *J. Am. Dent. Assoc.* **101**, 44–6.

Penarrocha M., Bagan J.V., Vilchez J. et al. (1990) Oral alterations in Steinert's myotonic dystrophy. *Oral Surg.* **69**, 698–78.

Pope F. M. and Nicholls A. C. (1984) Molecular abnormalities of collagen proteins and genes. In: Malcolm A. D. B. (ed.) *Molecular Medicine.* Lancaster, MTP Press, p. 117.

Prockop D.K. and Kivirikko K.I. (1981) Heritable diseases of collagen. *N. Engl. J. Med.* **311**, 376–86.

Prockop D.K. and Kuivaniemi H. (1986) Inborn errors of collagen. *Rheumatology* **10**, 246–71.

Ramsay A.N. (1986) *Post Viral Fatigue Syndrome - the saga of Royal Free Disease.* Gower, London.

Scully C. (1979/80) Orofacial manifestations of disease. 4: Fungal and viral infections, skeletal disorders and malignancies. *Dent. Update* **7**, 87: *Hosp. Update* **5**, 1119.

Scully C. and Cawson R. A. (eds) (1986) Oral medicine. *Med. Int.* **28**, 1129–51.

Seow W. K. and Latham S. C. (1986) The spectrum of dental manifestations in vitamin-D-resistant rickets and implications for management. *Pediatr. Dent.* **8**, 245–250.

Smith B. J. and Eveson J. W. (1981) Paget's disease of bone with particular reference to dentistry. *J. Oral Pathol.* **10**, 233–47.

Wenneberg B. and Kapp S. (1982) Clinical findings in the stomatognathic system in ankylosing spondylitis. *Scand. J. Dent. Res.* **90**, 373–81.

Wilkinson I. M. S. (1976) Giant cell arteritis. *Br. J. Hosp. Med.* **15**, 154–61.

Appendix to Chapter 11

SOME GENETICALLY DETERMINED SKELETAL DISORDERS

Achondroplasia	(p. 305)
Albers–Schönberg syndrome	(p. 307)
Albright's syndrome	(p. 315)
Apert's syndrome	Craniostenosis; syndactyly
Cheney syndrome	Osteoporosis; early loss of teeth
Cherubism	Familial symmetrical self-limiting soft tissue jaw lesions
Cleidocranial dysplasia	(p. 306)
Congenital hyperphosphatasia	Thickened calvarium; early loss of teeth; visual or hearing defects; blue sclerae
Crouzon's syndrome	Hypoplastic midface; proptosis; craniostenosis; hearing defects
Ellis–van Creveld syndrome	Atrial septal defect; dwarfism; polydactyly
Gardner's syndrome	(p. 201)
Gaucher's disease	(p. 301)
Goldenhar's syndrome	Same as Treacher Collins syndrome plus epibulbar dermoids
Gorlin's syndrome	(p. 527)
Hallermann–Streiff syndrome	Cataracts; mandibular retrognathism; scanty hair
Holt–Oram syndrome	Abnormalities of thumb, wrist and clavicle; atrial septal defect
Hypophosphataemia	Vitamin D resistant rickets; dentinal anomalies leading to early pulp involvement in caries
Klippel–Feil deformity	(Appendix to Chapter 19)
Maffuci's syndrome	(p. 157)
Mucopolysaccharidoses	(p. 302)
Noonan's syndrome	(Appendix to Chapter 19)
Odontomatosis	Multiple odontomas; cirrhosis; oesophageal stenosis
Ollier's disease	Multiple enchondromas
Orofacial digital syndromes	Facial anomalies; fraenal hyperplasia; tongue hamartomas; digital anomalies
Osteogenesis imperfecta	(p. 304)
Pierre Robin syndrome	Micrognathia; cleft palate; glossoptosis
Rubinstein–Taybi syndrome	Broad thumbs and toes; maxillary hypoplasia; patent ductus arteriosus

TAR syndrome	Thrombocytopenia, Absent Radius; atrial septal defect or tetralogy of Fallot
Treacher Collins syndrome	Hypoplastic malars and mandible; palpebral fissures slope down and out; colobomas; hearing defects
van Buchem's syndrome	Generalized cortical hyperostosis; facial palsy; optic atrophy; hearing defects

DIFFERENTIATION OF MARFAN'S SYNDROME FROM CONGENITAL CONTRACTURAL ARACHNODACTYLY (CCA) AND HOMOCYSTINURIA

	Marfan's	CCA	Homocystinuria
Inheritance	AD*	AD	AR†
Arachnodactyly	+	+	+
Loose joints	+	+contractures	±
Pectus excavatus	+	−	+
Ectopia lentis	+	−	+
Mental handicap	±	−	+
High palate	+	+	+
Crowding of teeth	+	−	+
Vacular	Dilatation of ascending aorta Dissecting aneurysm Aortic valve disease	−	Thromboses
Others	Blue sclerae Jaw cysts	Scoliosis Ear deformities Retrognathia	Malar flush Osteoporosis Prognathic mandible
Management problems	Risk of infective endocarditis	−	Postoperative thromboses

*AD, Autosomal dominant.
†AR, Atuosomal recessive.

Chapter 12

Neurological Disease and Facial Pain

The dentist frequently has to deal with pain or other symptoms from the mouth or face and may therefore have to recognize abnormalities involving the trigeminal, facial, glossopharyngeal, vagal or hypoglossal nerves. In addition, patients with maxillofacial or head injuries may have brain damage with impaired ocular movements or pupil reactions and loss of the sense of smell (anosmia).

The following is a brief synopsis of the examination of the cranial nerves. An outline of the investigation of diplopia, which is a common accompaniment of fractures of the middle third of the face, and of pupillary abnormalities is given later in this chapter.

The Olfactory Nerve (1st Cranial Nerve)

Unilateral anosmia is often unnoticed by the patient. Bilateral anosmia is common after head injuries, but in practice the patient may complain of loss of taste rather than sense of smell. An olfactory lesion is confirmed by inability to smell substances such as orange or peppermint oil. Ammoniacal solutions must not be used—they stimulate the trigeminal rather than the olfactory nerve.

The Optic Nerve (IInd Cranial Nerve)

Blindness or defects of visual fields are caused by ocular, optic nerve or cortical damage but the type of defect varies according to the site and extent of the lesion. If there is a complete lesion of one optic nerve that eye is totally blind there is no direct reaction of the pupil to light (loss of constriction) and, if a light is shone into the affected eye, the pupil of the *unaffected* eye also fails to respond (loss of the consensual reflex). However, the nerves to the affected eye that are responsible for pupil constriction, run in the IIIrd cranial nerve and should be intact. If, therefore, a light is shone into the unaffected eye, the pupil of the affected eye also constricts even though it is sightless. Lesions of the optic tract, chiasma, radiation or optic cortex cause various visual field defects involving both visual fields but without total field loss on either side. An ophthalmological opinion should always be obtained if there is any suggestion of a visual field defect.

The Oculomotor Nerve (IIIrd Cranial Nerve)

The oculomotor nerve supplies most of the orbital muscles that move the eye (but not the lateral rectus and superior oblique), and the muscle that raises the upper eyelid. The oculomotor also carries the nerve supply to the ciliary muscle and constrictor of the pupil. Normally the medial rectus (supplied by the IIIrd nerve) moves the eye medially (adducts). The lateral rectus (VIth nerve) abducts the eye. When the eye is abducted it is elevated by the superior rectus (IIIrd nerve) and depressed by the inferior rectus (IIIrd nerve). The adducted eye is depressed by the superior oblique muscle (IVth nerve) and elevated by the inferior oblique (IIIrd nerve). Disruption of the IIIrd nerve therefore causes:

1. Paralysis of internal, upward and downward rotation of the eye.
2. Double vision and divergent squint. The affected eye points downwards and laterally—'down and out' in all directions except when looking towards the affected side.
3. Ptosis (drooping upper eyelid).
4. A dilated pupil which fails to constrict on accommodation or when light is shone either onto the affected eye (negative direct light reaction) or into the unaffected eye (negative consensual light reaction).

The Trochlear Nerve (IVth Cranial Nerve)

The trochlear nerve supplies only the superior oblique muscle which moves the eye downwards and medially towards the nose. Damage to this nerve causes serious disability, because there is diplopia maximal on looking down and the patient may have difficulty reading, going downstairs or seeing obstructions on the ground. The lesion is characterized by:

1. The head tilted away from the affected side.
2. Diplopia, maximal on looking downwards and inwards.
3. Normal pupils.

There is often damage to the IIIrd and VIth nerves as well.

The Trigeminal Nerve (Vth Cranial Nerve)

The trigeminal nerve supplies sensation over the whole face apart from the angle of the jaw, and the front of the scalp back to a line drawn across the vertex, between the ears. It also supplies sensation to most of the mucosa of the oral cavity, conjunctivae, nose, tympanic membrane and sinuses. The motor division of the trigeminal nerve supplies the muscles of mastication (masseter, pterygoids, temporalis, myloyoid and anterior belly of the digastric). Taste fibres from the anterior two-thirds of the tongue, and secretomotor fibres to the submandibular and sublingual salivary glands and lacrimal glands, are also carried in branches of the trigeminal nerve.

Damage to a sensory branch of the trigeminal nerve causes hypoaesthesia in its area of distribution (see p. 352 for causes). Lesions involving the ophthalmic division also cause corneal anaesthesia: this is tested by *gently* touching the cornea with a wisp of cotton wool twisted to a point. Normally this procedure causes a blink, but not if the cornea is anaesthetic and the patient does not see the cotton wool. Lesions of the sensory part of the trigeminal nerve initially result in a diminishing response to pin-prick to the skin and, later, complete anaesthesia. It is important, with patients complaining of facial anaesthesia, to test all areas but particularly the corneal reflex with a wisp of cotton wool, and the reaction to pin-prick over the angle of the mandible. If, however, the patient complains of complete facial or hemifacial anaesthesia, but the corneal reflex is retained or there is anaesthesia over the angle of the mandible, then the symptoms are probably functional rather than organic.

Taste can be tested with sweet, salt, sour or bitter substances carefully applied to the dorsum of the tongue, or by asking the patient to touch his tongue between the terminals of a pocket torch battery: this normally gives a tingling sensation and a characteristic metallic taste.

Damage to the motor part of the trigeminal nerve can be difficult to detect and is usually asymptomatic if unilateral but the jaw may deviate towards the affected side on opening. It is easier to detect motor weakness by asking the patient to open the jaw against resistance, rather than by trying to test the strength of closure.

The Abducens Nerve (VIth Cranial Nerve)

The abducens nerve supplies only a single eye muscle, the lateral rectus. Lesions are characterized by (*Fig.* 12.1):

1. Paralysis of abduction of the eye.
2. Deviation of the affected eye towards the nose, and convergent squint with diplopia maximal on looking laterally towards the affected side.
3. Normal pupils.

Lesions of the abducens can be surprisingly disabling.

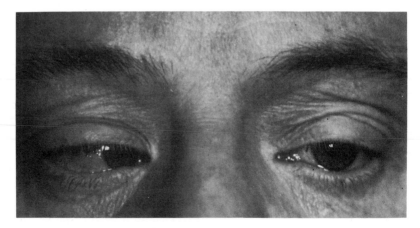

Fig. 12.1. Lesion of the abducens nerve: with the patient looking directly ahead, the affected eye deviates medially as the lateral rectus muscle is functionless.

The Facial Nerve (VIIth Cranial Nerve)

The facial nerve is the motor supply to the muscles of facial expression and also carries taste sensation from the anterior two-thirds of the tongue (via the chorda tympani), secretomotor fibres to the submandibular and sublingual salivary glands and to the lacrimal glands, and branches to the stapedius muscle in the middle ear.

The neurones supplying the lower face receive upper motor neurones from the contralateral motor cortex, whereas the neurones to the upper face receive bilateral upper motor neurone (UMN) innervation. An upper motor neurone lesion is characterized by unilateral facial palsy with some sparing of the frontalis and orbicularis oculi muscles because of the bilateral cortical representation. Furthermore, although voluntary facial movements are impaired, the face may still move with emotional responses, for example on laughing. Paresis of the ipsilateral arm (monoparesis) or arm and leg (hemiparesis), or dysphasia may be associated because of more extensive cerebrocortical damage.

Lower motor neurone (LMN) facial palsy is characterized by unilateral paralysis of all muscles of facial expression for both voluntary and emotional responses. The forehead is unfurrowed and the patient unable to close the eye on that side. Attempted closure causes the eye to roll upwards (Bell's sign). Tears tend to overflow on to the cheek (epiphora), the corner of the mouth droops and the nasolabial fold is obliterated. Saliva may dribble from the commissure and may cause angular stomatitis. Food collects in the vestibule and plaque accumulates on the teeth on the affected side. Depending on the site of the lesion, other defects such as loss of taste or hyperacusis may be associated.

Facial weakness is demonstrated by asking the patient to close the eyes against resistance, to raise the eyebrows, to whistle or to raise the lips to show his teeth. Schirmer's test for lacrimation, carried out by gently placing a strip of filter paper on the lower conjunctival sac and comparing the wetting of the paper with that on the other side, may be helpful. Lacrimation is decreased in a VIIth nerve lesion. Taste is tested by applying sugar, salt, lemon juice or vinegar on the tongue and asking the patient to identify each of them.

The Vestibulocochlear Nerve (VIIIth Cranial Nerve)

The auditory nerve has two components, the vestibular (concerned with appreciation of the movements and position of the head) and the cochlear (hearing). Lesions of this nerve may cause loss of hearing, vertigo or ringing in the ears (tinnitus). An otological opinion should be obtained if a lesion of the vestibulocochlear nerve is suspected, as special tests are needed for diagnosis.

The Glossopharyngeal Nerve (IXth Cranial Nerve)

The glossopharyngeal nerve is the sensory supply to the posterior third of the tongue and pharynx, carries taste sensation from the posterior third of the tongue, and the motor supply to the stylopharyngeus. It also carries secretomotor fibres to the parotid. Lesions of the glossopharyngeal are usually associated with lesions of the vagus, accessory and hypoglossal nerves (bulbar palsy,

p. 358). Symptoms resulting from a IXth nerve lesion include impaired pharyngeal sensation so that the gag reflex may be impaired; the two sides should always be compared.

The Vagus Nerve (Xth Cranial Nerve)

The vagus has a wide parasympathetic distribution to the viscera of the thorax and upper abdomen but is also the motor supply to some soft palate, pharyngeal and laryngeal muscles.

Lesions of the vagus are rare in isolation but have the followig effects:

1. Impaired gag reflex.
2. The soft palate moves towards the unaffected side when the patient is asked to say 'aah'.
3. Hoarse voice.
4. Bovine cough.

The Accessory Nerve (XIth Cranial Nerve)

The accessory nerve is the motor supply to the sternomastoid and trapezius muscles. Lesions are often associated with damage to the IXth and Xth nerves and cause:

1. Weakness of the sternomastoid (weakness on turning the head away from the affected side).
2. Weakness of the trapezius on shrugging the shoulders.

Testing this nerve is useful in differentiating patients with genuine palsies from those with functional complaints. In an accessory nerve lesion there is weakness on turning the head away from the affected side. Those shamming paralysis often simulate weakness when turning the head towards the 'affected' side.

The Hypoglossal Nerve (XIIth Cranial Nerve)

The hypoglossal nerve is the motor supply to the muscles of the tongue. Lesions cause:

1. Dysarthria (difficulty in speaking)—particularly for lingual sounds.
2. Deviation of the tongue towards the affected side, on protrusion.

In an upper motor neurone lesion the tongue is spastic but not wasted; in a lower motor neurone lesion there is wasting and fibrillation of the affected side of the tongue (*Fig.* 12.2).

Cranial nerve lesions are not, of course, necessarily seen in isolation and several may be affected at the same time. Multiple cranial nerve palsies are a feature of intracranial HIV infection, as discussed below. Various other syndromes, some of which are rare, are recognised, and these are tabulated in the Appendix to this chapter.

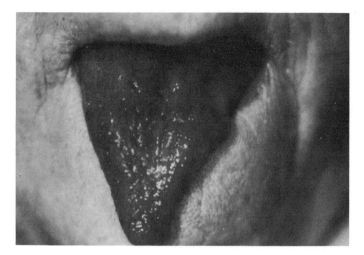

Fig. 12.2. Lesion of the hypoglossal nerve with wasting of the left side of the tongue (lower motor neurone lesion).

HEADACHE AND FACIAL PAIN

Headache and facial pain are common symptoms mainly caused by (*see also Table 12.1*):

1. Oral or perioral lesions, or diseases of the nose, sinuses, eye, ear or neck.
2. Neurological disease.
3. Psychogenic causes.
4. Vascular causes.
5. Pain referred from a distance.
6. Drugs such as vinca alkaloids.

Local Causes of Facial Pain

The Mouth

The oral causes of facial pain such as dental caries and its sequelae, periodontal abscesses, pericoronitis and various intraosseous lesions are fully discussed in other texts.

The Sinuses and Nasopharynx

Sinusitis can cause localized pain. In acute maxillary or frontal sinusitis local pain and tenderness (but not swelling), and radio-opacity of the affected sinuses, usually follow a cold.

Table 12.1. Causes of facial pain and headache

Local causes
    Dental or oral disease
    Infections or tumours of paranasal sinuses and nasopharynx
    Neck lesions
    Ocular lesions
Neurological causes
    Trigeminal neuralgia (benign paroxysmal trigeminal neuralgia)
    Glossopharyngeal neuralgia
    Herpetic neuralgia
    Raeder's neuralgia
    Intracranial disease
Psychogenic causes
    Tension headaches
    Atypical facial pain
    Temporomandibular-pain-dysfunction syndrome
Vascular causes
    Migraine
    Migrainous neuralgia
    Temporal arteritis
Other causes
    Referred pain
    Raised intracranial pressure
    Meningeal irritation
    Diseases of the skull
    Medical diseases (e.g. severe hypertension)
    Trauma
    Drugs (e.g. vinca alkaloids, nitrites or dapsone)

With maxillary sinusitis pain may be felt in related upper molars, several of which may be tender to percussion. The pain of ethmoidal or sphenoidal sinusitis is felt deeply in the nose, but may cause headache while frontal sinusitis causes an anterior headache.

Tumours of the sinuses or nasopharynx can also cause facial pain. These tumours are often carcinomas which involve various branches of the trigeminal nerve and can remain undetected until late. Some may cause pain simulating pain dysfunction syndrome.

Eagle's syndrome, a rare disorder due to an elongated styloid process, due to calcification of the stylohoid process, may cause pain on chewing, swallowing or turning the head. The elongated styloid process may be visualized radiographically, and palpation of it in the wall of the pharynx causes intense pain.

The elongated stylohyoid process can be shortened surgically, but regrowth and relapse is common.

The Eyes

Disorders of refraction can cause frontal headaches. Retrobulbar neuritis (for example in multiple sclerosis), or glaucoma (raised intraocular pressure), may cause pain in and around the orbit.

The Ears

Pharyngeal or middle ear disease may cause headaches. Oral disease can also cause pain referred to the ear; a classic picture is that of the elderly person with cancer of the tongue who complains of earache.

The Neck

Cervical vertebral disease, especially cervical spondylosis, occasionally causes pain referred to the face.

Neurological Causes of Facial Pain

Sensory innervation of the face and scalp depends on the trigeminal nerve, so that involvement of this nerve at any stage from its nuclei along its course from the pons can cause facial pain or sensory loss—sometimes with serious implications.

Idiopathic trigeminal neuralgia (tic douloureux)

Trigeminal neuralgia usually afflicts women over the age of 50. The pain has the following characteristics:

1. Pain is usually confined to the trigeminal area of one side, usually the maxillary or mandibular division or both.
2. The pain is severe and sharply stabbing (lancinating). It is of only a few seconds' duration, but paroxysms may follow in quick succession.
3. Mild stimuli, such as touch or cold, applied to trigger zones within the trigeminal area typically provoke an attack.
4. There is no objective sensory loss in the area, or other defined neurological deficit.

The pain of trigeminal neuralgia is typically remarkably severe and a patient seen crying with pain during an attack is not easily forgotten.

Characteristic trigger zones are near the ala nasae, near the commissure, or on the gingivae and are not necessarily situated in the sensory area where the pain is felt. Touching, washing, toothbrushing or chewing may trigger an attack.

Patients with idiopathic trigeminal neuralgia show no abnormal neurological signs. Neurological assessment is needed because similar pain may be secondary to multiple sclerosis, to posterior cerebral fossa lesions (particularly tumours) to neurosyphilis or to other lesions. Young patients who develop trigeminal neuralgia are likely to have multiple sclerosis.

Classic trigeminal neuralgia has been described and some purists dispute the existence of atypical variants. However, patients occasionally complain of unusual symptoms such as more continuous rather than lightning attacks of pain, or triggering by warmth rather than cold. The response of many such cases to carbamazepine strongly suggests that trigeminal neuralgia may produce a slightly variable clinical picture.

Management of trigeminal neuralgia.   It must be confirmed that no abnormal neurological signs are present before drug treatment is started. Spontaneous remissions of a month or two are relatively common and may make the assessment of treatment difficult.

Carbamazepine is the main treatment for trigeminal neuralgia. Starting with 100 mg twice or three times daily, the dose should be increased until symptoms are controlled or side-effects become excessive. Most patients respond to 200–400 mg three times daily. Side-effects include gastrointestinal upsets and in a few, rashes. Ataxia and drowsiness are dose-related and may be dose-limiting. There are many other possible toxic effects but are uncommon: leucopenia has been reported but is exceedingly rare. In high dosage, carbamazepine, which is sometimes also used for the treatment of diabetes insipidus, may cause the syndrome of inappropriate antidiuretic hormone secretion (Chapter 10), fluid retention and hyponatraemia particularly in the elderly or those with heart failure. Blood pressure, blood urea and electrolytes should therefore be monitored.

It is essential to appreciate that carbamazepine is not an analgesic and, if given when an attack starts, will not relieve the pain. Absorption is slow and its antineuralgic activity depends on its metabolites. Carbamazepine must therefore be given continuously for long periods. It is also important to note that if a patient has pain suggestive of trigeminal neuralgia, but has no benefit from carbamazepine, it is essential to ask the nature of the dosage regimen, as the drug is often taken intermittently under the impression that it is an analgesic. Should carbamazepine in tolerated dosage fail to control neuralgia then phenytoin can be given in addition, oxcarbazine tried, or surgery may be required.

Local cryosurgery to the trigeminal nerve branches involved can produce analgesia without permanent anaesthesia but the benefit may only be temporary.

If this treatment fails neurosurgery may be needed. Anaesthesia is then exchanged for the pain and can cause such problems as anaesthesia of, and risk of damage to, the cornea and occasionally continuous pain (anaesthesia dolorosa).

Glossopharyngeal neuralgia

Glossopharyngeal neuralgia is rare. The pain is equally severe, but affects the throat and ear, and is typically triggered by swallowing or coughing. Carbamazepine is usually less effective than for trigeminal neuralgia and adequate relief of pain can be difficult. Occasionally glossopharyngeal neuralgia is secondary to lesions (often tumours) in the posterior cranial fossa or jugular foramen (jugular foramen syndrome), and there are then often lesions of the vagus (X) and accessory (XI) nerves (*see* Appendix to this chapter).

Herpetic and post-herpetic facial neuralgia

Herpes zoster (shingles) is often preceded and accompanied by neuralgia (Chapter 17). Neuralgia may also persist after the rash has resolved. Post-herpetic neuralgia (unlike trigeminal neuralgia) causes continuous burning pain.

It mainly affects elderly patients and may be so intolerable that suicide can become a risk. Treatment is difficult but antidepressants, particularly desipramine or chlorpromazine, or transcutaneous electrical stimulation may sometimes help if analgesics are not effective. However, spontaneous improvement may follow after about 18 months in some patients.

Raeder' paratrigeminal neuralgia

Severe, persistent pain in and around the eye with an associated Horner's syndrome, is often caused by a lesion at the base of the skull and requires neurological attention.

Facial pain caused by intracranial tumours or other lesions

Any lesion affecting the trigeminal nerve from the nuclei to the pons, through the posterior and middle cranial fossae, to the foramen ovale and rotundum, and to the superior orbital fissure can cause facial pain. The clinical features vary with the site and extent of the lesion. Commonly, there is facial pain associated with a facial sensory deficit and impaired corneal reflex on the affected side. Anatomically closely related cranial nerves are frequently involved (see Appendix to this chapter).

Pontine ischaemia may be due to bilateral ventral pontine infarction and has been reported to cause burning orofacial pain. This needs to be recognized as it may be an early symptom of bilateral ventral pontine infarction causing the syndrome of quadriplegia, lower cranial nerve palsies but preservation of movement of the upper eyelids and vertical gaze. This constellation of effects is termed the *locked-in syndrome* because the patient, though able to understand what is being said or what is happening, is imprisoned by his inability to speak or move anything apart from his eyes. The prognosis is poor. Lateral medullary infarction may cause a similar but unilateral burning sensation.

Lesions in the posterior cranial fossa, such as cerebellopontine angle tumours (acoustic neuroma or meningioma), can cause facial pain associated with an absent corneal reflex (Vth nerve), deafness, tinnitus and vertigo (from involvement of the VIIIth nerve), facial palsy (VIIth nerve involvement), ataxia, intention tremor and nystagmus (cerebellar involvement) and spasticity of the leg (prramidal tract involvement).

Middle cranial fossa lesions can involve the Vth and VIth nerves, causing also a lateral rectus palsy. Carotid aneurysms, especially those in the cavernous sinus, or cavernous sinus thrombosis, may also cause facial pain and associated cranial nerve lesions (IIIrd, IVth and VIth nerves).

Cavernous sinus thrombosis is a life-threatening complication that may rarely result from infection spreading back through the emissary veins from the maxillary or nasal region, or upper teeth. Infected thrombi in the anterior facial vein or less commonly the pterygoid plexus can reach the cavernous sinus via either the ophthalmic veins or the foramen ovale.

Clinically, cavernous sinus thrombosis causes gross oedema of the eyelids, ipsilateral pulsatile exophthalmos and cyanosis due to venous obstruction. The superior orbital fissure syndrome (proptosis, fixed dilated pupil and limitation of eye movements) rapidly develops. Rigors and a high swinging pyrexia are associated. In the absence of effective treatment, similar signs rapidly develop on the opposite side.

Vigorous use of anticoagulants, antibiotics, drainage and elimination of the source of infection is essential. There is a mortality of up to 50 per cent and a further 50 per cent of those that survive are likely to lose the sight of one or both eyes.

Severe facial pain suggestive of trigeminal neuralgia but with physical signs such as facial sensory or motor impairment can result from brain stem ischaemia or infarction in cerebrovascular disease. Involvement of the posterior inferior cerebellar artery is often responsible.

Bell's palsy

Bell's (facial) palsy is preceded or accompanied by pain in the region of the ear and spreading down the jaw in about half the cases. However, the appearance of the typical facial paralysis leaves little doubt as to the diagnosis (*Fig.* 12.3).

Facial pain caused by extracranial lesions

Branches of the trigeminal nerve may be affected by inflammatory, traumatic or neoplastic lesions causing pain or sensory loss in their distribution.

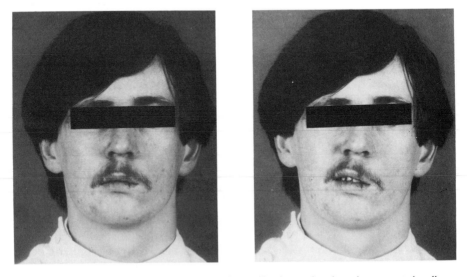

Fig. 12.3. Bell's palsy: the left side of the face is completely paralysed, as demonstrated well when the patient tries to smile.

Psychogenic Causes of Facial Pain

Tension headaches

Bilateral tension headaches are very common, especially in young adults. The pain, which is caused by muscle tension, affects the frontal, occipital or temporal muscles, and is felt as a constant ache or band-like pressure. The pain is often worse in the evening and at night, lasts a few hours, but does not waken the patient.

Reassurance may be effective but may be helped by a short course of diazepam 2 – 5 mg, three times daily, as this is both anxiolytic and a mild muscle relaxant.

Patients with tension headaches are frequently adamant that they suffer from migraine, as migraine is a more important-sounding diagnosis, is supposed to affect highly intelligent people, and has fewer neurotic connotations. The possibility of associated depression should also be considered.

Atypical facial pain (*see* Chapter 14).

Temporomandibular-pain-dysfunction syndrome (*see* Chapter 14).

Vascular Causes of Facial Pain

Migraine

Migraine is a recurrent headache affecting over 5 per cent of women. The number, frequency, intensity and duration of attacks vary widely but they tend to diminish in frequency and intensity with increasing age. Spontaneous remissions are not uncommon. Migraine appears to be related to arterial dilatation. Attacks may be precipitated by various foods, such as ripe bananas or chocolate, or the contraceptive pill. Stress often seems to be a precipitating factor in migraine as in many other disorders. The fact that attacks are more frequent at weekends, for example, should not be interpreted as excluding stress, as there is no doubt that some find the company and demands of their families more stressful than their work. Going away on holiday (Freud's 'reise fieber—travel fever') is also highly stressful for many. The belief that migraine is caused by occlusal dysharmony is unsubstantiated.

Several types of migraine are recognized (*Table 12.2*). Classic migraine is not the most frequent type, but is the most readily recognized by the following features:

1. The headache is preceded by warning symptoms (an aura).
2. The headache is severe, usually unilateral (hemicrania) and lasts for hours or days.
3. Photophobia, nausea or vomiting are typically associated.

The aura may last about 15 minutes and consists of visual, sensory, motor or speech disturbances. Visual phenomena are typically of zig-zag flickering light (fortification spectra) or transient visual defects. Sensory phenomena include paraesthesia or anaesthesia—usually of the contralateral upper limb, or face

Table 12.2. Migraine Variants

Type	Clinical features
Classic migraine	Unilateral headache preceded by an aura*
Migrainous neuralgia	Pain typically around the eye often with visible effects of vasodilatation
Facial migraine	Variant of migrainous neuralgia, but affects lower face (lower-half migraine)
Hemiplegic migraine	Rare Often familial; hemiparesis may outlast headache by several days; may rarely cause facial palsy
Ophthalmoplegic migraine	Rare Affects children (boys) mainly; pain around eye with impaired eye movement
Vertebrobasiliar migraine	Affects adolescent girls mainly Similar to classic migraine but aura includes ataxia, vertigo, diplopia; headache usually occipital; may be loss of consciousness at the onset
Complicated migraine	Term applied to any form of migraine complicated by residual neurological defect after attack

Note. Migraine frequently lacks the 'classic' features and may not be strictly unilateral or there may be no aura – it is then difficult to distinguish from non-migrainous headache.

and mouth. Obvious vascular phenomena may be associated but are variable in character, and range from flushing and oedema of the face on the affected side to temporary hemiplegia. Motor symptoms are mainly weakness—again of the contralateral upper limb. The headache often becomes throbbing and generalized and may be associated with facial pallor. The patient may complain of photophobia and nausea. Epilepsy is slightly more common in migraine sufferers than in the general population.

Management of migraine

Migraine is usually managed with drugs and avoidance of precipitating factors. If attacks are frequent, prophylaxis with propranolol is the treatment of choice but sometimes a serotonin antagonist (pizotifen or methysergide) is used. Methysergide has dangerous toxic effects, in particular, retroperitoneal fibrosis and fibrosis of the heart valves and pleura. It is only therefore given for refractory cases under specialist supervision. More recent evidence suggests that calcium channel blockers such as verapamil or nifedipine may be useful alternatives and low-dose aspirin (300 mg on alternate days) may reduce attacks by 20 per cent, probably by blocking prostaglandin production in response to stimulation of a 5-HT (serotonin) receptor. Sumatriptan, a 5-HT receptor against, has recently been introduced: it is effective, but contraindicated in cardiac disease.

In acute attacks, patients usually prefer to lie in a quiet, dark room. Effervescent aspirin or paracetamol are frequently effective. If not, ergotamine (1–2 mg) given early during the aura, may abort an attack, but in many cases absorption by mouth is too slow to be effective and a better alternative therefore is to use it by inhalation from a Medihaler. Even so, the use of ergotamine at the earliest possible moment must be emphasized. Ergotamine can also be given as a suppository and overcomes the problem of poor absorption if the patient is vomiting. In severe cases an anti-emetic such as metoclopramide may also be required. Modifications to the occlusion are unlikely to produce anything more than a placebo effect.

Migrainous neuralgia

Synonyms include periodic migrainous neuralgia, cluster headaches, Horton's neuralgia, superficial petrosal neuralgia, histamine cephalgia and others.

Migrainous neuralgia is less common than migraine and causes pain localized round the eye, forehead, cheek and temple (*Table 12.3*). Males are mainly affected and typical features are the onset of pain at night, or the clustering of attacks at the same time, night or day, for several weeks, flushing of the affected side of the face and features such as lacrimation, conjunctival injection and nasal congestion. Horner's syndrome (p. 361) may be associated.

Table 12.3. Differentiation between migraine and migrainous neuralgia

	Migraine	*Migrainous neuralgia*
Sex mainly affected	Females	Males
Family history	+ ve often	- ve
Pain unilateral	Usually	Always
Frequency of attacks	Less than 3 per week	May be daily
Time of attacks	Usually daytime	Often at night
Duration of attacks	Hours to days	Minutes to a few hours
Other features	May be aura, nausea and vomiting	May be nasal congestion and lacrimation

Adapted from Greenhall R. C. D. (1980) *Medicine (UK)* **31**, 1606.

Attacks are sometimes precipitated by alcohol and, if so, it should be avoided. Migrainous neuralgia is managed with ergotamine, pizotifen, beta-blockers, sumatriptan or rarely, methysergide prophylactically. Sometimes corticosteroids or lithium carbonate are used.

Cranial arteritis (*see* Chapter 11).

Other Causes of Headache and Facial Pain

Raised intracranial pressure: one of the most serious but also the least common cause of headache. It may be caused by malignant hypertension, a tumour, abscess or haematoma.

The headache is severe and often worse on waking but decreases during the day. Nausea and vomiting are common and the headache is aggravated by straining, coughing, sneezing or lying down. Neurological attention is essential.

Meningeal irritation: severe headache with nausea, vomiting, neck pain or stiffness (inability to kiss the knees) or pain on raising the straightened legs (Kernig's sign) implies meningeal irritation as in meningitis or subarachnoid haemorrhage.

Urgent neurological attention is needed.

Trauma: headaches are common after most head injuries. These headaches do not normally persist, but if they do, neurological advice must be sought to exclude intracranial haemorrhage. In the absence of neurological complications, persistent post-traumatic headaches may be due to compensation neurosis (Chapter 14).

Diseases of the skull: headache is occasionally the presenting feature of diseases such as bony metastases or Paget's disease (Chapter 11).

Systemic diseases: headache can be a feature of any fever, hypertension, chronic obstructive airways disease or some endocrinopathies. Facial pain may occasionally be drug-induced, for example by vinca alkaloids, phenothiazines (see Appendix to Chapter 19) or may be referred from the chest, particularly in ischaemic heart disease. Epstein–Barr virus appears to be associated with some headaches in young adults that recur daily but resolve spontaneously within a year (new daily persistent headache).

FACIAL SENSORY LOSS

Facial sensation is mediated through the trigeminal nerve; the skin over the angle of the mandible is supplied by cervical nerves.

Facial sensory loss may be caused by intracranial, or much more frequently by extracranial lesions of the trigeminal nerve.

Intracranial Cause of Facial Sensory Loss

Some intracranial causes of facial sensory loss are shown in *Table 12.4*. Important causes are stroke, multiple sclerosis, cerebral tumours (especially acoustic neuroma), collagen diseases, and infections. Syringomyelia is a rare cause.

In posterior cranial fossa lesions, facial sensory loss predominates, but is associated with an absent corneal reflex and other features such as:

1. Facial weakness (VIIth nerve involvement).
2. Deafness or vertigo (VIIIth nerve involvement).
3. Nystagmus and ataxia (cerebellar involvement).
4. Extensor plantar response with spastic weakness of the leg (pyramidal tract involvement).

Middle cranial fossa lesions tend to cause a trigeminal sensory deficit and there may also be:

1. Weakness or atrophy of the masticatory muscles (Vth nerve).
2. Extraocular palsies (IIIrd, IVth or VIth nerves affected).

Table 12.4. Causes of sensory loss in the trigeminal area

Intracranial		
Congenital	Syringobulbia	
Acquired	Inflammatory	—multiple sclerosis
		neurosyphilis
		sarcoidosis
		tuberculosis
		connective tissue diseases
		AIDS
	Neoplastic	—cerebral tumours
	Vascular	—cerebrovascular disease
		aneurysms
	Drugs	—stilbamidine
	Occupational	—trilene (dry cleaning)
	Idiopathic	—benign trigeminal neuropathy
		Paget's disease
Extracranial		
Acquired	Trauma	—to infraorbital, inferior dental or mental nerves or middle cranial fossa fracture
	Inflammatory	—osteomyelitis
	Neoplastic	—carcinoma of antrum or nasopharynx
		metastatic tumours
		leukaemic deposits

Extracranial Causes of Sensory Loss

Common extracranial causes of facial sensory loss are shown in *Table 12.4*. Damage to branches of the maxillary division of the trigeminal nerve may be caused by trauma (middle-third facial fractures) or a tumour such as carcinoma of the antrum. The mandibular division may be traumatized by inferior dental local anaesthetic injections, or surgery (particularly osteotomies or surgical extraction of lower third molars). Occasionally the mental foramen lies beneath a lower denture and there is labial anaesthesia as a result of pressure on the labial nerve. Labial gland biopsies can sometimes cause limited labial anaesthesia.

Nasopharyngeal carcinomas may invade the pharyngeal wall to infiltrate the madibular division of the trigeminal nerve, causing pain and sensory loss and, by occluding the Eustachian tube, deafness (Trotter's syndrome). Osteomyelitis or tumour deposits in the mandible may involve the inferior dental nerve to cause labial paraesthesia or anaesthesia.

FACIAL PARALYSIS

The motor nerve to the facial muscles is the VIIth cranial nerve and common causes of facial paralysis are strokes (upper motor neurone lesion) and Bell's palsy (lower motor neurone lesion). Other causes are shown in *Table 12.5* and features differentiating upper motor neurone from lower motor neurone lesions are outlined in *Table 12.6*. Facial palsy in Kawasaki's disease (Chapter 2) is rare, but particularly unusual in that it is seen in infancy (often at only 6 to 9 months) and is self-limiting.

Table 12.5. Facial palsy

Site of lesion	Causes	Muscles paralysed	Lacrimation	Hyperacusis	Taste	Other features
Upper motor neurone (UMN)	Cerebrovascular accident Cerebral tumour Trauma	Lower face	N	—	N	Emotional movement retained ± mono or hemiparesis ± aphasia
Lower motor neurone (LMN) Facial nucleus	Cerebrovascular disease Moebius syndrome Multiple sclerosis Syphilis HIV infection Lyme disease	All facial muscles	→	+	→	+ VIIth nerve damage
Between nucleus and geniculate ganglion	Fractured base of skull Posterior cranial fossa tumours Sarcoidosis	All facial muscles	→	+	→	+ VIIIth nerve damage
Between geniculate ganglion and stylomastoid canal	Middle ear infection Cholesteatoma Ramsay–Hunt syndrome Mastoiditis	All facial muscles	N	±	N or ↓	—
In stylomastoid canal or extracranially	Bell's palsy Trauma Misplaced inferior dental anaesthetic Parotid tumour Sarcoidosis Leprosy	All facial muscles	N	—	N	—
Branch of facial nerve extracranially	Trauma Local anaesthesia	Isolated facial muscles	N	—	N	—

N = normal. ↓ = reduced.

Table 12.6. Differentiation of upper from lower motor neurone lesions of the facial nerve

	UMN lesion	LMN lesion
Emotional movements of face	Retained	Lost
Blink reflex	Retained	Lost
Ability to wrinkle forehead	Retained	Lost
Drooling from commissure	Uncommon	Common
Lacrimation, taste and hearing	Unaffected	May be affected
Tongue protrusion	Normal	Deviates to unaffected side

Management of facial palsy

Clinical assessment should include a full neurological examination for possible causes, as shown in *Table 12.5*, but the primary distinction needed is between upper motor neurone and lower motor neurone lesions. Facial nerve stimulation or needle electromyography may be useful, as may electrogustometry, skull radiography, CT or MR scans or occasionally, lumbar puncture.

Cerebrovascular Accidents (*see* p. 378)

Bell's Palsy

Lower motor neurone paralysis of the face may be a symptom of serious disease but in at least two-thirds of cases no cause can be identified. The condition is then termed Bell's palsy, where there is inflammation in the stylomastoid canal. This may be immunologically mediated and associated with the herpes simplex or another virus, or Lyme disease. The onset of paralysis is acute over a few hours, although pain in the region of the ear or in the jaw may precede the palsy by a day or two. There is usually only unilateral facial palsy, but occasionally hyperacusis (loss of function of nerve to stapedius), or loss of taste (chorda tympani), are noted. Eighty per cent of patients recover within a few weeks but some have residual permanent palsy.

If paralysis persists and function remains incomplete the palpebral fissure may narrow and the nasolabial fold deepen; facial spasm may develop. Rare complications include irregular or anomalous lacrimation (crocodile tears) when the facial muscles are used, and permanent disfigurement.

Management of Bell's palsy

All patients with partial palsy and about three-quarters of those with total palsy recover quickly spontaneously. A favourable prognostic sign is persistence of the stapedial reflex, measured by electroneurography if possible. Bad prognostic signs are hyperacusis, severe taste impairment and/or diminished lacrimation or salivation, especially in older patients. Although most patients recover spontaneously, the after-effects in the remaining 10 – 20 per cent can be so severe and distressing that there is a strong argument for treating all patients with corticosteroids. Prednisolone 20 mg four times a day for 5 days, then tailed off over the succeeding 4 days is recommended but doubt has been cast on its effectiveness.

During the period of the palsy, the cornea should be protected with an eye pad. In chronic cases surgical decompression of the nerve in the stylomastoid canal may be attempted; alternatively, it may be necessary to use a splint to prevent drooping at the commisure, or to use a facial graft or other manoeuvres such as facial–hypoglossal nerve anastomosis in an attempt to overcome the cosmetic deformity. The results are, however, rarely entirely satisfactory.

In progressive facial palsy, radiographic evaluation of the internal acoustic canal, cerebellopontine angle and mastoid may be needed to exclude an organic lesion.

Dental aspects of facial palsy

Facial palsy may result in poor soft tissue cleansing and accumulation of food debris in the vestibules and of plaque on the teeth on the affected side. Saliva may leak from the affected side and cause angular stomatitis.

Construction of a splint to support the angle of the mouth may improve the aesthetics to some degree.

Most patients with Bell's palsy are otherwise healthy and present no other dental management difficulties than those discussed above, but facial palsy is also a feature of Melkersson–Rosenthal syndrome. HIV infecton, Lyme disease and a variety of other disorders (Table 12.5) and there are occasional (possibly coincidental) associations with diabetes mellitus, hypertension and lymphoma.

Ramsay–Hunt Syndrome

Severe facial palsy with vesicles in the ipsilateral pharynx and external auditory canal (Ramsay–Hunt syndrome) may be due to herpes zoster of the geniculate ganglion of the facial nerve.

Bilateral Facial Palsy

Bilateral facial palsy is rare but may be seen in acute idiopathic polyneuritis (Guillain–Barrè syndrome); sarcoidosis (Heerfordt's syndrome—uveoparotid fever, Chapter 6), arachnoiditis and posterior cranial fossa tumours.

Other Causes of Facial Weakness

An apparent facial palsy may be caused by myasthenia gravis, some myopathies (Chapter 11) or facial hemiatrophy.

Facial Dyskinesias and Dystonias

Facial dyskinesias are abnormal movements of the tongue or facial muscles, sometimes with abnormal jaw movements, bruxism or dysphagia. Involuntary tongue protrusion and retraction, and facial grimacing are frequent presentations.

Dystonias are a group of diseases, estimated to affect 20 000 people in Great Britain and characterized by abnormal movements (dyskinesias) associated with muscle spasm; they may be localized or generalized. Dystonias differ from dyskinesias mainly in that muscle spasm is more prominent, but they may be difficult to differentiate clinically. Examples of localized dystonias are torticollis and writer's cramp. The last is now included in a group of related disorders termed *repetitive strain injury*, but there is some evidence that a psychogenic element is involved in the latter. Otherwise, dystonias result from organic diseases affecting the brain (secondary dystonias), but despite the fact that a neurological disorder cannot always be identified (primary dystonias) it seems likely that there is a lesion in the basal ganglia. Support for this idea is given by the fact that many dystonias respond to antimuscarinics or levodopa.

Oromandibular dystonia refers to recurrent spasmodic episodes of lip movement, tongue protrusion and retraction, and jaw clenching or opening. This may be associated with blepharospasm and is then sometimes termed Meige's syndrome. Over one-third of patients may suffer from depression. Treatment is difficult but benzodiazepines may be helpful.

Acute cromandibular dystonia (drug-induced parkinsonism) can be caused by treatment within a short time (hours or days) of starting treatment with neuroleptics such as phenothiazines and butyrophenones (*see* Appendix to Chapter 19). It may resolve after withdrawal of the drug or be improved with antimuscarinic drugs such as benztropine. However, it is made worse by levodopa, which can itself also cause involuntary spasmodic movements if the dose is too great.

Oromandibular dystonia must be distinguished from the clinically somewhat similar *tardive dyskinesia* which is usually a late (hence *tardive)* complication of long-term treatment with neuroleptics such as the phenothiazines or butyrophenones. It rarely responds to their withdrawal, is usually made worse by giving anticholinergics and may be resistant to any form of treatment.

Facial tics

Facial tics are benign spasms (habit spasms), often involving the eyelids and usually affecting children. Common tics are blinking, grimacing, shaking the head, clearing the throat, coughing or shrugging. Emotion or fatique intensify tics but the natural history is of spontaneous remission. If persistent, haloperidol may be helpful. Rarely, botulinum toxin is used to control hemifacial spasm.

Gilles de la Tourette syndrome

In this syndrome, tics are associated with compulsive swearing. Self-mutilation such as tongue biting may be associated and tongue thrusting is common. The condition is familial and usually appears before the age of 15.

The dopamine receptor blocker, haloperidol is usually effective and this suggests that there is overactivity in the basal ganglia.

Hemifacial spasm

Hemifacial spasm (clonic facial spasm) mainly affects adults, particularly the elderly. The spasm affects especially the angle of the mouth or the eyelid and worsens towards evening. Some cases herald a cerebellopontine angle lesion but many are idiopathic. Occasionally facial paralysis or trigeminal neuralgia follow hemifacial spasm.

Facial myokymia

Facial myokymia is a rare condition in which there are continuous fine, worm-like contractions of one or more of the facial muscles—especially the perioral or periorbital muscles. Facial myokymia starts suddenly, lasts for variable periods and is unaffected by voluntary movements. Facial myokymia is frequently associated with multiple sclerosis, brain stem or posterior cranial fossa tumours or other neurological disorders. Patients must therefore be referred for a neurological opinion. Facial myokymia must be distinguished from facial hemispasm, facial tics or blepharospasm, which involves several muscles synchronously, and from benign fasciculation and myokymia of the lower eyelid, which are quite innocuous.

Bulbar palsy

Bulbar palsy is the term given to weakness or paralysis of muscles supplied by the medulla, namely the tongue, pharynx, larynx, sternomastoid and upper trapezius (cranial nerves IX–XII inclusive). Poliomyelitis or diphtheria can cause acute bulbar palsy. Chronic causes are progressive bulbar palsy, tumours or aneurysms of the posterior cranial fossa or nasopharynx, or strokes.

Trigeminal motor neuropathy

Trigeminal motor neuropathy may occasionally be seen in isolation and is possibly related to a viral infection. More frequently it is associated with trigeminal sensory neuropathy or found in lesions affecting the motor division of the trigeminal nerve when there are usually other cranial nerve deficits. Weakness and sometimes wasting of the masseter and temporalis muscles may be found.

Other cranial neuropathies affecting the orofacial region

The hypoglossal nerve may be affected in its intra- or extracranial course. Intracranial lesions typically cause bulbar palsy (*see below*). Disease in the condylar canals, such as Paget's disease or bone tumours, and peripheral lesions, such as glomus jugulare, carotid body or other tumours, trauma or radiation damage, can cause an isolated deficit.

DIPLOPIA

Double vision (diplopia) is not uncommon after maxillofacial trauma but usually resolves spontaneously within a few days. Persistent diplopia after trauma can be caused by blow-out fractures of the floor of the orbit, entrapment of, or damage to the orbital muscles or damage to the suspensory ligament to the frontal process or the zygomatic bone. Later fibrous adhesions between the orbital periosteum and coverings of the eye may cause permanent limitation of movement as may injury to cranial nerves III, IV and VI (*Table 12.7*). Diplopia may also be an occasional transient complication of dental local anaesthetic injections, presumably because the anaesthetic tracks to the inferior orbital fissure, where it can block orbital nerves.

Table 12. 7. Diplopia

Structure involved	Site	Causes	Features that may be associated
Extraocular muscles	Orbit	Trauma Exophthalmos Myasthenia gravis	Middle-third facial fracture Thyrotoxicosis Myopathy elsewhere
Cranial nerves III, IV and VI	Orbit	Trauma Tumour Sarcoid	Middle-third facial fracture
	Superior orbital fissure	Trauma Tumour Sarcoid	Often several muscles paralysed Involvement of ophthalmic division of trigeminal Pupil often normal
	Cavernous sinus	Aneurysms Infection Fistula Trauma	Similar to superior orbital fissure syndrome
	Skull base	Aneurysms Tumours Meningitis Fractures	May be involvement of single nerves: may be pupil dilatation
Cranial nerve nuclei	Brain stem	Vascular lesions Tumours Multiple sclerosis	May be involvement of trigeminal or facial nerves or complicated neurological disorders

Paralytic strabismus is characterized by variable deviation of the ocular axes according to the position of gaze and is the usual type of strabismus that follows maxillofacial injuries.

The eye affected can be identified by noting in which direction of gaze diplopia is maximal and then, while the patient looks in that direction, covering each eye in turn. The outermost image disappears when the affected eye is covered. Occasionally drugs such as carbamazepine, cause diplopia.

PUPILLARY ABNORMALITIES

The pupils are normally equal in size and constrict on exposure to bright light and on accommodation for near objects. Light shone in one eye causes pupillary constriction in that eye (direct light reflex) and also in the unexposed eye (indirect or consensual reflex). Pupil size is determined by dilator fibres (the sympathetic supply from the superior cervical ganglion runs along the internal carotid artery and joins the ophthalmic division of the trigeminal nerve and the long ciliary nerves) and constrictor fibres (the parasympathetic supply runs with the oculomotor nerve). The sympathetic nerve supply is also partially responsible for contraction of the levator palpebrae superioris muscle (raising the upper eyelid).

Pupil constriction (miosis) can be caused by a lesion of the sympathetic supply, and dilatation (mydriasis) by a IIIrd nerve lesion. The most important cause of a dilating pupil is a rise in intracranial pressure when the pupil also becomes non-reactive owing to pressure on the oculomotor nerve. Other causes of unequal pupils are shown in *Table 12.8*: they include drugs, trauma (traumatic mydriasis, *Fig. 12.4*) and the following:

Table 12.8. Causes of pupillary abnormalities

	Pupils	Other signs	Significance
Argyll-Robertson pupils	Small, unequal React to accommodation but not light	—	Neurosyphilis Multiple sclerosis Diabetes mellitus
Horner's syndrome	Constricted	Ptosis Absence of facial sweating Enophthalmos sometimes	Trauma, bronchial carcinoma or other causes of damage to sympathetic fibres in neck
Adie's (Holmes-Adie) pupil	One pupil dilated and reacts very slowly to light or convergence	Ankle or knee jerks may be absent	Benign

Adie's (Holmes–Adie) pupil

Adie's pupil is usually a benign condition and typically affects females. One pupil is dilated and reacts only very slowly to light or convergence and there may be associated loss of knee or ankle jerks. Occasionally this condition, like the Argyll–Robertson pupil, is associated with advanced syphilis.

Argyll–Robertson pupil

This is characterized by small, irregular, unequal pupils which fail to dilate in response to light but still react, by dilating, to accommodation. An Argyll–Robertson pupil is characteristically caused by neurosyphilis, but may sometimes also be seen in other conditions affecting the Edinger–Westphal nucleus, such as diabetes mellitus, sarcoidosis, Wernicke's encephalopathy, midbrain tumours, trauma, Lyme disease, amyloidois or multiple sclerosis.

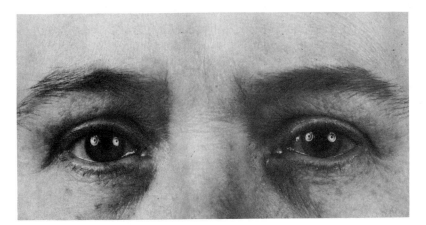

Fig. 12.4. Mydriasis: a unilateral fixed dilated pupil on the left, caused by trauma.

Horner's syndrome

Horner's syndrome comprises:

1. Miosis (constricted pupil), unreative to mydriatics.
2. Ptosis (drooping eyelid).
3. Loss of sweating of the face.
4. Enophthalmos (sometimes).

It is usually unilateral and caused by interruption of sympathetic nerve fibres peripherally, usually at the cervical sympathetic trunk, as a result, for example, of trauma to the neck, or bronchogenic or metastatic breast carcinoma infiltrating the superior cervical sympathetic ganglion.

NYSTAGMUS

A few irregular eye jerks are normal in some individuals when the eyes are deviated far to one side. However, involuntary rhythmic eye movements (nystagmus) may be a sign of disease.

Oscillating (pendular) nystagmus may result from ocular disease and is characterized by rapid oscillation of the eyes, increased on looking upwards. More common is rhythmic (jerk) nystagmus which is usually lateral, but can be vertical or rotary, and results from:

1. Drug intoxication (e.g. barbiturates).
2. Internal ear disease.
3. Cerebellar disease.
4. Brain stem disease.

EPILEPSY

Epilepsy is a disorder of brain function which causes episodic disturbances of consciousness and usually of motor or sensory function. It affects over 1 per cent of the general population but is more prevalent in the young and in the mentally or physically handicapped. Most cases of epilepsy have no identifiable cause (idiopathic epilepsy) but in a few patients it is secondary to local or generalized brain disease, drug addiction or metabolic disorders (symptomatic epilepsy) (*Table 12.9*).

Epilepsy has a variety of clinical patterns. The main types of epilepsy are major, minor or focal convulsions but there are many variants.

Tonic–Clonic (Grand Mal) Epilepsy

Tonic–clonic epilepsy usually begins in the pre-school child, or sometimes at about puberty. A typical seizure consists of a defined sequence beginning with a warning (aura) followed by loss of consciousness, tonic and the clonic convulsions and finally a variably prolonged recovery. This full sequence is, however, not always completed.

The aura may consist of a mood change, irritability, brief hallucination or headache. The attack then begins suddenly with total body tonic spasm and loss of consciousness. The sufferer falls to the ground and is in danger of injury. Initially the face becomes pale and the pupils dilate, the head and spine are thrown into extension (opisthotonous) and glottic and respiratory muscle spasm may cause an initial brief cry and cyanosis. There may also be incontinence and biting of the tongue or lips.

The tonic phase passes, after less than a minute, into the clonic phase. Then there are repetitive jerking movements of trunk, limbs, tongue and lips. Salivation is profuse with bruxism, sometimes tongue-biting and occasionally, vomiting. There may be autonomic phenomena such as tachycardia, hypervension and flushing. Clonus is followed by a state of flaccid semi-coma for a further 10 – 15 minutes.

Table 12.9. Causes of fits

1. *Idiopathic epilepsy*
2. *Symptomatic or secondary epilepsy*
   Febrile convulsions

Intracranial causes:	Space-occupying lesions
	Trauma
	Vascular defects
	Infections
	Cerebral palsy
	Rubella syndrome
	Phakomatoses (neurofibromatosis, epiloia)
	AIDS meningitis
Systemic causes:	Anoxia
	Hypoglycaemia
	Inborn errors of metabolism
	Drug withdrawal (anticonvulsants, barbiturates, alcohol, opioids, benzodiazepines)

Confusion and headaches are common afterwards and the patient may sleep for up to 12 hours before full recovery. The attack may occasionally be followed by a transient residual paralysis (Todd's palsy) or by automatic or aggressive behaviour.

Major convulsions can cause trauma, respiratory embarrassment or brain damage, or may pass into status epilepticus, but most seizures end without mishap.

A major fit is so dramatic an event that it sems to be of longer duration than it in fact is. If, however, it lasts more than 5 minutes (by the clock) or starts again after apparently ceasing, the patient must be regarded as being in *status epilepticus*.

Status epilepticus

In this dangerous form of epilepsy the tonic and clonic phases alternate repeatedly without consciousness being regained. Inhalation of vomit and saliva, or brain damage due to cerebral hypoxia, may result and cause a mortality of up to 20 per cent.

Syndromes associated with epilepsy

Epilepsy is usually an isolated problem in otherwise normal individuals but may be associated with other diseases. Five per cent of epileptics are mentally subnormal, while more than 50 per cent of patients with cerebral palsy and 50 per cent of phenylketonurics suffer from epilepsy.

Other Forms of Epilepsy

Petit mal (absence seizures) is the other common form of epilepsy and restricted to children. It consists of sudden but usually transient arrest of movement, attention and speech, often graphically described as absences, and may be precipitated by overbreathing. Absence seizures can be controlled with ethosuximide or sodium valproate (*Table 12.10*).

It is important not to mistake petit mal for uncooperative behaviour or for mental handicap in the affected child, and to appreciate that petit mal very occasionally precedes grand mal epilepsy.

Temporal lobe epilepsy (psychomotor epilepsy) is characterized by hallucinations, illusions of taste, smell, sight and hearing, disorientation, confusion and amnesia. Lip smacking and chewing movements may be seen. It is controlled by many of the anticonvulsants used in tonic–clonic epilepsy, particularly carbamazepine.

Ictal facial pain is an unusual manifestation of sensory epilepsy. It usually affects women of late middle age and consists of a throbbing diffuse pain which may

Table 12.10. Anticonvulsant drugs: uses and side-effects

Drug	Use	Systemic side-effects	Oral side-effects
Carbamazepine	TLE GM	Ataxia Drowsiness Leucopenia Lupoid syndrome	Dry mouth Erythema multiforme Dyskinesias
Valproate	GM PM	Drowsiness Bleeding diathesis	
Phenytoin	GM TLE PM	Cerebellar damage Hirsutes Nephrotic syndrome Hyperglycaemia	Gingival hyperplasia Dental anomalies Erythema multiforme Lupoid syndrome Cervical Lymphadenopathy
Ethosuximide	PM	Lupoid syndrome Renal damage Eosinophilia	
Primidone	GM TLE PM	Drowsiness Ataxia Oculomotor palsy	Megaloblastic anaemia
Phenobarbitone (virtually obsolete)	GM TLE PM	Lethargy Irritability Depression Rashes Ataxia	Erythema multiforme Bullae Fixed eruptions

GM, Grand mal; TLE, temporal lobe epilepsy; PM, petit mal.

be associated with facial or masticatory muscle twitches or generalized convulsions. It is usually controllable with phenytoin.

*Localized motor seizure*s (focal motor epilepsy) may take the form of clonic movements of a limb or group of muscles usually in the face, arm or leg. The clonus may spread (march) to adjacent muscles on the same side of the body (Jacksonian epilepsy).

General management of tonic–clonic epilepsy

Major epilepsy is frequently idiopathic but it is necessary, especially if fits begin in adult life, to exclude brain disease, such as a cerebral tumour (*Table 12.11*).

Most patients with major epilepsy are maintained on prophylactic anticonvulsants. Anticonvulsant medication is of such a long-term nature that side-effects are common. Carbamazepine usually is the first choice for the management of tonic—clonic epilepsy and, though capable of causing a variety of side-effects, these are fewer than those caused by phenytoin and uncommon in relation to the scale of use.

Alternatively, sodium valproate may be used, particularly when major fits are associated with absence seizures. Phenobarbitone is effective but undesirably sedating in adults and can cause behavioural disturbances in children.

Table 12.11. Causes of fits at different ages of onset

Age at onset	More common causes
Young child	Birth trauma, fevers, metabolic disease, congenital disease or idiopathic
Adolescent	Idiopathic or traumatic
Young adult	Traumatic, neoplastic, idiopathic, alcoholism or barbiturate abuse, AIDS
Middle age	Neoplastic, traumatic, cerebrovascular disease or drug abuse
Elderly	Cerebrovascular disease or neoplasm

Plasma anticonvulsant levels may sometimes need to be monitored, particularly with phenytoin where small changes in dosage can cause disproportionally great changes in plasma levels and toxic effects. Saliva may be used for this purpose.

Combined treatment may sometimes cause more toxic effects or interactions than a single drug in adequate doses. A second drug should only be given if a single agent in maximal dosage fails to control fits or causes undesirable toxic effects.

In pregnancy, drug treatment should follow the same principles as for non–pregnant patients but plasma levels need to be monitored as they may fall during the later stages. Antiepileptic drugs, particularly phenytoin are potentially teratogenic, but there is a greater risk to the fetus from uncontrolled epilepsy. Antiepileptic drugs, apart from barbiturates should also be continued during breast–feeding. Some interfere with the oral contraceptive.

Oro-dental complications of epilepsy or its treatment

I. Injuries caused by the fit:
    Laceration of tongue or buccal mucosa.
    Injuries to the face from falling (lacerations, haematomas, fractures of the facial skeleton).
    Fractures, devitalization, subluxation or loss of teeth (a chest radiograph may be required).
    Subluxation of the TMJ.
II. Complications of treatment (see also Table 12.10):
    Phenytoin—gingival fibrous hyperplasia (of interdental papillae particularly).
    Folate deficiency (rarely) megaloblastic anaemia and recurrent aphthae.
    Dental anomalies (small, late-erupting teeth).
    Cervical lymphadenopathy.
    Phenobarbitone—bullous erythema multiforme (exceptionally rarely).

Dental treatment

It is essential to appreciate that epileptics have good and bad phases and that various factors can precipitate seizures in susceptible patients (*Table 12.12*).

Table 12.12. Factors precipitating fits in susceptible subjects

1. Withdrawal of anticonvulsant medication
2. Epileptogenic drugs
       Methohexitone (and some other anaesthetics)
       Sympathomimetic amines
       Tricyclics
       Phenothiazines
       Alcohol
3. Fatigue
4. Infection
5. Stress
6. Starvation
7. Menstruation
8. Flickering lights (television; strobe lights)

Dental treatment should preferably be carried out in good phases when attacks are infrequent.

Large doses of lignocaine given intravenously for severe dysrhythmias may occasionally cause convulsions. An over-enthusiastic casualty officer may therefore blame a dental local anaesthetic for causing a fit. There is no evidence that this can happen, especially as intravenous lignocaine has also been advocated for the *control* of status epilepticus.

Those who have infrequent seizures, or who are dependent upon others (such as the mentally handicapped) may fail to take regular medication and thus be poorly controlled.

The main problems in the dental care of epileptic patients are:

1. Convulsions and their sequelae.
2. Drug reactions.
3. Psychiatric disorders.
4. Associated handicaps (Chapter 15).
5. Bleeding tendency caused by sodium valproate.

Convulsions and their sequelae. Trauma frequently results from a grand mal attack when the patient falls unconscious or from the muscle spasm. Such injuries include fractures of the vertebrae or limbs, dislocations, or periorbital subcutaneous haematomas in the absence of facial fractures.

When carrying out dental treatment in a known epileptic, a strong mouth prop should be kept in position and the oral cavity kept as free as possible of debris. As much apparatus as possible should be kept away from the area around the patient.

Drug reactions. Methohexitone, enflurane and ketamine are epileptogenic. Chlorpromazine, alcohol and tricyclic antidepressants may be epileptogenic and should be avoided.

Psychiatric problems in the epileptic. Psychomotor epilepsy in particular is associated with paranoid and schizophrenic features; antisocial and psychopathic behaviour may then make dental management difficult (Chapter 14).

Management of a fit in the dental surgery. Fits in the dental surgery are usually in known epileptics but it should be remembered that fits can also result from cerebral hypoxia when, for example, a normal patient faints but is not laid flat.

When a fit starts the patient should be constantly attended and should be laid on his side in the head injury position to maintain the airway. The face is rotated down to allow vomit to be expelled from the mouth and not inhaled. It is probably impractical to hold the traditional padded spatula between the teeth; the patient must, however, be placed away from equipment or furniture so that he cannot damage himself.

In an uncomplicated seizure no other treatment is necessary. If, however, the seizure persists or status epilepticus develops diazepam 10 mg or clonazepam 2 mg should be given slowly intravenously or intramuscularly and repeated if the episode is not terminated. Oxygen may also be needed.

FEBRILE CONVULSIONS

Febrile convulsions result from a rise in body temperature usually caused by infection. These convulsions usually affect children, about 3 per cent of whom go on in later life to develop epilepsy. Severe febrile convulsions can cause brain damage. Those under 18 months should be admitted to hospital since the fit may be due to meningitis.

Children who develop high fevers (above 38°C) should be put in a cool environment and bathed with tepid water and given paracetamol elixir.

SYNCOPE

Syncope is transient loss of consciousness caused by a sudden decrease in cerebral blood flow. The main causes include:

1. Vasovagal attack (fainting——*see below*).
2. Respiratory syncope (severe coughing).
3. Cardiac syncope (dysrhythmias, heart block, aortic stenosis).
4. Paralytic syncope. In the elderly, especially those taking drugs such as phenothiazines, levodopa, hypotensive agents, tricyclics or benzodiazepines.
5. Brain stem syncope. Migraine or vertebrobasilar disease, usually in the elderly.

Vasovagal Syncope (Fainting)

Vasovagal syncope is a reflex mediated by autonomic nerves in which there is splanchnic and skeletal muscle vasodilatation, bradycardia and loss of consciousness. Fainting can be precipitated by psychological factors such as pain, or fear at the sight of an injection needle or blood.

Fainting may also be caused by postural changes, anoxia or the carotid sinus syndrome. The latter is usually seen in elderly patients in whom mild pressure on the neck causes syncope with bradycardia or cardiac arrest— a vagal effect.

Management of syncope

Syncope is dangerous if the patient is not laid flat, since cerebral anoxia can result and the patient may then have a convulsion and suffer from hypoxic encephalopathy.

RAISED INTRACRANIAL PRESSURE

Raised intracranial pressure can be a complication of head injury and be fatal. As a result of the rigidity of the cranium any expansion of its contents causes a rise of intracranial pressure which, in turn, tends to impede the venous return from the brain and further to increase the pressure. Cerebral blood flow is thus reduced even though the increased CSF pressure causes a reflex rise in systemic blood pressure in an attempt to improve cerebral blood flow. Examples of causes of raised intracranial pressure include the following:

1. Intracranial haemorrhage (after head injury).
2. Space-occupying lesions (abscess or tumour).
3. Oedema of the brain (often a consequence of trauma, malignant hypertension, vascular lesions or tumours of the brain).
4. Obstruction to the flow of CSF (blockage of the aqueduct of Sylvius or subarachnoid adhesions due to meningitis).

Intracranial haematomas are a major cause of mortality following head injuries and it is therefore essential to recognize signs of raised intracranial pressure and cerebral compression which include:

1. Papilloedema (bulging of the optic disc with engorgement of its vessels seen by ophthalmoscopy).
2. Headache (in the conscious patient).
3. Restlessness (in the unconscious patient).
4. Vomiting.
5. Decreasing consciousness.
6. Rising blood pressure and slowing of the pulse.
7. Dilatation of the pupil on the side of the lesion and reduced reaction to light.

Lumbar puncture is contraindicated if intracranial pressure is raised as it can precipitate brain herniation and death by coning of the brain stem and medullary compression.

HERNIATION OF THE BRAIN

Herniation is the displacement of part of the brain from one dural compartment to another and is a serious consequence of raised intracranial pressure. The effects depend on the direction of displacement.

The possibility of herniation is suggested by signs of raised intracranial pressure, particularly pupil dilatation and reduced reactivity to light caused by stretching of the oculomotor nerves.

HYPOXIC ENCEPHALOPATHY

Acute cerebral hypoxia is particularly important in dental practice as it can readily follow head injuries or impaired oxygenation during general anaesthesia, particularly with intravenous barbiturates. There is often then a combination of contributory factors. The anaesthetic agent can depress respiration but there may also be partial, often unnoticed, respiratory obstruction. The patient may also have cerebrovascular disease which impairs the cerebral circulation and if there is anaemia the situation is even worse. As a consequence, some patients can die and others can suffer severe brain damage. Cerebral hypoxia can remain unrecognized because the patient is already unconscious from the anaesthetic. The main causes of cerebral hypoxia include:

1. Hypoxia— airways obstruction, respiratory failure or anaesthetic accidents.
2. Severe hypotension— cardiac arrest, shock syndrome, severe bradycardia.

Cerebral hypoxia causes loss of consciousness in less than a minute but, if the circulation and oxygenation of the blood are restored within about 3 minutes, recovery should be complete.

More prolonged hypoxia causes coma with dilated pupils unresponsive to light, inert or rigid limbs, unresponsiveness to all stimuli, abolition of brain stem reflexes and no electrical activity on electroencephalography (brain death).

The most vigilant supervision of all patients with head injuries or undergoing general anaesthesia is, therefore, essential. Special care must be taken to ensure that the patient is respiring fully and effectively, that oxygen supplies are adequate and maintained and that no signs of hypoxia, however slight, develop (Chapter 13).

CONGENITAL NEUROLOGICAL DISORDERS

Syringomyelia

Syringomyelia is of unknown aetiology and characterized by cavitation of the central part of the spinal cord, causing disruption of pain and temperature neurones of the anterior commissure of the cord. This leads to loss of pain and temperature sense, but preservation of the sense of touch.

Symptoms begin in adolescence or adult life and progress erratically. There is segmental loss of pain and temperature sense leading to painless ulcers, injuries or burns, and deranged (Charcot's) joints. Touch sensation is retained. Damage to the sympathetic neurones in the intermediolateral column of the spinal cord can cause Horner's syndrome and, late in the disease, the pyramidal tracts may be involved with signs of spasticity in the legs. Kyphoscoliosis develops at an early stage.

If the condition affects the brain stem it is known as *syringobulbia* and may cause facial or oral sensory changes or paralyses.

Syringobulbia can cause facial sensory loss with unilateral palatal and vocal cord palsies, nystagmus, weakness and atrophy of the tongue, dysphagia and dysarthria.

Damage to the medulla in syringobulbia does not usually, however, significantly affect the respiratory or cardiovascular centres.

There is no effective treatment.

Huntington's Chorea

Huntington's chorea is an autosomal dominant condition characterized by dementia and involuntary movements.

Clinically, Huntington's chorea is characterized by the appearance in early to middle age of irregular involuntary movements causing gross disturbances of speech and gait, usually associated with progressive dementia. Progress of the disease is slow, but life is often ended by intercurrent infection, or sometimes suicide, since patients are often aware of the family history and prognosis.

Other causes of tremor in addition to Huntington's chorea, Parkinson's disease and cerebellar disease, are shown in *Table 12.13.*

Table 12.13. Causes of involuntary movements

Disease	Features
Cerebellar disease	Ataxia and nystagmus
Parkinsonism	Rigidity and akinesia
Athetoid cerebral palsy	Writhing movements and deafness
Huntington's chorea	Chorea and dementia
Sydenham's chorea	Complication of rheumatic fever
Wilson's disease	Copper overload and cirrhosis
Tardive dyskinesia	Facial grimacing and jaw clenching
Essential tremor	Worse with anxiety; better with alcohol, benzodiazepines or beta-blockers
Alcoholism	Delirium tremens

Friedreich's Ataxia

Friedreich's ataxia, usually an autosomal recessive trait, is characterized by degeneration of many tracts of the spinal cord extending up to the brain stem, causing severe ataxia, loss of reflexes and secondary deformities. Degenerative heart disease with dysrhythmias may be associated. Treatment is symptomatic only.

INFECTIONS OF THE NERVOUS SYSTEM

Suppurative Meningitis

The chief causes are *Haemophilus influenzae, Neisseria meningitidis* (meningo-coccus), *N. gonorrhoeae, Streptococcus pneumoniae* (pneumococcus) and less frequently *Listeria monocytogenes*. The causative organisms differ in different age groups.

In adult life, the pneumococcus becomes increasingly important, particularly in those with impaired resistance as a result of such causes as alcoholism or sickle cell disease.

The meningococcus is carried in the nasopharynx and sometimes causes epidemics. Recent outbreaks in Britain have been of group B and C meningo-cocci. Group B, type 15 meningococcus in particular causes a severe form of the disease. Spread of the bacteria to the meninges is by the bloodstream or occasionally as a result of a maxillofacial fracture involving the cribriform plate of the ethmoid (Chapter 13).

The onset of meningitis is marked by severe headache, nausea or vomiting, drowsiness, stupor or coma and occasionally, convulsions. An important clini-cal sign is pain and stiffness of the neck.

A purpuric rash is characteristic of meningococcal septicaema which can go on to adrenocortical failure as a result of bleeding into the adrenal cortex, with vasomotor collapse, shock and death (Waterhouse–Friderichsen syndrome).

Diagnosis is confirmed with a Gram-stained smear and culturing the organ-ism from a lumbar puncture specimen of CSF. However, antibiotic treatment should started before the results are available. If treatment is prompt, the overall mortality is low, but about 20 per cent of patients have permanent neurological damage such as cranial nerve injuries (blindness, deafness or palsies), epilepsy, or mental retardation.

Patients with maxillofacial injuries involving the middle third of the face should be given prophylactic antimicrobials because of the danger of meningi-tis (Chapter 13).

There have been rare cases of meningitis caused by viridans streptococci which may have originated from the mouth.

Brain Abscess

Brain abscesses are usually secondary to chronic middle ear, sinus or pulmonary infections. Patients with congenital heart disease, particularly those with right-to-left shunts, are also at risk. Cerebral abscess can also be a complication of infective endocarditis.

Bacteria from periodontal pockets, particularly anaerobes, are a recognized but rare cause of cerebral abscess directly or as a complication of a lung abscess. Inhalation of a tooth fragment or materials used in dentistry can cause a lung abscess which can metastasize to the brain with serious consequences.

An established cerebral abscess characteristically causes signs and symptoms similar to other space-occupying lesions of the brain. Immediately after the diagnosis has been confirmed, treatment is by high doses of antibiotics followed, where necessary, by aspiration or drainage. The mortality is still between 30 and 40 per cent.

Viral Meningitis

Meningitis can be caused by several different viruses, particularly Coxsackie viruses and echoviruses. In viral meningitis there is little involvement of brain tissue and the infections are generally mild and self-limiting. No specific treatment is available.

Herpetic Encephalitis

Herpes simplex infection of the mouth or genitals is common but herpetic encephalitis is rare, though still the most frequent cause of encephalitis in temperate climates. Evidence as to whether it is a primary or reactivation infection is conflicting.

The clinical effects are highly variable. Early symptoms such as disorientation, personality changes, hallucinations and ataxia can be mistaken for drunkenness or psychosis. Other effects include stupor, fits, paralyses and sensory loss. Coma is often pre-terminal.

The disease. has often been fatal, particularly because confirmation of the diagnosis by brain biopsy is slow. However, the prognosis has improved greatly as a result of treatment with acyclovir, which is frequently given now, on suspicion. The incidence of neurological damage among survivors has also been reduced.

Neurosyphilis

Syphilis can affect the nervous system in the tertiary stage but is exceedingly rare, as a result of early treatment (Chapter 17). Neurosyphilis can take any of the following forms:

Meningovascular neurosyphilis has highly variable early symptoms but late effects may be hydrocephalus or lesions of the IInd, IIIrd and VIIIth cranial nerves. Pupils are also unequal and unresponsive to light (Argyll–Robertson pupils).

Paretic neurosyphilis begins insidiously with subtle mental disturbance going on to severe personality changes, complete dementia and widespread paralyses (general paresis of the insane, GPI).

Tabes dorsalis (*locomotor ataxia*) is mainly characterized by atrophy of the lumbar posterior nerve roots and sometimes of the optic nerves. Clinically, tabes dorsalis is characterized by sudden attacks of lightning-like pain and paraesthesiae of the leg or trunk. There is also loss of normal pain sensation and of deep proprioceptive reflexes. These cause the peculiar tabetic gait in which the feet are slapped on to the ground as a result of loss of sense of their position. These neuropathic joints then become disorganized (Charcot's joints).

Syphilis is frequently associated with HIV infection and then takes an atypical, accelerated course. Progress to the tertiary stage may be rapid and gummata may develop while the secondary stage is still active. Relapse is common despite treatment or the response to penicillin may be poor. The antibody response is also atypical and unpredictable

Dental aspects

Neurosyphilis is a rare cause of atypical trigeminal neuralgia but is now of little dental significance. Its presence should, however, be suspected in a patient with a gumma or syphilitic leucoplakia, which typically involves the dorsum of the tongue.

AIDS-ASSOCIATED NEUROLOGICAL DISEASE

Intracranial infections of many kinds and also brain tumours, particularly lymphomas, are common complications of AIDS. In addition, the virus itself can attack the brain to cause a wide variety of neurological symptoms culminating in dementia and death. These effects are not necessarily associated with the typical picture of immunodeficiency.

Neurological manifestations of AIDS can be acute, subacute or chronic. Acute disease can include such features as fever, malaise, mood changes resembling depression, fits, facial palsy and neuropathy of the extremities. Recovery usually, however, follows after several months.

Subacute encephalopathy affects about 30 per cent of AIDS patients. Typical features are gradual development of a confusional state associated with fever and symptoms that mimic depression. The patient may eventually become bedridden and incontinent.

Myelopathy or neuropathy associated with AIDS can cause weakness of the legs, sometimes paraesthesiae and in severe cases ataxia and incontinence. Alternatively, a form of meningitis may precede more typical features of AIDS and be characterized by headache, fever, meningeal signs and cranial nerve palsies most commonly affecting V, VII and VIII.

In brief, therefore, the neurological effects of HIV infection are so varied that it should be suspected in any high risk patient who develops unexpected behavioural or mood changes and neurological signs such as cranial nerve palsies.

MULTIPLE SCLEROSIS

Multiple (disseminated) sclerosis (MS) is the most common neurological disease affecting young adults, and is characterized by symptoms disseminated in both site and time. There is a high prevalence of multiple sclerosis particularly in Northern Europe and Northern America.

The aetiology is unknown but may perhaps be viral, possibly with immuno-logically mediated damage resulting in demyelination.

Typical clinical features are as follows:

1. The onset is characteristically highly capricious: transient visual disturbance or blindness (optic neuritis), or weakness or paralysis of a limb with complete though temporary recovery, are common features.

2. Later nystagmus, ataxia, jerky (scanning) speech, tremors and loss of muscular coordination develop as a result of cerebellar involvement.

3. Ultimately, widespread paralysis and often loss of sphincter control and urinary incontinence, can develop.

4. Depression can be a feature but, perhaps fortunately, euphoria also.

General management

There is no specific laboratory diagnostic aid nor specific treatment. Courses of ACTH or corticosteroids may be used during acute episodes, while diazepam or other relaxants may be needed to control muscle spasm.

Dental aspects

There are no specific oral manifestations but this diagnosis should always be considered in a young patient presenting with trigeminal neuralgia, particularly if there have been other neurological disturbances. Abnormal perioral sensa-tion, such as extreme hypersensitivity or facial anaesthesia, may develop especially in advanced MS, as may tremor. In addition to abnormalities of speech, cerebellar involvement may cause tremor and spasm of the muscles of the head and neck. Atropinics used in the treatment of bladder dysfunction may cause dry mouth.

Dental preventive care and treatment is important since oral hygiene may be poor, as in other handicapping conditions (Chapter 15). Limited mobility and psychological disorders may interfere with routine dental treatment. Some patients are on corticosteroids, with their attendant complications.

Guillain–Barré Syndrome (Infective or Idiopathic Polyneuritis)

The Guillain–Barré syndrome appears to be an immunologically mediated disorder resulting from various infections, especially viral, or vaccination.

Any age group can be affected and the clinical features are highly variable. Symptoms range from bilateral facial palsy with minor motor and sensory loss in the limbs, to fulminating disease with raised intracranial pressure, quadriple-gia and respiratory paralysis. Sudden respiratory paralysis develops in 10–20 per cent of cases and is lethal unless immediate mechanical ventilation can be given, sometimes with plasmapheresis. The disease usually reaches a peak within about a week, then gradually subsides after about 3 weeks. The majority recover slowly—but between 10 and 30 per cent have severe residual disabilities after a year.

MERCURY INTOXICATION

Mercury is neurotoxic in its metallic form and as salts, particularly methyl mercury. Mercury salts are also nephrotoxic and renal damage can be caused by the diuretic, mersalyl, which as a consequence is virtually obsolete. Metal mercury can be absorbed by inhalation of its vapour or through the skin and mucous membranes. Mercury salts are absorbed after ingestion.

Environmental poisoning from methyl mercury was widespread in Minimata Bay and Nigata, Japan, between 1953 and 1960, as a result of eating fish contaminated by mercury from industrial discharge. Many persons suffered neurological damage, some died, and later there was a high incidence of cerebral palsy in newborn children. It is now a problem in Brazil.

Acute poisoning by massive inhalation of mercury vapour is very rare but can cause potentially fatal pneumonitis and neurological symptoms, particularly tremor and excitability.

Chronic poisoning by inhalation of mercury vapour primarily affects the CNS. It is highly lipid-soluble rapidly penetrates the blood-brain barrier and infiltrates neurons. However, initial symptoms include not merely lassitude, but gastrointestinal disturbances, anorexia and weight loss. More prolonged exposure can cause tremor, memory loss, timidity and excitability (*erethism*). This syndrome was well recognized, particularly in the previous century, among workers with mercury such as thermometer makers and felt hat makers—hence, 'mad as a hatter'.

Other effects of chronic mercury poisoning include hypersalivation, accelerated periodontitis and a characteristic black gingival line due to deposition of sulphides of mercury along the line of the gingival crevice. Rarely, necrosis of the jaw could follow, but such manifestations are now only of historical interest.

Dental Aspects

There are three main considerations, namely:

1. Occupational exposure of dental staff to mercury
2. Alleged mercury–related neurological symptoms ('mercury allergy') in patients.
3. Local effects of mercury–containing amalgam fillings.

Mercury as an occupational hazard. The metal is highly volatile and readily absorbed through the respiratory tract and skin. In addition some mercury can be absorbed from foods, particularly fish and it is also an environmental pollutant.

Dentists are far more heavily exposed to mercury than the general population. On average up to 1.5 kg of mercury are used by a dental practitioner annually and, when little attention was paid to mercury hygiene, mercury vapour in the surgery atmosphere and its levels in the blood, hair, nails and urine in dentists were frequently above controls. Up to 45 per cent of dental personnel had higher levels of mercury in hair than controls and the median blood mercury concentration in a study of 130 Danish dentists was significantly raised. However, none of the latter blood levels of mercury were over the recognized 'safe' limit of 35 µg/l. Levels were highest in fish eaters, indicating that at least part of the mercury burden was from non-dental sources and as with the rest of the population some would have come from the environment.

Recent studies of dentists and dental surgery assistants have not shown excessively high urinary mercury levels where good mercury hygiene was practised and urinary mercury levels appear to be lower in dentists in 1986 than in 1983.

The greatest hazard is from inhalation of mercury vapour as a result of spillage, particularly when in proximity to an autoclave or other source of heat. Droplets of mercury can also accumulate in significant amounts in surgery carpeting or crevices in the floor. Mercury is also absorbed during hand trituration of amalgam or other skin contact. Removal of old amalgams from teeth with an air-rotor produces traces of mercury vapour but not if adequate water-cooling and aspiration are used.

In the past, after decades of practice, a few dentists and surgery assistants have suffered from chronic mercury toxicity with tremor, incoordination, polyneuropathies, and accelerated senility. Rarely, deaths have been reported after prolonged heavy exposure. Autopsy studies have shown mercury deposits particularly in the pituitary glands and occipital lobes in dentists. In another study, of female dentists and dental surgery assistants, a history of reproductive failures, menstrual disorders and spina bifida in their children appeared to be related to mercury levels in hair, but this has not been widely confirmed and other larger studies have no such correlation. Indeed the perinatal death and birth defects rate for infants born of dentists is lower than normal.

Objective investigation of neurological and psychological function, in 1982, showed evidence of a polyneuropathy in dentists with high tissue mercury levels. However, neurological defects were not evident clinically and it seems unlikely that these findings would apply now to dentists who apply high standards of mercury hygiene.

Mercury and its salts are also potential sensitizing agents and exposure to them can occasionally lead to contact dermatitis. As a consequence the frequency of positive patch tests increases as dental students progress through their course. Nevertheless, contact dermatitis to mercury surprisingly rarely restricts dental practice.

In summary therefore, mercury presents an occupational threat to the health of dentists and dental assistants, but provided that reasonable care is taken in its use, does not appear to represent a significant hazard. Indeed, dentists, despite exposure to mercury, have one of the lowest mortality rates of any profession.

'*Mercury allergy*'. A few patients have genuine contact sensitivity to mercury. Nevertheless they can tolerate the insertion of amalgams, provided that none is spilt onto the skin.

Another group of patients have symptoms such as headache, lassitude, a general feeling of ill–health which they ascribe to mercury toxicity or allergy. Unfortunately this belief has been encouraged by unscrupulous practitioners who carry out expensive but spurious tests to detect alleged effects of dental amalgams. However, there is no evidence that sufficient mercury is absorbed from amalgams to cause neurological damage.

It has also been shown that patients who complain of amalgam–related symptoms also suffer more frequently from other, unrelated complaints, such as chronic craniofacial pain, than controls. It was noteworthy in that in this same study, out of 20 patients who complained of amalgam-related symptoms and were offered blood tests for mercury concentrations, only 5 were willing to be tested.

Because of this concern about possible mercury toxicity from dental amalgams, the American Dental Association has carried out extensive investigation of the data available and in 1989, their Council on Dental Therapeutics concluded that 'there is insufficient evidence to justify claims that mercury from dental amalgams has an adverse effect on the health of patients'. In view of the claims that could result from litigation if this information was shown to be incorrect and in view of the strong financial stimulus to use more expensive materials, such a statement was certainly not lightly made.

Local effects of mercury–containing restorations. See Chapter 17.

MOTOR NEURONE DISEASE

Motor neurone disease (MND) comprises a group of uncommon diseases affecting motor neurones (especially anterior horn cells) at various levels in the nervous system. MND mainly affects males, especially in old age. The aetiology is unclear but may be viral. There are three subtypes:

1. Progressive muscular atrophy— lesions limited to the anterior horn below the foramen magnum.
2. Progressive bulbar palsy— anterior horn affections of the brain stem.
3. Amyotrophic (primary) lateral sclerosis— lesions of the anterior horn and pyramidal tract.

Progressive muscular atrophy is characterized by wasting and weakness which starts in the small muscles of the hands and spreads proximally.

Progressive bulbar palsy is characterized by wasting, weakness and fasciculation of the muscles of the pharynx, tongue, palate, sternomastoid and trapezius which result from involvement of cranial nerve motor neurones arising in the medulla (IX–XII inclusive).

Amyotrophic lateral sclerosis involves upper and lower motor neurones with wasting and weakness of the hands and spasticity of the legs. Involvement of the brain stem leads to *pseudobulbar palsy* with bulbar paralysis and emotional lability.

Dental aspects of motor neurone disease

Motor neurone disease is only important in dentistry in so far as oral hygiene may be impaired as in other handicapping conditions, and weakness or paralysis of the neck and head and oral musculature can lead to dysphagia. Protection of the airway may also be impaired but patients with this degree of disability, however, are likely to be hospitalized.

CEREBROVASCULAR ACCIDENTS (STROKES)

Strokes are a common cause of disability and death, especially in the elderly. Strokes result from acute destruction of part of the brain caused by cerebral haemorrhage or ischaemia. The main types of stroke are:

1. Subarachnoid haemorrhage.
2. Cerebral haemorrhage thrombosis and embolism.

Subarachnoid Haemorrhage

Rupture of a congenital berry aneurysm of the circle of Willis accounts for about 10 per cent of strokes. Hypertension, atherosclerosis and acute physical or emotional stress are contributory.

Blood from the ruptured aneurysm spreads into the subarachnoid space but can burst through the brain into a cerebral ventricle causing death within a few minutes.

Clinically, subarachnoid haemorrhage can affect any age group from the twenties onwards, and is characterized by the sudden onset of excruciatingly severe headache, quickly followed by coma. In some cases slow leakage from the aneurysm causes headache or minor neurological dysfunction before the acute attack.

Unlike other types of stroke, localizing signs, such as hemiplegia, are typically absent. The prognosis is poor and about 30 per cent of patients die from the initial haemorrhage. Neurosurgery can be curative, but many of the survivors have a fatal recurrence within 6–12 months.

Cerebral Haemorrhage, Thrombosis and Embolism

Cerebral haemorrhage is the most lethal type of stroke and mainly affects those past middle age. Predisposing factors are hypertension and atherosclerosis and, in general, the higher the blood pressure the greater the risk of cerebral haemorrhage. Bleeding into the brain destroys and tears apart the tissue, forming an expanding lesion, distorting the brain and causing gross cerebral oedema.

Cerebral thrombosis is the most common cause of stroke. Atherosclerosis is the main contributory factor to thrombosis, which then cuts off the blood supply to part of the brain.

Cerebral emboli originate from such sources as a fibrillating atrium or intracardiac thrombosis secondary to a myocardial infarct, and are relatively uncommon.

These different types of stroke may not be distinguishable clinically. Embolism, however, is typically of dramatic suddenness and may affect a younger person, in whom a source of the embolus should be identifiable. Thrombosis tends to be the least rapid in its development but, like haemorrhage, is most frequently associated with hypertension and atherosclerosis in the middle-aged and elderly (*Table 12.14*).

Table 12.14. Clinical features of strokes

	Haemorrhage	*Thrombosis*	*Embolism*
Prodromal signs	—	Transient ischaemic attacks	—
Onset	Acute	Gradual	Sudden
First symptom	Headache (50%)	Ill-defined	Headache
Progression	Hemiplegia and aphasia	Gradual and intermittent	Immediate
Underlying disease	Hypertension Atherosclerosis	Hypertension Atherosclerosis	Atrial fibrillation
Prognosis	75% die in a month	Range from minimal dysfunction to death in a week	Recurrence in 80%

Typical features of a stroke are as follows:

1. Sudden loss of consciousness, often going on to coma or death.

2. Hemiplegia (loss of voluntary movement of the opposite side of the body to the lesion).

3. Loss of speech (aphasia) is usually the result of a lesion on the left side of the brain, so that most patients are also deprived of the ability to write.

General management of a cerebrovascular accident

The airway must be protected during the acute attack and the usual precautions must be taken later in the care of the comatose patient. These include prevention of pressure sores and care of bladder and bowel. Anticoagulation may be used only if it has been established with certainty that the stroke is thrombotic or embolic.

Dental aspects

Patients after a stroke may have unilateral (upper motor neurone) facial palsy. This differs from Bell's palsy in that the lower face is mainly affected and emotional facial responses may be retained. Oral hygiene tends to deteriorate on the paralysed side and impaired manual dexterity may interfere with toothbrushing. An electric toothbrush may therefore help. Communication is often difficult as a result of aphasia.

Subarachnoid or cerebral haemorrhage can be precipitated by acute hypertension and fatal subarachnoid haemorrhage has resulted from the use of noradrenaline in local anaesthetic solutions. Cerebral haemorrhage can also result from hypertension caused by interactions of monoamine oxidase inhibitors with other drugs, particularly pethidine. On the other hand, opiates and barbiturates are best avoided in strokes as they may cause severe hypotension.

Strokes are also a possible cause of sudden loss of consciousness in the dental surgery and should be recognizable by the features already described, especially the sudden loss of consciousness and, usually, signs of one-sided paralysis. Protection of the airway and a call for an ambulance are the only useful measures.

Difficulties in dental management may include:
1. Communication difficulties.
2. Impaired mobility.
3. Hypertension.
4. Cardiovascular disease.
5. Diabetes mellitus.
6. Anticoagulation.
7. Old age.

PARKINSON'S DISEASE

Idiopathic Parkinson's disease (paralysis agitans) is a common disorder, due to degeneration of the pigmented cells of the substantia nigra, leading to deficiency of the neurotransmitter, dopamine. Its prevalence increases with age and there is no sex predilection.

Parkinsonism may also be caused by cerebrovascular disease, head injury, encephalitis lethargica, some toxins (such as heavy metals or carbon monoxide) or drugs, particularly the phenothiazine and butyrophenone neuroleptics, which are dopamine receptor blockers. Severe Parkinsonism has followed the use of an illicitly manufactured opioid (MPTP); this has led to better understanding of the pathogenesis and the suggestion that many cases of apparently idiopathic disease are due to unidentified environmental toxins.

The main features of Parkinson's disease are:

1. Tremor—mainly affecting the hands (pill rolling) and arms, and worst at rest.
2. Rigidity—the arms are flexed and held stiffly at the sides. Limb movement has a so-called cog-wheel rigidity.
3. Abnormal posture—the neck and shoulders are rigid, causing a stooping posture.
4. Bradykinesia—slowness in the initiation and execution of movements and poverty of spontaneous movements. Speech and swallowing may be affected. The patient may be slow at starting to walk but then runs forwards (festinant gait) or shuffles with slow short steps. Bradykinesia may progress to akinesia and total rigidity.
5. Akathisia—restlessness.

Complications include subtle psychiatric disorders, deformities of the hands and feet, ocular abnormalities and urinary and gastrointestinal disturbances. Autonomic dysfunction may cause mild postural hypotension, disordered respiratory control and hypersalivation which with the movement defect, may result in drooling. The face in Parkinsonism is often expressionless and there is a loss of the blink reflex as a response gentle tapping of the bridge of the nose. Oculogyric crises may be seen in drug-induced or post–encephalitic disease.

General management

If the diagnosis can be made sufficiently early, the monoamine oxidase B inhibitor, selegiline, by decreasing the breakdown of dopamine in the basal ganglia, may delay progress of the disease slightly. Antimuscarinic drugs such as orphenadrine or benzhexol give some help to nearly 60 per cent of patients with mild symptoms, particularly tremor. For disabling idiopathic Parkinson's disease, levodopa is the most effective drug but has many toxic effects. It is usually given in combination with an inhibitor of the degradative enzyme, dopa decarboxylase such as carbidopa (co–beneldopa; Sinemet) or benserazide (co–careldopa; Madopar), to increase the concentration of dopamine centrally. In such combinations, levodopa is effective at lower doses and side-effects (such as nausea, vomiting and cardiovascular disorders) are lessened. Bromocriptine (Parlodel) is a direct dopamine agonist and is useful particularly when levodopa cannot be tolerated.

Antimuscarinics (or selegiline) may be given with levodopa in severe cases. Antimuscarinics are also given for post-encephalitic and drug-associated Parkinsonism which may be made worse by levodopa.

A major disadvantage of levodopa is that its major benefits persist for only a few years and then the duration of control from each dose diminishes. Many combinations of drugs have been used in the attempt to overcome this problem but as yet there is no practical alternative to giving levodopa to maintain mobility but at the cost of increasing dyskinesias. Experimentally, brain grafts of fetal adrenal or nigral tissue have been given. The latter has been more succesful but the value of this procedure is as yet unclear.

Dental aspects

The main problems are tremor and drooling. It is also essential, in patients with Parkinson's disease, not to let the blankness of expression and apparent unresponsiveness be mistaken for stupidity. Sympathetic handling is therefore particularly important, as anxiety increases tremor.

Drooling of saliva may be troublesome, though treatment with antimuscarinic drugs reduces both the tremor and salivation to some degree.

Orofacial involuntary movements (dyskinesia) such as `flycatcher tongue'and lip pursing are side-effects of levodopa and bromocriptine (*see* Appendix to Chapter 19).

The monamine oxidase inhibitor, selegeline, differs from the antidepressives of this group in that it should not cause acute hypertensive episodes. However, a serious interaction with pethidine has been reported. Pethidine should therefore be avoided in patients receiving selegeline or other MAOIs.

The neuroleptic malignant syndrome

This is a rare complication of treatment particularly with neuroleptics such as chlorpromazine, haloperidol or flupenthixol, or abrupt withdrawal of levodopa. The syndrome is characterized by hyperthermia, muscular rigidity, fluctuating consciousness and autonomic dysfunction. The last causes pallor, sweating, tachycardia, labile blood pressure and incontinence. Symptoms may persist for several days or death can result from renal failure.

To avoid this hazard, phenothiazines should be avoided for patients who have stopped their levodopa before a general anaesthetic. Levodopa can be given before a general anaesthetic apart from the fact that it may cause vomiting.

TUMOURS OF THE CENTRAL NERVOUS SYSTEM

Brain tumours account for approximately 2 per cent of all cancer deaths but are second only to leukaemia as a cause of death in children.

A possible relationship between brain tumours and dental radiography has been reported but not as yet confirmed.

Cerebral tumours are usually metastatic: most primary cerebral tumours are malignant but even histologically benign tumours have a poor prognosis because they are often not amenable to surgery. Intracranial lymphomas are a well recognized feature of HIV disease and are increasing in prevalence.

Typical features of cerebral tumours are:

1. Localizing signs dependent on the site: examples are convulsions or paralysis.
2. Signs of raised intracranial pressure: these include headache, vomiting, papilloedema, disturbance of consciousness, a rising blood pressure and slowing of the pulse.

Epileptiform fits developing for the first time in an adult are strongly suggestive of a cerebral tumour.

Metastatic Tumours

Metastatic tumours are second only to cerebrovascular lesions as a cause of neurological disease. The main sources are carcinomas of the lung, breast, gastrointestinal tract and kidney, of which a cerebral tumour is sometimes the first indication.

Acoustic Neuroma (Neurofibroma)

This is a benign tumour arising from the neural axonal or neural sheath in the cerebellopontine angle, at the root of the vestibular part of the VIIIth cranial nerve, where it leaves the brain stem. Bilateral acoustic neuromas are the characteristic feature of neurofibromatosis type II.

Clinically, an acoustic neuroma produces a highly characteristic picture as the trigeminal, facial, glossopharyngeal and vagus nerves become stretched over the growth. Typical early results are tinnitus (ringing in the ears), deafness and rotational vertigo (a sensation of spinning). Further growth of the tumour causes postauricular pain, disturbance of balance, facial twitching or weakness and paraesthesia, together with difficulty in speaking and swallowing.

The growth can be completely removed, though with difficulty, in about 60 per cent of cases.

Pituitary Tumours

Adenomas are the most common pituitary tumours but their endocrine effects dominate the clinical picture and they are discussed in Chapter 10. Non-functional pituitary tumours compress the gland and can cause hypopituitarism, but can also produce signs common to other cerebral tumours. The most important non-functional tumours are adenomas and the craniopharyngioma. The latter arises from Rathke's pouch, an upgrowth from the primitive stomatodeum, and may resemble an ameloblastoma microscopically.

Dental aspects

Cerebral tumours rarely have important dental implications, but an acoustic neuroma and occasionally other tumours can cause impaired sensation or motor function in the trigeminal or facial nerves, as discussed earlier, and pituitary adenomas may cause acromegaly, Cushing's disease or Nelson's syndrome (Chapter 10).

MYASTHENIA GRAVIS

Myasthenia gravis is a rare cause of muscle weakness. In this disease, the response of the muscle to the neurotransmitter acetylcholine (ACh) is weak and circulating autoantibodies to ACh receptor proteins can be detected in at least 85 per cent of patients. These autoantibodies are associated in 75 per cent of cases with thymic hyperplasia and, in the remainder, a thymoma. Removal of the thymus typically cures the disorder. Occasional cases are associated with carcinoma elsewhere (Eaton–Lambert syndrome) or other diseases.

Thymic disease can also depress immunological responses and there is an uncommon syndrome of thymoma, myasthenia gravis, depressed cell mediated immunity, chronic mucocutaneous candidosis and haematological disease (Good's syndrome, Chapter 16).

Women between 20 and 30 are usually affected and the main feature is rapid and severe fatigue of muscles, particularly of those in most active use. The extraocular muscles and the muscles of face, tongue, neck and extremities are therefore severely affected. Weakness of the masticatory muscles causing the mouth to hang open (hanging or lantern jaw sign) is a characteristic feature and patients typically tend to support the jaw with their hand. Ptosis, diplopia, squinting and difficulties in speech and swallowing may also develop. Disability is worsened by fatigue of the muscles particularly towards the end of the day. A potentially lethal complication is involvement of the respiratory muscles, particularly in the elderly. Respiratory insufficiency may result either from the disease itself (myasthenic crisis), or treatment (cholinergic crisis).

General management

The disease very occasionally remits spontaneously but in those with thymomas the prognosis is poor. An anticholinesterase such as pyridostigmine, given orally, restores muscle strength in the majority of patients, but is not curative. Atropine is often also required to counteract parasympathomimetic effects such as diarrhoea or bradycardia.

Corticosteroids, preferably in combination with azathioprine, are effective when there is a thymoma but thymectomy is contraindicated.

Dental aspects

Masticatory muscle fatigue is often conspicuous; occasionally there is also furrowing of the tongue. Salivation is increased if an anticholinesterase, alone, is being taken. Occasionally, Sjögren's syndrome or other autoimmune disorders, particularly pemphigus, may be associated. If there is a thymoma there may be chronic candidosis.

Dental treatment is best carried out during a remission. Weakness increases during the day. Fatigue or emotional stress may precipitate a myasthenic crisis and, therefore, treatment is best carried out early in the day, within 1 to 2 hours of routine medication with anticholinesterases. A small dose of a benzodiazepine may be given if the patient is anxious. Local anaesthesia is preferred but minimal doses should be given. Lignocaine, prilocaine or mepivicaine can safely be used, but the older ester types (such as procaine) are contraindicated.

General anaesthesia or intravenous sedation must not be given in the dental surgery since bulbar or respiratory involvement impairs respiration. Postoperative respiratory infection can result and may also cause myasthenia to worsen. Many drugs used in general anaesthesia, such as opioids, barbiturates, suxamethonium, curare or anaesthetic agents are potentiated by or aggravate the myasthenic state.

Other drugs to be avoided since they increase weakness include tetracyclines, clindamycin, lincomycin, sulphonamides and aminoglycosides. Penicillin or erythromycin can safely be used.

Corticosteroids, other immunosuppressants, or emotional lability may also complicate dental treatment. Occasionally, aspirin has produced a cholinergic crisis in those on anticholinesterases. Paracetamol and codeine do not have this potential disadvantage.

MÉNIÈRE'S DISEASE

Labyrinthine dysfunction underlies this syndrome which comprises vertigo, tinnitus and sensorineural hearing loss, with nausea and sometimes nystagmus. Betahistine and cinnarizine have been promoted as specific treatments but phenothiazines, prochlorperazine or thiethylperazine may be required.

PERIPHERAL NEUROPATHIES

The peripheral neuropathy of greatest relevance in dentistry is Bell's palsy. Peripheral neuropathies may also be seen in vitamin B_{12} deficiency (Chapter 4), diabetes mellitus (Chapter 10), alcoholism and abuse of nitrous oxide (Chapter 19). Less common causes are summarized in the Appendix to this chapter.

Bibliography

Bayer D. B. and Stenger T. G. (1979) Trigeminal neuralgia: an overview. *Oral Surg.* **48**, 393–9.

Brooke R. I. (1978) Periodic migrainous neuralgia: a cause of dental pain. *Oral Surg.* **46**, 511–17.

Caplan L. and Gorelick P. (1983) 'Salt and pepper on the face' pain in acute brainstem ischemia. *Ann. Neurol.* **13**, 344–34

Cawson R.A., McCracken A.W., Marcus P.B. et al. (1989) *Pathology: the Mechanisms of Disease.* 2nd edn. St Louis, CV Mosby.

Cawson R.A. and Spector R.G. (1989) *Clinical Pharmacology in Dentistry.* 5th edn. Edinburgh, Churchill Livingstone.

Chia L.G. (1988) Pure trigeminal motor neuropathy. *Br. Med. J.* **296**, 609–11.

Cnossen M. W. (1985) Considerations in the dental treatment of patients with multiple sclerosis. *Oral Med.* **37**, 62–4.

Dacso C.C. and Bortz D.L. (1989) Significance of the Argyll–Robertson pupil in clinical medicine. *Am. J. Med.* **86**, 199–202.

Dalessio D.J. (1990) Aspirin prophylaxis for migraine. *JAMA* **264**, 1721.

Diaz-Mitoma F., Vanast W. J. and Tyrrell D. L. J. (1987) Increased frequency of Epstein–Barr virus excretion in patients with new daily persistent headaches. *Lancet* **i**, 411–15.

Drachman D. B. (1978) Myasthenia gravis. *N. Engl.J. Med.* **298**, 186.

Editorial (1975) Involuntary facial movements. *Br. Med. J.* **1**, 476.

Fernando I.N. and Phipps J.S.K. (1988) Dangers of an uncomplicated tooth extraction: a case of Streptococcus sanguis meningitis. *Brit. Dent. J.* **165**, 220.

Flint S. and Scully C. (1990) Isolated trigeminal sensory neuropathy: a heterogeneous group of disorders. *Oral Surg.* **69**, 153–6.

Greenhall R. C. D. (1980) Headache and facial pain. *Medicine (UK)* **31**, 1606–10.

Graham S.H., Sharp F.R. and Dillon W. (1988) Intraoral sensation in patients with brainstem lesions: role of the rostral spinal trigeminal nuclei in pons. *Neurology* **38**, 1529–33.

Havard C. W. H. (1977) Progress in myasthenia gravis. *Br. Med. J.* **2**, 1008–11.

Heloe B. and Heiberg A. N. (1980) A follow-up study of a group of female patients with myofascial-pain-dysfunction syndrome. *Acta Odontol. Scand.* **38**, 129–34.

Larner A. J. (1986) Aetiological role of viruses in multiple sclerosis. *J. R. Soc. Med.* **79**, 412–17.

Lazar M. L., Greenlee R. G. and Naarden A.L. (1980) Facial pain of neurologic origin mimicking oral pathologic conditions; some current concepts and treatment. *J. Am. Dent. Assoc.* **100**, 884–8.

Leading Article (1982) Bell's palsy. *Lancet* **i**, 663.

Leading Article (1989) Carbamazepine. *Update* **2**, 595–7.

Lowe O. (1986) Tourette's syndrome: management of oral complications. *J. Dent. Child* , 456–60.

Ludman H. (1981) Facial palsy. *Br. Med. J.* **282**, 545–7.

Luker J. and Scully C. (1990) The lateral medullary syndrome. *Oral Surg.* **69**, 322–4.

Marks P.V., Patel K.S. and Mee E.W. (1988) Multiple brain abscesses secondary to dental caries and severe periodontal disease. *Br. J. Oral Maxillofac. Surg.* **26**, 244–7.

Olesen J. (1988) Classification and diagnostic criteria of headache disorders, cranial neuralgia and facial pain. *Cephalgia* **8**, 1–96.

Preston-Martin S. and White S.C. (1990) Brain and salivary gland tumours related to prior dental radiography: implications for current practice. *J. Am. Dent. Assoc.* **120**

Raskin H. H. and Appenzeller O. (1980) Headache. *Major Probl. Intern. Med.* **19**.

Reutens, D.C. (1990) Burning oral and mid-facial pain in ventral pontine infarction. *Aust. NZ Med. J.* **20**, 249-.

Robinson B. B., Harris M. and Harvey W. (1983) Abnormal skeletal and dental growth in epileptic children. *Br. Dent. J.* **154**, 9–13.

Rontal E. (1982) Lesions of the hypoglossal nerve—diagnosis, treatment and rehabilitation. *Laryngoscope* **92**, 927.

Scully C. (1980) Orofacial manifestations of disease. 6. Neurological. psychiatric and muscular disorders. *Hosp. Update 6, 135;* Dent. Update **7**, 375; **8**, 135.

Scully C. (1982) The mouth in general practice. 3. Oral and facial pain. *Dermatol. Practice* **1**, 16–18.

Scully C. (1987) *The Mouth in Health and Disease.* London, Heinemann Medical.

Scully C. and Cawson R. A. (ed.) (1986) Oral medicine. *Med. Int.* **28**, 1129–51.

Severn A.M. (1988) Parkinsonism and the anaesthetist. *Brit. J. Anaesth.* **61**, 761–70.

Shaw D. H., Cohen D. M. and Hoffman M. (1985) Dental treatment of patients with myasthenia gravis. *J. Oral Med.* **37**, 118–20.

Stevens, M.R., Wong, M.E. (1988) Meige syndrome: an unusual cause of involuntary facial movements. *Oral Surg.* **66**, 427–9.

Talako, A.A., Reade, P.C. (1990) Progressive bulbar palsy. *Oral Surg.* **69**, 182-4.

Tolosa, E.S. (1981) Clinical features of Meige's disease: idiopathic orofacial dystonia. *Arch. Neurol.* **36**, 147–51.

Appendix to Chapter 12

PERIPHERAL NEUROPATHIES

1. Hereditary
   Charcot–Marie–Tooth disease
   Refsum's disease
   Déjérine–Sottas disease
2. Acquired
   Infective: herpes zoster
               Guillain–Barré syndrome
               Leprosy
               Diphtheria
               Lyme disease
   Neoplasms: Various
   Trauma:
   Metabolic: Diabetes mellitus
               Vitamin deficiencies, especially B_{12}
   Toxic: Alcohol
        Heavy metals
        Gold
   Nitrous oxide abuse
   Idiopathic: Bell's palsy

CRANIAL NERVE SYNDROMES*

Syndrome	Cranial nerves involved	Site of lesion	Other features
Avellis'	X	Medulla	Hemiplegia
			Horner's syndrome
Benedikt's	III	Midbrain	Cerebellar ataxia
			Tremor
			Hemiplegia
Cerebellopontine angle	V, Vll, VIII and sometimes IX	Posterior cranial fossa	Cerebellar ataxia
Claude's	III	Midbrain	Cerebellar ataxia
			Tremor
Collet–Sicard	IX, X, XI, XII	Retroparotid space	
Foix's	III, IV, V (ophthalmic). VI	Cavernous sinus	Proptosis

Gradenigo's	V, VI	Petrous temporal	Pain
Jackson's	X, XII	Medulla	Hemiplegia Horner's syndrome
Jacob's	II, III, IV, V, VI	Middle cranial fossa	
Millard–Gubler	VII, VI	Pons	Hemiplegia
Nothnagel's	III	Midbrain	Cerebellar ataxia
Parinaud's	III, IV, VI	Midbrain	
Sphenoid fissure (superior orbital fissure)	III, IV, V (ophthalmic) VI and sometimes II	Superior orbital fissure	Proptosis
Vernet's	IX, X, XI	Jugular foramen Nasopharynx	
Villaret's	IX, X, XI, XII	Retroparotid space	Horner's syndrome

Wallenberg's
  (Posterior inferior
cerebellar artery
PICA)
	V, IX, X, XI	Medulla	Horner's syndrome
			Cerebellar ataxia
			Loss of pain and
			  temperature sense

Weber's	III	Midbrain	Hemiplegia

* Modified from: Victor M. and Adams R. D. (1980) In: Isselbacher K. J. et al. (ed.) *Principles of Internal Medicine*, 9th ed. Tokyo, McGraw-Hill Kogakusha, p. 2020.

Chapter 13

Medical Aspects of Maxillofacial Injuries

In Great Britain approximately 40 persons die each day from accidents which are also the most common cause of death in children and in men under the age of 35. Up to a third of these deaths are, theoretically at least, preventable.

Most maxillofacial injuries are in previously fit young men, usually from road accidents, assaults or fights. Alcohol is a frequent factor. Violence is increasing but trauma from road accidents is not. Industrial accidents, sport and epilepsy are other causes. Severe maxillofacial injuries are often seen by the oral or maxillofacial surgeon after the patient has been examined and major injuries treated by other specialists, but this is not invariable and dental surgeons may find themselves in charge of the whole initial care of such patients.

Medical complications of maxillofacial injuries can include hazards to the airway, head injuries and damage to the chest, liver, spleen, kidneys or bladder. Indeed, about 70 per cent of patients admitted with multiple injuries also have a head injury. The possibility of pre-existing disease must always also be considered. Road traffic accident victims admitted to a neurosurgical unit more frequently (40 per cent) have multiple injuries than those admitted for other reasons (11 per cent). Shock is most unusual in uncomplicated maxillofacial injuries or head injuries and its presence is often an indication of internal haemorrhage. Maxillofacial injuries may be associated with coma, the differential diagnosis of which is difficult and demands systematic examination.

Major complications with maxillofacial injuries may therefore include:

1. Head injuries.
2. Chest injuries.
3. Ruptured viscera with internal haemorrhage.
4. Eye injuries.
5. Fractures of the cervical or thoraco–lumbar spine.
6. Long bone fractures.

The management of these injuries and their complications takes precedence; *the most urgent attention is needed to maintain the airway* and control bleeding.

INITIAL MANAGEMENT OF MAXILLOFACIAL INJURIES (*Table 13.1*)

Airway and Breathing

Respiratory obstruction is the most important preventable cause of early death after maxillofacial trauma and many patients have died from neglect of the

Table 13.1. Maxillofacial trauma—early management

1. *Immediate care* (ABC)
   Airway
   Bleeding
   Chest injury
2. *General assessment*
   Pulse
   Blood pressure
   Respiratory rate
   Pupil size
   Pupil reaction
   State of consciousness
3. *Assessment of head injury*
   Skull examination
   Examination for cerebrospinal fluid leak
   Neurological assessment
   Skull radiography
   Blood analyses
4. *Assessment for other injuries*
   Chest
   Neck
   Spine
   Abdomen
   Perineum
   Limbs

airway before admission to hospital. Foreign bodies or the tongue can easily fall back to obstruct respiration, especially if there are bilateral fractures or comminution of the mandible, and the patient is unconscious.

Management

The patient must be laid semi-prone on his side, face towards the ground, to allow any potential obstruction to fall forwards. The mouth and pharynx must be quickly cleared of debris and sucked out. In the case of bilateral mandibular body fractures, a traction suture through the tongue will hold it forward, but frequently, medial displacement of the posterior fragments prevents the anterior fragment from falling backwards unless the bone is comminuted. Posterior displacement of the maxilla in middle third injuries may cause the soft palate to occlude the airway; obstruction can then be overcome by manual disimpaction of the maxilla and the insertion of a nasopharyngeal tube. In the unconscious patient a cuffed endotracheal tube is more satisfactory, but in gross trauma tracheostomy may be needed. All unconscious patients should also have a gastric tube passed to aid stomach aspiration and feeding.

If there is supraglottic airways obstruction an airway can be established by laryngotomy using a wide-bore (2–3 mm) needle inserted through the cricothyroid membrane. Tracheostomy can then be carried out. Indications for tracheostomy are summarized in *Table 13.2.*

There is special danger to the airway if there has been trauma to and oedema of the tongue, fauces, pharynx or larynx, or uncontrollable nasal haemorrhage.

Table 13.2. Indications for tracheostomy

1. Obstruction of the airway by—
   Gross retroposition of the middle third of the face
   Pharyngeal oedema
   Uncontrollable nasal haemorrhage
   Loss of tongue control
2. Where positive pressure ventilation is needed, e.g. crushed or flail chest
3. Where tracheobronchial suction is needed, e.g. chronic obstructive airways disease

Chest injuries, particularly those causing tension pneumothorax or flail chest, or inhalation of toxic or hot gases further impair respiration (*see* Burns).

Flail chest can be recognized by extreme difficulty in breathing, associated with paradoxical movements of the chest and cyanosis. Intermittent positive-pressure ventilation must be given via an endotracheal tube.

Haemorrhage

Severe haemorrhage or shock very rarely results from maxillofacial injuries alone, unless caused by gunshot wounds. Even a ruptured inferior dental artery usually stops bleeding spontaneously.

If bleeding recurs, the damaged vessel must be ligated, at open operation if necessary, and an intravenous infusion line should be set up in case blood transfusion is needed.

Severe nose bleeds that do not cease spontaneously after pressure or after packing with 1/2 inch ribbon gauze may be controlled using a Foley balloon catheter passed through the nose into the nasopharynx, softly inflated and then pulled gently forwards against the posterior nasal choanae.

It is essential to remember that bleeding may be concealed, or occasionally aggravated by disseminated intravascular coagulation (Chapter 3) secondary to the head injury. Internal haemorrhage, for example into the abdomen from a ruptured viscus, or into the thigh from a fractured femur, can cause life-threatening hypotension. Haemorrhage into the pleural cavity from fractured ribs can also embarrass respiration. Latent haemorrhage may be recognized by the following:

1. Increasing pulse rate.
2. Falling blood pressure.
3. Increasing pallor.
4. Air hunger.
5. Restlessness.

Severe haemorrhage can lead to cardiac or renal failure or cause fatal cerebral hypoxia.

If haemorrhage is suspected a surgical opinion should be sought and the following quarter- or half-hourly observations should be recorded:

1. Pulse rate.
2. Blood pressure.
3. Respiratory rate.
4. Urine output and fluid balance (usually hourly).

A falling blood pressure with rising pulse rate suggests hypotension because of bleeding. If haemorrhage is persistent blood should be taken for grouping and cross-matching and an intravenous line established.

If, however, the blood pressure is found to be rising then cerebral oedema and increasing intracranial pressure must be suspected, as discussed later.

Blood transfusion

Blood may be needed to replace loss from acute haemorrhage. Blood transfusion is not needed to replace loss of less than 500 ml in an adult, unless there was pre-existing anaemia or deterioration of the general condition warrants transfusion. Since time is needed to obtain correctly cross-matched blood, normal saline, plasma or a plasma expander such as dextran 70 or 110 may be given initially. Dextran can interfere with blood-grouping and cross-matching so that samples should be collected before a dextran infusion is started (*see* Chapter 3). In view of the risks of infection with HIV and other agents, blood transfusion should be used only where the clinical condition genuinely warrants it.

HEAD INJURY

Head injuries are a major cause of death in patients with maxillofacial injuries. Even mild head injuries carry the risk of life-threatening complications such as intracranial haematoma or infection, or of post-traumatic epilepsy, and it is important to appreciate that the brain can be fatally damaged without fracture of the skull or even a blemish on the scalp.

Of those with brain damage, 12 per cent die within 2 days, while approximately 50 per cent have permanent after-effects such as paralyses, loss of speech, impaired vision, epilepsy, disturbances of personality or severe mental defects, rendering them disabled for life.

Almost 50 per cent of deaths from head injury happen before the patient reaches hospital and most of the remainder follow within the first few days of admission. It is important to recognize and to treat factors that can contribute to the morbidity and mortality and which include the following:

1. Airway obstruction.
2. Intracranial haematoma.
3. Hypotension.
4. Meningitis.
5. Uncontrolled epilepsy.
6. Stress-induced gastric bleeding (Cushing's ulcer).

History

Many patients are brought in confused or in coma and as good a history as possible must therefore be obtained from witnesses. Family or friends may be able to provide information about the patient's medical background. Consciousness is almost invariably impaired after diffuse brain damage, although the patient may lose consciousness only transiently. However, there is usually amnesia for the traumatic event, and afterwards (post-traumatic amnesia) for a period far exceeding that of coma. Consciousness is not, however, always lost if brain damage is local—when, for example, the skull is penetrated by a sharp object. Maintenance of consciousness does not therefore imply the absence of brain damage. Thirty per cent of patients with ultimately fatal head injuries may talk after injury and some are completely lucid for a time. Concussion is always associated with brain damage even if after-effects are not detectable.

The brain is, therefore, invariably damaged in those who have lost consciousness, for however brief a period, and sometimes in those who have not. Prolonged unconsciousness, when there are no complications such as haematomas and where there are no focal signs, is caused by severe brain damage or other unrelated disease (*see Table 13.4*).

Examination

Essential examination and investigations include the following:

1. Examination of the head.
2. Examination for cerebrospinal fluid leakage.
3. Assessment of neurological function.
4. Blood pressure estimation.
5. Radiographic examination.
6. Blood analyses.

Clinical examination

Lacerations of the scalp can cause severe loss of blood and provide a pathway for infection into the cranial cavity. They may also be associated with a depressed fracture, which may be palpable.

Leakage of cerebrospinal fluid

Particular care must be taken to look for signs of orbital or retromastoid haematomas (which may indicate fractures with dural tears) and cerebrospinal rhinorrhoea or otorrhoea, in all of which there is the risk of meningitis because of skull fracture. The mortality may ultimately reach 20 per cent. CSF rhinorrhoea is found in about 2 per cent of all head injuries, but is seen in 25 per cent of fractures of the middle facial third and of the nasoethmoidal complex. The leak usually persists for about a week and the risk of meningitis is greatest within the first fortnight. Occasionally the fistula may be occluded by herniated brain but the dural tear fails to heal. Meningitis may follow after some months or years and dural repair is desirable. A neurosurgical opinion should therefore be obtained.

In the early stages leakage of CSF may be obscured by haemorrhage, but any clear watery discharge from the nose is suspect. CSF contains sugar but little protein—which differentiates it from a serous nasal discharge. Lacrimal fluid, however, also contains small amounts of glucose and CSF must therefore be positively identified by protein electrophoresis and by accurate measurement of the glucose. Prophylactic antimicrobials are needed if there is a risk of meningitis and should therefore be given to all patients with a middle third injury. Penicillin does not adequately enter the cerebrospinal fluid. Sulphadiazine or co–trimoxazole 960 mg, 12 hourly for 5–7 days may be a suitable regimen and should be maintained if there is a CSF leak. Because of the danger of sulphonamide crystalluria, extra fluids may need to be given.

Many bacteria causing post-traumatic meningitis, such as meningococci, *Staphylococcus aureus* or *Streptococcus pneumoniae* are resistant to sulphonamides. Effective alternatives are rifampicin 600 mg b.d. for 4 days or minocycline 100 mg b.d. for 5 days: they readily reach the CSF and are well absorbed when given orally. Rifampicin is effective against *Neisseria meningitidis*, *S. aureus* and *S. pneumoniae* and may possibly be a more suitable drug than sulphonamides for prophylaxis of post–traumatic intracranial infection.

The main toxic effects of rifampicin are influenzal, abdominal and respiratory symptoms or rarely, renal failure or thrombocytopenia after prolonged treatment. Serious toxic effects are unlikely to complicate the short-term prophylaxis of meningitis. However, patients should be warned that their saliva and urine will turn orange.

Rifampicin may be contraindicated in those with liver disease and alcoholics—unfortunately a well-represented group amongst head injury cases.

Neurological function

Pupil size and reaction must be checked for localizing signs of neurological damage. A dilated fixed (unreactive to light) pupil often indicates rising intracranial pressure and is usually a serious sign. Severe facial oedema may, however, make examination of the eyes difficult and the eyelids should then be prised open. A fixed dilated pupil may also be caused by local damage to the optic or oculomotor nerves and must be differentiated by clinical examination, radiographs (including, if necessary, tomography) and by the absence of signs associated with brain damage or of rising intracranial pressure.

Rising intracranial pressure is typically associated with bradycardia and rising blood pressure, but these may sometimes be absent. Limb reflexes should be tested. Convulsions early on considerably increase the likelihood of late epilepsy.

The level of consciousness is assessed by three features:

1. Opening the eyes spontaneously (*a*) in response to command, (*b*) in response to pain, (*c*) not at all.

2. Verbal response which may be (*a*) rational, (*b*) confused, (*c*) inappropriate, (*d*) incomprehensible, or (*e*) lacking.

3. Motor responses. Limbs may (*a*) move precisely in response to command, (*b*) move to the site of pain, on command, (*c*) flex to painful stimuli, or (*d*) extend to painful stimuli (nail-bed pressure).

A scale for the assessment of brain damage due to various causes (Glasgow Coma Scale) is now widely used (*Table 13.3*). The degree of brain damage is assessed by the level of consciousness and, later, by the duration of coma and of post-traumatic amnesia. All patients who score less than the full 15 points should be admitted to hospital for observation even if drugs or alcohol are the suspected causes of depressed consciousness.

Table 13.3. Glasgow Coma or Responsiveness Scale

		Score
Eye opening	spontaneous	E4
	to speech	3
	to pain	2
	nil	1
Motor response	obeys	M6
	localizes	5
	withdraws	4
	abnormal flexion	3
	extends	2
	nil	1
Verbal response	orientated	V5
	confused conversation	4
	inappropriate words	3
	incomprehensible sounds	2
	nil	1
EMV score or responsiveness sum		3–15

7 or less = coma in 100 per cent.
9 or more = absence of coma.

Up to 60 per cent of all patients admitted in coma are alcoholics who have often had a head injury. Toxic and metabolic disorders cause no focal or localizing neurological signs. However, when there is disease of the CNS itself sensory or motor disturbances may indicate the site of the lesion. In some of these diseases white cells and bacteria or blood may also appear in the CSF.

Intoxications, whether the result of exogenous agents or disorders of metabolism and severe infections, all have essentially similar effects and will not be discussed further here.

Estimation of blood urea and electrolyte levels are needed in case there has been renal failure secondary to loss of blood, and as a baseline to monitor progress and the effects of intravenous fluid replacement. A full blood picture is also needed as a baseline for possible effects of transfusion and for any coincidental haematological disease. As described earlier (Chapter 3), early haemoglobin levels give no useful indication of the amount of blood lost.

Observation

Patients must be carefully and regularly observed to detect the development of complications, especially intracranial haematomas which need immediate neurosurgical attention. The most important sign is deterioration of consciousness, sometimes with increasing restlessness, headache and vomiting. Focal signs such as hemiparesis, dysphasia or focal epilepsy are uncommon.

Patients with severe head injuries fall into three main groups:

1. Most are stable neurologically with gradual improvement in consciousness.

2. Rising intracranial pressure causing progressive deterioration in level of consciousness in the absence of localizing signs. Cerebral oedema may be reduced by ensuring adequate oxygenation and by giving mannitol and/or dexamethasone.

3. Progressive deterioration in level of consciousness with localizing signs. However, localized intracranial bleeding with or without cerebral oedema, contusions or lacerations may be manageable, if the bleeding can be evacuated by craniotomy.

Dilatation of the pupil on the side of the fracture and decerebrate rigidity—late signs caused by raised intracranial pressure and brain shift—are soon followed by bilateral pupil dilatation, periodic respiration, respiratory arrest and death, unless there is immediate neurosurgical intervention.

The level of consciousness is depressed further by sedatives and many analgesics. Morphine and its analogues are especially dangerous because they both depress respiration and disguise eye signs of rising intracranial pressure by causing pupillary constriction. Pentazocine is also contraindicated. If analgesia is essential, codeine or buprenorphine can be used.

Benzodiazepines should not be given for such purposes as controlling fits or to allow suturing of head wounds. In patients with head injuries, benzodiazepines can cause respiratory depression which can be fatal, unless ventilation is given. If there are repeated fits, phenytoin by intravenous infusion is less likely to depress respiration.

In deep coma there are no verbal or motor responses but in less severe cases the eyes may open transiently from time to time and there may be vague or weak responses to stimuli. The level of consciousness should be charted regularly half-hourly, or even more frequently, along with the pulse, blood pressure, respiration and pupil reactivity.

Blood pressure

Regular monitoring of the blood pressure is essential. A low or falling blood pressure with rising pulse rate is indicative of haemorrhage or shock which can lead to fatal cerebral anoxia or renal failure. A systolic blood pressure lower than 60 mmHg brings with it a risk of brain damage. A high or rising blood pressure with bradycardia, by contrast, is indicative of raised intracranial pressure secondary to cerebral oedema or haemorrhage as a result of the injury.

Radiography

Radiography (typically AP, lateral and Towne's views) and sometimes CT scans, are essential to exclude fractures of the skull and brain lesions. They should be carried out early before infection can reach the cranial cavity. Radiography may also reveal a depressed fracture involving the paranasal sinuses; this suggests a meningeal tear which is occasionally confirmed by seeing intracranial air (aerocoele). A linear fracture indicates the possibility of intracranial haematoma but even normal radiographs do not exclude brain damage.

About 50 per cent of patients with intracranial injuries have no skull fracture, but approximately 90 per cent of patients with fractures of the skull have no resulting intracranial injury.

Table 13.4. Some causes of coma

1. *Local disease of the central nervous system*
   Trauma
   Haemorrhage (subarachnoid, epidural or subdural)
   Infarction (thrombosis or embolism)
   Infections (abscess, meningitis or meningo-encephalitis)
   Tumours (metastatic or primary)
   Epilepsy
   Raised intracranial pressure from any cause
2. *Systemic causes (toxic and metabolic)*
   Intoxication (alcohol, barbiturates, opiates, etc.)
   Metabolic disorders (diabetic hypo- or hyperglycaemia, Addisonian crisis, hypothyroidism, hypoglycaemia from any cause, uraemia, hepatic coma)
   Severe systemic infections (pneumonia, typhoid fever, malaria)
   Hypoxia
   Acute hypotension (circulatory collapse from any cause)
   Hypertensive encephalopathy
   Hypo- or hyperthermia
   Reye's syndrome

Blood analyses

Some of the many causes of coma are listed in *Table 13.4.* Coma from various causes differs in the nature of the associated signs, which are discussed in more detail in this and other chapters. More than one cause may be operative. Blood and urine samples should therefore be collected for analysis for alcohol, drugs and metabolic disorders, particularly diabetes. Transient glycosuria unrelated to diabetes may, however, follow the stress of head injuries.

COMPLICATIONS OF MAXILLOFACIAL INJURIES

Cranial Nerve Injuries

Cranial nerve lesions in patients with head injuries may indicate a basal skull fracture or other lesion. Cranial nerves I, II, III, V, VII and VIII are most vulnerable to damage (*Table 13.5* and Chapter 12).

Table 13.5. Cranial nerve lesions complicating head injuries

Nerve lesion	Usual site of injury	Comments
I (Olfactory)	Ethmoidal complex (may be no fracture)	Anosmia (usually permanent); apparent loss of taste
II (Optic)	Orbit* or sphenoid	Pupil dilated, unreactive to light, but consensual reflex retained†; partial or complete blindness
III (Oculomotor)	Orbit*	Affected eye looks down and out. Pupil dilated, unreactive to light. No consensual reflex. Loss of medial and vertical movement of eye. Divergent squint
IV (Trochlear)	Orbit*	Diplopia only on looking down . Similar features result if superior oblique muscle is entrapped. Pupil; normal reactivity
V (Trigeminal)	Middle fossa, orbit,* maxilla or mandible	Commonly extracranially. Anaesthesia or paraesthesia in sensory area
VI (Abducens)	Orbit * or petrous temporal	Diplopia. Loss or lateral movement of eye Convergent squint. Pupil reacts normally
VII (Facial)	Direct trauma to nerve or basal skull fracture	Facial palsy which may be delayed for a few days (*see* Facial palsy)
VIII (Vestibulo-cochlear)	Petrous temporal	Deafness, vertigo and nystagmus alone or together. Deafness after head injury may also be caused by ruptured ear drum or blood in middle ear
IX-XII		Uncommon as a result of head injuries

*May be damage to orbital contents with or without fracture. These nerves are often injured together and urgent neurosurgery may be indicated since nerve dysfunction if caused by haemorrhage or oedema within the optic canal or other confined space may be reversible.
†Consensual reflex is the constriction of the pupil as a normal response when a light is shone into the other eye.

Anosmia

Sense of smell is disturbed or lost (anosmia) in 5–10 per cent of patients with head injuries. The olfactory nerves can be damaged in frontal bone injuries and fractures involving the cribriform plate of the ethmoid. There is often also cerebrospinal fluid rhinorrhoea.

Traumatic anosmia improves in only about 10 per cent of cases and perversion of the sense of smell may develop during recovery. These effects are remarkably troublesome or even disabling, but untreatable.

Orbital Injuries

Ocular or orbital injuries may need the attention of an ophthalmological surgeon; zygomatic fractures or isolated orbital injuries may hazard vision. Diplopia (double vision) is often present early because of oedema and haemorrhage within the confined space of the orbit; circumorbital and subconjunctival ecchymoses are usually associated. Occasionally periorbital emphysema is present.

Diplopia can also result from enophthalmos associated with orbital floor or wall fractures, from muscle or nerve injury, or from muscle entrapment. Orbital blowout fractures also depress the level of the eye and limit ocular movement, especially upwards.

Disruption of the bony margins of the superior orbital fissure, haematoma or traumatic aneurysm at this site may cause the superior orbital fissure syndrome of ophthalmoplegia, ptosis, exophthalmos, a fixed dilated pupil or absence of consensual reflex, and some sensory loss over the distribution of the ophthalmic division of the trigeminal nerve. These signs are caused by injury to cranial nerves III, IV, V and VI, where they pass through the orbital fissure.

The diagnosis of diplopia is discussed in Chapter 12.

Atlanto-axial Subluxation

Dislocation at the atlanto-axial joint or fracture of the odontoid peg may follow trauma or other factors such as congenital anomalies of the odontoid process (as in Down's syndrome), rheumatoid arthritis or ankylosing spondylitis.

Traumatic dislocation may be lethal. If not, there may only be weakness of the legs or even no immediate neurological sequelae. Transient blackouts, weakness of the limbs, sensory loss, facial paraesthesia, nystagmus, ataxia and dysarthria may be complaints and sudden movement of the neck may cause spastic quadriplegia or death. Patients should therefore be moved with great care not to extend the neck after maxillofacial injuries to avoid this complication.

Burns

Burns can be serious injuries, especially where more than 10 per cent of the body surface area is involved. First–aid care includes maintenance of an adequate airway, the administration of oxygen if there has been exposure to hot air or smoke, and lessening pain by cooling the burn and giving analgesics. Morphine 5–15 mg for an adult may be indicated. Subsequent treatment should be in a Burns or Plastic Surgery Unit.

After receiving burns in a closed or confined space, a change in voice, hoarseness, dysphonia, stridor or the coughing of sooty sputum are all danger signs suggesting inhalation injury. Endotracheal intubation or tracheostomy may be indicated. The reader is referred to Wachtel, Frank and Frank (1981) for further details.

Adult Respiratory Distress Syndrome

This is a sequel to pulmonary injury, characterized by diffuse alveolar damage, pulmonary oedema and hyaline membrane formation. It may culminate in respiratory failure and the mortality is high. Patients showing the suggestive signs of dyspnoea, increased respiratory rate, abnormal breath sounds (râles) with bilateral diffuse interstitial and intra-alveolar oedema on radiography, should be admitted to Intensive Care.

Injuries to the Spinal Cord

Spinal cord injuries can accompany maxillofacial injuries and are an all too common result of road traffic or sports injuries. The resulting disability can be appallingly severe.

Cord injury is usually the result of vertical compression, sometimes with flexion or extension of the neck, or violently sudden extension of the neck (whiplash injury) as when a vehicle is hit from behind.

Most vertebral injuries affect the C1–2, C4–7 and T11–L2 vertebrae. The clinical effects are determined largely by the level of the cord damage (*Table 13.6, 13.7*). Paraplegia is common.

Fracture-dislocation or dislocations of the cervical spine are potentially lethal. The possibility of such damage should always be considered in patients involved in road traffic accidents since movement of the neck may then cause serious cord damage.

The clinical effects of spinal cord injury develop in two main stages: (*a*) spinal shock; (*b*) reflex activity (*Table 13.7*).

If movement can be elicited or any sensation is retained during the first 2–3 days the prognosis is more favourable. Any symptoms persisting after 6 months are likely to be permanent.

Table 13. 6. Spinal cord damage

Level of damage	Features
C1–C5	Quadriplegia (tetraplegia) or death
C5–C6	Paraplegia
	Arms paralysed except for abduction and flexion
C6–C7	Paraplegia
	Hands, but not arms, paralysed
T11–T12	Paraplegia
	Sensory loss T12 and below
T12–L1	Legs paralysed below knees

Table 13. 7. Effects of spinal cord damage

Early (spinal shock)
1. Loss of motor function
    (quadriplegia if damage at C4–C5;
    paraplegia if damage in thoracic cord)
2. Loss of sensation—
    below lesion, leading to skin pressure ulcers
3. Loss of reflexes—
    below lesion, with muscle flaccidity
4. Bladder and bowel sphincter paralysis
    leading to urinary or faecal retention

Delayed (after 2–3 weeks)
1. Loss of motor function—
    may improve if cord not completely transected
2. Loss of sensation—
    may improve if cord not completely transected
3. Reflexes—
    involuntary flexor, then extensor spasms below level of lesion
4. Bladder and bowel sphincter paralysis—
    irregular reflex micturition and defaecation

General management of paraplegics

Treatment in general is supportive and symptomatic, and is mainly directed toward the prevention of complications such as:

1. Muscle wasting or contractures.
2. Pressure sores.
3. Postural hypotension.
4. Urinary infections.
5. Constipation.
6. Psychological problems.

Physiotherapy is essential to reduce muscle wasting and to maintain function in unparalysed or partly paralysed muscles. Joints must be regularly passively moved and the position of the patient carefully checked, to prevent soft tissue contractures and pressure sores.

Postural hypotension and autonomic dysreflexia can complicate high level spinal cord lesions. Intense vasoconstriction below the level of the cord injury follows certain stimuli such as bladder contraction. The vasoconstriction is associated with rapid onset of hypertension, facial sweating and headache.

Urinary retention invariably complicates acute spinal cord lesions, and aseptic catheterization is needed. Infections must be treated promptly—recurrent urinary infections were previously the main factor in renal disease and amyloidosis complicating paraplegia.

Dental management of paraplegics

Dental management may be uncomplicated, although postural hypotension in the early stages may necessitate treatment in the supine position. Paraplegics have impaired mobility. Quadriplegics are at risk from respiratory infections and general anaesthesia should be avoided if possible and never carried out in the dental surgery. Other problems are dealt with in Chapter 15.

Admission of Conscious Patients to Hospital

Ideally, every patient who has a head injury should be admitted for observation but this is impractical. However, the following categories of patients should be admitted:

1. Children, the mentally handicapped or those with psychiatric disease.
2. Patients living alone or without a responsible companion.
3. If there is fracture of the skull.
4. If there is post-traumatic amnesia.
5. If there are other injuries.

If there is evidence of a depressed skull fracture, debridement and elevation of the fracture is needed within 24 hours.

Late Sequelae of Head Injury

Late sequelae that may complicate head injuries include the following:

1. Chronic extra- or subdural haematomas.
2. Post-traumatic syndrome.
3. Epilepsy (Chapter 12).
4. Infection (see above).
5. Diabetes insipidus (Chapter 10).
6. Mental handicap.
7. Physical handicap.
8. Compensation neurosis (Chapter 14).

Extradural haematoma

Extradural haematoma is a consequence of bleeding between the skull and dura. The usual cause is a fracture tearing the middle meningeal artery or one of its branches. The haematoma forms a tumour-like mass which compresses part of the brain and causes increasing intracranial pressure as it expands.

Clinically the typical story is of a heavy blow followed by loss of consciousness. There is usually then a period of apparent recovery (lucid interval) followed by signs of increasing intracranial pressure. If the clot is not removed, death from respiratory arrest follows.

A radiograph showing a fracture line crossing the line of the middle meningeal artery strongly suggests extradural haemorrhage. CT scanning will confirm the diagnosis. The neurosurgical treatment is to drill bur holes through the skull to drain the clot and ligate the bleeding vessel.

Subdural haematoma

Bleeding between the dura mater and the leptomeninges (pia-arachnoid) maybe acute or chronic.

Acute subdural haematoma is often the result of an injury causing a tear in the arachnoid and may be associated with laceration or contusion of the brain.

Clinically, there is a latent interval after the injury, followed by progressive deterioration of consciousness and development of symptoms somewhat similar to those of an extradural haematoma. Once coma has developed, up to 50 per cent of patients die.

The main principles of management are to localize the lesion and to evacuate the clot through bur holes. The results are variable and depend on the degree of cerebral damage.

Chronic subdural haematoma can be caused by very mild injury. Nevertheless, the veins between the pia and the dura mater are torn.

Leakage of blood into the subdural space is very slow. There is a fibroblastic response and eventually the haematoma becomes enclosed in scar tissue or, occasionally, resorbed.

Clinically, the head injury, especially in an elderly person, may be so slight as to have been forgotten but, after several weeks, or even months, symptoms such as headache, dizziness, slowness of thinking, or confusion and disturbance of consciousness develop. There may be localizing signs such as hemiparesis or aphasia; the patient may have ptosis and be unable to look upwards (pressure on the IIIrd nerve). Urgent neurosurgical intervention is needed to evacuate the haematoma.

Post-traumatic syndrome

The post-traumatic syndrome may be caused by mild brain damage or damage to the cochlear–vestibular apparatus and frequently follows severe head injuries. Complaints include temporary headache, irritability, inability to concentrate, short temper, loss of confidence, vertigo and hyperacusis. If symptoms persist psychiatric advice should be sought.

Diabetes insipidus

Diabetes insipidus may follow a head injury as a result of traction on the pituitary stalk, especially where there is a basal skull fracture (*see* Chapter 10).

Syndrome of Inappropriate ADH Secretion (see Chapter 10)

STAB WOUNDS

A small entrance wound may well hide injuries to deeper structures. Wounds caused by stabbing or glass fragments must always be explored before closure.

GUNSHOT WOUNDS

Hand guns usually inflict low velocity bullet wounds that damage only the tissues they hit and such wounds can be managed by conventional surgical-methods. In contrast, high velocity missiles (explosive blast fragments or rifle bullets) produce extensive tissue damage and contamination, though the entrance wounds may be minute. To avoid gas gangrene, necrotic tissue should be excised and antibiotics given (see below).

PREVENTION OF INFECTION

Four main infective problems can complicate maxillofacial injuries:

1. Meningitis.
2. Local wound infection and osteomyelitis.
3. Tetanus.
4. Actinomycosis (rarely).

Meningitis

Meningitis is an important complication of opening the cranial cavity (shown by leakage of CSF), as discussed earlier. It is by far the most important infective complication of maxillofacial injuries and can also result from lacerations of the scalp when infection can reach the brain via the emissary veins.

Wound Infection

The risk of infection of lacerated or contused soft tissues, or osteomyelitis, is increased when there is:

1. Inadequate wound toilet.
2. Foreign bodies in the wound or teeth in the fracture line.
3. Gross delay in treatment.
4. Systemic disease with decreased resistance to infection, particularly alcoholism.

Intramuscular benzyl penicillin 600 mg 6-hourly or cephazolin is usually an effective prophylactic for compound fractures. Gross debris, broken teeth, detached bone and foreign bodies should be removed.

Extreme care must be taken to identify foreign material within the tissues. Some types of glass and plastic are radiolucent and may be missed unless the wound is systematically probed. After preliminary wound toilet, lacerations can usually be sutured under local anaesthesia, but larger lacerations can be covered with tulle gras and dry dressings for closure as soon as possible under general anaesthesia.

Teeth in the fracture line may need to be extracted unless required for stabilization of a bone fragment.

Tetanus

Tetanus is an uncommon, infectious but non-communicable disease caused by contamination of wounds by the sporing bacterium *Clostridium tetani*. Tetanus is a dangerous infection with a mortality still between 10 and 60 per cent. About 10–15 cases of tetanus are reported each year in the United Kingdom.

Spores of *C. tetani* are ubiquitous in soil or dust, particularly where there is faecal contamination (for example in agricultural land). Tetanus is most likely to follow contaminated deep wounds, such as puncture wounds, especially if there is necrosis.

Clostridium tetani produces tetanospasmin, a neurotoxin, responsible for the violent muscular spasms characteristic of the disease. Trismus (lockjaw) due to masseteric spasm is the single most common early sign. Facial spasm produces a so-called sardonic smile (risus sardonicus) where the eyebrows are raised with eyes closed and the lips are drawn back over clenched teeth. Spasm of spinal muscles causes arching of the back (opisthotonos), while laryngeal spasm leads to asphyxiation. Autonomic dysfunction can cause cardiac dysrhythmias and fluctuations in blood pressure.

Death may follow within 10 days of the onset of tetanus, usually from asphyxia, bronchopneumonia or autonomic dysfunction.

General management

Prophylaxis.   Active immunization in childhood is given as triple vaccine (diphtheria, pertussis and tetanus antigens) starting at the age of 12 weeks, followed by further injections 6–8 weeks later and then after a further 4–6 months. Booster immunization (diphtheria plus tetanus) is given on starting primary school and at 15–19 years (Appendix to Chapter 17).

The duration of immunity after such an immunization schedule is not known but current practice is to boost it every 10 years. Groups at risk, for example farm workers, should be given boosters every 5 years. It is not, however, good practice always to give tetanus toxoid after every minor injury, as severe allergic reactions can occasionally follow.

Management of the wounded patient.   Patients who have contaminated wounds, such as those associated with maxillofacial injuries caused by road traffic or riding accidents, are at risk from tetanus. An outline for the management of patients with such injuries is shown in *Table 13.8.*

Table 13.8. Management of wounded patients at risk from tetanus

	Immune status of patient	*Course of action**
Superficial wound or abrasion	Immune	—
	Not known to be immune	Start active immunization with toxoid
Deep wounds Puncture wounds Bites	Immune	Give toxoid booster†
	Not known to be immune	Give antibiotics and start immunization with toxoid and (a) if seen after 4 h give 250 units HTIG; (1) if seen after 24 h give 500 units HTIG

* Wound débridement in all.
† Unneccessary if toxoid given within the previous 5 years.
HTIG, Human antitetanus immunoglobulin

Treatment of tetanus.   The patient should be admitted to an Intensive Care unit. The main principles are as follows:

1. Protection of the airway.
2. Antitetanus immunoglobulin injection.
3. Control of muscle spasms.
4. Wound débridement.

The airway. Tracheostomy should be carried out if the airway is endangered and to facilitate artificial respiration if it becomes necessary.

Antiserum. Antiserum must be given early as it is ineffective after the toxin has become bound to nervous tissue. Human antitetanus immunoglobulin (ATG, Humotet 500 or more units) should be given. If this is not available animal antitetanus serum (ATS) can be given after testing for hypersensitivity and with adrenaline and corticosteroids available in case a severe reaction develops.

Control of muscle spasms. Spasms are controlled by heavy sedation or, in severe cases, with general anaesthesia, muscle relaxants and mechanical ventilation.

Wound débridement. The purpose of wound débridement is to remove the source of toxin as antibiotics alone are ineffective.

Survivors recover completely but should have active immunization with toxoid. The mortality is high especially among the elderly.

Dental aspects

Trismus is usually caused by local irritation such as pericoronitis or temporo-mandibular-pain-dysfunction syndrome. Tetanus must always, however, be considered in the differential diagnosis of trismus in the absence of a local cause. Such patients should therefore be asked whether they have had any recent wounds, particularly if farm workers or gardeners. Dyskinesias due to phenothiazines include facial grimacing but rarely trismus—the mouth is usually forcefully opened.

Actinomycosis

Actinomycosis is rare. It usually affects the soft tissues at the angle of the mandible (*see* Oral Surgery texts).

SPORTS INJURIES

Injuries to the teeth and oral soft tissues are common particularly in football, ice hockey, basket ball and boxing. Those involved in these sports as well as wrestling, karate, judo and gymnastics should wear a mouth shield. These are usually made of vinyl or acrylic and three types are available:

1. Stock protectors. These are cheap and easily adjusted but less comfortable.
2. Mouth–formed protectors moulded onto the teeth.
3. Custom–made protectors.

Child abuse (see Chapter 14)

SUMMARY

The priorities of early management of a patient with maxillofacial and other injuries, especially if in coma, are as follows:

1. Ensure a clear airway.
2. Look for and control bleeding, whether intra- or extracranial.
3. Look for other serious injuries, particularly to the cervical spine, thorax and abdomen.
4. Look for fractures of other bones.
5. Look for leakage of cerebrospinal fluid.
6. Look for injuries to the eyes.
7. Establish a neurological base-line for future reference.
8. Reduce and immobilize a fracture only if it threatens the airway. Definitive treatment must be delayed until the patient is out of danger.
9. Debride and suture facial lacerations.
10. Give prophylactic antibiotics and tetanus prophylaxis as necessary.

In the general assessment of the patient the 'five Bs' may serve as a reminder of the practical sequence of the main investigations of the seriously injured or comatose patient. These comprise attention to:

1. Breathing.
2. Bleeding.
3. Blood pressure.
4. Brain function.
5. Blood analyses.

Bibliography

Brady F. A., Roser S. M. and Hieshima G. B. (1976) Orbital emphysema. *Br. J. Oral Surg.* **1**, 67–71.
Brockehurst G., Gooding M. and James J. (1987) Comprehensive care of patients with head injuries. *Br. Med. J.* **294**, 345–7.
Cawson R.A., McCracken A.W., Marcus P.B. et al. (1989) *Pathology: the Mechanisms of Disease.* 2nd edn. St Louis, Mosby.
Cawson R.A. and Spector, R.G. (1989) *Clinical Pharmacology in Dentistry.* 5th edn. Edinburgh, Churchill Livingstone.
Commission on the Provision of Surgical Services 1988. Response of the Working Party on the Management of Patients with Major Injuries. London, Royal College of Surgeons.
Evans A. S. (1979) The treatment of burns in infancy and childhood. In: Mustarde J. C. (ed.) *Plastic Surgery in Infancy and Childhood.* Edinburgh, Churchill Livingstone, p. 578.
Evans R. F. (1979) Major disasters: the patient with multiple injuries. *Br. J. Hosp. Med.* **22**, 329–32.
Gentleman D., Teasdale G. and Murray L. (1986) Cause of severe head injury and risk of complications. *Br. Med. J.* **292**, 449.
Goubran G. F. (1977-78) Traumatic bilateral abducent nerve palsies. *Br. J. Oral Surg.* **15**, 268–75.
Hindle J. F. (1978) The management of multiple injuries. *Br. J. Hosp. Med.* **19**, 219.
Horton J. M. (1980) Care of the unconscious. *Br. Med. J.* **28**, 638–40.
Jamieson K. G. (1971) *A First Notebook of Head Injury.* London, Butterworths.
Jennett B. (1980) Medical aspects of head injury. *Medicine (UK)* 1641–8.
Kaltman S. I. and Sladen A. (1977) Current concepts of the adult respiratory distress syndrome. *J. Oral Surg.* **35**, 652–9.

Kerr L. (1983) Dental problems in atheletes. *Clinics in Sports Medicine* **2**, 115–22.
Leading Article (1980) CSF rhinorrhoea. *Lancet* **i**, 408–9.
Leading Article (1989) Abnormal blood clotting after head injury. *Lancet* **ii**, 957
Lewis A. F. (1983) *The Management of Acute Head Injury.* London, HMSO.
Lishman W. A. (1973) The psychiatric sequelae of head injury. *Psychol. Med.* **3**, 304–18.
Mason J. K. (1978) *The Pathology of Violent Injury.* London, Arnold.
Masters S. J. et al. (1987) Skull x-ray examinations after head trauma. *N. Engl. J. Med.* **316**, 84–91.
Miller J.D. (1990) Assessing patients with head injuries. *Br. J. Surg.* **77**, 241–2.
Rowe N. L. (1975) Fractures of the facial skeleton. *Br. J. Hosp. Med.* **13**, 319–42.
Schultz R. C. and de Camera D. L. (1984) Athletic facial injuries. *JAMA* **252**, 3395–8.
Scully C. (1985) *Hospital Dental Surgeons Guide.* London, British Dental Journal.
Wachtel T. L., Frank D. H.and Frank H.A. (1981) Management of burns of the head and neck. *Head Neck Surg.* **3**, 458–74.
Williams J. G. P. and Sperryn P. N. (1976) *Sports Medicine.* London, Arnold.
Yates D. W. (1979) Major disasters: surgical triage. *Br. J. Hosp. Med.* **22**, 323–8.
Zook E. G. (1980) *The Primary Care of Facial Injuries.* Littleton, Mass., PSG.

Chapter 14

Psychiatric Disease

Most patients who come for dental treatment are anxious—a normal reaction to an unpleasant experience. It is essential, therefore, not to dismiss patients who will not accept a proposed treatment as simply being 'uncooperative'. Anxious patients may genuinely want dental care but be unable to cooperate, often be unaware of their anxiety and, as a consequence, may be hostile in their responses or behaviour.

Also it is important to be aware that psychiatric disorders are exceedingly common and often under-diagnosed. Some patients are difficult or even impossible to manage because of personality disorders or psychiatric disease but age, cultural and other factors can also cause difficulties in communication and, as a consequence, of management.

In addition to behavioural problems there may be self-induced lesions or other oral symptoms caused by the psychiatric disease or its treatment. Drugs such as monoamine oxidase inhibitors, tricyclic antidepressants, phenothiazines, lithium or barbiturates may influence dental care (Appendix to Chapter 19).

Psychiatric Disorders Caused by Organic Brain Disease

Relatively few patients with psychiatric disorders have recognizable organic brain disease. The clinical features of organic disease differ somewhat from those caused by non-organic mental disorders. Acute organic brain disease is characterized by disorientation and impairment of consciousness. In chronic organic brain disease, amnesia (especially for recent events), inability to concentrate, disorientation in time, place or person and intellectual impairment (including loss of normal social awareness) are common. Other less specific symptoms include mood changes or paranoia.

Anxiety, fear, hallucinations and delusions can be features of either chronic or acute organic brain damage.

DEMENTIA

Dementia is loss of intelligence, memory and cognitive functions.

Dementia is usually associated with ageing but there are many possible causes (*Table 14.1*). Dementia is frequently of unknown or untreatable causes such as

Table 14.1. Organic causes of psychiatric disease

Cerebral infection
  Neurosyphilis
  AIDS
Connective tissue disease
  Systemic lupus erythematosus
  Giant cell arteritis
Neoplasms
  Cerebral tumours
Subdural haematoma
Cerebral degenerative disorders
  Alzheimer's disease
  Cerebrovascular disease
  Multiple sclerosis
  Huntington's chorea
  Parkinson's disease
  Wilson's disease
Systemic disease
  Endocrinopathies
  Alcoholism
  Porphyria
  Vitamin B_{12} deficiency
  Severe liver disease
  Renal dialysis
Drugs (see Table 14.3)
Heavy metal poisoning

Alzheimer's or vascular (multi–infarct) disease, but increasingly now in young persons is caused by HIV infection. Occasionally, dementia is treatable.

Alzheimer's disease

Alzheimer's disease is the most common cause of presenile and senile dementia and is estimated to affect 10–15 per cent of those over 65 and 20 per cent of those over 80. The current attention to it results from the increasing numbers of the elderly and the fact that cerebral atrophy can be recognized by MRI. The characteristic lesions are neurofibrillary tangles and neuritic plaques consisting of dying nerve fibres clustered round deposits of amyloid. Similar changes can be seen in the brains of persons over 40 with Down's syndrome and both have a defect in a gene on chromosome 21 where the amyloid protein gene is located. In Alzheimer's disease there may also be increased amounts of aluminium in the brain.

Clinically, Alzheimer's disease is characterized by gradual, progressive loss of memory and other cognitive activity, leading to inability to recognize family or friends, or carry out the simplest tasks such as combing the hair, general deterioration of motor skills, disorientation and grossly inappropriate or bizarre behaviour. Personality changes, delusions, mood swings or depression and disordered behaviour of many kinds, may be associated.

Diagnosis depends on evidence of progressive dementia in the absence of focal neurological deficits and exclusion of other organic dementing diseases.

Currently there is hope that the chelating agent, desferrioxamine, may reduce the amount of aluminium deposited in the brain and possibly delay the progress of Alzheimer's disease.

Dental aspects. The chief problems of those with Alzheimer's and many other types of dementia are behavioural. In the early stages, dental appointments and instructions are forgotten. Later, there is progressive neglect of oral health as a result of forgetting the need or even how to brush the teeth or clean dentures. Dentures are also frequently lost or broken. Later, deterioration of dental care may lead to destruction of the dentition by caries and periodontal disease and increase the problems of management because of difficulty in eating and halitosis.

While it is still possible to give dental treatment, it should be planned with the knowledge that the patient will sooner or later become unmanageable. Treatment should, as far as possible carried out in a familiar environment with care to explain every procedure before it is carried out and to avoid discomfort. Attention to oral hygiene and preventive care is important but after a time may no longer be practicable.

Creutzfeld–Jacob Disease (CJD)

Creutzfeld–Jacob disease (CJD) is a rare transmissible type of dementia, probably caused by a prion ('slow virus'). The chief risk of CJD is that it can be transmitted by transplantation of human cranial tissue, such as pituitary extracts of human growth hormone. It has also been transmitted by human dura mater which was formerly used for antral repairs and for which it is now banned.

Systemic Disease Causing Psychiatric Disorders

Many endocrine diseases can be complicated by psychiatric disturbances (*Table 14.2*), as may alcoholism, drug abuse or therapy (*Table 14.3*).

Major trauma, surgery or severe life-threatening disease can also frequently cause emotional reactions such as anxiety or depression, or conditions such as compensation neurosis (p. 426).

Table 14.2. Psychiatric complications of endocrine diseases

Endocrine disorder	Psychiatric disorder that may result
Acromegaly	Emotional lability
Addison's disease	Apathy, mild recent amnesia
Corticosteroid therapy	Euphoria or depression. Psychoses with delusions or hallucinations
Cushing's syndrome and disease	Depression, paranoia
Hypoglycaemia (in treated diabetes mellitus)	Confusion, dementia
Hypothyroidism	Impaired concentration, amnesia, depression, paranoia, acute confusion
Hyperparathyroidism with hypercalcaemia	Apathy, depression
Thyrotoxicosis	Anxiety and agitation, depression

Table 14.3. Some drug-induced psychiatric disorders

Disorder	Drugs sometimes responsible	
	Used in medicine	Used in dentistry also
Confusion	Antihypertensives Antihistamines Tricyclics	Benzodiazepines
Aggressive behaviour	Dopa derivatives	Benzodiazepines (in children)
Nightmares or hallucinations	Some antihypertensives	Pentazocine Ketamine
Mania	Levodopa	Aspirin Corticosteroids
Depression	Antihypertensives Contraceptive pill	Pentazocine Corticosteroids
Delirium	Antihypertensives Antitubercular drugs Anticonvulsants Oral hypoglycaemics	Procaine penicillin Sulphonamides
Paranoia	Antihypertensives Anticonvulsants Amphetamines	Ephedrine Corticosteroids

Personality Disorders

Personality disorders are chronic peculiarities of character or maladaptation to life. These disorders shade into neuroses or psychoses, but insight is not lost and most patients manage to pursue a fairly normal lifestyle, though they are frequently made unhappy by the fact that their inadequacies prevent them from forming satisfactory relationships or cause them to be in frequent conflict with others. Severe personality disorders can lead to grossly antisocial criminal behaviour (*Table 14.4*).

Handling patients with personality disorders requires patience and tolerance, and the exercise of tact and skills which only come with appreciation of the

Table 14.4. Personality disorders

Disorder	Characteristics
Antisocial	Selfish, callous, disloyal, in conflict with everyone and everything
Asthenic	Tired all the time
Cyclothymic	Rapid alternation between depression and elation
Explosive	Rage or aggression on minor provocation
Hysterical	Immature, manipulative, attention-seeking, shallow interpersonal relationships
Inadequate	Continually dependent on others, often anxious and depressed
Obsessive	Chronically worried about standards and self-image; unable to relax and often depressed
Paranoid	Suspicious, litigious, lacking humour, blames others
Passive–aggressive	Stubborn, obstructive, awkward, anti-authority
Schizoid	Secretive, isolated, lacks friends

Adapted from: Adams R. D. (1980) In: Isselbacher K. J. et al. (ed.) *Harrison's Principles of Internal Medicine*, 9th ed. Tokyo, McGraw Hill-Kogakusha, p. 68.

existence of these disorders and with experience. Even then, little progress may be possible. A dental surgeon may also have a personality disorder and find himself in conflict with others including colleagues—often to his disadvantage—and may find it difficult not to antagonize patients and staff.

Psychosomatic Diseases (Psychogenic Disorders)

Psychosomatic diseases are bodily (somatic) disorders thought to be initiated or aggravated by psychological factors. Chronic emotional problems such as anxiety and depression may be contributory.

Typical examples of disorders in which there is often a psychosomatic element are asthma and migraine. Disorders such as anorexia nervosa, psychogenic vomiting and, sometimes, obesity, may be psychosomatic or hysterical in nature, and depression may be responsible for oral complaints such as atypical facial pain and burning mouth.

Functional and Other Disorders

'Functional disorders' is a term used for those that have no demonstrable organic cause. There are two broad groups, the neuroses and the psychoses. A neurosis is a disease in which contact with reality and insight are retained and there are no bizarre symptoms such as delusions or hallucinations. A psychosis, by contrast, is characterized by impairment of contact with reality and sometimes phenomena such as delusions or hallucinations.

There are, however, no defects of memory, intellect or consciousness—features which suggest organic disease.

NEUROSES

Neurotic illnesses, particularly anxiety and depressive states, are by far the most common types of psychiatric disease (*Table 14.5*), but frequently remain unrecognized or untreated. Nearly everyone becomes anxious or depressed at some time and these mood changes must be accepted as part of life. However, if the symptoms or signs are out of proportion in severity or duration, to an adverse event, they suggest psychiatric disease.

Depressive Neurosis

The main manifestations of depression appear to relate to changes in the hypothalamic centres that govern food intake, libido, circadian rhythms and various thalamic hormones. Hypercortisolism is common. However, the immediate mechanism of depression appears to be the result of depleted cerebral amine levels. The latter are raised by antidepressant drugs and, more rapidly, by electroconvulsive therapy.

Table 14.5. Neuroses and psychoses

	Features
Neurosis	
Depressive neurosis	Pessimism, excessive self-criticism, low self-regard, depression of mood, sleep disturbances and physical complaints, misery
Anxiety neurosis	Diffuse anxiety, irritability and physical complaints e.g. palpitations
Phobic neurosis	Intense irrational fears of particular situations or objects
Obsessional neurosis	Preoccupation with thoughts or acts
Hysterical neurosis	Conversion type—physical symptoms; dissociative type— alterationin consciousness not associated with organic disease
Hypochondriacal neurosis	Morbid preoccupation with disease and physical complaints
Psychosis	
Manic-depressive psychosis	Mainly depression but may be manic episodes for weeks, months or years
Schizophrenia	Disorder of thought, behaviour and affect with hallucinations, delusions and illusions
Korsakoff's psychosis	Recent amnesia and confabulation

Adapted from: Adams R. D. (1980) In: Isselbacher K. J. et al. (ed.) *Harrison's Principles of Internal Medicine*, 9th ed. Tokyo, McGraw Hill-Kogakusha, p. 68.

Approximately 5 per cent of adults suffer from depression at some stage in their life. The illness is characterized by lowering of mood (affect) and can range from complete apathy towards the normal more pleasurable aspects of life, to utter despair or misery so extreme that death is sought as a release. Disturbances of bodily functions such as sleep, appetite or sexual activity and slowing of thought and action (psychomotor retardation) are frequently associated. Agitation, anxiety or crying attacks may be prominent, but symptoms often vary in severity from day to day, or in less severe cases may be relatively effectively repressed. In the latter case, drugs that have a releasing effect often allow latent depression to become apparent. Thus, the tearful drunk is a well known phenomenon but depression following the taking of diazepam is usually ascribed, unfairly, to an effect of the drug itself. In other cases relief from depression is sought in alcohol and leads to alcoholism (Chapter 19).

Reactive depression follows some unpleasant experience, such as a bereavement, but symptoms are disproportionate in intensity or duration.

Endogenous depression is characterized by depressive symptoms unrelated to environmental stress, but many now believe that these are artificial distinctions. A few patients with depression have repeated mood swings from depression to mania (manic-depressive psychosis, p. 428) and are sometimes classified as having bipolar depression. 'Unipolar depression' is the term used when mania is absent.

The features of major depressive illness are shown in *Table 14.5*, but it must be appreciated that the clinical manifestations of depression are frequently atypical. It is widely believed for example that so–called myalgic encephalitis (ME) is largely due to depression and may respond to antidepressant drugs if patients can be persuaded to take them. A swing to a manic phase after antidepressant treatment has also been reported in a patient with ME.

Involutional melancholia, which is often characterized by severe anxiety and hypochondriasis, is a depressive illness beginning in later life and mainly affects women.

Depression may also accompany other psychiatric diseases such as schizophrenia or be caused by drugs such as reserpine, methyldopa, fenfluramine, corticosteroids or oral contraceptives; by withdrawal of drugs such as amphetamines or antidepressants; by Parkinsonism; by endocrinopathies; by viral infections such as influenza, viral hepatitis or infectious mononucleosis; or by various malignant diseases.

Seasonal Affective Disorder (SAD) is a type of winter depression, recently recognized by psychiatrists. It is apparently related to deprivation of sunlight and characterized particularly by lethargy, excessive desire for sleep and craving for carbohydrates. However, long before this complaint was given a name, most people recognized that long periods of grey weather were likely to make them miserable.

General management of depressive illness (*Fig.* 14.1)

Treatment of depression should be carried out by specialists, especially as there may be a risk of suicide and the level of risk is frequently difficult to assess. If

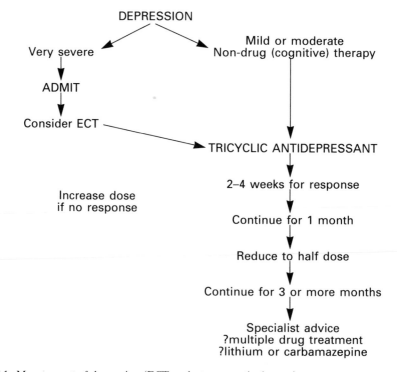

Fig. 14.1. Management of depression (ECT = electromagnetic therapy).

there is a risk of suicide or there are psychotic features such as delusions or hallucination, admission to hospital is desirable. However, it is frequently difficult to persuade a depressed patient of the need for psychiatric treatment.

The monoamine oxidase inhibitors (MAOIs) were the first effective antidepressants but, though many newer agents have been introduced, still have a place in treatment. The MAOIs are thought by some to be particularly useful in specific cases and are used, either alone or in combination with tricyclic antidepressants, in spite of possible interactions between these two groups of drugs. The commonly used MAOIs are phenelzine and tranylcypromine.

The most serious adverse effects of MAOIs are liver damage (particularly with iproniazid) and drug or food interactions. Hypertensive crises have resulted from interaction of MAOIs with foods containing tyramine, particularly cheese, but also with yeast products, chocolate, bananas, broad beans, some red wines and beer, pickled herring or caviar. Drugs such as pethidine and other opioids are potentiated (*see* Appendix to Chapter 19). Interactions of MAOIs with pethidine are the most dangerous and have sometimes been fatal. Ephedrine and similar drugs often present in nasal decongestants or cold remedies, may cause severe hypertension. Dry mouth and hypotension are not uncommon side-effects of MAOIs.

Tricyclic derivatives despite their undesirable side-effects are probably the most effective antidepressants and have stood the test of time. Their onset of action is, however, slow and they may take 4 weeks to exert their full effect. The action of tricyclic antidepressants is dose-dependent and lack of effect is often the result of failure to achieve adequate plasma levels.

The most commonly used tricyclic antidepressives are amitriptyline, dothiepin and imipramine. Sedation is a common side-effect, particularly with amitriptyline, but this may be an advantage if the patient is agitated (*Table 14.6*). Various other tricyclics have particular advantages: imipramine for

Table 14.6. Tricylic antidepressants

Drug	Specialist comments*
Amitriptyline	More sedative and anti-muscarinic than many. Caution with general anaesthesia
Amoxapine	May cause tardive dyskinesia
Butriptyline	Less sedative than some
Clomipramine	Possibly less sedative
Desipramine	Possibly less sedative and antimuscarinic effects
Dothiepin	Sedative
Doxepin	Sedative
Imipramine	Possibly less sedative than most but more antimuscarinic
Lofepramine	Avoid in renal or hepatic disease
Nortriptyline	Like desipramine
Protriptyline	Has a stimulant effect
	Photosensitive rashes
Trimipramine	

*Up to 4 weeks are required before symptom control can be expected. Reduce doses in the elderly. Dysrhythmias and heart block may be seen as well as drowsiness, dry mouth, urinary retention and constipation (antimuscarinic actions)

example, is mildly stimulating and clomipramine appears to be useful where there are obsessional or phobic problems. Tricyclic antidepressants have strong antimuscarinic effects and therefore cause dry mouth, constipation, impaired visual accommodation and sometimes postural hypotension. More serious side-effects include dysrhythmias, and tricyclics are absolutely contraindicated if the patient has had a recent myocardial infarct. Doxepin (similar to imipramine) is the drug of choice if there is evidence of cardiovascular disease. Side-effects of the tricyclics are more serious in the elderly.

Mianserin causes less antimuscarinic effects, but frequently causes dizziness or, occasionally, marrow depression and is thought by many to be less effective.

Newer agents include maprotiline, trazodone, viloxazine, fluoxetine and fluvoxamine, but full assessment of their effectiveness and toxicity takes a considerable time. Fluoxetine for example, is regarded by some in Britain as a valuable drug, but in the USA its use has allegedly been associated with aggressive behaviour, including murders. Flupenthixol, a neuroleptic, also has antidepressant activity.

Electroconvulsive therapy (ECT) is sometimes given, where drugs have been ineffective, or where there is strong risk of suicide. Amnesia is the main side-effect.

Lithium is used mainly for the prophylaxis of manic–depressive illness, but carbamazepine is increasingly used when there is no response to lithium. Either may sometimes also be used for unipolar depression.

Dental aspects of depression

Oral symptoms associated with depression or its treatment.   The most common complaint of depressed patients under treatment is of dry mouth, especially as a result of the use of tricyclic antidepressants. This may predispose to oral candidosis and increased caries activity. The effect can occasionally result in ascending suppurative parotitis. The most effective treatment is to change the antidepressant to another, such as mianserin which has little anticholinergic activity, but if this is not acceptable the dry mouth should be managed as in Sjögren's syndrome (Chapter 7). Other drugs which may add to the xerostomia, such as antihistamines, hyoscine or other atropine-like drugs, should therefore be avoided. Both MAOIs and tricyclics have been reported occasionally to cause facial dyskinesias (*see* Appendix to Chapter 19) and prolonged use of flupenthixol can lead to intractable tardive dyskinesia.

Bodily complaints, often related to the mouth, are common in depression and the dental surgeon should appreciate the possibility of a psychiatric basis for such oral complaints.

Depression is associated especially with the following painful disorders of the orofacial region:

1. Atypical facial pain.
2. Burning mouth or sore tongue (oral dysaesthesia).
3. Temporomandibular pain-dysfunction syndrome may occasionally be associated with depression and is also discussed here.

Other oral complaints may be delusional and include:

Discharges (of fluid, slime or powder coming into the mouth)
Dry mouth
Spots or lumps
Sialorrhoea
Halitosis
Disturbed taste sensation

It must be emphasized that the recognition of psychogenic symptoms is usually diagnosis by exclusion, but it is important to try to recognize them, however limited and subjective the methods may be. The symptoms cause real enough suffering to the patient and should, if possible, be relieved. Unnecessary surgery must also be avoided.

Features that may suggest that symptoms are psychogenic but not necessarily depressive may include any of the following.

1. *Absence of organic cause or physical signs:* The affected area typically appears normal and if, for example, a putatively diseased tooth is extracted, the symptoms are unaffected.

2. *Character and duration of the symptoms:* Many complain of persistence of pain or other symptoms for very long periods, sometimes for years. Clearly, after such periods any organic cause would have become apparent.

3. *Character of the pain:* The symptoms may be bizarre, such as 'drawing' or 'gripping' sensations or apparently exaggerated 'unbearable' pain in spite of normal physical health or often sleep. The symptom is often also of fixed and unchangeable character, often for very long periods.

4. *Distribution of the pain:* The site of the pain or other symptom is often somewhat vague and the patient may be unable to put a finger precisely upon the painful area. Alternatively the distribution of the pain may not follow an anatomical pattern. Very frequently, however, atypical facial pain is in the general region of the maxilla.

5. *Provocation of symptoms:* Symptoms are usually not provoked by recognizable stimuli such as hot or cold foods, or mastication. However, psychogenic sore tongue is often said to be aggravated by sharp flavoured foods.

6. *Use of analgesics:* In contrast to patients with severe organic pain who typically reach for analgesics, occasionally to the extent of analgesic abuse, many patients with atypical facial pain make little attempt to get relief from analgesics. Alternatively analgesics, after a brief trial, are said to be totally ineffective.

7. *Other signs or symptoms of psychiatric disturbance:* Patients' personality and manner are highly variable. Some appear obviously neurotic but few are overtly depressed. Indeed the organic symptoms can be regarded as more acceptable substitutes ('depressive equivalents') for more typical manifestations

of depression. These varied clinical pictures are discussed more fully below. Patients may have several so–called psychosomatic complaints at the same time.

8. *Response to psychoactive drugs:* In some patients the response to antidepressant drugs is dramatic, with relief of symptoms and striking general improvement in mood, after the drug has had time to take effect. However, effective dosage varies widely and in the case of tricyclic antidepressants the response is generally related to the plasma levels achieved. Thus doses may sometimes have to be very large before an effect is evident.

Nevertheless, it is clear that there is a hard core of patients who over the course of years go from specialist to specialist without positive results from innumerable investigations or response to any form of treatment. Indeed, the patient may seem to take a sort of perverse pride in the resistance of the pain to the challenge of medical science.

Psychogenic symptoms can generally be regarded as a patient's plea for help or attention. This occasionally becomes distressingly apparent in a patient who at the start appears well-balanced and self-controlled—even occasionally joking about the symptoms—but after a little while is crying uncontrollably. At the other extreme there are patients who reject the possibility of mental illness and aggressively assert that *'It is not due to nerves'* (even if no such suggestion has been made) and typically also reject the idea of specialist psychiatric help, however obliquely and sympathetically this is suggested.

Examples of these varied clinical pictures therefore include the following:

1. The patient may be overtly depressed and cries readily or is obviously having difficulty in restraining tears. Alternatively, initial self-control is followed by unrestrainable crying.

2. The patient may complain (in effect) of depression by saying that the pain or other symptom makes them miserable.

3. Some when allowed to discuss their symptoms relate them to trouble with the family or at work.

4. A few are already having, or have had, antidepressant drugs but the atypical symptoms have not been controlled.

5. A few have associated bizarre (delusional) symptoms such as 'powder' or 'slime' coming out of the sore or painful area as mentioned earlier.

6. Some, given the chance of a sympathetic hearing, gratefully expand on their problems and welcome the suggestion of psychiatric help.

7. The most difficult and relatively common group is the rejectors, who are unable to accept the idea of psychiatric disturbance and refuse to have the possibility investigated or to accept that drug—which they equate with drugs of dependence—may be helpful.

It should not need to be emphasized that, where psychogenic symptoms are suspected, discussion with the patient must be conducted patiently, gently and sympathetically. Surprisingly, this may perhaps be the first opportunity that patients have had to unburden themselves. Unfortunately some doctors are at least as intolerant of 'neurotic' patients as many members of the public. This is not to suggest that the dentist should attempt to be an amateur psychiatrist but an effort must be made to distinguish psychogenic symptoms from organic disease. It is probably unnecessary to inquire into details of family relationships or broken homes. If a patient is depressed, the cause is often as much the patient's susceptibility to depression as the so–called life situation. In any case, amelioration of the life situation is unlikely to be feasible, and it is only too common for those so affected to be unable to overcome their difficulties without help.

Finally, it is essential to appreciate that, however neurotic a patient's manner may be, the symptoms may have an organic cause. The concurrence of emotional and physical disease is one of the most difficult problems in medicine. The organic basis of the symptoms in many cases remains undiscovered until severe manifestations become obvious later. A striking example is the transient and apparently hysterical signs and symptoms of early multiple sclerosis. The most careful investigation is therefore essential to exclude possible organic causes before the diagnosis of psychogenic disorder is made (*Fig.* 14.2).

Atypical facial pain (psychogenic facial pain).   Headache and facial pain are common symptoms most frequently caused by dental or other local infections (Chapter 12). However, there is a group of patients, mainly women, who have continuous pain, particularly in the maxillary region, in the absence of any detectable organic cause. The pain is usually a dull ache, albeit with intermittent episodic exacerbations. The pain has no obvious precipitating factors, although it may be attributed to dental disease or treatment, and is rarely completely relieved by analgesics. The pain may waken the patient in the early morning. Sometimes the pain may appear as a hysterical conversion neurosis and many patients have obsessional personality traits.

Organic causes for the pain must be excluded; psychiatric assistance and antidepressant treatment are then needed. Since many of these patients have already rejected the idea of mental illness, it may be difficult to persuade them of the need for psychiatric help. In some cases it is helpful to make it clear that depression is both common and is an illness like any other—indeed worse than many—and, like other illnesses, can also cause physical symptoms. Tricyclic

Psoriasis from head to in between toes
Perpetual scream in left ear
Spasmodic pressure above left ear
Constant ulcers in mouth and on tongue
Asthma bronchitis severe bouts of indigestion
Sore mouth due to grinding of bottom right molar
Severe pain under crutch after any exertion
Constant irritation around back passage
Spasmodic bleeding piles

Medicines taken internally
Predicalone
Ventolin
Asilone suspension
Bronchipax

Fig. 14.2. Note as presented by a patient. Such histories vary in length, detail and imagination and sometimes suggest that the patient is disturbed (*maladie du petit papier*).

antidepressants such as imipramine, amitriptyline, or dothiepin may be effective, but monoamine oxidase inhibitors may be needed.

Idiopathic odontalgia may be a variant of atypical facial pain and is characterized by complaint of severe throbbing pain in one or several teeth which are hypersensitive to any stimulus. Extractions typically lead to transference of the symptoms to adjacent teeth.

Oral dysaesthesia. A complaint of a burning tongue or mouth is the common type of oral dysaesthesia, although any part of the mouth may be involved. Patients are mostly middle-aged or elderly women who have a burning sensation that comes on after waking and increases in intensity during the day. The symptoms may sometimes be relieved by chewing or drinking.

Dry mouth, disturbed taste sensations, or delusions of halitosis are other dysaesthesias and are often also manifestations of a depressive neurosis. There is often cancerphobia, or anxiety about the possibility, for example, of venereal disease.

Organic causes, particularly deficiency states, candidosis and diabetes, must be excluded by investigation. Once this has been done antidepressants may be helpful.

Temporomandibular pain-dysfunction syndrome. This syndrome (with its many synonyms, such as *facial pain-dysfunction, myofascial pain-dysfunction* or *facial arthromyalgia),* is a common problem predominantly affecting young women. Some believe that depression may be a contributory factor and there may be a greater frequency of migraine, rhinitis, peptic ulcer and irritable bowel syndrome associated.

There is typically dull pain, usually in front of the temporomandibular joint, and sometimes joint clicking, alone or in various combinations. The pain tends to radiate over the masseter and temporalis muscles and sometimes occipitally or cervically, and there may be tenderness in the masticatory muscles including the pterygoids. The mandible often deviates towards the affected side on opening and there may be trismus ('locking'). There may be an audible click or palpable crepitus in the joint but radiography shows no significant abnormality. Nevertheless, organic disease must be excluded.

Patients frequently grind or clench their teeth or develop various (parafunctional) habits, such as pencil chewing, and there is often faceting on the teeth, ridging of the tongue margins and buccal mucosa at the occlusal line, and sometimes signs of lip-chewing. Occlusal anomalies, especially loss of molars, may be present, as in normal persons.

The psychiatric basis of the temporomandibular pain-dysfunction syndrome is controversial, but it may be seen in ambitious obsessional personalities, in anxiety states, or in agitated depression. Treatment consists of reassurance and use of a bite–raising appliance to provide a free, sliding occlusion. Mild anxiolytics such as diazepam (also a muscle relaxant) may be helpful but should only be given for a limited period and may need to be supplemented with analgesics. If there is evidence of depression, tricyclic antidepressants such as dothiepin may be of more use. Overall, however, a temporary bite guard, providing free, sliding occlusion, alone is likely to relieve symptoms effectively.

In summary, the diagnosis of depression when manifested as orofacial symptoms is difficult, as the patients often have no typical depressive symptoms. This is often the result of repression of symptoms caused in turn by shame or guilt at the idea of mental illness—a particularly British and puritanical attitude where 'keeping a stiff upper lip' and 'pulling oneself together' in adversity, are traditional and valued attributes.

Dental aspects. The features aiding recognition of depression have been suggested above and the dental surgeon should be alert to this possibility, particularly where the patient appears withdrawn, difficult or aggressive, or where there are oral complaints of the types described earlier. Great tact, patience and a sympathetic but unpatronizing manner are needed in handling depressed patients. Dental treatment is preferably deferred until the depression is under control.

Patients on MAOIs are at risk from general anaesthesia since prolonged respiratory depression may result. Any CNS depressant, especially opioids and phenothiazines, given to patients on MAOIs (or within 21 days of their withdrawal) may precipitate coma. Pethidine is particularly dangerous (*see* Appendix to Chapter 19).

Indirectly acting sympathomimetic agents such as ephedrine or cocaine can interact with MAOIs to cause hypertension, and must therefore not be used.

MAOIs and tricyclics can cause postural hypotension and the patient should not be stood immediately upright if he has been lying flat during dental treatment, but the chair should slowly be brought upright.

In the case of tricyclic antidepressants *intravenous* adrenaline and noradrenaline have been shown experimentally to cause hypertension. Severe hypertension can also result from high concentrations (1:20000) of noradrenaline in local anaesthetic agents, whether or not the patient is receiving antidepressants. However, no clinical evidence has been found to confirm that adrenaline in local anaesthetics causes either hypertension or significant dysrhythmias in patients receiving tricyclic antidepressants.

In spite of reported statements to the contrary there is no clinical evidence of interactions between either MAOIs or tricyclic antidepressants and adrenaline in local anaesthetic agents used in dentistry. However, atropinics are potentiated by tricyclic antidepressants.

Chronic Fatigue Syndrome ('Myalgic Encephalomyelitis')

Chronic fatigue syndrome is a non-specific disorder characterized by lack of energy, tiredness or muscle and joint pains after minimal effort, emotional lability, poor concentration and memory and often other symptoms. Though it is widely thought to be a new disease this clinical picture was described by Beard in 1867 and termed by him 'neurasthenia'. However, the symptoms in many ways resemble those of the recovery phase of a viral infection such as influenza. In the US a in particular, a viral cause is still being sought and the complaint is termed *postviral fatigue syndrome* . Claims for EBV, herpesvirus 6 and Coxsackie B having a causative role, have not been substantiated and no consistent association with any virus has yet been found. Nevertheless most patients insist that 'ME' is a viral infection, even though this is of no help to them as there is no effective treatment for most viral infections or their after–effects.

Tests showing disorders of muscle function or any other organic lesion have also not been substantiated. By contrast, those with organic neuromuscular diseases do not have the mental symptoms characteristic of 'ME'. In Britain most authorities believe that most cases are due, as the symptoms suggest, to depression. Fifty to eighty per cent of patients, on rigorous psychiatric assessment, have been found to fulfil the criteria for psychiatric disorder and depression in particular. Though the complaint may be heterogeneous and have a variety of causes, a typical characteristic is these patients, like many patients with more obvious depression, strongly reject any suggestion that they are depressed and the idea that depression is a 'real diagnosis'. For this reason, patients prefer to be said to have the more glamorous sounding 'myalgic encephalomyelitis', even though there is no evidence of a neurological lesion. Most also refuse to take antidepressives, but those who have been persuaded to do so frequently improve. One patient is even on record as having undergone reversal into mania as a result.

Though fatigue may persist for a long period it is ultimately self–limiting. In the interim, patients need emotional support and one authority has suggested that this need is the basis for the complaint. Controversy persists as to whether exercise or rest is better for the myalgia. When assessment indicates that depression is present, patients should be persuaded to have antidepressive treatment and are likely to benefit from it.

Other Psychogenic Syndromes Related to Dentistry

So-called chronic candidosis syndromeis discussed on p. 492 and mercury allergy syndrome in Chapter 10.

Anxiety States

Anxiety can be generated by such ordeals as public speaking or solo musical performances, examinations or interviews. Anxiety can cause severe physical effects as a result of overwhelming sympathetic activity: thus public speakers have been shown to develop severe pre-ischaemic ECG changes, while instrumental soloists may freeze and be unable to perform. These patients respond better to beta-blocking agents (for example propranolol) than to benzodiazepines.

Anxiety Neuroses

Although fear and anxiety are normal reactions to stressful situations, excessive anxiety, often amounting to panic, characterizes the anxiety neuroses. These may develop from long-standing personality disorders. Sometimes the anxiety is centred about a specific situation and is then known as a 'phobia'. Tension, agitation, hypochondriasis, rapid breathing, palpitations, giddiness, tremor, sweating, flushing and dry mouth are common features, while hostility readily develops if the anxious patient is forced to face threats such as unwelcome dental treatment.

General management of anxiety neuroses

As a broad generalization, anxiety can be characterized by agitation and a diffuse sense of dread. Physical signs as described earlier may be associated but are usually not the chief problem. It is important to exclude organic causes such as hyperthyroidism or hypoglycaemia. Anxiety may also develop as a consequence of withdrawal of alcohol, other drugs of abuse, benzodiazepines or other sedatives (Chapter 19), but also abuse of such drugs may, in part at least, result from an attempt to gain relief from an anxiety neurosis. Reassurance, explanation and the encouragement of family support are therefore the first lines of treatment.

Benzodiazepines are the drugs most frequently given for the relief of anxiety since they are safer and more effective than most. However, they should only be given for a short period because of development of tolerance and the risk of dependence.

There are no great differences between the various benzodiazepines, apart from their duration of action, but lorazepam is sometimes useful for its briefer activity than diazepam. Newer drugs such as clobazam appear to have advantages over diazepam and may cause less impairment of judgement. Beta-blockers are preferred if there are severe somatic symptoms (for example palpitations) and some patients benefit from low doses of phenothiazines (chlorpromazine), butyrophenones (haloperidol) or thioxanthenes (flupenthixol). Antidepressants, especially MAOI, can lessen anxiety, and have the advantage of less risk of inducing drug dependence than the benzodiazepines.

Dental aspects of anxiety states

Oral manifestations such as a complaint of dry mouth, lip-chewing or bruxism may be seen and sometimes cancerphobia is an indication of an anxiety state. Anxiety is a normal reaction to dental treatment; diazepam or preferably, temazepam 10 mg orally on the night before and 1 hour before dental treatment can be used to supplement gentle sympathetic handling and reassurance of the anxious patient. Intravenous sedation with midazolam, or relative analgesia using nitrous oxide and oxygen, are also useful.

Dental treatment is otherwise usually straightforward unless there are difficulties as a result of: (a) alcoholism or drug dependence, (b) drug treatment with major tranquillizers, MAOIs or tricyclics.

Phobias (Phobic Neuroses)

A phobia is a morbid fear or anxiety out of all proportion to the threat. Phobic neuroses differ from anxiety neuroses in that the phobic anxiety arises only in specific circumstances, whereas patients with anxiety neuroses are generally anxious. Most patients are female. Phobias may also be a minor part of a more severe disorder such as depression, obsessive neurosis, anxiety state, personality disorder or schizophrenia.

Agoraphobia (fear of leaving sheltered familiar places) and claustrophobia (fear of closed spaces) are probably the most common phobic disorders. Social phobias (such as fear of performing social duties in public) can severely limit normal activities. Most phobias are, however, centred on more understandable threats such as flying or anaesthetics and, under these circumstances, normal life is possible if such threats are avoided.

General management of phobic states

Phobias can sometimes be controlled by anxiolytic drugs. Behaviour therapy aims at desensitization by slow and gradual exposure to the frightening situation. Implosion is a technique where patients are asked to imagine a persistently frightening situation for 1 or 2 hours. Antidepressants, especially tricyclics, are used if there is a significant depressive component.

Dental aspects of phobias

Patients with a true phobic neurosis about dental treatment are uncommon, but when seen demand great patience on the part of the dentist. The main aids are the use of anxiolytics such as oral diazepam, supplemented if necessary with intravenous or inhalational sedation during dental treatment. Most of the comments above, concerning anxiety states, apply to the phobic states.

Obsessional Neuroses (Obsessive–Compulsive Neuroses)

Obsessional personality traits are not uncommon, especially amongst dental and medical personnel, and are often salutary. However, the obsessional neuroses can cause significant disruption of normal life—for example, the dental surgeon who felt compelled to telephone his patients late at night because he was obsessed with the notion that, having prepared the cavity, he might have forgotten to place the filling.

Obsessional thoughts are those that come repeatedly into consciousness against the patient's will, are usually unpleasant, but are always recognized as the patient's own thoughts. Such thoughts are not, however, accepted by the patients as harmless or inevitable and an internal struggle against them leads to obsessional symptoms. To counteract the thoughts, secondary ritualistic thought or behaviour patterns (compulsions) are developed (for example, continually checking that doors are locked). The obsessional thoughts may also in turn generate depression.

Typical obsessions are the repeated questioning of decisions, the fear of harm or harming, or the fear of dirtiness or contamination. Obsessional symptoms are also associated with disorders such as depression, schizophrenia or, rarely, organic brain disease.

Obsessional patients are often intelligent, many are unmarried and many have a premorbid state such as an uncertain and vacillating, or alternatively, a stubborn, rigid, morose and irritable personality.

General management of obsessional states

Treatment is often difficult. Antidepressants, especially the tricyclics, are useful when there is also depression, and clomipramine in particular seems to be effective. The benzodiazepines may be useful when anxiety is predominant.

Dental aspects of obsessional states

It is questionable whether true obsessions become centred on the mouth but they may, for example, result in compulsive toothbrushing or excessive use of antiseptic mouthwashes. Occasional patients become obsessed with the possibility of infections in the mouth (as for example a patient who was obsessed with the idea that his Fordyce spots were thrush) and refuse to be reassured.

Hysterical States

Three main hysterical states exist: hysterical personality disorders, hysterical neuroses and acute hysterical psychoses.

Hysterical neuroses

Hysterical conversion neurosis is characterized by physical complaints that have no demonstrable organic basis, such as pain, anaesthesia, dysphagia, fainting, fits, paralysis or tremor. Dissociative states are characterized by disturbances of consciousness or identity (but no physical symptoms) in the absence of demonstrable organic disease. Amnesia, states of fugue (when the patient wanders aimlessly away), or (rarely) multiple personalities are examples of dissociative states. There are, however, no basic differences between these two types of hysterical neurosis and most patients at some time exhibit both.

Hysterical neuroses mainly affect females—sometimes those working in medical or paramedical occupations. Conversion symptoms frequently result in patients being submitted to operation and may as a result have multiple scars. It is often difficult to establish that the patient is gaining something by the illness, although in compensation neurosis the nature of the potential gain is easily recognized.

Munchausen syndrome is the term given to a disorder in which patients go to considerable length to fabricate histories and simulate symptoms apparently for the sake of undergoing operations. This may be done repeatedly, even occasionally, by assuming false names and travelling to many hospitals scattered about the country. Ultimately the patient may become extensively scarred and develop abdominal adhesions or other complications. Munchausen syndrome is categorized as a conversion syndrome by some but may be a delusional state.

Munchausen syndrome–by–proxy is the term given to a parent who invents symptoms in and demands medical or surgical treatment for a child.

Compensation neurosis usually follows an accident (especially a head injury), or operation, and is characterized by paralysis, chronic pain (often headache) or other symptoms of obscure origin and of no obvious organic cause. Men and women are equally susceptible, there is no previous history and the lack of insight is less convincing than in hysteria. Settlement of the claim for compensation typically results in rapid disappearance of the symptoms.

Panic disorder is the term given to recurrent, unpredictable attacks of severe anxiety with physical symptoms such as palpitations, chest pain, dyspnoea, paraesthesiae and sweating. Many or most of the symptoms may result from hyperventilation (Chapter 18) but mitral valve prolapse (Chapter 2) may be found in up to 50 per cent of these patients.

Eating Disorders

The main eating disorders apart from obesity are (a) *anorexia nervosa* and (b) *bulimia.* These disorders are relatively common, particularly among white females in the higher socioeconomic groups. Obesity (Chapter 10) may be consequence of another type of eating disorder.

Anorexia Nervosa

Anorexia nervosa is characterized by severe weight loss due to self-starvation and is mainly a disease of previously healthy adolescent girls. The incidence may be as high as 1 per cent of all schoolgirls in the United Kingdom.

The disorder, which is regarded as an hysterical neurosis, is associated with a preoccupation to be thin. The body image appears to be so distorted that, even when emaciated, the patient still regards herself as too fat.

Anorectic patients usually refuse to eat or, if forced to do so, often induce vomiting. Some patients cannot control their voluntary food restriction and have episodes in which they gorge food (bulimia) and then induce vomiting. Menstrual upset is an early feature. Peripheral cyanosis and coldness with bradycardia and amenorrhoea are common, as are depression which lacks the classic features of depression in adults, and obsessional features (*Table 14.7*).

Anorexia nervosa may be complicated by anaemia, endocrine disturbances, peripheral oedema and electrolyte depletion (especially hypokalaemia).

General management

Some 2–5 per cent of cases may be fatal. However, if treatment is initiated early, prognosis is usually good. Anorexia nervosa must be distinguished from nutritional disorders, depression and Turner's syndrome. There is no specific treatment. Patients are usually admitted to hospital if weight loss is rapid or persistent. Psychiatric care is required: anxiolytics may be useful.

Table 14.7. Features of anorexia nervosa

1. Females under 25 years, mainly
2. Pronounced anorexia overriding hunger
3. Weight loss
4. No other organic or psychiatric disease
5. Sometimes self-induced vomiting (especially after orgies of eating)*
6. Amenorrhoea
7. Bradycardia

*Regarded as a different disorder from anorexia nervosa by some (bulimia), but having the same effects.

Dental aspects

Parotid enlargement (sialosis) and angular stomatitis may develop, as in other forms of starvation. The parotid swellings tend to subside if the patient returns to a normal diet. Erosion of teeth (perimylolysis) may result from repeated vomiting. The erosion is usually most severe on lingual, palatal and occlusal surfaces. Oral ulcers or abrasions, particularly in the soft palate, may be caused by fingers or other objects used to induce vomiting. Full-coverage plastic splints may be needed to protect the teeth and it may help to fill these splints with magnesium hydroxide. Topical daily sodium fluoride applications or a 0.05 per cent sodium fluoride mouthwash combined with bicarbonate after each vomiting incident may lessen dental damage.

Anaemia and the possibility of hypokalaemia and consequent dysrhythmias must be remembered if a general anaesthetic is considered necessary for dental treatment.

Bulimia ('ox-hunger')

Bulimia has been reported in up to 10 per cent of young adult women. Bulimics, in contrast to anorectics, may be of normal or near-normal weight. Uncontrolled and unpredictable ingestion of huge amounts of foods (usually soft sweet or starchy foods) is followed by vomiting. Bulimia may be seen in isolation, or in anorexia nervosa, and appears to be stress-related. Erosion of the teeth, sore throat, angular stomatitis and painless swelling of the parotid glands may be seen and there may be severe caries. Dental care is as described above for anorexia nervosa.

Hypochondriacal Neuroses

Minor degrees of hypochondriasis are common, especially among the elderly. However, hypochondriacal neurosis is a morbid preoccupation with physical symptoms or bodily functions, in which minute details are related incessantly.

There is no organic disease or physiological disturbance. Most patients are depressed and some are deluded.

428 MEDICAL PROBLEMS IN DENTISTRY

General management

Organic disease should always be excluded, as should schizophrenia. Reassurance and supportive care are then needed and antidepressant drugs may be helpful.

Dental aspects

The common oral hypochondriacal symptoms are dry or burning mouth, disturbed taste and oral or facial pain.

PSYCHOSES

Manic-depressive Psychosis

Mania is a recurrent disorder in which most patients also have depressive (*bipolar*) episodes (manic-depression). Between attacks the patient is usually normal, but episodes last for months or years. The disorder usually appears first in young adults and its onset in the elderly may indicate organic disease such as a neoplasm, or an effect of drugs, such as corticosteroids, cocaine or alcohol. The manic state is characterized by elation, irritability, belligerence, over-confidence, generalized hyperactivity, decreased sleep, flight of ideas and lack of restraint in financial matters or social behaviour.

General management

Psychiatric care is required and lithium is the most effective drug, but blood levels must be monitored and patients with cardiovascular, renal or thyroid disorders are at risk. Lithium may induce dysrhythmias or frank myxoedema. Carbamazepine is used for patients unresponsive to lithium and appears to be particularly effective in patients with rapid cycling manic–depressive illness. In the depressive phases there is a danger of suicide and antidepressant treatment needs to be given.

Dental aspects

Lithium very occasionally causes a dry mouth or impaired taste, as a result of dehydration (*see* Appendix to Chapter 19) and may increase caries. Interactions with neuroleptics such as droperidol may precipitate facial dyskinesias, while lithium with diazepam may induce hypothermia. Lithium may also interact with suxamethonium and other muscle relaxants to prolong muscle relaxation. Many non-steroidal anti-inflammatory analgesics reduce the excretion of lithium and may cause toxicity but aspirin, paracetamol or codeine are safe to use.

Lithium treatment should be monitored by the regular assay of plasma concentrations since dysrhythmias may be precipitated, particularly during general anaesthesia. It may be advisable to stop lithium treatment 2–3 days before general anaesthesia.

Manic-depressive patients may also be treated with antidepressant drugs with oral side effects such as xerostomia.

Schizophrenia

Schizophrenia is a common psychosis with its onset in early adult life. Unlike most psychiatric disorders where the complaints are recognizable exaggerations of normal emotions or related disturbances, schizophrenia corresponds with the lay idea of madness. However, schizophrenia is not, as popularly believed, a splitting of the personality—Doctor Jekyll and Mister Hyde are the creation of a novelist of genius—but a disintegration of the personality, causing thoughts and behaviour to be totally inappropriate and incomprehensible. Moods, thoughts and actions are, as a result, disorganized and irrational. Intelligence is, however, unimpaired and insight may even be retained, with the result that occasionally the patient may be aware that his behaviour is bizarre and even of the consternation that such behaviour creates in others.

Acute schizophrenia may develop in previously normal individuals and is often precipitated by organic disorders or external stress. Affective symptoms such as depression may be associated.

Chronic schizophrenia is more common and characterized by inappropriate affect, disordered thought processes, delusions, and hallucinations. Some patients are strikingly paranoid, others have mainly motor symptoms (catatonia), a bizarre mixture of emotional, behavioural and thought disturbances (hebephrenia), or neuroses.

Schizophrenic thought disorder causes loss of cohesion between logical thought sequences, and speech may include non-existent words (neologisms) or be inconsequential ('word salad'). There may be disruption of the stream of speech (thought-blocking), together with inappropriate affect and withdrawal from social contact.

Delusions are often bizarre, while catatonia with abnormalities of movement, posture and speech, negativism, echolalia, mannerisms and stereotypia may also be features.

The best known schizophrenic delusion, in the past at least, was of being Napoleon, but schizophrenic delusions are highly variable in character. Hallucinations are frequently auditory, when mysterious voices constantly whisper frightening or unpleasant things to the patient. The bizarre nature of the patient's disorder may be made obvious when he shouts back at the unheard voices.

Paranoia is a projection of the patient's internal disturbance which, as a consequence, is believed to be the result of the hostility of others, such as neighbours, secret agents or foreign powers who, for example, may be projecting mysterious rays to achieve their malign objectives.

There is considerable variation in the diagnostic criteria of schizophrenia, but auditory hallucinations and ideas of a passive or irresistible response to external influences which may control or block the patient's thoughts, dictate or control his behaviour to conspire to do him harm, are features most suggestive of this disorder.

General management

Psychiatric care is essential and admission to hospital is necessary if behaviour causes disturbance in the home. If there is considerable anxiety or hyperactivity, a phenothiazine with sedative activity (for example chloropromazine or methotrimeprazine) is needed. Butyrophenones such as haloperidol are useful for violent patients. If no sedation is needed piperazine phenothiazines such as trifluoperazine or fluphenazine may be given, but these are more likely to cause extrapyramidal (Parkinsonian) symptoms and may worsen depression. Maintenance therapy is conveniently carried out with long-acting preparations such as fluphenazine, pipothiazine, perphenazine or flupenthixol. Anti-Parkinsonian drugs such as benzhexol or orphenadrine are required to control extrapyramidal symptoms, which sometimes develop after only a few doses. Prolonged administration of neuroleptics can cause intractable tardive dyskinesia. ECT may be given if there is poor response to medication or if there is catatonia.

Dental aspects

Mild schizophrenic features (which are often unrecognized), include loss of social contact, flatness of mood or inappropriate social behaviour, which may appear at first as mere tactlessness or stupidity. Thus the patient, when asked to sit down in the surgery, sits in the operator's rather than the dental chair; the response to attempts at communication indicate a failure to get through, or are interrupted by totally irrelevant remarks. Such patients may have delusional oral symptoms, the treatment of which is beyond the expertise of the dental surgeon. Psychiatric help must be sought.

Schizophrenics controlled by drugs may appear quite normal and have no complaints related to their disorder or to the treatment. However, drugs used for the treatment of schizophrenia can have severe side-effects. The long-term use of neuroleptics (phenothiazines, butyrophenones, thioxanthines and others) can lead to complications such as xerostomia (with an increased susceptibility to candidosis and caries), oral pigmentation and severe extrapyramidal symptoms. Muscular rigidity or tonic spasms (facial dyskinesias: Chapter 12) frequently involve the bulbar or neck muscles with subsequent difficulties in speech or swallowing. Alternatively, there may be uncontrollable facial grimacing (orofacial dystonia) which may start after only a few doses. This may be controlled by stopping the neuroleptic and giving anti-Parkinsonian antimuscarinic drugs. Tardive dyskinesia (uncontrollable face, jaw and tongue movements) can develop, particularly after prolonged use of neuroleptics. It does not respond to withdrawal of the neuroleptic and is frequently unresponsive to any form of treatment. Haloperidol occasionally increases salivation.

Phenothiazines can cause dose–related hypotension and interfere with temperature regulation. They may occasionally cause obstructive jaundice, leucopenia, or ECG changes which can influence dental management. General anaesthesia, especially with intravenous barbiturates, may lead to severe hypotension and should therefore be avoided if possible.

Korsakoff's Psychosis

Korsakoff's psychosis is characterized by amnesia for recent events, impaired ability to learn new facts and fabricated descriptions of recent events (confabulation). Nevertheless the patient is alert, responsible, and behaves in an otherwise apparently normal manner. Chronic alcoholism, associated with thiamine deficiency is an important cause, though relatively few alcoholics develop the syndrome; other possible causes include cerebrovascular disease, tumours or degenerative disorders. The disease results from a symmetrical lesion in the periaqueductal area, thalamus, mamillary bodies and cerebellar vermis.

Other Psychoses

Psychoses can complicate various endocrine disturbances, the puerperium or drugs such as alcohol, amphetamine or psychotomimetics (*see Tables 14.1–14.3*).

THE OVERACTIVE (HYPERKINETIC) CHILD

Although parents not infrequently describe their badly behaved child as 'overactive', the term should be limited to those who demonstrate gross behavioural abnormalities including:

1. Uncontrolled activity.
2. Impulsiveness.
3. Impaired concentration.
4. Motor restlessness and extreme fidgeting.

These activities are seen particularly when orderliness is required, for example in the dental waiting room or surgery. Mischievous children are not, of course, abnormal and overactivity applies to gross misbehaviour such as reckless escapes from parents while on public transport.

Overactivity can be caused by external factors, or factors affecting parents, the child or the child–parent relationship (*Table 14.8*). Overactivity is often associated with low intelligence. Extreme overactivity (hyperkinetic syndrome) usually begins in infancy, almost invariably before the age of 5 years.

It is especially common in the mentally handicapped, those with neurological disease, and epileptics (especially in temporal lobe epilepsy). Autism (Chapter 15), mania and anxiety states may cause similar abnormal behaviour.

General management of the overactive child

Psychiatric care, and counselling of the parents are usually necessary. Impaired concentration may respond to stimulants such as amphetamines, pemoline or methylphenidate, but little is known of the adverse effects and dependence is a possibility, although it seems rare.

Sedatives and tranquillizers should be avoided as they may impair learning ability, or cause paradoxical reactions such as aggressive behaviour.

Table 14.8. Causes of overactivity

---

1. External
    Institutionalization
    Excessive demands at school

2. Parental
    Marital disharmony
    Depression

3. Child
    Hyperkinetic syndrome
    Brain damage
    Low intelligence
    Tartrazine sensitivity
    Anxiety states
    Drug abuse

4. Child-parent relationship
    Rejection or overprotection
    Inconsistent discipline
    Lack of parental love

Dental aspects of the overactive child

Overactive children are often impossible to manage in the dental surgery, and frequently succeed in frustrating all concerned. Any dental treatment is unlikely to be possible unless general anaesthesia is used and such patients are therefore best referred to hospital for dental care. Tranquillizers such as diazepam should be avoided as they usually increase rather than depress overactivity.

JUVENILE DELINQUENCY

Various orofacial lesions appear to be more common in juvenile delinquents than in the general population: facial and oral tattoos; smoking-related lesions such as keratoses; fellatio lesions on the palate; lip and cheek-chewing and scars are seen more frequently.

THE ACUTELY DISTURBED OR HOSTILE PATIENT

The acutely disturbed patient can totally disrupt his environment and harm those with whom he comes into contact. Frequently the cause is drunkenness or an acute psychosis. In other cases, the disorder may be due to organic disease such as infections, drugs such as psychotomimetics or amphetamines, or the withdrawal of drugs such as alcohol or barbiturates.

Management of the acutely disturbed patient

If the patient appears unresponsive to normal reasoning, no dental treatment should be attempted but the general practitioner or psychiatrist should be contacted. If the patient becomes violent the police have to be called; ambulance personnel cannot usually manage such cases.

No attempt should be made to sedate the patient. Benzodiazepines usually worsen violently psychotic behaviour and adequate doses of phenothiazines such as chlorpromazine can cause severe hypotension. The usual treatment, once the patient has been forcibly restrained is to give haloperidol by injection.

Patients can only be compulsorily admitted to hospital for psychiatric care if the requirements of the appropriate sections of the Mental Health Act (England and Wales 1983) or Mental Health Act (Scotland 1960) are fulfilled (*see* Appendix to Chapter 14).

THE CONFUSED PATIENT

The confused patient has fluctuating consciousness, impaired orientation and short-term memory. Delusions or hallucinations can cause severe agitation. Patients are usually more confused at night. Confusional states need to be differentiated from dementia, in which there are similar disturbances of orientation and memory, but consciousness is not impaired. The confused patient should receive immediate medical attention since brain damage may result from many of the causes, which include:

1. Alcohol or drug intoxication (or withdrawal).
2. Head injury.
3. Cardiac, respiratory, hepatic or renal failure.
4. Fever.
5. Cerebral infection (encephalitis) and AIDS encephalopathy.
6. Other causes (*see Table 14.1*).

SELF-INFLICTED (FACTITIOUS) ORAL LESIONS

Minor, subconsciously self-induced oral lesions are common, the classic examples being bruxism and cheek-biting (morsicatio buccarum). Other lesions may be self–inflicted when the oral mucosa is anaesthetized such as after a local anaesthetic or surgery to the trigeminal nerve.

Serious deliberate self-inflicted lesions in the mouth are considerably less common than on the skin. This may be due to an underlying need or desire for attention and oral lesions are insufficiently obvious.

Stewart and Kernohan (1972) have studied these lesions in children and adolescents in detail. They classify such lesions as follows: (*a*) Injuries superimposed on a pre-existing lesion; (*b*) Injuries secondary to another established habit; and (*c*) Injuries of unknown and/or of complex aetiology.

This last group mainly comprised patients who were emotionally disturbed. Though serious psychiatric disease is less common in children, an indication of the severity of the disorder which may underlie trivial oral injuries is the fact that one of Stewart and Kernohan's patients later committed suicide in adolescence.

The most common type of self-inflicted oral injuries reported in the past has been so-called self-extraction of teeth. Soft-tissue lesions can be produced, however, typically by picking at the gingivae with the fingernails. In adults injuries may be produced by the use of the pointed end of a nail file, often also at the gingival margins. Other types of injury include the application of caustic substances to the lips or injuries from attempts at suicide.

The diagnosis of self-inflicted injury may be difficult. They should be suspected when the lesions:

1. Do not correspond with those of any recognized disease.
2. Are of bizarre configuration with sharp outlines and in an otherwise healthy mouth.
3. Are in sites accessible to the patient.

In addition the patient may show signs that suggest mental handicap, emotional disturbance or may be known to be under psychiatric treatment (*Fig.* 14.3).

In spite of such a background, a few patients will admit to injuring themselves. More frequently the diagnosis can be confirmed only by discreet observation after admission of the patient to hospital. However, even when seen to cause the injuries the patient may still deny having made them.

Once the diagnosis has been made the patient's family doctor should be told of the necessity for specialist psychiatric assessment.

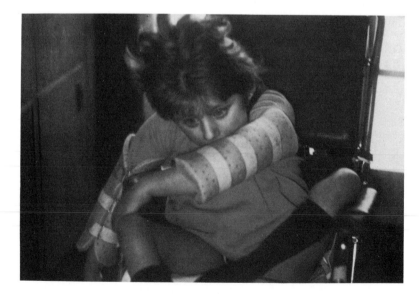

Fig. 14.3. Self-mutilation may be a manifestation of psychiatric disease, mental handicap, disorders of sensation or, rarely, the Lesch–Nyhan syndrome (Appendix, Chapter 10). This mentally handicapped child managed to bite through to her biceps.

Rare causes of self–injury include the Lesch–Nyhan syndrome (Chapter 10), and Gilles de la Tourette's syndrome of multiple tics which may affect the face and coprolalia (involuntary uttering of obscenities).

Child Abuse (Battered Child Syndrome; Non-accidental Injury)

Child abuse is any act of omission or commission that endangers or impairs the physical or emotional health or development of a child.

Battered children frequently have facial and oral lesions. It is an important condition to be recognized by the dental surgeon, since there is a high risk of further assaults on or death of the child and of siblings. Some 35–60 per cent of physically abused children suffer further injury, with a 5–10 per cent mortality. Most affected children are less than 3 years of age and usually less than 1 year of age. Affected families are predominantly of classes IV and V.

The injuries are varied and often multiple. Lacerations, bruising, pinching, bites, abrasions or burns are the main soft-tissue lesions, involve the head and face in over 65 per cent, but can be found in any part of the body. Lacerations of the upper labial mucosa and tearing of the lip from the gingiva are found in about 45 per cent of victims. Other injuries include fractured, missing, displaced or discoloured (dead) teeth, bruising or scars of lips or tongue, binding marks from a gag or lacerations. Fractures of any bone may be seen, but over 33 per cent have fractured ribs or long bones and there may be jaw or head injuries. Most suffer significant neurological, intellectual or emotional damage. The child may also be malnourished and generally neglected.

The injuries are usually inflicted by an adult, often a parent, or by an older sibling. The person responsible may be supported by an inactive partner. Causal factors may be related either to those affecting the parent, or to those affecting the child—often both (*Table 14.9*). It is noteworthy that the person responsible is only rarely psychotic, but the mothers are often emotionally immature or depressed and the fathers often have a psychopathic personality and either or both are frequently of low intelligence.

Child abuse should be suspected if any injuries are incompatible with the history and if any of the features in *Table 14.10* are noted. After genuine accidents, children are usually immediately taken for medical or dental attention; when children are abused, there is often considerable delay.

Table 14.9. Child abuse: associated factors

1. Marital disharmony
2. Chronic physical illness in parent
3. Emotionally deprived, inadequate or impulsive parent
4. Parents of low intelligence
5. Unwanted child
6. Abnormal pregnancy or delivery
7. Neonatal separation
8. Hyperactive or aggressive child
9. Ill child

Table 14.10. Findings suggestive of child abuse

1. Cowed child
2. Long interval before attendance for treatment
3. Injuries often committed at night
4. Multiple injuries
5. Injuries incompatible with history
6. Injuries at unusual sites
7. Evidence of previous injury (or a previous history of injury)

Management of child abuse

The child must be fully examined to exclude serious injury, especially subdural haematomas or intraocular bleeding, and must therefore be admitted to hospital. Full records *must* be kept. A skeletal radiographic survey should be undertaken to reveal both new and old injuries and a paediatrician should be consulted. Facial and oral injuries must be carefully recorded, preferably with photographs, and treated appropriately. The differential diagnosis may include osteogenesis imperfecta.

Patients are kept in hospital until the diagnosis is confirmed, since there is a high risk of further injury which may be fatal. If this problem is suspected, the medical practitioner, social services and a child protection society must be involved early on, but strict confidentiality must be observed. Social work departments now keep registers of non-accidental injuries which help identify known offenders.

The dentist should also inform his protection society as there may be legal involvement later.

Sexual Abuse

Sexual abuse can take a variety of forms but in addition to physical and psychological injury, the victim may acquire one or more sexually transmitted disease, including HIV infection.

Bibliography

Abrams R. A. and Ruff J. C. (1986) Oral signs and symptoms in the diagnosis of bulimia. *J. Am. Dent. Assoc.* **113**, 761–64.

Badger G. R. (1986) Child abuse: Symposium. *Paediatr. Dent.* Special issue 1.

Beck F.M., Kaul T. J. and Weaver J. M. (1979) Recognition and management of the depressed dental patient. *J. Am. Dent. Assoc.* **99**, 967–71.

Bick P.A. (1986) Seasonal major affected disorder. *Am. J. Psychiatry* **143**, 90–1.

Blanton P. L., Hurt W. C. and Largent M. D. (1977) Oral factitious injuries. *J. Periodontol.* **48**, 33.

Brady F. A. (1979) Gilles de la Tourette's syndrome. *J. Oral Med.* **34**, 69–72.

Brady W. F. (1980) The anorexia nervosa syndrome. *Oral Surg.* **50**, 509–16.

Brown G. W. (1977) Depression and loss. *Br.J. Psychiatry* **130**, 1–18.

Cawson R. A. (1969) Sore tongue. *Br. J. Dermatol.* **82**, 462.

Cawson R.A. and Spector R.G. (1989) *Clinical Pharmacology in Dentistry.* 5th edn. Edinburgh, Churchill Livingstone.

Clark D. C. (1985) Oral complications of anorexia nervosa and/or bulimia. *J. Oral Med.* **40**, 134–8.

Davies G. R., Domoto P. K. and Levy R. L. (1979) The dentist's role in child abuse and neglect. *Dent. Children* **46**, 185–92.

Editorial (1981) Child abuse: the swing of the pendulum. *Br. Med. J.* **283**, 170.

Feinmann C. and Harris M. (1984) Psychogenic facial pain. *Br. Dent. J.* **156**, 165-9, 205–9.

Fiske J. (1990) Alzheimer's disease. *Br. Dent. J.* **169**, 188.

Freeman R.E. (1985) Dental anxiety: a multifactorial aetiology. *Br. Dent. J.* **159**, 406–8.

Friedlander A.H. and Gorelick D.A. (1987) Panic disorder: its association with mitral valve prolapse and appropriate dental management. *Oral Surg.* **63**, 309–12.

Friedlander A.H. and Jarvik L.F. (1987) The dental management of the patient with dementia. *Oral Surg.* **64**, 549–-53.

Gross K.B.W., Brough K.M. and Randolph P.M. (1986) Eating disorders: anorexia and bulimia nervosa. *J. Dent. Child.* Sept, 378–81.

Hamilton J. R. (1983) Mental Health Act 1983. *Br. Med. J.* **286**, 1720–5.

Harris M. (1975) Psychosomatic disorders of the mouth and face. *Practitioner* **214**, 372–9.

Harris M. and Davies G. (1990) Psychiatric disorders. In: Jones J. H. and Mason D. K. (ed.) *Oral Manifestations of Systemic Disease*, 2nd edn. London, Ballière Tindall Cox.

Johnson G.F.S. and Wilson P. (1989) The management of depression: a review of pharmacological and non-pharmacological treatments. *Med. J. Aust.* **151**, 397–406.

Kiloh L. G. (1980) The diagnosis and management of depressive illness. *Medicine (UK)* **35**, 1773–6.

Kleier D. J., Aragon S. B. and Averback R. E. (1984) Dental management of the chronic vomiting patient. *J. Am. Dent. Assoc.* **108**, 618–21.

Leading Article (1987) Child abuse and osteogenesis imperfecta. *Br. Med. J.* **295**, 1082–3.

Moody G.H., Drummond J.R. and Newton J.P. (1990) Alzheimer's disease. *Br. Dent. J.* **169**, 45–7.

Niessen L.C., Jones J.A., Zocchi M. et al. (1985) Dental care for the patient with Alzheimer's disease. *J. Am. Dent. Assoc.* **110**, 207–9.

Scully C. (1982) Orofacial manifestations of the Lesch–Nyhan syndrome. *Int. J. Oral Surg.* **10**, 180–3.

Scully C. and Cawson R. A. (ed.) (1986) Oral medicine. *Med. Int.* 1129–56.

Short P. W. (1981) The psychiatrically violent patient. *Br. Med. J.* **282**, 279.

Stewart D. J. (1976) Minor self-inflicted injuries to the gingivae. *J. Clin. Periodontol.* **3**, 128.

Stewart D. J. and Kernohan D. C. (1972) Self-inflicted gingival injuries–gingivitis, factitial gingivitis. *Dent. Pract. Dent. Rec.* **22**, (11), 418.

Symons A.L., Rowe P.V. and Romanink K. (1987) Dental aspects of child abuse: review and case reports. *Aust. Dent. J.* **32**, 42–7.

van Wyck C. W. (1983) An oral pathology profile of a group of juvenile delinquents. *J. Forensic Odonto-Stomatol.* **1**, 3–10.

Walsh B. T., Croft C. B. and Katz J. L. (1981) Anorexia nervosa and salivary gland enlargement. *Int. Psychiatry Med.* **11**, 255–61.

Appendix to Chapter 14*

COMPULSORY PROCEDURES (MENTAL HEALTH ACT 1983) FOR THE MANAGEMENT OF PATIENTS WITH PSYCHIATRIC DISEASE

Section	Purpose	Duration	Persons making application	Medical recommendations
2	Hospital admission for observation	28 days	Nearest relative or authorized social worker	Both 1. Registered medical practitioner and 2. Recognized psychiatrist
3	Hospital admission for treatment	1 yr. May be renewed if appropriate. Patient may appeal to a Mental Health Tribunal in the first 6 mth	Nearest relative or authorized social worker (the latter must, where practicable, first consult the nearest relative)	Both 1. Registered medical practitioner who knows patient and 2. Recognized psychiatrist
4	Hospital admission for observation in emergency (when only one doctor is available and the degree of urgency does not permit delay to obtain a second medical opinion)	72 hours	Any relative or authorized social worker	Registered medical practitioner
5	Emergency detention of an informal patient already in hospital	3 days beginning on the day on which report furnished		The responsible consultant psychiatrist in charge of the case. His deputy may act on direct instructions

COMPULSORY PROCEDURES (MENTAL HEALTH ACT SCOTLAND 1960) FOR THE MANAGEMENT OF PATIENTS WITH PSYCHIATRIC DISEASE

Section	Purpose	Duration	Persons making applications	Medical recommendations
136	Removal by police to a place of safety. Persons who appear to be mentally disordered in a place to which public have access, if in immediate need of care or control, may be taken by police to a place of safety to await examination by doctor and authorized social worker	72 hours	Police officer	
24	Hospital admission for observation	28 days	Nearest relative or authorized social worker	Both 1. Registered medical practitioner and 2. Medical practitioner recognized under s. 27
31	Hospital admission for observation in emergency (where s. 24 is not applicable) or emergency detention of an informal patient already in hospital	7 days	Any relative or authorized social worker	Registered medical practitioner who has examined the patient on that day
104	Removal by police to a place of safety	72 hours	Police officer	

*Adapted from Morgan H. G. (1979) In: Read A. E., Barritt D. W. and Hewer R. L. (ed.) *Modern Medicine*. Tunbridge Wells, Pitman Medical.

Chapter 15

The Handicapped and the Elderly

THE HANDICAPPED

Handicapping conditions are disorders that impair normal social, educational or recreational activities. Handicapped patients need dental attention and treatment to at least the same standard as non-handicapped patients and frequently have a greater predisposition to dental disease. Nevertheless there is evidence of much neglect of handicapped patients by the dental profession.

It is important to appreciate, however, that treatment of handicapped patients is not necessarily more difficult than with normal children, but can be highly rewarding. The sad fact is that the institutionalized patient may lead an existence so dreary and emotionally isolated that any sort of friendly personal attention—which must be the essence of dental care—becomes a delightful event to be eagerly anticipated and touchingly gratefully received.

Only patients with mental, neurological and related handicaps will be considered here. Patients with other specific handicapping diseases, such as haemophilia and muscular dystrophies, are discussed in other chapters.

Some patients with neurological disorders, notably cerebral palsy (spasticity), have severe physical disorders of neuromuscular function and, though many of them are mentally defective, some are highly intelligent but have such severely impaired speech as to appear subnormal.

In addition to obvious disabilities such as mental defect, others such as congenital heart disease are frequently associated.

The main causes of handicapping disorders are shown in *Table 15.1.*

Table 15.1. Important handicapping conditions

Mental handicap
Chromosomal anomalies, especially Down's syndrome
Cerebral palsy
Spinal cord damage (especially paraplegia) and spina bifida
Thalidomide deformities
Hydrocephalus
Cleft deformities
Autism
Visual defects and hearing defects
Cardiac disease
Cystic fibrosis
Juvenile arthritis
Muscle diseases

MENTAL HANDICAP

Mental handicap is a state of incomplete development of mind, particularly of intelligence, to such a degree that medical treatment or special care or training of the patient is needed. An intelligence quotient of less than 70 is the arbitrary dividing line that distinguishes the mentally handicapped from the educationally subnormal.

Approximately 3 per cent of the population are mentally handicapped, often with multiple handicaps. The cause of subnormality is usually unknown; the main definable causes are outlined in *Table 15.2*.

Table 15.2. Causes of mental handicap

1. *Congenital*
    Chromosome anomalies
        Fragile X syndrome
        Autosomal trisomies Edwards' syndrome
                                  Patau's syndrome
                                  Down's syndrome
        Deletions 5, short arm: Cri du chat syndrome
        Deletions 4, short arm: Wolf syndrome
        Sex XO   Turner's syndrome
            XXX   Superfemale
            XXY   Klinefelter's syndrome
            XYY   XYY syndrome
    Inborn errors of metabolism

Protein	Hypothyroidism (cretinism)
	Phenylketonuria
	Homocystinuria
	Wilson's disease
Carbohydrate	Galactosaemia
	Mucopolysaccharidosis
Lipids	Tay–Sachs disease
	Gaucher's disease
Purines	Lesch–Nyhan syndrome

    Phakomatoses
            Neurofibromatosis (von Recklinghausen's disease)
            Encephalofacial angiomatosis (Sturge–Weber syndrome)
            Tuberous sclerosis (epiloia)
        Microcephaly
            Primary or secondary
        Intrauterine damage
            Anoxia
            Prematurity

Infections	Cytomegalovirus
	HIV
	Rubella
	Syphilis
	Toxoplasma gondii

        Prematurity
            Radiation
2. *Acquired*
            Trauma
            Alzheimer's disease
            Meningitis, encephalitis
            Metabolic disorders
            Poisons
            Rhesus incompatibility

Mental handicap is frequently the result of brain damage of many types but genetic causes, birth trauma and, later, road traffic accidents are particularly important.

Brain damage causes not only mental but also physical handicaps. Most patients are 'high grade' (IQ between 50 and 75) and frequently live at home. More severely subnormal patients (IQ below 50), who are totally dependent on others, usually have to be admitted to a long-stay hospital. There are often associated problems such as epilepsy, visual defects, hearing, speech or behavioural disorders, facial deformities or cardiac defects.

Mental handicap has three main aspects, namely:

1. Subnormal intelligence.
2. Social incapacities.
3. Abnormal behaviour.

Crime and sexual promiscuity are common, especially in the higher grades. Retribution often follows because the mentally handicapped lack the resources to evade detection and often find themselves pregnant or in court, or both at an early age. Psychiatric disorders are qualitatively little different from those in the non-handicapped, but the symptoms are often modified by poor language development and other defects. However, problems such as hyperkinesis, autism, and stereotyped movements are more frequent. Body-rocking and self–mutilation are common in the severely retarded, especially in the barren environment of an institution. Pica (the ingestion of inedible substances) is also common.

Self-mutilation may involve the oral or orofacial tissues, as in Lesch–Nyhan syndrome (*see* Appendix to Chapter 10) where the lips or tongue may be chewed almost to destruction. Rarely, oral self-mutilation is accidental in patients with congenital indifference to pain, including Riley–Day syndrome (*see* Appendix to Chapter 10).

General management of the mentally handicapped

Mental handicap is so varied in severity and character that it is impossible to generalize about management. Many patients can be cared for adequately by committed parents or guardians; others are admitted to hostels or institutions at an early age.

Complications may result from over-indulgence by parents, with consequent obesity and its sequelae. Institutionalized patients may develop behavioural disturbances and are prone to infections, particularly viral hepatitis, gastrointestinal infections or infestations, or tuberculosis. Prolonged medication with tranquillizers or anticonvulsants often causes adverse effects.

Dental aspects of mental handicap

Preventive dental care is of paramount importance for the handicapped.

Dental caries. Most of the mentally handicapped, particularly those with Down's syndrome, have low caries activity unless over-indulged with sweets by parents or others. Nevertheless, when caries develops it is frequently untreated or inadequately treated, and the teeth are lost prematurely.

Periodontal disease.   Poor oral hygiene is the most common problem in handicapped patients and it is frequently impossible for these patients to improve their level of plaque control because of lack of understanding or motivation, associated physical handicaps or other disabilities.

The main questions that must be answered in assessing the possibilities for the dental management of mentally handicapped patients are as follows:

1. Can the patient understand how to maintain oral hygiene?
2. Is oral hygiene by the patient impossible because of low intelligence, physical disability or personality disorder?
3. Is the patient able to sit still and cooperate sufficiently to allow conventional dental treatment under local anaesthesia?
4. Is the patient always so unmanageable that dental treatment can only be carried out under general anaesthesia or sedation?
5. Are there any other associated disorders, particularly epilepsy, which need to be anticipated?
6. Can special means be devised to overcome minor physical handicaps to allow maintenance of oral hygiene?
7. Can the patient's interest in maintaining oral hygiene be stimulated in any way such as by simple rewards of various sorts?
8. Has the patient a speech or other communication disorder rather than defective intelligence and is it possible to overcome this communication disorder?

Having solved these problems and decided which patients can be treated by conventional means it is important to appreciate that this is not necessarily more difficult than normal. Preventive dental care is particularly important, but as mentioned earlier it is frequently impossible to maintain good routine oral hygiene.

Restorative dentistry.   Routine, simple conservative dental treatment should be carried out wherever possible to preserve the teeth. For this purpose, local anaesthesia (if necessary with intravenous or inhalational sedation) is preferable and is usually satisfactory. General anaesthesia certainly makes the work easier for the operator, may permit a higher technical standard of dentistry, and by saving time, may enable more patients to be treated. It is therefore used for most handicapped patients by some operators. However, to do so presupposes the absence of medical contraindications, the assistance of an anaesthetist, as intubation is usually necessary, and other essential facilities.

Periodontal treatment.   In the higher grades of mental defect, electric toothbrushes may be easier to use and effective, and chlorhexidine rinses may also control plaque accumulation to some degree. Regular, routine scaling usually improves the gingival state considerably but there is no indication for sophisticated periodontal surgery.

Other factors contributing to periodontal disease include gingival hyperplasia caused by phenytoin or by one of the genetic syndromes, where gingivectomy may sometimes be justifiable.

Surgical treatment. Minor oral surgical procedures are usually limited to extractions. If there are cardiac defects, antibiotic cover may be indicated (Chapter 2).

Prosthetics. Handicapped patients are often made prematurely edentulous. Dentures are often impractical since many patients are incapable of managing them. Poor oral hygiene also predisposes to periodontal disease of any remaining teeth.

Prostheses may also be contraindicated in severe epileptics, who may inhale foreign bodies during a convulsion; certainly any prosthesis for an epileptic should be constructed of radio-opaque materials.

Clinical prosthetic work can be very difficult. Impression-taking is facilitated by using a viscous material (such as composition or a putty-type material such as Optosil) which, if the patient objects violently, can be readily removed without leaving unset material in the oropharynx. If patients will not keep their mouths open, a mouth prop on alternate sides and sectional impressions may overcome the difficulty. Registration of occlusal records can be very trying, but with patience can usually be effected. Those patients who are incapable of managing full dentures become dental cripples in addition to their other disabilities.

Dentures should be marked with the patient's name typed onto a paper strip. This can be added to the fitting surface at flasking and covered with clear acrylic before processing.

CHROMOSOMAL ANOMALIES

Chromosomal abnormalities are a common cause of spontaneous abortions and of natal and early neonatal deaths. The sex chromosomes and autosomes are equally frequently affected. Sex chromosome anomalies are usually compatible with life and rarely associated with severe physical disability but autosomal abnormalities are often lethal. Abnormalities of the smaller chromosomes may be compatible with life but can cause multiple handicaps, as in Down's syndrome.

The most common source of major chromosomal anomalies is an error in meiosis (non-disjunction) such that one chromosome too few, or one too many, enters a gamete and subsequently the zygote.

Most of the chromosomal anomalies are rare and many affected individuals survive only for a few years. The most common anomaly of significance indentistry is Down's syndrome. Medical problems and the main oral manifestations of other chromosomal anomalies are summarized in Appendix to this chapter.

Down's Syndrome (Mongolism or Trisomy 21)

Down's syndrome is the most common autosomal chromosome abnormality and also the most common of the clinically classifiable categories of mental handicap. With an incidence of approximately 1 in 700 live births, Down's syndrome accounts for 5–10 per cent of institutionalized mentally handicapped patients, and about one-third of severely mentally handicapped children. The trisomic mongol is usually born of an elderly mother: there is a 1 in 2000 chance for a 25-year-old, rising to 1 in 100 at 45 years of age. The other important variant is the translocation type who is born to a younger mother. In about 50 per cent of the latter patients the condition is inherited from a parent, usually the mother. The risk to these mothers of having a further Down's syndrome baby is 1 in 3 to 6, so that genetic counselling is important.

Congenital cardiac anomalies are found in up to 50 per cent. The main types are atrial septal defect, mitral valve prolapse or, less often, atrioventricular canal and ventricular septal defect. About one-third die in the first few years of life from cardiac disease.

There are typically multiple immunological defects so that infections of the skin, gastrointestinal and respiratory tracts are common, especially in institutionalized patients who are also liable to be hepatitis B carriers.

The risk of acute leukaemia (usually acute lymphoblastic) in Down's syndrome is 20 times greater than in the general population.

Dental aspects of Down's syndrome

All are mentally subnormal to some degree, but are usually amiable and cooperative most of the time. Epilepsy or cerebral palsy are rare. There are many oral abnormalities, the most obvious being an open-mouth posture with a protrusive tongue. The tongue may be absolutely or relatively large and is often scrotal, more especially after the age of about 4 years. The circumvallate papillae enlarge but the filiform papillae may be absent. The lips tend to be thick, dry and fissured. There is a poor anterior oral seal and also a strong tongue thrust. Anterior open bite, posterior crossbite and other types of malocclusion are common. The maxillae and malars are small and the mandible is somewhat protrusive. Class III malocclusion is common, but 46 per cent are class I. The orthodontic prognosis is poor because of mental handicap, parafunctional habits and severe periodontal disease. Although the palate often appears to be high, with horizontal palatal shelves (the omega palate), a short palate is more characteristic. There is also an increased incidence of bifid uvula, cleft lip and cleft palate.

As in all other aspects of their development, mongols have retarded tooth formation and eruption. The first dentition may begin to appear only after 9 months and may take 5 years to complete, if ever. The deciduous molars may erupt before the deciduous incisors and deciduous lateral incisors are absent in about 15 per cent. The eruption of the permanent teeth is often also irregular. Missing teeth are common, although, as in the general population, the third molars and lateral incisors are most often absent. Up to 30 per cent have morphological abnormalities in both dentitions, particularly teeth with short, small crowns and roots. The occlusal surfaces of the deciduous molars may be hypoplastic and both dentitions may be hypocalcified.

The most important dental disorder is severe early onset periodontal disease. Lower anterior teeth are usually severely affected and lost early. Acute ulcerative gingivitis is also seen. In contrast, caries incidence is usually low in both dentitions. The cause of the low incidence of caries is unknown but may be related to such factors as the high salivary pH and bicarbonate content.

Mongols are generally more easily managed than many other types of mentally handicapped patients. If general anaesthesia is needed, it must be administered by a specialist anaesthetist. Most can, however, be treated under local anaesthesia with sedation if necessary.

General anaesthesia is best avoided where possible in view of management difficulties which include:

1. Cardiac defects.
2. Respiratory disease. There may be difficulty in intubation because of the hypoplastic midface; congenital anomalies of the respiratory tract may be present and there is increased susceptibility to chest infections (*Fig.* 15.1).
3. Anaemia.
4. Possible atlanto-axial subluxation (care when extending neck).

Additional points to be considered include:

5. Cardiac defects predisposing to infective endocarditis (rarely).
6. Hepatitis B carriage.
7. Mental handicap.

Fragile X Syndrome

Fragile X syndrome is so named because the tip of the X chromosome is susceptible to breakage and appears as a thin thread of chromatin joining two

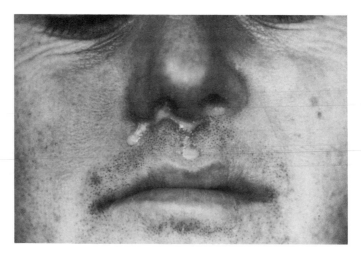

Fig. 15.1. Respiratory infection is one contraindication to general anaesthesia in Down's syndrome. Others include cardiac disease, atlanto-axial instability and anaemia.

chromosome bands in appropriate preparations of metaphase nuclei. It was earlier thought to be a typical sex–linked recessive disorder but approximately 30 per cent of carrier females are mentally retarded and there are a few pheno-typically normal carrier males. Fragile X syndrome therefore appears to be a sex–linked dominant trait with variable penetrance.

Fragile X syndrome affects 1 in 1000 to 1500 of the population and is the second most common chromosomal defect associated with mental deficiency, after Down's syndrome. In addition to mental handicap, patients have large testes, a long face and prominent ears.

Dental aspects

Earlier descriptions of palatal anomalies in fragile X syndrome have not been confirmed but cross–bite and open bite are abnormally frequent. Unlike Down's syndrome, there is no special pattern of frequency of dental caries or periodontal disease.

Hyperactivity, a short attention span and behavioural disorders similar to those of autism, make dental management difficult.

OTHER HANDICAPPING SYNDROMES

See Appendix 2 to this chapter and Appendix to Chapter 10 for inborn errors of metabolism.

CEREBRAL PALSY

Cerebral palsy (CP) is the most common congenital physical handicap and patients are often loosely referred to as 'spastics'. CP is the motor manifesta-tion of cerebral damage or defect, causing disordered movement and posture, but because of the many types of brain damage there is no uniform pattern of CP defects (*Table 15.3*). Many patients with CP are mentally normal but about 50 per cent have additional disorders such as mental handicap, epilepsy, defects of hearing, vision or speech, or emotional disturbances. CP in the infant usually causes poor feeding, delayed development and abnormal muscle tone.

Spastic Cerebral Palsy

Fifty per cent of CP patients are spastic and have excessive muscle tone, contractures, pathological reflexes and hyperactive tendon reflexes as a result of an upper motor neurone lesion (*Fig. 15.2*).

Hemiplegia is the most common form of spastic CP. Mental handicap is not usual but associated neurological disorders such as visual field defects, epilepsy or sensory deficits are common.

Table 15.3. Types of cerebral palsy

1. *Spastic*	Monoplegic	—involves only one limb
	Paraplegic	—involves lower etremities
	Hemiplegic	—involves one upper and lover limb on same side
	Double hemiplegic	—involves all limbs, but mainly the arms
	Diplegic	—involves all limbs, but mainly the legs
	Quadriplegic (tetraplegic)	—involves all limbs equally
2. *Athetoid*	Athetosis	
	Chorea	
	Choreoathetosis	
3. *Ataxic*		
4. *Rigid*		
5. *Mixed*		

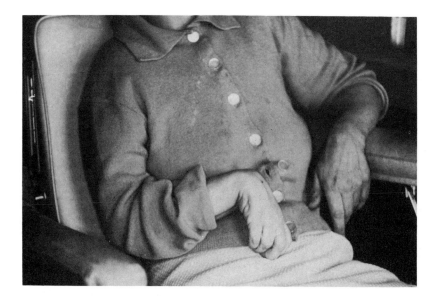

Fig. 15.2. Cerebral palsy: the limbs assume characteristic deformities, with flexion at all joints in the upper limbs and scissoring of the lower limbs if physiotherapy is neglected.

Quadriplegics with CP are usually more frequently mentally handicapped than hemiplegics but are less often epileptic.

Paraplegics and diplegics with CP have an IQ intermediate in level between quadriplegics and hemiplegics, but are the least likely to have epilepsy.

Athetoid Cerebral Palsy

From 15 to 20 per cent of CP is athetoid and caused by an extrapyramidal lesion, usually in the basal ganglia. There is increased muscle tone (of 'lead pipe' type) but normal tendon reflexes and no contractures.

Unlike most spastic CP, athetoid CP usually involves all four limbs—especially the arms. Smooth worm-like movements of the distal parts of the extremities are characteristic and become exaggerated if the patient is anxious. Mental retardation is less common than in spastic CP but epilepsy can be associated. Athetoid CP is often accompanied by high tone deafness and is caused mainly by intrauterine rubella (the rubella syndrome, Chapter 17) and by hyperbilirubinaemia (kernicterus, e.g. in Rhesus incompatibility).

Ataxic Cerebral Palsy

Ataxic cerebral palsy is characterized by disturbance of balance. It accounts for about 10 per cent of all CP and is caused by a cerebellar lesion.

Dental aspects of cerebral palsy

There is no dental disease unique to CP, but there may be delayed eruption of the primary dentition and enamel hypoplasia is common. Caries incidence appears normal, unless there is over-indulgence by parents, but lack of treatment frequently leads to premature loss of primary teeth, and earlier eruption of premolars and permanent canines.

Most dental disease is more common when the arms are severely involved. Periodontal disease is common, especially in the older child because soft tissue movement is abnormal and oral cleansing is impaired. Mouth breathing worsens the periodontal state. A papillary hyperplastic gingivitis may be seen, even in the absence of treatment with phenytoin.

Malocclusion is common and thought to be caused by abnormal muscle behaviour. The maxillary arch is frequently tapered or ovoid, with a high palate. The upper teeth are often labially inclined, due to the pressure of the tongue against the anterior teeth during abnormal swallowing. Most, however, have skeletal patterns within normal limits.

Bruxism, abnormal attrition and spontaneous dislocation or subluxation of the temporomandibular joint are common. Certain lesions are more prevalent in different types of cerebral palsy (*Table 15.4*).

In cerebral palsy, preventive dental care is important. Parental counselling about diet, oral hygiene procedures and the use of fluorides should be started

Table 15.4. Oral complications of cerebral palsy

Spastic CP	Athetoid CP
Class II division 2	Class II division I
Anterior open bite	Anterior open bite
Narrow arches	High palate
High palate	
Periodontal disease	Bruxism
	Hypoplasia. Green teeth of kernicterus

early. Manual dexterity is usually poor but favourable results are often possible with an electric toothbrush or a modified handle to the normal brush.

Dental management may be difficult for the following reasons:

1. Epilepsy.
2. Communication difficulties, which may give a misleading impression of low intelligence.
3. Anxiety.
4. Cooperation; concentration is often poor.
5. Posture and mobility. Manual support is often required and ataxic patients may need the chair to be tilted backwards. Many of the handicapped, however, become apprehensive when this is done.
6. Mental handicap in some patients.
7. Drooling. Poor control of the oral tissues and of head posture often leads to drooling.
8. Abnormal swallowing.

Anxiety may increase athetosis or spasticity, so that anxiolytic drugs such as diazepam are useful as premedication. Patients restricted to wheelchairs can sometimes be treated in their chair but it is often better to transfer them to the dental chair by carrying them or by sliding them across a board placed between the wheelchair and dental chair.

In uncomplicated CP, where oral hygiene can be maintained, routine dental procedures can be carried out.

SPINAL CORD DISEASE

Spinal cord damage is most frequently caused by trauma, particularly road traffic accidents, when it may be associated with maxillofacial injuries, as discussed in Chapter 13. Both children and adults frequently suffer severe and permanent disablement as a result.

Other causes of spinal cord disease such as infarction, haemorrhage, myelitis or tumours are mainly diseases of adults, but spina bifida is an important cause of spinal cord disease and severe physical handicap in children.

Neural Tube Defects (Spina Bifida)

Spina bifida is the failure of fusion of vertebral arches, of unknown aetiology, and may be associated with neurological defects and other complications leading to severe handicap.

Spina bifida occulta

There is rarely any obvious clinical or neurological disorder but the defect can be detected radiographically in about 50 per cent of normal children. The most obvious sign is a small naevus or tuft of hair over the lumbar spine in some patients.

Spina bifida cystica

There is an extensive vertebral defect through which the spinal cord or its coverings protrude. The incidence of this severe form of spinal bifida is about 2 per 1000 live births in the United Kingdom: there are two main types:

Meningocele is protrusion of the meninges as a sac covered by skin. Neurological defect is rare but 20 per cent have hydrocephalus.

Myelomeningocele is a protrusion of meninges and nerve tissue which are exposed and liable to infection, particularly meningitis. It is ten times more common than meningocele.

Myelomeningocele causes severe neurological defects. The usual pattern is complete paralysis of and loss of sensation and reflexes in the lower limbs. Deformities of the lower limbs follow. Patients with myelomeningocele therefore tend to suffer from paraplegia and hence they have

1. Inability to walk:
2. Pressure sores.
3. Urinary incontinence.
4. Faecal retention
5. Meningitis.
6. Other problems such as hydrocephalus, cerebral complications (epilepsy or mental handicap), other vertebral or renal anomalies.

General management of spina bifida cystica

Surgical closure of myelomeningocele and decompression of hydrocephalus is often carried out, usually in early infancy. These patients are severely handicapped and require specialist paediatric attention to manage urinary tract, bowel and locomotion disabilities.

Dental aspects of spina bifida cystica

Children with spina bifida must be managed in consultation with the physician and with due regard to the possible problems outlined earlier.

THALIDOMIDE DEFECT

The teratogenic effects of the hypnotic, thalidomide, include reduction deformities of the limbs (phocomelia, *Fig.* 15.3) and defects of the eyes and ears, cardiac defects, renal and gastrointestinal defects, facial anomalies but normal intelligence. Many affected persons have a globular head with hypertelorism (widely spaced eyes), depressed nasal bridge and a central facial naevus extending from the forehead down to the nose.

Since the withdrawal of thalidomide, those affected are now adults and phocomelia in children is currently a congenital defect of unknown cause.

Oral effects include enamel hypoplasia, cleft palate and abnormalities in tongue morphology.

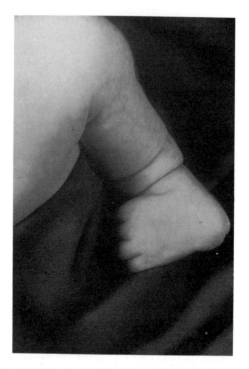

Fig. 15.3. Phocomelia (seal limb) in the thalidomide syndrome.

HYDROCEPHALUS

In the most common type of hydrocephalus, dilatation of the cerebral ventricles is caused by obstruction to the circulation of cerebrospinal fluid and results in compression and atrophy of the brain, and enlargement of the skull. Myelomeningocele may be associated. The main features are outlined in *Table 15.5*. A short-circuit operation with the insertion of a ventriculo-atrial or ventriculo-peritoneal shunt may relieve the intracranial pressure. The cerebrospinal fluid is drained from the cerebral ventricles via a catheter with one-way valves to the right atrium or the peritoneal cavity (*Fig.* 15.4).

Although effective, the valve may become blocked or detached and is susceptible to infection if there is bacteraemia.

Dental aspects of hydrocephalus

The weight of the head may be a problem, especially in the anaesthetized patient, and there may be many associated handicaps (*Table 15.5*). Management difficulties in hydrocephalus may also include:

1. Infection of ventriculo-atrial shunt.
2. Spina bifida (frequently associated).

3. Epilepsy.
4. Mental handicap.
5. Visual impairment.

Table 15.5. Hydrocephalus

Mechanisms
Congenital blockage of aqueducts or foramina in Arnold–Chiari[1] malformation or Dandy–Walker[2] syndrome
Acquired blockage of subarachnoid space or cerebral cisterns, e.g. meningitis, haemorrhage, tumour

Signs
Large head and bulging fontanelles in children
Headache, vomiting, mental changes, papilloedema

Complications
Epilepsy
Visual impairment
Spasticity
Mental handicap or dementia

Notes
1 Downward displacement of medulla and part of cerebellum through the foramen magnum blocking escape of CSF from fourth ventricle.
2 Congenital obstruction of the foramina of Magendie and Luschka.

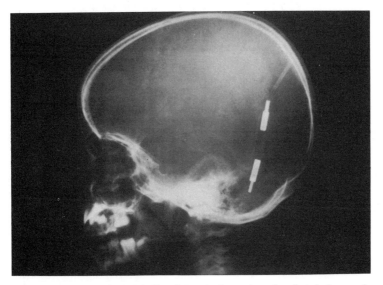

Fig. 15.4. Hydrocephalus: the lateral skull radiograph shows the valve that drains cerebrospinal fluid from the cerebral ventricles to the venous system.

Dental procedures occasionally cause infection of the valve and antibiotic cover should therefore be given, as for prevention of infective endocarditis, though infection is rarely from a dental source.

CLEFT LIP AND PALATE

The total incidence of cleft deformities is between 2 and 3 per 1000 live births. Cleft lip is more prevalent in males, cleft palate more prevalent in females. No teratogens causing clefts have been positively identified in man although thalidomide was and steroids may be associated with an increased incidence. Cleft palate is associated with a wide range of congenital defects, especially with chromosome anomalies (Down's syndrome, Edward's syndrome), and in the Pierre–Robin, Treacher–Collins and Klippel–Feil syndromes (Appendix to this Chapter).

Surgical and other technical aspects of management are covered in specialist texts but the usual classification is shown in *Fig.* 15.5. In general, when the lip alone is cleft, initial cosmetic repair is carried out at about 3 to 6 months of age, while a cleft palate is repaired before the child speaks, between 6 and 18 months, but usually at about 15 months of age. Orthodontic and restorative dental procedures are discussed elsewhere but, as in many other handicapped patients, preventive and continuity of care is of utmost importance and a high rate of success can be achieved.

In addition to hearing and speech defects, systemic complications are more frequent in patients with cleft palate than in those with cleft lip alone. They include especially skeletal, cardiac, renal and central nervous systemdefects. Up to 20 per cent of patients with clefts have additional abnormalities which can affect dental management in various ways. These include cardiovascular and renal defects in particular.

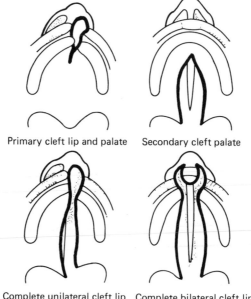

Primary cleft lip and palate   Secondary cleft palate

Complete unilateral cleft lip   Complete bilateral cleft lip
and palate   and palate

Fig. 15.5. Clefts of the lip and palate. (Adapted from Poswillo D. E. (1986). In *Clinical Dentistry* (Rowe A. H. R., Alexander A. G. and Johns R. B. (eds)), London, Blackwell Scientific Publications p. 132.)

Submucous cleft palate

In this condition, the palatal shelves may fail to join but the overlying mucous membranes are intact and the muscle attachments of the soft palate are abnormal. About 1 in 1200 births are affected and the defect can be recognized by a notched posterior nasal spine, a translucent zone in the midline of the soft palate and a bifid uvula. However, not all these features are necessarily present and a bifid uvula may be seen in isolation.

Feeding difficulties, speech defects and middle ear infections may develop in 90 per cent of affected children. They should therefore, be referred to a specialist.

AUTISM

Autism is a disorder beginning in the first 30 months of life, in which there is failure to develop interpersonal relationships, delayed development of speech and language, and ritualistic or compulsive behaviour. Autism is seen mainly in first-born males, possibly as a result of some abnormality of pregnancy.

The three main clinical features are:

1. Onset within the first 2 to 3 years of life.
2. Autism (profound aloneness).
3. Obsessional desire for maintaining an unchanging environment.

These children appear to be isolated from everyone around them and fail to respond to any stimuli, even to being lifted by the parents. They show complete lack of interest in people but are often fascinated with inanimate objects. Some display a combination of lack of response to stimuli, including pain, with abnormal fearlessness. Autistics wander aimlessly about with little creative or imaginative activity. Rages, tantrums and self-directed aggression (which may be reactions to boredom or frustration) are common, or there may be inappropriate giggling.

Most characteristic of the motor abnormalities are finger flicking near the eyes and hand flipping. Facial grimaces, jumping and toe walking are also common and all mannerisms are exaggerated if the autistic is distressed or excited.

Communication disorders such as delayed or immediate echolalia (repetition of words heard) are common. The autistic child rarely uses the pronoun 'I' and frequently uses meaningless words or phrases in a generally immature speech. Some remain mute. Seventy per cent of autistics have an IQ below 70 but some are highly intelligent. Temporal lobe epilepsy develops in about 30 per cent.

Dental aspects

There are no specific dental lesions or medical problems in autism, although there may be trauma from head-banging, and epilepsy. Parental concern is usually above average. An essential consideration is to ensure that a routine is developed in which the child is not kept waiting, has a short quiet visit, and sees the same dental staff. Autistics may be disturbed by noise such as a high-speed aspirator or air rotor and it may be necessary to avoid their use.

Many autistics manage to make dental treatment under local anaesthesia impossible by their lack of response to requests or commands. General anaesthesia or relative analgesia may then be needed, but some may be on medication, such as monoamine oxidase inhibitors or tricyclic antidepressants, which can complicate treatment.

VISUAL DEFECTS

Impaired vision is an important handicap and invariably restricts the activity of the patient to some degree. Visual defects are among the most common genetic disorders. Many of them, such as short-sightedness, though a nuisance or worse to those afflicted, present no difficulties in management. The main visual defects associated with significant systemic disorders which may complicate management are shown in *Table 15.6.*

Table 15.6. Causes of impaired vision

Congenital
  Cerebral lipidoses
  Laurence–Moon–Biedl syndrome
  Various inborn errors of metabolism
  Marfan's syndrome*
  Ehlers–Danlos syndrome*
Acquired
  Infections
    Herpes simplex*
    Herpes zoster*
    Congenital syphilis*
    Toxoplasmosis
    Cytomegalovirus
  Inflammatory
    Behçet's syndrome*
    Reiter's syndrome*
    Stevens–Johnson syndrome*
    Multiple sclerosis
    Temporal arteritis*
    Sjögren's syndrome*
    Mucous membrane pemphigoid*
    Ulcerative colitis
  Glaucoma
  Trauma*
  Metabolic
    Diabetes mellitus
    Acromegaly*
    Malignant hypertension
  Drugs
    Methanol
    Quinine
    Phenothiazines*

*May be oral lesions.

Dental aspects of patients with visual defects

Visual defects do not, in themselves, directly affect dental management or routine oral hygiene. However, constant gentle explanation and reassurance about every phase of dental treatment is needed to prevent a sightless patient from being frightened by unexpected noises or unpleasant sensations such as injection of a local anaesthetic.

Maintenance of oral hygiene may be difficult when the patient is unable to see whether or not toothbrushing has been effective.

It is also important to emphasize that visual defects or blindness can be complications of diseases which may appear to be mainly oral or mucocutaneous. Referral to an ophthalmologist may, paradoxically, therefore be the most important aspect of the investigation of a patient with oral disease, such as Sjögren's syndrome or mucous membrane pemphigoid. Patients with visual defects following maxillofacial or head injuries must be seen early by an ophthalmologist as loss of sight is a serious handicap.

Several causes of late-onset disturbance or loss of vision are severe systemic diseases, such as diabetes mellitus or atherosclerosis, which may complicate dental treatment in various ways so that, from the dental viewpoint, the visual defects should prompt consideration of the underlying causes and consideration of their practical implications. In many cases, however, damage to sight is a late complication and many such patients are edentulous.

HEARING DEFECTS

Deafness is common and, in over 30 per cent of cases, is hereditary. Deafness is caused by conductive disorders involving the middle or external ear or by neural disorders such as defects of the cochlear nerve or its central connections. Dental management may be complicated by difficulty in communication, but associated medical problems are infrequent. X-rays do not damage hearing aids.

Deafness may occasionally be associated with congenital malformations such as first arch syndromes (Treacher–Collins syndrome, Apert's syndrome) with associated facial anomalies, or rarely with cardiac disease or mental handicap.

THE ELDERLY

An increasing proportion of the population is over the age of 65 and the elderly now account for some 15 per cent of the population. The sex differences in life expectancy are resulting in an increase in the proportion of elderly females, many of whom are widows.

Very many elderly patients are edentulous and some problems of dental management are thereby greatly reduced. It seems, however, that the proportion of edentulous elderly patients is gradually decreasing and, as a consequence, more of them need restorative dentistry or surgery of various types. Many physical disorders affect the elderly, particularly an increase in the incidence and severity of cardiovascular disease, which can affect their dental management. Also important, however, are mental and emotional problems and defects of hearing or sight, as these affect all aspects of treatment, even prosthetic procedures. Dementia from such causes as Alzheimer's disease becomes increasingly common with age. On the other hand, it must not be assumed that an elderly patient is stupid merely because responses are slow.

Remember always to treat the elderly with sympathy and respect and that, while it may be difficult to find the patience to deal with their disabilities, these same ageing processes are operating in us all.

Of about 65 million persons in the United Kingdom some 15 per cent are over the age of 65 years, some 3 per cent are bedridden, 8 per cent walk with difficulty and 11 per cent are house-bound. Thus more than one million elderly persons have great difficulty in reaching any facilities for health care. Many of the elderly receive no dental attention whatsoever, despite much evidence of their need. It has been reported, for example, that oral disease of some kind was found in 81 per cent of a group of elderly patients and 20 per cent needed further investigation to exclude serious oral disease.

Nevertheless, elderly patients are often reluctant to demand attention, especially if they fear consequent hospitalization.

Multiple Disease

There is a rising prevalence with age of many diseases (*Table 15.7*), particularly cardiovascular disease, thromboembolic disease and malignant disease. Up to 75 per cent of those over 65 years of age have one or more chronic diseases. Multiple diseases, atypical symptomatology, polypharmacy and abnormal reactivity towards many drugs further complicate the situation.

Many disorders in the elderly cause non-specific effects such as general malaise, social incompetence, a tendency to fall and mild amnesia. Important causes include Alzheimer's disease, hypothyroidism, anaemia, diabetes, malignant disease and chronic renal failure.

Ataxia, fainting and falls may be due to transient cerebral ischaemic attacks, Parkinsonism, postural hypotension, cardiac dysrhythmias or epilepsy.

Intellectual Failure

Dementia, particularly as a result of Alzheimer's disease (Chapter 12) is common in the elderly. Mental symptoms in the elderly are often also caused by underlying physical disease, especially if the symptoms are of recent onset. An acute confusional state may result from disorders as widely different as minor cerebrovascular accidents, respiratory or urinary tract infections, or left ventricular failure. A chronic confusional state may result from conditions such as diabetes mellitus, hypothyroidism, carcinomatosis, anaemia, uraemia or drug therapy.

Table 15. 7. Diseases especially affecting the elderly

1. *Oral orpredominantly oral*
   Lichen planus
   Mucous membrane pemphigoid
   Trigeminal herpes zoster and post-herpetic neuralgia
   Carcinoma, premalignant and other white lesions
   Sore tongue
   Sjögren's syndrome
   Candidosis (denture stomatitis and angular stomatitis)
2. *Cardiovascular disease*
   Hypertensive and ischaemic heart disease
   Cardiac failure
   Temporal arteritis
3. *Neurological disease*
   Alzheimer's disease
   Multi-infarct (cerebrovascular) dementia
   Parkinsonism
   Strokes
   Ataxia
   Trigeminal neuralgia
4. *Respiratory*
   Chronic bronchitis and emphysema
   Pneumonia
5. *Musculoskeletal*
   Osteoarthritis
   Osteoporosis
   Paget's disease
6. *Haematological*
   Anaemia (especially pernicious anaemia)
   Chronic leukaemia
7. *Genitourinary*
   Urinary retention or incontinence
   Prostatic hypertrophy
   Renal failure
8. *Psychiatric*
   Insomnia
   Paranoia
   Dementia
   Acute confusional states
   Dependence on hypnotics
   Loneliness and depression
   Atypical facial pain
9. *Miscellaneous*
   Cancer
   Nutritional deficiencies
   Deafness
   Poor vision
   Accidents

Depression may be an important feature in hypothyroidism or with some drugs. Nutrition may be defective due to poverty, apathy, mental disease or dental defects. Nutritional defects may in turn lead to poor tissue healing and predispose to ill health. Ageing is often also associated with reduced acuity of many of the senses. Hearing and sight are frequently impaired (*Fig.* 15.6) as may the sense of smell and taste.

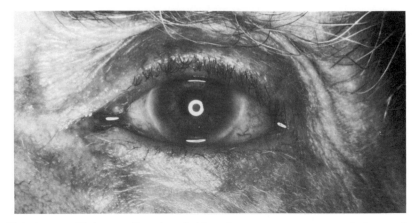

Fig. 15.6. Arcus senilis is a manifestation of old age but may appear prematurely in some hyper-lipidaemias.

Social disabilities are common as a result of such causes as loss of the spouse, isolation from the family, poverty and lack of mobility. Psychological disorders such as loss of morale are therefore common.

Temperature regulation may be disturbed so that respiratory, urinary infections or even more serious infections, often fail to cause fever. The elderly also readily become hypothermic especially if thyroid function is poor.

Drug treatment is more hazardous. The extent of this problem is reflected by the finding that 10 per cent of admissions to geriatric units were caused partly or wholly by drug reactions. Inappropriate treatment, poor supervision, excessive dosage, drug interactions and polypharmacy, or impaired drug metabolism may all contribute to adverse drug reactions. A further complication is that some drugs may precipitate or aggravate the physical disorders that are more frequent in the elderly. For example, drugs with antimuscarinic activity, such as atropine or antidepressants, may cause urinary retention if there is prostatic enlargement, or may precipitate glaucoma. Phenothiazines may worsen or precipitate Parkinsonism, or may cause hypotension, hypothermia, apathy, excessive sedation or confusion.

Drowsiness, excessive sedation or confusional states may also be caused by the benzodiazepines, barbiturates, or tricyclic antidepressants, while depression and postural hypotension not uncommonly follow the use of hypotensive agents. Other drug-induced disorders in the elderly are outlined below.

Altered presentation of disease

Disease may present in a less florid and dramatic way in elderly people. Even severe infections, for example, may cause no fever.

Dental aspects of care of the elderly

Many of the elderly are edentulous and of those with remaining teeth, at least 75 per cent have periodontal disease. Dental caries is usually, however, less acute but root caries is more common. Caries may become active if there is xerostomia, especially if there is overindulgence in sweet foods.

Reduced salivation may contribute to a high prevalence of oral candidosis, which especially affects hospitalized patients. Xerostomia is even more likely if there is medication with neuroleptics or antidepressants. Other oral infections that may affect the elderly include herpes zoster, while some such as herpes simplex or other viral infections are less common.

Some studies have demonstrated mucosal lesions in up to 40 per cent of elderly patients. Most of these are fibrous lumps or ulcers, with a minority of potentially premalignant lesions such as keratoses. Oral malignant disease is mainly a problem of the elderly and is a further reason for regular oral examination of these patients. Atypical facial pain (often related to depressive illness), migraine, trigeminal neuralgia, and oral dysaesthesias are not uncommon.

By no means all patients complain of oral symptoms or denture-related difficulties but many of the elderly are edentulous with little alveolar bone to support dentures, a dry mouth and a frail, atrophic mucosa. Inability to cope with dentures, or a sore mouth for any reason, readily demoralizes the elderly patient, and may tip the balance between health and disease. The dentist therefore has an important role in supporting morale and contributing to adequate nutrition.

The transformation from a dentate to edentulous state and adaptation to the wearing of dentures can present great difficulties. Sound teeth should therefore be conserved if they can serve, at least for a few years, as abutments or retainers for prostheses. It may also be unwise to alter radically the shape or occlusion of dentures where they have been worn for years.

Attrition and brittleness of the teeth may complicate treatment, and it may be necessary to provide cuspal coverage in complex or large restorations. Endodontic therapy may be more difficult in view of secondary dentine deposition. Hypercementosis, brittle dentine, low bone elasticity and reduced tissue healing may also complicate surgical procedures.

Delivery of dental care.   Access to dental care can be a major difficulty for the elderly who may be frail and have limited mobility. Domiciliary care may be more appropriate and avoids the physical and psychological problems of a hospital or clinic visit.

Handling of elderly patients may demand immense patience on the part of the operator. Elderly patients are often extremely anxious about treatment and should therefore be sympathetically reassured and if necessary, sedated. Treatment is best carried out using local anaesthesia where possible, since the risks of general anaesthesia are greater than in the young patient, not least because of associated medical problems. Benzodiazepines are preferable to opioids for sedation, but intravenous sedation in the dental chair is best avoided if there is any evidence of cerebrovascular disease, as a hypotensive episode may cause cerebral ischaemia. Relative analgesia is therefore preferable.

Benzodiazepines are preferable for the induction of general anaesthesia, which may be continued with nitrous oxide–oxygen supplemented with halothane, but the choice of agents depends on the anaesthetist.   Postoperatively, elderly patients are prone to pulmonary complications, such as atelectasis, and to deep vein thrombosis and pulmonary embolism.

The possibility of physical or mental disorders that may complicate management should always be considered (see *Table 15.7*) and drug treatment should be carefully controlled, with the possibility of adverse reactions always in mind. If it appears possible that there is hepatic or renal disease likely to impair drug metabolism or excretion, drug dosage should be reduced appropriately.

Polypharmacy must be avoided, not only because of the danger of drug interactions but also because of the practical difficulties that the patient may have in taking the correct doses at the correct times. Elderly patients frequently have difficulties in understanding the medication and in remembering to keep to a regimen.

Bibliography

Benington I. C., Watson I. B., Jenkins W. M. M. et al. (1979) Restorative treatment of the cleft palate patient. *Br. Dent. J.* **146**, 14–17.

Benington I. C., Watson I. B., Jenkins W. M. M. et al. (1979) Restorative treatment of the cleft palate patient. *Br. Dent. J.* **146**, 47–50.

Braff M. H.and Nealon L. (1979) Sedation of the autistic patient for dental procedures. *J. Dent. Child.* **46**, 404–6.

Cawson R.A. and Spector R.G. (1989) *Clinical Pharmacology in Dentistry.* 5th edn. Edinburgh, Churchill Livingstone.

Cohen B. and Thomson N. (eds) (1986) *Dental Care of the Elderly.* London, Heinemann Medical.

Croll T. P., Greiner D. G. and Schut L. (1979) Antibiotic prophylaxis for the hydrocephalic dental patient with a shunt. *Pediatr. Dent.* **1**, 2, 81–6.

Fleishman R., Peles D. B. and Pisanti S. (1985) Oral mucosal lesions among elderly in Israel. *J. Dent. Res.* **64**, 831–6.

Fontaine A. J. (1985) Managing the cerebral palsy patient. *Dentistry* **85, 5**, 27–8.

Giles D. L. and Murphy W. M. (1980) Dental treatment of the elderly inpatient. *J. Dent.* **8**, 341–8.

Hodkinson H. M. (1976) *Common Symptoms of Disease in the Elderly.* Oxford, Blackwell.

Jones A. A. et al. (1986) Dental x-rays found to have no effect on hearing aids. *J. Am. Dent. Assoc.* **113**, 912–3.

Kanar H. L (1986) Pharmacologic considerations for patients with disabilities. *Compend. Contin. Educ. Dent.* **7**, 210–21.

Moore R.S. and Hobson P. (1989) A classification of medically handicapping conditions and the health risks they present in the dental care of children. Part I—Cardiovascular, haematological and respiratory disorders. *J. Paediatr. Dent.* **5**, 73–83.

Moore R.S. and Hobson P. (1989) A classification of medically handicapping conditions and the health risks they present in the dental care of children. Part II—neoplastic, renal, endocrine, metabolic, hepatic, musculoskeletal, neuromuscular, central nervous system and skin disorders. *J. Paediatr. Dent.* **6**, 1–14.

Moss A.L.H., Piggott R.W. and Jones K.J. (1988) Submucous cleft palate. *Br. Med. J.* **297**, 85.

Peak J., Eveson J. and Scully C. (1992) Oral Manifestations of Rett's syndrome. *Br. Dent. J.* **172**, 248–9.

Robertson N. R. E. (1978) The orthodontic management of cleft lip and palate patients. *Br. Dent. J.* **145**, 204–6; 236-40; 269–72.

Scully C. (1973) Down's syndrome. *Br. J. Hosp. Med.* **10**, 89.

Scully C. (1976) *Something to Bite on: Dental Care for Mentally Handicapped Children.* London, National Society for Mentally Handicapped Children.

Scully C. (1976) Down's syndrome: aspects of dental care. *J. Dent.* **4**, 167–74.

Scully C. (1976) Dentistry for the handicapped in general dental practice. Part 1: General problems. *Dent. Practice* **14**, 11.

Scully C. (1976) Dentistry for the handicapped in general dental practice. Part 2: Mongolism and cerebral palsy. *Dent. Practice* **14**, 7.

Scully C (1976) Down's syndrome and dentistry. *Dent. Update* **3**, 193.

Scully C. (1977) Dentistry for the handicapped in general dental practice. Part 3: Autism and epilepsy. *Dent. Practice* **19**, 5.

Scully C. (1977) Down's syndrome. In: Chamberlain E. V. (ed.) *Contemporary Obstetrics and Gynaecology.* London, Northwood Publications, p. 231.

Scully C. (1980) The de Lange syndrome. *J. Oral Med.* **35**, 32–4.

Scully C. (1981) Down's syndrome. In: Crown 5. (ed.) *Practical Psychiatry.* London, Northwood Publications, p. 208.

Scully C. (1981) Oral mucosal lesions in association with epilepsy and cutaneous lesions: Pringle–Bourneville syndrome. *Int. J. Oral Surg.* **10**, 68–72.

Scully C. (1981) Special patient. In: Manning J. (ed.) *General Dental Practice. London, Kluwer, A.* 5(9–01)–(9–06).

Scully C. (1987) The Mouth in Health and Disease. London, Heinemann.

Scully C. and Davison M. F. (1980) Orofacial manifestations of the Cri du chat (5p-) syndrome. *J. Dent.* **7**, 313–32.

Shellhart W.C., Casamassimo P.S. Hagerman, R.J. et al. (1986) Oral findings in fragile X syndrome. *Am. J. Med. Genet.* **23**, 179–87.

Steele L. (1982) The delivery of dental care for elderly handicapped patients. *J. Dent.* **10**, 281–8.

Townsend G. C. (1983) Tooth size in children and young adults with Trisomy 21 (Downs syndrome). *Arch Oral Biol.* **28**, 159–66.

Turner G., Daniel A. and Frost M. (1980) X-linked mental retardation, macroorchidism and the (X) (q27) fragile state. *J. Pediatr.* **96**, 836–41.

Van der Waal I. (1983) Disease of the oral mucosa in the aged patient. *Int. Dent. J.* **33**, 319–24.

M. (ed.) *Dentistry for the Special Patient: The Aged and Chronically Handicapped.* Philadelphia, Saunders.

Appendix 1 to Chapter 15

CHROMOSOMAL ANOMALIES

Abnormality	Oral manifestations	Possible management problems
Trisomy 21 (Down's syndrome)	Cranial abnormalities Maxillary hypoplasia Dental abnormalities	Mental handicap Cardiac defects in 40% Infections Hepatitis B carriage
Trisomy 13 (Patau's syndrome)	Cranial abnormalities Cleft lip or palate in 75%	Mental handicap Cardiac defects in 80% Deafness Epilepsy
Trisomy 18 (Edwards' syndrome)	Cranial abnormalities Microstomia Hypoplastic parotids Gingival cysts	Mental handicap Cardiac defects in most Renal disease
Deletion of short arm of chromosome 5 (Cri du chat syndrome)	Cranial abnormalities Malocclusions	Mental handicap Cardiac defects Respiratory infections
Deletion of short arm of chromosome 4 (Wolf's syndrome)	Hypodontia	Mental handicap
Monosomy X (Turner's syndrome	Small mandible Malocclusions	Cardiae defects Diabetes Keloid formation Renal malformations Mental handicap
Trisomy X (Superfemale)	—	Mental handicap
Klinefelter's syndrome (XXY)	Taurodontism	Personality defects Diabetes mellitus Asthma

Appendix 2 to Chapter 15

MISCELLANEOUS SYNDROMES AND OTHER UNCOMMON DISORDERS OF POSSIBLE RELEVANCE TO DENTISTRY NOT INCLUDED ELSEWHERE

Disorders	Manifestations	Oral features	Management problems
Acanthosis nigricans	Pigmented papillomatous skin lesions	Papillomatous lesions	Adenocarcinoma (usually gastrointestinal)
Acrodermatitis enteropathica	Skin vesicles, Hair loss, Diarrhoea	Perioral or oral erosions, Candidosis	Malabsorption syndrome
Alstrom's syndrome	Nerve deafness, Retinitis pigmentosa	—	Diabetes mellitus
Ataxia telangiectasia	Mental handicap, Ataxia, Immunodeficiency	Occasional telangiectasia	Mental handicap, Diabetes mellitus, Hypoadrenocorticism, Hypoglycaemia, Hyperlipidaemia
Beckwith's syndrome	Gigantism, Omphalocoele or umbilical hernia	Macroglossia, Hypoplastic middle third of face	Diabetes mellitus, Obesity, Anaemia
Biemond's syndrome	Obesity, Hypogonadism	—	
Blackfan–Diamond syndrome	Red cell aplasia	—	
Bloom's syndrome	Telangiectasia, Depigmentation, Short stature	Chronic cheilitis, Carcinoma	50% develop neoplasia, particularly lymphoreticular

Chapter 16

Immunodeficiency and Immunologically Mediated Disease

The Normal Immune Response

The main activity of the immune response is protection against infections, but occasionally it may be directed towards the host and mediate tissue damage. Immune responses are dependent on lymphocytes and macrophages and may be *humoral* (antibody) or *cell-mediated,* or often both. Other components of the immune response include complement and polymorphonuclear leucocytes.

Humoral immunity

Antibodies are produced by plasma cells derived from B-lymphocytes. T-lymphocytes either assist (T-helper cells) or moderate (T-suppressor cells) antibody production.

Antibodies are immunoglobulins of five main classes. IgA is secreted by exocrine glands and helps to protect mucosal surfaces. IgG and IgM are essential for protection against bacterial infections, by such functions as neutralizing toxins, activating complement, or promoting phagocytosis (opsonization). Recovery from infections rarely, however, depends on antibodies alone: cell-mediated responses are usually also involved. IgE is important in the mediation of atopic allergy but has a role in defence against parasites. The function of IgD is unclear.

Cell-mediated immunity

Cell-mediated immunity is dependent on T-lymphocytes. These lymphocytes originate, as do B-lymphocytes, in bone marrow but T-lymphocytes differentiate within, and are under the control of the thymus. Immunological competence is normally acquired within the thymus and requires the normal functioning of purine metabolism. When activated by antigens, T-lymphocytes produce soluble mediators (lymphokines) which can modulate the activity of nearby cells, particularly macrophages, and have a variety of other activities. Cell-mediated immunity is particularly important in defence against some intracellular bacteria, such as mycobacteria, viruses and fungi.

Complement

The complement system comprises at least nine plasma proteins, which are activated in sequence (comparable to the blood clotting cascade) by a variety of triggering agents, especially immune (antigen/antibody) complexes. Many biologically active products, including important mediators of inflammation, compounds capable of attracting leucocytes, and others causing cell membrane damage, are liberated. Complement activation is controlled by a variety of inhibitors.

Polymorphonuclear leucocytes and macrophages

These are the dedicated phagocytes which are attracted towards antigens by activated complement following an antigen–antibody reaction. They can ingest and often kill micro-organisms coated by specific antibody and activated complement components. Macrophages are intimately involved in antigen-processing and the transference of information to lymphocytes. Polymorphs and macrophages may discharge degradative enzymes (lysosomal enzymes) during phagocytosis or attempted phagocytosis of, for example, immune complexes. Lysosomal enzymes may then cause local tissue damage.

Abnormal Immunological Function

Immune responses may be inadequate (in the immunodeficiency diseases) or control of the immune response may be disturbed and lead to immunologically mediated disease. Four types of immunologically mediated (hypersensitivity) reactions which may cause disease are summarized in *Table 16.1*.

HLA Typing and Disease

Compatible blood transfusion depends mainly on ensuring that donors' and recipients' blood are of compatible ABO groups. Tissue transplantation, by contrast, involves a much more complex system of antigens, namely the HLA (human lymphocyte antigen) system. The genes for these histocompatibility antigens are identified by a letter (A to D) and a number.

A genetically determined susceptibility to many immunologically mediated diseases is often suggested by a positive family history, and also by the finding that there is a significant association between certain histocompatibility antigens and several immunologically mediated diseases.

It is often assumed that HLA specificities determine the pattern of susceptibility to disease, particularly to autoimmune disease, and further that since the HLA specificities are determined by the appropriate genes, such diseases must be genetically determined. However, the strongest associations are between HLA D2 and narcolepsy and HLA B27 and ankylosing spondylitis, which are not known to be immunologically mediated. Rheumatoid arthritis by contrast has some association with HLA DR4, but any genetic predisposition is controversial. Many of the organ-specific autoimmune diseases are

Table 16.1. Hypersensitivity reactions

Type of reaction*	Mechanism	Examples
I. Immediate (anaphylactic)	Free Ag binds to IgE fixed on mast cells and basophils, causing release of histamine, etc.	Anaphylaxis Asthma Hay fever
II. Cytotoxic	Free IgG or IgM Ab binds to Ag on cell membranes to cause complement activation, cell damage or phagocytosis	Transfusion reactions. Idiopathic thrombocytopenic purpura Pemphigus
III. Immune-complex	Persistence of Ag/Ab complexes may lead to activation of complement, inflammation and tissue damage, particularly vasculitis and arthritis	Serum sickness Rheumatoid arthritis Lupus erythematosus
IV. Cell-mediated	Ag activates sensitized T-cells to become cytotoxic and to release factors (lymphokines) that stimulate other leucocytes	Contact dermatitis Graft rejection

Ag, Antigen; Ab, antibody.
*Some recognise Type V (immunostimulatory IgG) e.g. Grave's disease.

associated with HLA B8 and DR3, but the association is not sufficiently strong to help in the diagnosis. In contrast, HLA associations are rare in immunodeficiency states.

The significance of the association of different HLA specificities with particular diseases is, therefore, as yet unknown. HLA specificities are also of little value in diagnosis because of the inconstancy of their association with individual diseases, apart from narcolepsy and ankylosing spondylitis.

INVESTIGATIONS OF ABNORMAL IMMUNOLOGICAL FUNCTION

An adequate history together with the physical findings will frequently suggest the nature of disease resulting from abnormal immunological function. Thus, as discussed later, recurrent infections are particularly suggestive of immunodeficiency which may result from a primary abnormality of the immune system or be secondary to lymphoproliferative or other diseases.

Investigation of Immunodeficiencies

Preliminary screening comprises:

1. Full blood picture including a differential leucocyte count.
2. Total serum protein levels.

These are straightforward, routine investigations which can identify gross abnormalities such as neutropenia or leukaemia and show whether total immunoglobulin levels are depressed.

More specific investigation may include the following:

1. Serum levels of individual immunoglobulins and antibodies and electrophoresis.

2. Total numbers of circulating B- and T-lymphocytes and the helper to suppressor T-cell ratio (CD4 : CD8 cell ratio).

3. Blastogenic response (lymphocyte transformation) in response to non-specific mitogens and to specific antigens of interest.

4. Skin testing for delayed hypersensitivity (cell-mediated immunity) in response to: (a) natural antigens (such as tuberculin or Candida albicans) and (b) synthetic substances such as dinitrochlorobenzene (DNCB) to detect ability to respond to primary sensitization.

5. In vitro tests of cell-mediated immunity, namely macrophage migration inhibition factor (MIF) production in response to particular antigens.

6. Assays of complement components.

7. Assessment of polymorph function.

8. HIV antibody test.

Primary complement component deficiencies are so rare as to come low in the order of priorities, but a broad idea of the integrity of the complement system is provided by the haemolytic complement level (CH_{50}). The value of in vitro neutrophil function tests is limited and mainly of value for uncommon but well-defined disorders such as chronic granulomatous disease. Estimation of C1 esterase inhibitor may be needed for the diagnosis of hereditary angio-oedema.

Investigation of Immunologically Mediated Disease

The clinical features (Table 16.2) are often suggestive but preliminary screening comprises:

1. Full blood picture including erythrocyte sedimentation rate (ESR) or plasma viscosity.

2. Serum protein levels.

The blood picture will show haematological abnormalities such as haemolytic anaemia, thrombocytopenia or leucopenia that may result from autoantibody production. Alternatively, there may be leucocytosis associated with inflammatory processes. The ESR, a non-specific test, is raised as a result of hypergammaglobulinaemia or secondarily to inflammation.

Serum protein levels are typically raised in autoimmune diseases as a result of over-production of immunoglobulins

More specific tests for auto-immune disease include the following:

1. Autoantibody profile.

2. Tissue immunofluorescence or immunoperoxidase staining to detect immunoglobulin or complement deposits.

3. Serum complement levels.

4. Tests for circulating immune complexes.

Table 16.2. Typical features of autoimmune disease

1. More common in women
2. Family history frequently positive
3. Hypergammaglobulinaemia
4. Autoantibodies specific to tissue under attack sometimes present in the circulation
5. Multiple autoantibodies frequently detectable but often without clinical effect
6. Circulating autoantibodies often detectable in unaffected relatives
7. Immunoglobulin and complement sometimes detectable by immunofluorescence microscopy at sites of tissue damage, e.g. damaged blood vessels
8. Some associated with HLA B8 and DR3
9. May respond to immunosuppressive treatment

Auto-antibody profiles usually include the most commonly found abnormalities, namely rheumatoid and antinuclear factors and thyroid microsomal, gastric parietal cell, mitochondrial, smooth muscle and reticulin antibodies. Other specific autoantibodies can be identified by special tests.

Tissue immunofluorescence is carried out as described later (p. 506).

Complement levels (CH_{50}) are often depressed as complement is consumed when the cascade is activated by antigen/antibody reactions or other triggering factors.

Many tests have been used for detecting circulating immune complexes but there is no consensus yet as to which is most useful. Detection of cryoglobulins may be used for this purpose. The mere presence of circulating immune complexes alone does not establish that there is immune complex-mediated tissue damage. However, biopsy may show (for example) vasculitis with deposits of immunoglobulins and complement in the damaged vessel walls, as in polyarteritis nodosa, and is strongly suggestive of immune complex injury.

Lymphocyte transformation is a blastogenic response of sensitized lymphocytes to specific antigens of interest which include antigens of common microorganisms such as *Mycobacterium tuberculosis* or *Candida albicans*. Greater numbers of lymphocytes are stimulated by non-specific plant substances known as 'mitogens' (phytohaemagglutinin, PHA; poke-weed mitogen, PWM; concanavalin A, con-A) which can be selected to examine B- or T-lymphocyte responses. The ability of lymphocytes to transform to lymphoblasts (to become activated) when exposed to an antigen is a normal and essential immune response. Lymphocyte transformation in response to plaque bacteria or drugs, for example, therefore means only that the latter are antigenic and reaching immunocompetent lymphocytes. Lymphocyte transformation does not mean that such bacteria or drugs are provoking immunologically mediated disease. Thus penicillin provokes lymphocyte transformation and antibody production in over 50 per cent of patients to whom the drug has been given, but only a few of the latter are prone to adverse reactions.

Macrophage migration inhibition factor (MIF) is a lymphokine produced by T-lymphocytes and is used as an *in vitro* test of one aspect of cell-mediated immune function. As with lymphocyte transformation and delayed hypersensitivity, MIF production is a normal response to certain antigens. Failure of MIF production, on the other hand, is significant as it may indicate an immunological deficiency.

For example, isolated failure of MIF production to *Candida albicans* is a recognized but rare limited immune defect found in a few patients with chronic mucocutaneous candidosis.

Skin testing for delayed hypersensitivity measures not only T-lymphocyte responses but also the afferent (receptor) arc of the cell-mediated immune response. Thus, the majority of adults show delayed hypersensitivity to tuberculin in the tuberculin (Mantoux) test, since they have had previous contact with *Mycobacterium tuberculosis* or BCG. A positive response is generally an index of immunity to the disease and certainly does not mean that mycobacteria are actively causing cell-mediated tissue damage. By contrast, a negative reaction to tuberculin indicates susceptibility to infection or occasionally that there is overwhelming infection.

Cell-mediated immune mechanisms are, however, responsible for rejection of organ grafts, contact dermatitis and possibly for tissue damage in some other diseases. The basic problem is therefore to distinguish between cell-mediated 'immunity' (resistance to infection) and cell-mediated 'hypersensitivity' (tissue damage), since both are dependent on the same mechanism. This complex problem remains largely unresolved and the two terms tend to be used interchangeably.

Failure of lymphocyte transformation or absence of delayed hypersensitivity reactions after sensitization with appropriate antigens are typical features of immunodeficiency states.

Paraproteinaemias

In the paraproteinaemias, particularly multiple myeloma, there is proliferation of a single clone of plasma cells, overproduction of a single specific immunoglobulin and often susceptibility to infection. The abnormal immunoglobulin and its light or heavy chains (paraproteins) are identified by immunoelectrophoresis which supplements routine examinations such as a full blood picture, haemostatic function, blood chemistry, marrow or other tissue biopsy and skeletal radiographic survey (Chapter 5).

The importance of most of these diseases is that they are malignant. The immunological abnormalities are secondary but must be identified for diagnostic purposes.

IMMUNODEFICIENCY DISEASES

Immunodeficiency diseases can be:

1. Primary (genetically determined or the result of developmental anomalies), which are uncommon, or

2. Secondary and caused by disease or immunosuppressive treatment. These are by far the most common and the acquired immune deficiency syndrome (AIDS) is an increasing public health problem worldwide (see p. 477).

A patient with immunodeficiency of any of these types is often somewhat grandiloquently referred to as an 'immunocompromised host'.

Immunodeficiency diseases can affect any component of the immune system but often do not produce clinical pictures precisely predictable from the immune defect. Thus in T-cell disorders, antibody production as well as cell-mediated immunity may be impaired, while B-cell disorders have a variety of effects on antibody production. Either type of immune defect can be caused by intrinsic leucocyte defects, disorders affecting leucocytes, serum inhibitors of leucocyte function or immunoregulatory cell defects or disorders.

The most important effect of immunodeficiency is increased susceptibility to infections, frequently caused by organisms of such low pathogenicity as rarely to affect the normal individual (opportunistic infections).

Infections vary in character (*Table 16.3*) as a consequence of:

1. The nature of the immune defect.
2. The kinds of micro-organisms to which the patient is exposed.
3. Attempts at treatment.

Table 16.3. Important causes of opportunistic infections in immunodeficient or immunosuppressed patients

1. *Viral*
      Herpes simplex
      Varicella zoster virus
      Hepatitis viruses
      Cytomegalovirus
      Epstein–Barr virus
      Human herpes virus 6
2. *Bacterial*
      Staphylococci (especially *S. epidermidis*)
      Pseudomonas spp.
      Klebsiella spp.
      Escherichia coli
      Serratia spp.
      Nocardia
3. *Fungal*
      Candida albicans and other species
      Aspergillus spp.
      Mucormycosis
      Histoplasma capsulatum
      Cryptococcus neoformans
4. *Parasitic*
      Pneumocystis carinii
      Toxoplasma gondii

Thus broad-spectrum antibiotics used to control bacterial infections increase the hazard of fungal infections. Oral infections in patients with immunological defects can also be opportunistic and be caused by unusual microbes.

PRIMARY (CONGENITAL) IMMUNODEFICIENCY DISEASES

Congenital immunodeficiency diseases can be categorized according to the main type of immune defect as shown in *Table 16.4*. Their main features are summarized in *Table 16.5*. Immune defects are also common in Down's syndrome (Chapter 15).

Table 16. 4. Main categories of primary immunodeficiencies

B-cell defects predominantly
    X-linked infantile hypogammaglobulinaemia (Bruton's syndrome)
    Common variable immunodeficiency
    Transient hypogammaglobulinaemia of infancy
    Hypogammaglobulinaemia after intrauterine infection
T-cell defects predominantly
    Congenital thymic aplasia (Di George's syndrome)
    Late onset immunodeficiency (thymoma syndrome)*
Combined B- and T-cell defects
    Severe combined immunodeficiency
    Cellular immunodeficiency with abnormal immunoglobulin
      synthesis
    Ataxia-telangiectasia
    Immunodeficiency with thrombocytopenia and eczema
      (Wiskott–Aldrich syndrome)
Selective immunodeficiencies
    IgA deficiency
    Complement component deficiencies

---

*Variable type of immunological defect but usually T-cell predominantly.

The more severe diseases are all uncommon and often cause early death, so that they are not relevant to dental practice except in so far as some are now treated by marrow transplantation: in this way some patients can survive.

IgA deficiency is considerably more prevalent than most other immunodeficiency disorders and is considered in some detail. The only defects in the complement system of relevance are C1 esterase deficiency (hereditary angio-oedema) and C2 deficiency associated with lupus erythematosus.

Selective IgA Deficiency

Selective IgA deficiency is the most common natural immunodeficiency disorder and the prevalence in the normal population may be about 1 in 600.

IgA is deficient in both serum and secretions; the levels of other classes of immunoglobulin are normal or raised. Autoantibodies frequently, however, form against IgA, and can sometimes cause anaphylactic reactions when blood transfusions or immune globulins are given.

IgA deficiency is compatible with normal health but in others IgA deficiency may be associated with any of the following types of disease:

Table 16.5. Primary (genetically determined) immunodeficiency diseases

Type or name of syndrome	Immunological function	Clinical effects	Possible oral features
X-linked infantile hypogammaglobulinaemia (Bruton syndrome)	Immunoglobulins of all classes deficient or absent	Recurrent pyogenic infections starting in infancy. Hepatitis, CNS viral infections	Sinusitis, absent tonsils, cervical lymph node enlargement, oral ulceration
X-linked lymphoproliferative disease (Duncan's disease)	Deficiency of anti-EBV nuclear antigen	Lymphomas	Lymphomas
Common variable immunodeficiency	Variable deficiency of different immunoglobulins	Respiratory infections starting in childhood	Sinusitis, hyperplastic tonsils, cervical lymph node enlargement, oral ulceration
Wiskott–Aldrich syndrome	Deficiency mainly of IgM, IgA and IgE may be increased	Recurrent infections especially by pneumococci, meningococci and *H. influenzae*. Thrombocytopenia, eczema	Purpura, candidosis, herpetic infections
Transient hypogammaglobulinaemia of infancy	Hypogammaglobulinaemia in early childhood only	Eczema, food allergies	NR
Hypogammaglobulinaemia after intrauterine viral infections, e.g. rubella	Deficiency usually of only one Ig class (e.g. IgA)	Occasionally increased susceptibility to infection	Enamel hypoplasia
Congenital thymic aplasia (Di George syndrome)	Defective cell-mediated immunity. Ig production also impaired	Viral and fungal infections starting in infancy. Cardiovascular defects. Hypoparathyroidism	Abnormal facies. Bifid uvula. Candidosis. Herpetic infections
Severe combined immunodeficiency*	Defective cell-mediated immunity and agammaglobulinaemia	Lack of resistance to all types of infection	Candidosis, viral infections. Oral ulceration
Cellular immunodeficiency with abnormal immunoglobulin production	Defective cell-mediated immunity. Little antibody response	Lack of resistance to all types of infection	Candidosis. Herpetic infections

Immunodeficiency with ataxia telangiectasia	Defective cell-mediated immunity. Ig production impaired	Respiratory infections starting in infancy. Ataxia telangiectasia, mental handicap	Sinusitis, oral ulceration
Late onset immunodeficiency	Defective cell-mediated immunity or hypo-gammaglobulinaemia	Susceptibility to various infections starting late in life. Myasthenia gravis, anaemia	Chronic candidosis
IgA deficiency	Variable. Deficient IgA and sometimes IgE or IgG_2	Recurrent respiratory infections or atopic allergy or auto-immune disease or normal health	Tonsillar hyperplasia, possibly oral ulceration, herpetic infections
IgG_2 subclass deficiency	Defective humoral immunity	Recurrent respiratory infections	Sinusitis
Complement deficiencies C1, C2 or C4	Defects in complement pathways	Tend to be associated with autoimmune disease, especially lupus erythematosus	Possibly oral lesions of lupus erythematosus
C1, C3 or C5 deficiencies		Increased susceptibility to infection	NR
C1 esterase inhibitor deficiency	Abnormal complement activation	Swelling of face and neck Airway obstruction	Swellings
Cyclical neutropenia	Depression of neutrophil count at 21-day intervals	Periodic infections—especially bacterial	Recurrent oral ulceration. Periodontitis
Chronic granulomatous disease	Leucocyte killing defect	Infections with catalase-positive bacteria. Lymph node abscesses	Cervical lymph node enlargement and suppuration, enamel hypoplasia
Myeloperoxidase deficiency	Leucocyte killing defect	Candidosis	Candidosis
Chediak–Higashi syndrome	Leucocyte defect of chemotaxis and phagocytosis	Albinism, recurrent infections, hepato-splenomegaly, thrombocytopenia	Cervical lymph node enlargement, oral ulceration, periodontitis

NR, Not recorded.
*Sub-types are caused by deficiencies of enzymes adenosine deaminase or purine nucleoside phosphorylase, involved in purine metabolism.
†To *Haemophilus influenzae* in particular.

1. Recurrent respiratory infections.
2. Atopic disease.
3. Autoimmune disease.

Recurrent bacterial or viral infections of the respiratory tract are the most common manifestations of IgA deficiency, particularly if there is an associated deficiency of IgG_2. IgA-deficient patients also have an abnormally high incidence of allergic disease. Almost any type of autoimmune disease, but particularly lupus erythematosus, rheumatoid arthritis and Sjögren's syndrome are significantly more common in IgA-deficient patients. Coeliac disease is also more frequent and, as a consequence, malabsorption is sometimes the main clinical manifestation of IgA deficiency.

Dental aspects of IgA deficiency

Despite the fact that IgA is the main salivary antibody, reported effects of IgA deficiency on dental caries are conflicting and there is no convincing evidence that caries or periodontal disease are more frequent or severe. Part of the reason for this apparently anomalous situation is that other immunoglobulins may be secreted in saliva in place of IgA. However, it is noteworthy that dental caries is the only infective disease that is *not* promoted by the severe immune deficiency of AIDS, though it may be a complication of xerostomia that develops in a minority of these patients.

IgA deficiency may be occasionally associated with oral ulcers and herpes labialis but firm evidence is scanty.

Mucociliary Syndromes

Cilia in the respiratory tract normally clear mucus and act as a defence mechanism. Impairment of this mechanism in some genetic and acquired disorders may lead to chronic sinusitis or other respiratory infections. Examples are Kartagener's syndrome (mucociliary disease and dextrocardia) and intolerance of non-steroidal anti–inflammatory drugs in the Fernand–Widal syndrome.

Graft-versus-host Disease

Graft-versus-host (GVH) disease is an immunologically mediated reaction wherein lymphocytes contained in a donor graft mount an immunological response against the recipient. GVH disease is now seen with increasing frequency since bone-marrow transplants are being given to an increasing number of patients. A characteristic feature of GVHD is a lichenoid reaction that may involve skin and/or the oral mucosa. Sicca syndrome may also occasionally result.

ACQUIRED IMMUNODEFICIENCIES

Diseases causing Immunological Defects

Immune responses can be impaired in a wide range of diseases but particularly in cancers of lymphoid or haemopoietic tissues as shown in *Table 16.6*. In some of these diseases, infections such as herpes zoster or candidosis may be the first sign of the underlying immunodeficiency. In others, the immune defect is demonstrable only by specific tests. Thus in active tuberculosis the tuberculin test may become negative (anergy).

The most common disease associated with weakened resistance to infection is diabetes mellitus where defective phagocytosis is probably a main factor. Neutropenia from any cause is also an important determinant of abnormal susceptibility to infection.

THE ACQUIRED IMMUNE DEFICIENCY SYNDROME (AIDS)

The acquired immune deficiency syndrome is an increasingly common disease characterized by a severe defect particularly of cell-mediated immunity, susceptibility to an enormous variety of infections, otherwise rare tumours and neurological disease. The disease is particularly unusual in that it is a *transmissible* form of immunodeficiency and many hundreds of thousands of cases have now been reported worldwide, but it is particularly common in Africa, New York and San Francisco. Worldwide, many millions of people, especially in the developing world, have become infected.

1. Acquired immune deficiency syndrome can be defined as the constellation of opportunistic infections, particularly by *Pneumocystis carinii*, and/or Kaposi's sarcoma or other tumours (particularly lymphomas), associated with severe immunodeficiency developing in previously healthy persons who have not had immunosuppressive treatment.

2. AIDS was first recognized in 1981 among promiscuous male homosexuals in the USA (gay-plague). However, AIDS has now spread across the world. In the USA alone there had been 100 000 cases by August 1990 and over 200 000 by the end of 1992. It is also epidemic in Africa, in some areas of which it is the main cause of death among adults, and in many other developing countries.

3. A virus originally termed the Human T-cell Lymphotropic Virus type III (HTLV-III) and some closely related viruses are the aetiological agents. These viruses are now termed Human Immunodeficiency Viruses (HIV) of which there are HIV-1 and HIV-2. HIV–2 is widespread in West Africa. At the time of writing only 12 cases of HIV–2 infection have been reported in Britain, all but one of these patients came from or became infected in higher risk countries, particularly Africa.

4. HIV specifically attacks T helper lymphocytes (CD4 cells) and typically leads eventually to progressively more severe immunodeficiency. In fully developed AIDS, the unusually severe defect, predominantly of cell-mediated immunity, includes particularly:

Table 16.6. Secondary immunodeficiencies

Disease	Main defect		
	T-cell	B-cell	Phagocyte
Malignant disease			
Hodgkin's disease	+	—	—
Acute leukaemia	+	—	—
Non-lymphoid cancers	+	—	—
Thymoma	+	+	—
Infections			
AIDS	+	—	—
Severe tuberculosis	+	—	—
Leprosy (lepromatous type)	+	—	—
Congenital viral infections	+	—	—
Acute severe viral infections	+	—	—
Deficiency states			
Malnutrition	+	—	+
Iron deficiency	+	—	—
Protein loss	—	+	—
Autoimmune disease			
Systemic lupus erythematosus ⎤			
Rheumatoid arthritis ⎬	+	—	—
Chronic autoimmune hepatitis ⎦			
Miscellaneous			
Neutropenia	—	—	+
Diabetes mellitus	—	—	+
Chronic renal failure	+	—	—
Sickle cell disease	—	—	+
Severe burns	+	+	—

Lymphopenia.

Reduced numbers of CD 4 (T4: T-helper) cells and abnormally low T-helper/suppressor ratio.

Reduced mitogenic responses

Anergy to skin testing.

5. Exposure to HIV or related viruses usually also results in production of antibodies but these do not protect against the diseases, and virus can be carried simultaneously with antibody and remain infective. All HIV antibody-positive individuals are probably therefore, potentially infective and must not be allowed to donate blood, organs for transplantation or semen for artificial insemination. A few patients with AIDS have no detectable HIV antibody. Absence of HIV antibody does not therefore necessarily exclude infection with HIV.

6. Virtually all persons who are HIV antibody-positive will develop AIDS.

7. HIV has been detected in blood, plasma, semen, saliva, tears and cerebrospinal fluid. The chief mode of transmission of the disease was receptive anal intercourse among promiscuous male homosexuals (75 per cent of patients), but there is increasing transmission by normal heterosexual intercourse.

Table 16. 7. Major risk groups for HIV infection and HIV-related diseases

Risk group	Percentage of AIDS patients*
Male homosexual/bisexual	80.5
i.v. drug abuser	4.3**
Transfusion recipients	1.0
Haemophiliacs	0.6
Heterosexual contacts of above groups	0.5
Others (such as immigrants from tropical Africa)	0.2

*UK figures (1990).
**May also be homo-/bisexual

8. AIDS can also be transmitted by blood and blood products; intravenous drug abusers are an increasing risk group (*Table 16. 7*). Fortunately, haemophiliacs form only a small proportion of AIDS patients; blood for transfusions is now routinely screened for HIV antibody as an indicator of possible infectivity.

9. The incubation period of AIDS is highly variable, but can be as long as 10–15 years. This is mainly because depression of the immune system, though detectable by appropriate tests, may take a considerable time to become clinically apparent as opportunistic infections.

10. Infection by HIV can lead to a variety of clinical syndromes, any of which can culminate in full-blown AIDS. Many may remain asymptomatic for some time (though they may be able to transmit the disease) but probably most eventually develop full-blown AIDS. However, this hazard cannot be excluded until after a long period of observation has excluded signs of declining immune responsiveness, as the virus appears to persist in the body.

11. Kaposi's sarcoma (an otherwise exceedingly rare tumour of endothelial cells among elderly persons) is common mainly in male homosexuals with AIDS, but atypical in its early age of onset, distribution (particularly in the head and neck area) and greater malignancy. Lymphomas are also common in AIDS and frequently affect the brain.

12. In addition to its effects on the immune system, the AIDS virus also attacks the brain and patients can develop increasing encephalopathy and ultimately dementia sometimes in the absence of significant immunodeficiency.

13. Autoimmune disease may be associated and thrombocytopenic purpura is relatively common (*Table 16. 8*).

14. AIDS in Africans has spread rapidly especially in central Africa and is often characterized by a diarrhoea-wasting syndrome ('slim disease'), opportunistic infections such as tuberculosis, cryptococcosis and cryptosporidiosis, or disseminated Kaposi's sarcoma. *Pneumocystis carinii* pneumonia is less common than in AIDS patients from the West, but tuberculosis is more common.

Diagnosis

Diagnosis of HIV disease is based on the clinical features as outlined above, together with immunological findings indicative of a severe immune defect

Table 16. 8. Opportunistic infections, neoplasms and other features of HIV-related diseases and AIDS

Opportunistic infections*	
Pneumonia, sinusitis	*Pneumocystis carinii*
	Aspergillosis
	Candidosis
	Cryptococcosis
	Zygomycosis (mucormycosis)
	Strongyloidosis
	Toxoplasmosis
	Non-tubercular mycobacterioses
	Cytomegalovirus
	Legionellosis
	Pseudomonas aeruginosa
	Staphylococcus aureus
	Streptococcus pneumoniae
	Haemophilus influenzae
Gastrointestinal	Cryptosporidiosis
	Microsporidiosis
	Isosporiasis
	Giardiasis
Meningitis; encephalitis	JC virus and other papova viruses*
	Toxoplasma gondii
	Papovavirus
Mucocutaneous	Herpes simplex
	Herpes zoster
	Human papilloma virus
	Non-tuberculous mycobacteria
	Candida albicans
	Staphylococcus aureus
	Histoplasmosis
Disseminated	*Mycobacterium fortuitum and avium-intracellulare*
	Cryptococcus neoformans
	Histoplasma capsulatum
	Cytomegalovirus
	Adenoviruses
Neoplasms	
Kaposi's sarcoma	
Lymphoma (especially of the central nervous system)	
Squamous cell carcinoma (of anus and rectum)	
Leukaemia	
Other complications	
Encephalopathy†	
Thrombocytopenic purpura†	
Lupus erythematosus	
Seborrhoeic dermatitis	

*See *Table 16.9* for oral infections. ªJC = Jacob Creutzfeld.
† These are as common clinical features of AIDS; up to 60 per cent of patients may manifest symptoms of encephalopathy.

characterized by a striking lymphopenia with a uniquely severe reduction in CD4 lymphocytes and usually, a positive HIV antibody test (*see below*).The reduction in CD4 cells leads to an irreversible fall in the ratio of helper to suppressor (CD8) cells: the CD4/CD8 (T4/T8) ratio falls from a normal of about 2 to about 0.5 in AIDS.

Patients with AIDS-related complex have similar abnormalities, as do some asymptomatic individuals.

'The AIDS test'

Infection with HIV can result in an antibody response and most seroconvert within the first 6–12 weeks. However, there can sometimes be both false-positive and false-negative results. Moreover, some patients are infected with HIV but do not appear to produce antibody to it, or lose it as AIDS develops. The presence of antibody to HIV means that the patient has been infected with the virus; it implies a carrier state but does *not* indicate immunity to the AIDS virus. Conversely, the absence of antibody to HIV clearly does not always mean that infection is absent. There are reliable tests for HIV antigen and RNA, but their routine use does not appear to be justified as seronegative infected patients are so infrequent. In the meantime, indiscriminate screening is discouraged. Testing for HIV antibody is useful for the screening of blood and tissue donors or in women in high-risk groups who are contemplating pregnancy, but in other instances any potential advantages should be weighed carefully (with appropriate counselling of patients) against the potential psychological sequelae to patients on learning that they have a potentially life–threatening infection which they can transmit to others. In the UK, patients must be counselled before testing.

Management

There is no effective treatment yet for the underlying immune defect in AIDS. Antimicrobial and supportive treatment may prolong life but are not life-saving.

Drugs such as the thymic hormones; thymosin and thymopentin; interferon; and drugs active against retroviruses, such as ribavirin, interferon, dideoxyinosine and other agents are being examined. Currently, zidovudine (azidothymidine, AZT) is the main drug used: it may raise T4 levels, reduce HIV infection of mononuclear cells and give clinical improvement, but is not curative. Dideoxyinosine (DDI) is also being increasingly used but may sometimes cause optic neuritis.

As yet the only reliably effective prophylaxis is avoidance of sexual promiscuity (particularly in high–risk countries such as Africa) and dangerous sexual practices such as unprotected intercourse, especially anal intercourse. Also important is to avoid if possible, tranfusions or invasive surgical procedures in high–risk countries. Attempts are being made to produce a vaccine against HIV but, even if it can be made, it is unlikely to become available within at least the next 5 years. Giving zidovudine prophylactically after exposure to the virus may be beneficial but its value is uncertain.

Oral aspects

Oral manifestations: The majority of AIDS patients have head and neck manifestations. *Table 16. 9* shows the relative frequency of oral lesions.

Table 16. 9. Oral manifestations in HIV disease

Common	Less common
Cervical lymphadenopathy	Angular stomatitis
Candidosis	Herpes simplex or zoster
Kaposi's sarcoma	Venereal warts
'Hairy' leukoplakia	Recurrent ulcers
	Osteomyelitis
	Mycobacterial or histoplasmal ulcers
	Periodontitis and gingivitis
	Addisonian pigmentation
	Lymphoma
	Parotitis
	Xerostomia
	Cranial neuropathies

Cervical lymph node enlargement: Lymphadenopathy is an almost invariable feature of AIDS and AIDS-related complex.

Infections: Oral candidosis (usually thrush or erythematous candidosis) is common in AIDS and AIDS-related diseases, is often the initial manifestation, and is seen in 50 per cent of patients. Oral candidosis is frequently associated with oesophageal candidosis and is also a predictor of liability to systemic opportunistic infections. In a young adult male particularly, the development of thrush without a local cause, such as xerostomia or treatment with corticosteroids or antibiotics, is strongly suggestive of HIV infection. Conventional antifungal treatment is indicated initially, although ketoconazole or fluconazole may be required, especially if there is oesophageal infection.

Infections with herpes viruses—herpes simplex virus, varicella-zoster virus, Epstein–Barr virus, and cytomegalovirus—are also common in AIDS and AIDS-related syndromes. Herpesviruses, especially EBV, as well as human papilloma viruses (HPV) have been implicated in the hairy leukoplakia found in some patients (*see below*).

Herpes simplex infections are usually intraoral, sometimes severe and persistent but rarely disseminate: they usually respond well to acyclovir.

Less common oral and perioral complications include xerostomia, venereal warts, major aphthous ulceration, cranial neuropathies, mycobacterial oral ulcers and oral histoplasmosis or cryptococcosis, as well as sinusitis, gingivitis or periodontitis. Chronic parotitis is common mainly in children with HIV infection.

Saliva from affected patients contains CMV usually also contains HSV, herpesvirus 6 and EBV, as in other immunocompromised patients. The presence of HIV in saliva but lack of evidence of transmission are discussed below.

Hairy leukoplakia: Hairy leukoplakia (condyloma plana) is highly characteristic of HIV and seen only exceptionally rarely in other patients. It derives its name from the raised white areas of thickening, from which hair–like filaments of keratin may protrude. More frequently the surface is corrugated and usually affects the lateral borders of the tongue. Approximately 60 per cent of patients with hairy leukoplakia develop full-blown AIDS within 3 years. EBV is implicated it its etiology.

Neoplasms: Kaposi's sarcoma, an endothelial cell tumour, is the characteristic malignant neoplasm found in AIDS and in 50 per cent of patients is oral or peri-oral. Kaposi's sarcoma is often an early oral manifestation, presenting as a red or purple macule or a nodule, usually on the palate. Male homosexuals are predominantly affected. Kaposi's sarcoma in the mouth of a male who is not on immunosuppressive treatment is therefore virtually pathognomonic of AIDS.

Oral and salivary gland lymphomas also develop more frequently in patients with AIDS than in a normal population.

Transmission Routes and Risks

HIV is transmitted sexually, particularly by receptive anal intercourse, and by administration of blood or blood products including plasma. Semen, tears and breast milk may also contain HIV. Semen can transmit the infection, but evidence of transmission via the orogenital route is weak. Reports that HIV virions were present in a cell-free state in saliva, have not been confirmed. There is as yet *no* reliable evidence for transmission by saliva or by normal social contact.

From the viewpoint of dental practice, the chief occupational risk of acquiring the infection is as a result of injury by a sharp instrument, particularly a local anaesthetic needle which can contain a significant amount of contaminated fluid. The level of risk is also related to the numbers of infected patients that are treated.

The epidemiology of HIV infection is similar to that of hepatitis B. Homosexual or bisexual men are still the major risk groups, accounting for well over two-thirds of cases of AIDS in the western world, but there is increasing anxiety about the appearance of AIDS in heterosexual. Female consorts of infected individuals are at risk; HIV infection can also be sexually transmitted from females to males, and in Africa the disease appears to be transmitted *mainly* by promiscuous heterosexual activity. Both female and, particularly, male prostitutes in several areas are frequently HIV positive; in some areas of Europe and USA up to 40 per cent of female prostitutes are positive and in Africa, the prevalence is nearly 90 per cent in some areas. Condoms lessen the risk of transmission of HIV, but are by no means completely protective.

For British females, the greatest risk factor has been heterosexual intercourse abroad and this has accounted for nearly three times as many cases as intercourse with known 'high–risk' partners in Britain. However, recent (1991) anonymous testing in antenatal clinics has shown that approximately 1 in 500 pregnant women in inner London were HIV antibody positive. In one London teaching hospital, HIV antibody positivity among women attending antenatal clinics had increased ninefold between 1988 and 1990.

In other parts of Britain the frequency of antibody positivity in pregnant women was 1 in 16 000 or less. By contrast, among males attending genitourinary clinics in inner London, 1 in 100 heterosexuals and 1 in 5 homosexuals were antibody positive.

Dental treatment

Needle–stick injuries can transmit the AIDS virus, but despite reports of many such injuries, infection among health personnel caring for AIDS patients, is rare. By early 1991 (a decade after the disease was first recognized) only about 30 persons caring for HIV-infected individuals had been shown to have contracted HIV infection. In most health care workers who have acquired AIDS, the infection has been sexually transmitted.

The risk of transmission of HIV occupationally (less than 1 per cent) appears to be far lower than the nearly 26 per cent of persons who develop hepatitis B infection after a needle-stick injury. Hepatitis B virus is a less fragile and more infectious virus than HIV.

There has been, as yet only one report of dental staff contracting AIDS as a consequence of his occupation, even in endemic areas. By contrast a dentist with this infection in the USA appears to have transmitted it to at least 5 patients as a consequence of invasive dental procedures. That the dentist was the source of the infection was confirmed by the fact that the strain of the virus was the same and by the lack of other risk factors in the patients' lifestyles. The precise mode of transmission remains uncertain as the dentist has since died.

Sexual intercourse appears to be the only type of interpersonal contact likely to lead to transmission of HIV infection, and there are now several studies that have failed to demonstrate HIV transmission from infected patients to family members through normal social contact. Based on current evidence therefore, casual person-to-person contact, even within a family, appears to pose no risk.

Dental treatment should be carried out with the precautions outlined in Chapter 8 and additional attention given to the possibility, though small, of postoperative infection and haemorrhage.

Paediatric and neonatal aids

Children may acquire AIDS from exposure to blood or blood products, or occasionally in utero even as early as 20 weeks of intra-uterine life. Later they may be infected by intrapartum transmission from infected mothers. Children account for about 2 per cent of AIDS patients in the USA: nearly 2000 child cases in the USA had been diagnosed by late 1989.

HIV infection in children causes them to appear ill, stunts their growth, and causes staphylococcal and streptococcal infections such as otitis media, rashes and bouts of diarrhoea. AIDS in young children differs from the adult disease in such respects as the following:

1. Humoral immunity is more severely affected. Hypergammaglobulinaemia is also severe and 13 per cent of children have thrombocytopenic purpura.
2. Normal CD4/CD8 ratios may persist late in the disease and lymphopenia is uncommon.
3. Bacterial infections are relatively more common because of depressed humoral immunity and may long precede changes in T lymphocyte subsets.
4. Asymptomatic infection is less common.

5. Generalised lymphadenopathy and hepatosplenomegaly are often the first signs.

6. Neurological disease develops in the great majority.

7. Interstitial lymphoid pneumonitis is particularly characteristic.

8. B cell lymphomas are the most common AIDS–associated tumours. Kaposi's sarcoma is rare and particularly rarely affects the skin.

9. Other systemic effects of HIV infection in children include renal disease and cardiomyopathy.

10. Chronic parotitis is a more frequent clinical manifestation than in adults.

Oral features of childhood AIDS

Parotitis. As mentioned above, chronic parotitis is common in affected children and in those at risk from exposure to HIV, is reported to be virtually pathognomonic of AIDS.

Candidosis Chronic oral candidosis is present in 75 per cent and is the single most common mucocutaneous manifestation of HIV infection in children. Any type of oral candidosis may be seen but most frequently it is in the form of persistent thrush. Difficulties in swallowing usually indicate involvement of the oesophagus.

Herpetic stomatitis. Unlike normal children, those with AIDS are frequently subject to recurrent intraoral as well as labial herpetic infection. Initially the infection responds to intravenous acyclovir but becomes more resistant as AIDS progresses.

Herpes zoster. Shingles is rare in normal children, but can be an early sign of AIDS in child, and tends to be more severe and painful.

Immunosuppressive Treatment

Immunosuppressive treatment is used as an adjunct to renal transplantation and other organ grafts, and for the treatment of immunologically mediated disease. Immunosuppressive drugs include corticosteroids, azathioprine, cyclosporin and cyclophosphamide. The actions of immunosuppressive drugs are complex and by no means fully understood but most of them predominantly affect cell-mediated responses and autoantibody production more strongly than normal antibody production.

The most common complication of immunosuppressive treatment is infection, which is the main cause of death. An uncommon but important complication is a predisposition to lymphomas or less frequently, Kaposi's sarcoma after prolonged immunosuppressive treatment. The widespread use of immunosuppressive treatment is a factor contributing to the increasing problem of infectious diseases in hospitals today.

Dental aspects of acquired immunodeficiencies other than AIDS

If there are severe immunological defects, particularly deficiency or functional disorders of neutrophils, acute gingival infections or soft-tissue ulcers can be caused by bacteria. These oral infections are a recognized and troublesome complication of conditions such as acute leukaemia or severe neutropenia (agranulocytosis). In acute leukaemia the response to dental plaque may be gross gingival swelling caused by dense infiltration of the gingivae with leukaemic cells. If untreated, the gingival margins become necrotic and ulcerated, and the periodontal tissues are rapidly destroyed. Extensive mucosal ulceration can develop where the soft tissue of the cheek is in contact with plaque on a tooth or without any obvious cause for the site of localization. In agranulocytosis, infection can also lead to ulceration and necrosis of the gingivae, oral mucosa and pharynx (Chapter 5).

In immunosuppressed patients oral infections can be painful and a potential source of metastatic infections or septicaemia. Oral infections can be caused by a variety of organisms but can usually be controlled with topical or systemic antibiotic therapy or sometimes with antiseptics such as chlorhexidine. Mixed infections can often be controlled by a broad-spectrum antibiotic such as topical tetracycline, but this should be given together with an antifungal drug because of the risk of superinfection. Failure to respond to such treatment indicates that the causative bacteria are not sensitive and bacteriological investigation may show infection by bacteroides species, for example. Clindamycin may then be a more suitable choice.

In patients where the main defect is of cell-mediated immunity, mucosal infections by viruses or fungi are particularly common. In the immunodeficient patient, bacteria can produce plaques that clinically resemble thrush. Hairy leukoplakia can be a complication of immunosuppressive treatment. Oral Kaposi's sarcoma and lymphoma are rare, but squamous carcinoma of the lip is a recognized complication of immunosuppression if there is exposure to strong sunlight

Dental surgical procedures should therefore be covered with an antibiotic and particular attention should be paid to the possibility of thrombocytopenia with haemorrhagic tendencies and to the risks associated with corticosteroid treatment (Chapter 10).

An oral manifestation of particular note in patients on cyclosporin is gingival hyperplasia.

CANDIDOSIS

Thrush was aptly described in the nineteenth century as a 'disease of the diseased' and candidosis can certainly be a reflection of impaired immune responses. However, the common form of candidosis (denture–induced stomatitis) is seen in patients who are usually otherwise healthy.

Oral candidosis can produce a variety of clinical pictures and can sometimes be secondary to an underlying disorder. The main types which may be seen in dental practice are as follows.

1. Thrush.
2. Erythematous candidosis—usually denture–induced stomatitis, or generalized (*see below*)
3. Angular stomatitis.

4. Candidal leukoplakia (chronic hyperplastic candidosis). .
5. Rare mucocutaneous candidosis syndromes.

Angular stomatitis can be seen in association with any type of intraoral candidosis and is the only feature which they all share in common. Angular stomatitis is occasionally seen in isolation when it may be staphylococcal rather than candidal.

Thrush is the best known type of candidosis and produces the highly characteristic picture of soft, creamy-coloured, slightly raised patches which can be wiped off the mucosa leaving a red area. These lesions may form isolated flecks or large confluent areas. Typical sites are the buccal mucosa or the soft palate.

Thrush is common in the newborn in whom it may clear up spontaneously or in response to topical antifungal treatment. In adults, unless known to be having immunosuppressive treatment, thrush is rare and should prompt investigation for an underlying cause. Thrush in a young or middle-aged adult, particularly a male homosexual, must be regarded as a sign of HIV infection until proved otherwise. The other main possibilities are antibiotic treatment, anaemia, diabetes mellitus or an immunological defect, as shown in *Table 16. 6.*

The diagnosis can be readily confirmed by taking a Gram-stained smear which shows long tangled masses of candidal hyphae.

In addition to treatment of any underlying disorder the local infection should be manageable with topical antifungal drugs such as nystatin lozenges (500 000 u), nystatin pastilles (100 000 u) or amphotericin (10 mg) lozenges allowed to dissolve slowly in the mouth four times daily for a week or longer if necessary. Alternatively, a nystatin suspension (100 000 u/ml) or systemic fluconazole may be indicated.

Occasionally patches of thrush are present under a denture in association with denture stomatitis but if not unusually severe or widespread are unlikely to be the result of any underlying disorder.

Erythematous candidosis. Mucosal erythema due to candidal infection can result from antibiotic treatment, xerostomia or coverage of the mucosa with a denture. It is sometimes seen on the palate or tongue in HIV infection.

Antibiotic stomatitis occasionally follows the use of broad-spectrum antibiotics, particularly tetracycline used topically in the mouth. The whole of the oral mucosa is then typically red, oedematous and sore. One or two flecks of thrush may be found in protected situations such as the posterior upper buccal sulcus. As with any other type of candidosis, angular stomatitis may be associated.

The treatment is to stop the use of the antibiotic, if feasible, or alternatively to give topical antifungal drugs as described earlier.

A similar picture of generalized redness and soreness of the oral mucosa is the typical manifestation of candidosis associated with xerostomia.

Denture-induced stomatitis (denture sore mouth) is a common candidal infection secondary to long-standing occlusion of part of the oral mucosa by a denture. There is no convincing evidence that trauma is a factor and denture-induced stomatitis commonly develops beneath a well-fitting upper denture which effectively cuts off the mucous membrane from the normal oral defence mechanisms. As may be expected therefore, denture stomatitis is seen only rarely under a lower denture, in spite of the fact that the latter is a common cause of trauma.

The characteristic features are uniform bright erythema of the whole of the upper denture-bearing area and limited by the denture margin. Occasionally the erythema is patchy or there may be flecks of thrush. Symptoms are typically absent but occasionally there is associated soreness.

Angular stomatitis is frequently associated but may be intermittent and absent when the patient is first seen. In patients with deep folds at the angles of the mouth as a result of ageing, inflammation may spread for a centimetre or so along the fold, producing a conspicuous line of erythema. In other cases there may be cracking, bleeding or prominent crusting. In such cases there may be a mixed staphylococcal and candidal infection.

The vast majority of patients with denture stomatitis are healthy, as local factors determine the pathogenesis. Occasionally, patients may be iron deficient but less frequently than might be expected from the fact that angular stomatitis is often regarded as a typical sign of anaemia. Other occasional underlying factors are dry mouth, folate deficiency or diabetes mellitus. It is, however, unjustifiable to screen all patients with denture stomatitis but investigation should be considered if the patient has any other complaints suggestive of such disorders or if the infection is particularly severe or intractable.

Treatment includes leaving dentures out of the mouth at night and storing them in hypochlorite to clear the fungus from the denture surface. Topical antifungals should also be used, as suggested above.

Angular stomatitis (angular cheilitis) is probably most frequently seen in dental practice as a complication of denture-induced stomatitis but can be associated with any type of oral candidosis. In such cases, clearance of the intraoral infection with adequate antifungal treatment typically leads to healing of the lesions at the angles of the mouth without any local treatment.

Angular stomatitis can also sometimes be staphylococcal or a mixed infection. Bacteriological examination may therefore be necessary, but imidazoles such as miconazole or clotrimazole also have antibacterial activity and may be effective.

In addition, angular stomatitis is a 'classic' sign of iron deficiency anaemia, though, in practice, this is infrequently found in patients with denture stomatitis. However, angular stomatitis is very occasionally an isolated initial sign of anaemia, such as vitamin B_{12} deficiency, and clears up when the underlying disease has been treated. Treatment is outlined above, and miconazole cream applied to the lesion may be useful.

Candidal leukoplakia (chronic hyperplastic candidosis) appears as white plaques clinically indistinguishable from other types of keratotic lesions. These candidal plaques appear quite different from those of thrush in that they are tough and firmly adherent. Most patients are men of middle age or over, and many are heavy smokers. Typical sites are the buccal mucosa just within the commissures, or the dorsum or edges of the tongue. Long-standing angular stomatitis and occasionally also denture stomatitis may be associated. Patients are usually otherwise well.

Diagnosis of candidal leukoplakia depends on biopsy when hyphae of *Candida albicans* and a characteristic inflammatory reaction can be seen in the superficial epithelial plaque. Investigation should include a family history, haematological examination and, possibly, tests for cell-mediated responses to *C. albicans*. In the great majority of cases no abnormality is detectable but such investigations may be needed to exclude one of the rare mucocutaneous candidosis syndromes which show similar oral lesions as described below.

Treatment is difficult as the response to topical antifungal drugs such as nystatin or amphotericin is poor. Excision is also followed by recurrence, but newer antifungals such as miconazole topically or ketoconazole or fluconazole systemically appear to be more effective.

These lesions may account for up to 10 per cent of leukoplakias and several reports of apparent malignant transformation have appeared. However, the prevalence of candidal leukoplakia and its potentialities remain uncertain.

Candidosis in immune deficiency states

Carriage of oral *C. albicans* may be promoted by high numbers of suppressor T-lymphocytes. Persistent oral candidosis is a well-recognized complication of defective cell-mediated immunity and may be seen in the following circumstances:

1. As a complication of primary immunodeficiencies, especially severe combined (Swiss) type or Di George's syndrome. In these conditions candidosis is not the main feature of the disease and is only one of many complications. Such patients are unlikely to be seen in dental practice.

2. As a common complication of intense immunosuppression particularly for organ grafts. Both thrush and herpetic infection may be present together and produce confluent lesions. In most cases, the candidal infection responds eventually to antifungal drugs but sometimes the immunosuppressive treatment has to be moderated for a time.

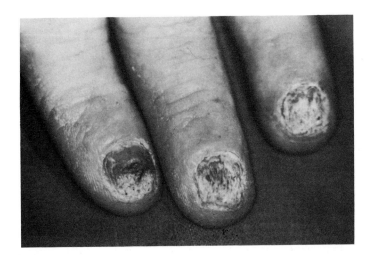

Fig. 16.1. Chronic candidosis affecting the nails in a patient with chronic mucocutaneous candidosis.

Patients on long-term corticosteroid treatment for any of the immunologically mediated diseases are also susceptible to oral candidosis but not often as a serious problem.

3. *HIV infection*

4. *Chronic mucocutaneous candidosis.* In this group of disorders candidosis is the main or a prominent feature (*Fig.* 16. 1). Various types of defects of cell-mediated immunity may be detected, particularly in the more severe cases, as discussed later, but are not, however, invariable.

Rare mucocutaneous candidosis syndromes

The main types of these rare disorders and their salient features are summarized in *Table 16. 10*. In all of them, candidosis even if relatively mild, is persistent and responds poorly to topical treatment with nystatin or amphotericin but may respond to ketoconazole or fluconazole. In general, the more severe the infection, the greater the likelihood that immunological defects (particularly of cell-mediated immunity) will be found. However in some cases these defects are secondary to the infection and so–called antigenic overload.

In the *diffuse type,* candidosis is particularly severe and can give rise to gross, proliferative and disfiguring lesions of the skin (so–called granulomas) as well as widespread oral lesions. Immunological defects are frequently found and there is also susceptibility to bacterial infections of the respiratory tract or elsewhere. Even in this unusually severe form of the disease, candidosis remains superficial and does not progress to candidal septicaemia or other types of disseminated infection.

There is also the possibility—though small—that a patient with chronic candidosis has one of the rare disorders such as the candidosis-endocrinopathy syndrome. In these diseases candidosis (when present) probably invariably involves the mouth which is often the most severely affected site.

The early-onset forms of CMCC (Types 1–3) typically have the following features in common:

1. Onset in infancy, often as persistent thrush.
2. Candidosis is mainly or entirely oral.
3. Immunological defects sometimes associated.

Table 16.10. Chronic mucocutaneous candidosis (CMCC) syndromes

Type	Clinical features
1. Familial	Persistent oral candidosis
	Often iron deficiency
2. Diffuse CMCC (*Candida granuloma*)	Severe chronic candidosis
	Susceptibility to bacterial infections
3. Candidosis-endocrinopathy syndrome	Mild chronic oral candidosis
	Hypoparathyroidism
	Hypoadrenocorticism
4. Candidosis-thymoma syndrome	Chronic oral candidosis
	Myasthenia gravis
	Haematological disorders

Candidosis-endocrinopathy syndrome has been the source of considerable misunderstanding. Candidosis is typically the initial feature and is usually mild but persistent. Endocrine disorders may not appear until 10 or 15 years later, but occasionally this sequence is reversed. There is no evidence that candidosis causes the endocrine disorders or vice versa. Hypoparathyroidism or Addison's disease or both are the most commonly associated endocrinopathies.

This purely coincidental association between chronic candidosis and hypoparathyroidism (Type I polyendocrinopathy syndrome), also seen in the Di George syndrome, has given rise to the myth that hypoparathyroidism predisposes to candidosis. However, treatment of hypoparathyroidism has no effect on candidosis and hypoparathyroidism from any other cause is not associated with candidosis.

The endocrine disorders in candidosis-endocrinopathy syndrome are associated with multiple organ-specific autoantibodies both in patients and unaffected relatives. The possible effects (in various combinations) are shown in *Table 16. 11*. Chronic candidosis appears to be an essential feature of Type I polyendocrinopathy syndrome, but frequently has not been noticed in the past as it is typically mild, or has been thought to be the result of the endocrine disease. The latter is the more important feature and, at one time, was an important cause of death.

Patients may for long appear to be quite well apart from chronic oral candidosis. If, therefore, a patient, particularly a child or adolescent with chronic oral candidosis, has a family history of any of the disorders shown in *Table 16. 11*, and autoantibodies (particularly to glandular tissues) are found, then it is probable that endocrine disease will develop at some time in the future. The patient should therefore be kept under observation. The candidosis can be treated with topical antifungal agents, particularly one of the imidazoles, such as miconazole, or systemically with oral ketoconazole or fluconazole.

An adult with chronic oral candidosis may have the familial form of the disease which can escape diagnosis until middle age unless inquiry is made as to whether siblings are affected and whether there was any parental consan-

Table 16.11. Polyglandular autoimmune disease* Type I and Type II

Entity	Type I	Type II
Addison's disease	100%	100%
Hypoparathyroidism	76%	—
Chronic mucocutaneous candidosis	73%	—
Alopecia	32%	0.5%
Malabsorption syndromes	22%	—
Gonadal failure	17%	3.6%
Pernicious anaemia	13%	0.5%
Chronic active hepatitis	13%	—
Insulin-dependent diabetes	4%	52%
Autoimmune thyroiditis	11%	69%
Female: male ratio	1:5:1	1:8:1
HLA associations	No constant findings	B8 (A1)

*Polyendocrine deficiency syndromes.

guinity, as the disease appears to be autosomal recessive. In familial candidosis, investigation for iron deficiency should be carried out, since treatment with
iron may improve the response to antifungal drugs.

Alternatively, chronic candidosis in the older patient can be the first manifestation of a thymic disorder (late onset chronic mucocutaneous candidosis).
Evidence of impaired cell-mediated immunity, particularly to C. albicans, may
then be found. In such a case, investigation for a thymoma should be carried
out, as early excision may improve the prognosis.

In summary therefore it may be helpful to know whether any patient with
chronic candidosis has any immunological defect, as the latter may sometimes
be indicative of underlying disease. However, isolated unresponsiveness to
antigens of C. albicans seems also to be a specific, limited immunological
deficiency compatible with otherwise normal health.

'Chronic Candidosis Syndrome'

Many normal persons harbour *Candida albicans* as part of their normal
microflora. This finding has been exploited, particularly in the USA, as a
supposed explanation of such symptoms as headaches, fatigue and lassitude,
rashes and gastrointestinal symptoms. This so–called syndrome has absolutely
no scientific basis. There is no evidence that antifungal treatment is warranted
and a controlled trial has shown that it has no effect on the symptoms.

OTHER ORAL FUNGAL INFECTIONS IN IMMUNOCOMPROMISED PATIENTS (*Table* 16.12)

Aspergillus spp. may infect the paranasal sinuses, palate or other sites in
immunocompromised patients. Infection spreads by direct extension and
haematogenously. Diagnosis is by demonstration of hyphae in a smear, serology and biopsy. Intravenous amphotericin may be effective.

Mucormycosis (zygomycosis: phycomycosis) is infection by *Mucor* or
Rhizopus spp., mainly of the paranasal sinuses and nose of poorly controlled
diabetic or leukaemic patients. Diagnosis is by biopsy and culture: treatment is
by control of diabetes or other underlying disease, debridement and intravenous
amphotericin. In the case of mucormycosis secondary to leukaemia, the prognosis is poor.

Other mycoses can affect the mouth, particularly in AIDS, as discussed
earlier (p. 185).

IMMUNOLOGICALLY MEDIATED DISEASES

Important immunologically mediated diseases are shown in *Table 16.13*.

ATOPIC DISEASE

Atopic disease is the term given to the group of allergic conditions (asthma, eczema, hay fever and others) which are by far the most common type of immunologically mediated disease and affect about 10 per cent of the population. Susceptibility is usually genetically determined. IgA deficiency (which is also common) is frequently associated with allergic disease.

Atopic disease depends on production of specific IgE antibody which binds to mast cells. Degranulation of mast cells, with release of mediators such as histamine, follows further exposure to the allergen. Cell-bound IgE is present, particularly in the bronchial tree, nasal mucosa, dermis and intestinal wall. The clinical types of atopic disease are therefore asthma, hay fever, urticaria, angiooedema, eczema and food allergies. Common allergens are grass pollens, mites in house dust, fungal spores and milk and egg proteins, but in many cases the allergen cannot be reliably identified. Patients with atopy were also thought to be more prone to develop allergy or anaphylaxis in response to drugs such as penicillin or intravenous anaesthetic agents but this does not appear to have been confirmed.

Normal individuals also produce IgE antibodies but without ill-effect and the reasons for the abnormal response of allergic individuals is unknown.

General management of atopic disorders

A history of 'allergy' to a variety of substances is common but may need to be confirmed by objective tests. True food allergy is rare while systemic 'allergy' to amalgam restorations and phenomena such as 'total allergy syndrome' are myths. The history should, however, indicate whether the allergy takes any of the recognized forms mentioned earlier and whether there is a positive family history. Confirmatory tests include the following:

Skin tests for allergens.   Allergy to individual substances may be detected by skin testing. This can be done either by pricking the allergen into the skin (intradermal or prick testing) or, less efficiently, by applying it in an absorbent dressing taped onto the skin (patch testing). A positive reaction is shown by a wheal and erythema which starts to appear within about 20 minutes. Adequate controls must be used. A complication of skin testing is that it can induce sensitivity to the test compound. Anaphylactic reactions can occasionally follow intradermal skin test doses of penicillin.

Laboratory tests.   These include:

1. Serum IgE levels (PRIST test; paper radio-immunosorbent test).
2. Radioallergosorbent test (RAST) for IgE antibodies to specific antigens.

IgE is present in very low concentration in the serum and its quantification depends on sensitive radio-immunoassay. In many cases of allergy, also, serum IgE levels are within the normal range.

Table 16.12. Orofacial lesions in important deep mycoses

Disease	Organism	Source	Main endemic areas	Orofacial lesions	Clinical forms	Pathology	Prognosis
Aspergillosis	*Aspergillus fumigatus, A. flavus, A. niger* and other *Aspergillus* species	Ubiquitous	Worldwide	Aspergilloma in paranasal sinuses. Invasive rhinocerebral type may invade palate	Allergic bronchopulmonary Pulmonary Disseminated Aspergilloma	Invasion of blood vessels causing infarcts	Variable Poor in invasive pulmonary or disseminated types or in immunocompromised
Blastomycosis	*Blastomyces dermatiditis*	Soil	Mississippi and Ohio valleys in USA, Canada, North Africa and Venezuela	Ulcers	Cavitary pulmonary Disseminated Others	Granulomatous inflammation Chronic suppuration, especially of skin lesions	Often good except in disseminated form
Coccidioido-myis	*Coccidioides immitis*	Soil	Southwestern USA, Mexico	Ulcers	Acute pulmonary Disseminated Chronic pulmonary Meningitis	Granulomatous inflammation Chronic suppuration	Often good except in meningeal forms or the immunocompromised
Cryptococcosis	*Cryptococcus neoformans*	Soil, pigeon droppings	Latin America Worldwide	Ulcers	Pneumonia Meningitis Disseminated Cryptococcoma	Granulomatous inflammation	Poor especially in meningeal forms or the immunocompromised

Histoplasmosis	Histoplasma capsulatum	Soil; bird and bat droppings	Ohio and Mississippi valleys in USA Latin America, Africa, India, Far East Australia	Ulcers or lumps	Benign pulmonary Disseminated Chronic pulmonary Cutaneous	Granulomatous inflammation Yeast cells in macrophages	Usually good except in disseminated form or immunocompromised
Mucormycosis	Mucor, Rhizopus and Absidia	Ubiquitous	Worldwide	Rhino-cerebral form may cause swelling, necrosis, or destruction of palate	Rhinocerebral Pulmonary Gastrointestinal	Invasion of blood vessels to cause thrombosis and infarction	Variable
Paracoccidioidomycosis (South American blastomycosis)	Paracoccidioides brasiliensis	Soil	South America, esp. Brazil	Ulcers Very common	Pulmonary Disseminated	Granulomatous inflammation	Usually good in young patients
Sporotrichosis	Sporothrix schenkii	Associated with thorny plants, wood, sphagnum moss	Worldwide especially in tropical countries	Rare	Lymphocutaneous Localized cutaneous Pulmonary Disseminated	Granulomatous inflammation and chronic suppuration	

Table 16.13. Examples of immunologically mediated diseases

I. *Reactions to foreign antigens*
    Allergic rhinitis (hayfever)
    Asthma
    Eczema
    Urticaria and angio-oedema (angioneurotic oedema)*
    Drug and food allergies
    Anaphylaxis
    Contact dermatitis
II. *Disorders with an autoimmune basis*
    1. *Rheumatoid (collagen) diseases*
        Systemic lupus erythematosus*
        Rheumatoid arthritis*
        Sjögren's syndrome*
        Systemic sclerosis*
        Polymyositis-dermatomyositis
        Polyarteritis nodosa*
    2. *Haematological disease*
        Pernicious anaemia*
        Autoimmune haemolytic anaemia
        Idiopathic and drug-associated thrombocytopenic purpura*
        Drug-induced neutropenia*
        Aplastic anaemia (some cases)*
    3. *Gastrointestinal and liver diseases*
        Chronic atrophic gastritis and pernicious anaemia*
        Gluten-sensitive enteropathy (coeliac disease)*
        Chronic autoimmune hepatitis
        Primary biliary cirrhosis
    4. *Cardiac diseases*
        Acute rheumatic fever
    5. *Renal diseases*
        Glomerulonephritis (various types)
        Goodpasture's syndrome
    6. *Cutaneous disease*
        Pemphigus*
        Pemphigoid*
        Dermatitis herpetiformis*
    7. *Endocrine diseases*
        Chronic (Hashimoto's) thyroiditis
        Hyperthyroidism
        Idiopathic adrenocortical insufficiency*
        Idiopathic hypoparathyroidism*
    8. *Neurological diseases*
        Guillain-Barré syndrome
        Myasthenia gravis
    9. *Eye diseases*
        Sympathetic ophthalmia
        Sjögren's syndrome*
        Pemphigus vulgaris*
        Mucous membrane pemphigoid*

*Also affect oral tissues.

In the RAST test, purified extracts of a wide range of allergens are coupled to cellulose or paper discs to which the patient's serum is applied. Its ability to react with one or more of these allergens is tested by adding rabbit anti-IgE labelled with radioactive iodine. The level of radioactivity then indicates the levels of specific IgE antibodies.

As discussed later, no tests will reliably predict the possibility of anaphylactic reactions in patients sensitized to penicillin and the history of the response to previous exposure is the main precaution.

Desensitization of patients is attempted by administering the allergen initially in minute but in progressively increasing doses. However, there is little objective evidence of the value of this procedure and there is a risk of fatal anaphylaxis or other severe reactions during the process. Since safe and effective drugs such as sodium cromoglycate or topically active corticosteroids are available, desensitization has few useful applications and is regarded as obsolete by many authorities.

Dental aspects of atopic disease

There is no evidence that immediate type hypersensitivity affects the oral mucosa and there is no oral counterpart of eczema. Denture stomatitis, for example, has been shown *not* be be caused by allergy to polymethylacrylate.

Other dental materials which accidentally come into contact with the patient's skin can very occasionally provoke an acute eczematous reaction or contact dermatitis.

No oral diseases have been proved to have any significant direct association with atopic disease, although patients with allergic rhinitis may be mouth-breathers and develop gingival hyperplasia.

In a few patients with aphthous stomatitis, ulceration appears to be precipitated by certain foods—especially walnuts, chocolate or citrus fruits. Although there may be a slightly increased prevalence of allergic diseases associated with aphthous stomatitis, there is little evidence for an allergic mechanism.

The main clinical implications of atopic disease in dental practice are therefore as follows:

1. Possibly an increased risk of sensitization or of acute allergic reactions to drugs used in dentistry.
2. Problems caused by drugs, particularly corticosteroids, used to control allergic disease.
3. Anaesthetic hazards in asthmatic patients (Chapter 6).
4. Management of severe asthma in the dental surgery (Chapter 18).
5. Dry mouth and drowsiness in patients taking antihistamines.

Hypersensitivity to drugs used in dentistry.   Those with atopic disease or from an affected family *may* be more likely to develop hypersensitivity to drugs. The drugs causing the most severe and potentially lethal reactions are the penicillins and intravenous anaesthetic agents, but in many cases these are in patients without any atopic tendency.

Hypersensitivity to penicillins: Allergic reactions are likely to follow parenteral rather than oral penicillin. The common reactions to penicillins are rashes which are typically urticarial and irritating, but sometimes a serum sickness type of reaction with joint pains and fever can follow some days or even weeks after administration.

The most dangerous type of reaction is acute anaphylaxis, which has been estimated to have caused approximately 300 deaths a year in the United States of America.

Mechanism of penicillin allergy. The major antigenic determinant appears to be the penicilloyl group which forms as a result of metabolic cleavage of the beta–lactam ring. This product acts as a hapten and binds to body proteins to become antigenic.

Most persons receiving penicillin develop IgG or IgM antibodies but these only occasionally cause reactions. Specific IgE antibodies to penicillin form rarely, but are the cause of anaphylactic reactions by binding to mast cells and triggering release of mediators. Contrary to traditional belief and surprisingly, there appears to be no association between penicillin anaphylaxis and atopic disease even though the latter is mediated by the same mechanisms.

On the very rare occasions when no other antibiotic than a penicillin is indicated for a life–threatening infection, it may be possible to predict the possibility of an IgE mediated response and an anaphylactic reaction, by skin testing with benzylpenicilloyl polylysine, which gives a wheal and flare reaction within 10 minutes. Only about 10 per cent of those who claim to be allergic to penillin react positively in this way. Anaphylaxis is virtually unknown in those who give negative reactions to this test.

A history of previous reactions to penicillin suggests a greater risk of acute anaphylaxis but there is no completely reliable method of prediction. From the practical and medicolegal viewpoints therefore, reliance has to be placed on the history and an alternative antimicrobial—but *not* one of the many penicillin derivatives—given, when the patient claims to be allergic to penicillin.

Unfortunately anaphylaxis can occasionally also be the first manifestation of sensitivity to penicillins and, rarely, a patient who has had penicillins on several occasions without ill-effect can suddenly develop acute anaphylaxis. A negative history therefore reduces the chances but does not totally exclude the possibility of anaphylaxis.

A patient should of course be lying down when injections are given as fainting after injections is common and may otherwise cause confusion with anaphylaxis.

Management of anaphylaxis.   An anaphylactic reaction can be recognized by the onset of symptoms within a few minutes of injection. Reactions after oral administration are delayed by the time taken for the drug to be absorbed.

The first symptoms are likely to be anxiety, usually followed by such changes as paraesthesiae around the mouth or of the extremities, and wheezing. Loss of consciousness and pallor caused by a precipitous and dangerous fall in blood pressure follow almost immediately. The blood pressure may fall so low as to be difficult to measure and the pulse may be impalpable. Ashen cyanosis quickly follows in severe cases. Oedema of the face or larynx may be associated. Death can follow within 5 minutes, and immediate treatment is essential. The patient should be laid flat with legs raised. Intramuscular adrenaline, 1 ml of 1:1000, is given and the plunger of the syringe withdrawn before injection to make sure that the needle is not in a vein. Although there is a risk of inducing dysrhythmias, the hazards from adrenaline are less than that of the acute hypotension which can precipitate cardiac arrest.

Intramuscular adrenaline should be followed by intravenous injection of hydrocortisone succinate 200 mg at least.

Cardiopulmonary resuscitation should be started if the heart stops. There is no evidence that antihistamines alone (by any route) are effective (*see* Chapter 18).

Medical assistance should be obtained and the patient should be removed to hospital as soon as possible for observation or further treatment if necessary.

Since a negative history of reactions to penicillin does not exclude the possibility of anaphylaxis it is arguable that penicillin should not be given immediately before a general anaesthetic. Admittedly the chances are small but acute anaphylactic reactions during anaesthesia have been reported and, clearly, their recognition under such circumstances could be difficult. If penicillin has to be given, half an hour should be allowed to elapse before induction of anaesthesia: after such a period a severe reaction is unlikely.

Sensitivity to any of the penicillins confers sensitivity to all members of this group of antibiotics. Depot penicillins, which are slowly excreted, can maintain the antigenic challenge so that treatment of a reaction may have to be continued until all the antigen is used up.

Cephalosporins have a somewhat similar chemical structure to penicillins and about 10 per cent of those sensitized to penicillin are also sensitive to the cephalosporins. Equally, a patient sensitive to penicillin is more likely to become sensitized to the cephalosporins than an unsensitized person. A cephalosporin should preferably not be given to a patient allergic to penicillin unless there is a specific bacteriological indication. However, this is rarely a consideration in dentistry.

Procaine penicillin can occasionally cause vertigo, hallucinations and acute anxiety reactions if given intravenously or if it accidentally enters a vein. Such reactions, though rare, may be mistaken for anaphylaxis.

Reactions to intravenous anaesthetic agents: Intravenous anaesthetic agents can cause anaphylactic-type reactions, either as a result of hypersensitivity or by inducing histamine release. These agents are, in order of risk, propanidid, Althesin, methohexitone and thiopentone. These reactions have sometimes been fatal, probably because of failure to recognize their nature, and both propanidid and Althesin have now been withdrawn in the UK because of this.

The level of risk is difficult to estimate, but it has been estimated that reactions complicated more than 1 per 1000 administrations of propanidid and fatalities from this cause have put this drug out of use. Althesin has been estimated to have caused reactions in 1 in 10 000–20 000 administrations. In one report it was estimated that allergic reactions to methohexitone developed in 1 per 7000 administrations but this is probably an overestimate. Similarly in a survey of 100 anaphylactic reactions to anaesthetic agents the only fatal cases (4 in number) were apparently caused by thiopentone. This, however, is probably more likely to be a reflection of the enormous scale of use of thiopentone than an indication of the true prevalence of allergy to this drug.

Allergic reactions to intravenous anaesthetic agents can take several forms. In the most severe type there is bronchospasm, flushing of the skin and a sharp fall in blood pressure. The loss of consciousness thus caused must be distinguished from the onset of anaesthesia.

Fatal reactions of this type have now been reported for all the intravenous agents in current use and one of the most important aspects of management is their recognition. Treatment is then by the same means as for penicillin anaphylaxis.

Halothane hepatitis. This reaction appears to be mediated at least in part by some form of hypersensitivity as discussed in Chapter 1.

Allergic reactions to muscle relaxants and related compounds: Certain muscle relaxants appear responsible for about 50 per cent of adverse reactions during general anaesthesia. Tachycardia, vascular collapse and skin reactions (flushing, oedema or urticaria) are the most frequent signs. Suxamethonium is the agent most commonly implicated but alcuronium, tubocurarine and other relaxants are sometimes implicated.

Allergic reactions to other drugs: Among dental drugs that might cause allergic reactions, lignocaine presents only a theoretical risk. It is estimated that at least 50 000 000 cartridges of lignocaine are used each year in Great Britain and *authenticated* allergic reactions or confirmation that lignocaine was the component responsible, have hardly ever been reported. The risk of hypersensitivity to other amide local anaesthetics such as prilocaine or mepivicaine is equally low.

The component of local anaesthetic solutions that is the most sensitizing agent is the methyl parabens preservative. As a consequence this has been replaced in some anaesthetic solutions. Amide local anaesthetics far more rarely cause contact dermatitis than the ester–type agents and fewer than 20 cases have been reported worldwide.

Investigation of putative allergy to local anaesthetics by skin testing is time–consuming, not always conclusively informative and rarely justified. In vitro tests depending on histamine release from sensitized basophils may be more informative but are not readily available.

Unlike lignocaine, amethocaine, sometimes used in surface anaesthetic preparations, is a potent sensitizer.

Aspirin can rarely also provoke allergic reactions. Aspirin-induced asthma is a recognized but rare side-effect, mainly in patients with nasal polyps ('triad asthma'— asthma, nasal polyps and aspirin sensitivity). Again, in relation to the scale of use of aspirin (an estimated 6 000 000 000 tablets annually) the incidence of such complications is almost negligible. If, however, there is a history of allergy to aspirin, it should not be given.

Even more rarely, other non-steroidal anti–inflammatory analgesics may induce allergic reactions. Morphine by contrast, directly triggers histamine release from mast cells and very occasionally causes anaphylactoid reactions.

Methylmethacrylate. Though it is virtually impossible to prove that any material is totally non-antigenic, there is little evidence that polymethylmethacrylate denture base causes contact sensitization. Occasionally there are isolated reports of persons who appear to have had allergic reactions to polymethylmethacrylate. However it is difficult to assess the significance of such cases in view of the widespread use of PMMA as a wool substitute (Acrylic) for clothing and as a denture base without trouble.

Drugs used in the treatment of allergic disease. The main drugs used in the treatment of allergic diseases include antihistamines, sympathomimetic agents, sodium cromoglycate (Intal; Rynacrom) and corticosteroids.

Food Intolerance

Allergy to foods is an emotive subject but far less common than the lay public believes. Adverse effects to foods may be due to intolerance, coeliac disease, reactions to food additives such as azo dyes or benzoic acid, or may be purely imaginary. Mothers have been known so to restrict the diet of their children because of alleged food allergy as to cause severe malnutrition.

Some children are hypersensitive to cow's milk protein for example, and this may cause diarrhoea. The effects of true food allergies are varied and in addition to gastrointestinal disturbances, can cause rhinorrhoea, bronchospasm, urticaria or angioedema. The last can be dangerous to those sensitive to egg protein, as discussed below, if they are given a vaccine derived from viruses grown on chick embryo.

Acute Allergic Angio-oedema

Angio-oedema (unjustifiably also called 'angioneurotic oedema') is characterized by rapid development of oedematous swelling, particularly of the head and neck region. The facial oedema, even though temporary, can cause embarrassment, but when oedema involves the neck and extends to the larynx, rapidly fatal respiratory obstruction can develop. Acute allergic oedema of this type can develop alone or may be associated with anaphylactic reactions as described earlier. Since minute amounts of allergen can trigger the reaction its nature may not be recognized. Thus patients sensitive to egg proteins have had dangerous reactions to viral vaccines when the virus had been grown on chick embryo tissues.

Mild angio-oedema may respond to antihistamines or to a sympathomimetic agent such as ephedrine which can be taken by mouth. In more severe cases,especially if there is a threat to the airway, the emergency should be managed in the same way as for an anaphylactic reaction. For intractable chronic cases corticosteroids may be required.

Hereditary angio-oedema (C1 esterase inhibitor deficiency)

Hereditary angio-oedema produces a clinically similar reaction to allergic angio-oedema but is caused by continued complement activation resulting from a genetically determined deficiency of C1 esterase inhibitor activity rather than an allergic reaction. In this reaction C4 is consumed and its plasma level falls. The level of C3, however is usually normal. Activation of kinin-like substances are the probable cause of the sudden increase in capillary permeability. In spite of its hereditary nature, usually as an autosomal dominant trait, the disease may not present until later childhood or adolescence.

Oedema typically affects the mouth, face and neck region, the extremities and gastrointestinal tract. Abdominal pain, nausea or vomiting, diarrhoea, rashes and peripheral oedema sometimes herald an attack. Involvement of the airway is a constant threat. The mortality has been estimated to be as high as 30 per cent in some families but the disease is compatible with prolonged survival if emergencies are effectively treated. Blunt injury is the most consistent precipitating event. The trauma of dental treatment is a potent trigger of attacks, and some attacks follow emotional stress.

Plasminogen inhibitors such as tranexamic acid have been used to mitigate attacks but currently the most effective agents are the androgenic steroids, danazol and, more recently, stanazolol, which raise plasma C1 esterase inhibitor levels to normal. The usual dose of stanazolol for an adult is 2.5–10 mg daily. It should not be given during pregnancy. Oligomenorrhoea may be induced in women and there may be acne, hirsutism, hypercalcaemia or headache.

Dental aspects of atopic disease

Antihistamines are useful only for minor manifestations of allergies, such as hay fever. Sedation usually accompanies effective doses of antihistamines, unless some of the newer agents, such as terphenadrine, are used. Therefore, these drugs normally have an additive effect with other sedating agents. Antihistamines also reduce salivary flow and can cause dry mouth.

Sympathomimetic agents such as ephedrine may be used as nasal drops to relieve congestion of the mucosa in hay fever or sinusitis, while others such as salbutamol or terbutaline are given by mouth or inhaler for the control of asthma. Sodium cromoglycate is widely used by inhalation for the long-term prophylaxis of asthma and hay fever. These drugs are unlikely to complicate dental treatment.

Corticosteroids used systemically for otherwise uncontrollable asthma can cause severe complications, but are usually now administered in aerosol form. Examples are beclomethasone dipropionate (Becotide) and betamethasone valerate (Bextasol) inhalers. The doses are very small and a Becotide inhaler for example, usually gives a total daily adult dose of only 300–400 µg. The only significant side-effect is to cause oropharyngeal thrush in a minority of patients and there is little evidence of systemic effects. Corticosteroids absorbed from ointments used for eczema can, however, cause adrenal suppression (Chapter 10).

Contact Dermatitis

Contact dermatitis causes an eczema-like, but cell-mediated reaction. It also differs from atopic eczema in that it is caused by some readily identifiable substance with which the susceptible individual comes into repeated contact and which produces a reaction restricted to the site of contact. A typical example is dermatitis of the hands of housewives using detergents, particularly those containing enzymes. A variety of dental materials, particularly mercury, are also potential causes.

Dental materials capable of causing contact dermatitis in susceptible individuals are shown in *Table 16.14*. Nevertheless, contact dermatitis affecting either dentist or patient is surprisingly uncommon. Like eczema, there is little convincing evidence for the existence of an oral equivalent of contact dermatitis. In

Table 16.14. Dental materials that may cause contact reactions

Mercury	Periodontal dressings
Methylmethacrylate monomer	Denture fixatives
Epoxy resins	Essential oils
Rubber base materials	Toothpastes

those sensitized to mercury, amalgam restorations can safely be inserted, provided that no stray amalgam is allowed to reach the patient's skin.

Dental amalgam has been reported to cause mucosal reactions, such as lichenoid lesions. However, the evidence is conflicting and mercury can be absorbed from amalgams into the mucosa without causing any reaction.

Illustrative of the difference in response between skin and mucosa to sensitizing agents is that occasionally a substance to which the patient is sensitized, when put in the mouth, can induce the typical rash on the skin. This has been reported in the case of nickel sensitivity when a nickel-containing denture caused a rash but not an oral reaction.

As mentioned earlier, methylmethacrylate monomer is sensitizing and irritant, but its low antigenicity is shown by the fact that even those who are habitually handling undiluted monomer rarely develop allergy to it. There is also little evidence that monomer leaks out of dentures but, if it does, rarely causes local irritation.

Contact dermatitis can occasionally affect the vermilion border of the lips or, more frequently, the perioral skin. Causes include components of lipsticks (such as fluorescein, oleyl alcohols and cinnamon or other essential oils), toothpastes and some foods, notably mangoes and oranges. Some food additives are thought occasionally to cause granulomatous oral reactions. Components of toothpastes can also cause inflammation of the gums or other parts of the oral mucosa but there is no convincing evidence that most such reactions are caused by hypersensitivity rather than chemical irritation.

Perioral dermatitis, cheilitis, gingivitis and other lesions have been described in patients using tartar control toothpastes which contain pyrophosphates or cinnamonaldehyde.

The main consideration in the management of contact dermatitis is strict avoidance of the sensitizing agent or, if it must be handled, gloves should be used.

AUTOIMMUNE DISEASE

Autoimmune disease can be broadly divided into two main groups (*Table 16.15*). There are, first, diseases such as pemphigus vulgaris where there are tissue or organ-specific auto-antibodies which appear to mediate the damage to the tissues. Second, there are the so-called connective tissue diseases, which are not caused by tissue-specific autoantibodies but probably mediated by immune complex reactions. The latter may be precipitated by other autoantibodies, such as anti-nuclear antibodies in systemic lupus erythematosus. These two groups of diseases are not entirely as clear-cut as this may imply and both

Table 16.15. Types of autoimmune disease

Organ or cell -specific autoantibodies	Non organ-specific autoantibodies— the collagen diseases*
Hashimoto's thyroiditis	Lupus erythematosus
Chronic atrophic gastritis (pernicious anaemia)[a]	Rheumatoid arthritis
Idiopathic Addison's disease	Sjögren's syndrome
Idiopathic hypoparathyroidism	Systemic sclerosis
Pemphigus vulgaris	Dermatomyositis
Pemphigoid	
Idiopathic thrombocytopenic purpura	
Autoimmune haemolytic anaemia	

*Probably mediated by immune complex reactions. [a]Not all chronic atrophic gastritis.
Note: 1. Only the more important and typical examples are given.
2. Even in the collagen diseases, cell-specific autoantibodies may also be produced but are incidental to the main disease processes.

types of phenomenon may be present in many cases especially in the connective tissue diseases. Patients with one autoimmune disease are especially liable to develop further autoimmune diseases; a few develop polyglandular autoimmune diseases (*Table 16.11*). Features suggestive of autoimmune disease are shown in *Table 16.2* and important examples are shown in *Table 16.15*. Several, such as rheumatoid arthritis or endocrine disorders are described in other, appropriate chapters. Only the remaining relevant diseases are therefore discussed here.

Pemphigus Vulgaris

There are several variants of pemphigus but pemphigus vulgaris is the most frequently seen. It is an uncommon disease which affects the skin and mucous membranes and, in the absence of treatment, is usually fatal. It has the most clearly defined autoimmune pathogenesis of any disease affecting the mouth. Pemphigus is characterized by widespread formation of vesicles and bullae followed by ulceration (*Fig.* 16.2). The majority of patients are middle-aged women.

The main immunological finding is circulating antibodies to the intercellular attachments of epithelial cells. These antibodies, and complement components, can also be localized by immunofluorescence along the intercellular junctions of epithelial cells. The loss of adherence of these cells to one another, with resulting destruction of the epithelium, is the essential feature of the disease. These changes can usually be abolished by immunosuppressive treatment.

Clinically, pemphigus vulgaris is characterized by thin-roofed vesicles or bullae which frequently first affect the oral mucosa. Stroking the mucosa with a finger may induce vesicle formation in an apparently unaffected area or cause

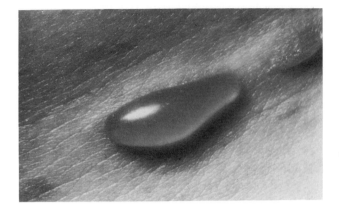

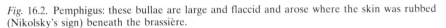

Fig. 16.2. Pemphigus: these bullae are large and flaccid and arose where the skin was rubbed (Nikolsky's sign) beneath the brassière.

a bulla to extend (Nikolsky's sign), but this is rarely positive in the mouth. The course of the disease varies from fulminating to relatively chronic but when initially affecting the oral mucosa can be expected to involve the skin within a few weeks or months at most. In the absence of treatment, pemphigus is fatal as a result of extensive skin damage leading to fluid and electrolyte loss, and often infection.

Management of pemphigus vulgaris

Acute cases need immediate immunosuppressive treatment. Rapid diagnosis is therefore essential and the following means are available.

Direct smears: Smears, preferably (but not easily) obtained from vesicle fluid or from a recently ruptured vesicle, should show acantholytic (Tzanck) cells which are detached epithelial cells, round in shape as a result of contraction of the cytoplasm. Acantholytic cells are isolated or seen in small clusters. Absence of Tzanck cells does not exclude the diagnosis of pemphigus.

Confirmation of the diagnosis can be made by immunofluorescence to demonstrate a coating of antibody (immunoglobulin) and/or complement around the acantholytic cells but biopsy should be carried out.

Biopsy is essential to confirm the diagnosis and for this purpose the specimen should be halved to enable both immunofluorescent and light microscopy to be carried out.

Immunofluorescent examination can be carried out by the direct method using fluorescein conjugated anti-human IgG and anti-complement (C3) sera on the frozen specimen or on exfoliated cells. In the indirect method, the patient's serum is incubated with normal mucosa, which is then labelled with fluorescein-conjugated, anti-human globulin. This method detects circulating antibodies but is more cumbersome and less sensitive than the direct method, and involves unecessary killing of an animal (*Table 16.16*).

Table 16.16. Immunostaining in oral mucosal diseases

Disease	Direct immuno-fluorescence	Epithelial location	Indirect immuno-fluorescence	Type of antibody*
Pemphigus vulgaris	Yes	Intercellular	Yes	IgG
Bullous pemphigoid	Yes	Basement membrane area	Yes	IgG
Mucous membrane pemphigoid	Yes	Basement membrane area	Rarely	IgG
Angina bullosa haemorrhagica	No	—	No	—
Dermatitis herpetiformis	Yes	Basement membrane area	No	IgA
Linear IgA disease	Yes	Basement membrane area	No	IgA
Systemic lupus erythematosus	Yes	Basement membrane area	Yes	ANA
Chronic discoid lupus erythematosus	Yes	Basement membrane area	No	ANA
Lichen planus	Frequently	Basement membrane area	No	— (usually fibrin)

* Usually with complement deposits, ANA = antinuclear antibody.

Light microscopy on a paraffin section is usually distinctive and shows supra-basal cleft formation and intra-epithelial vesicles containing free-floating acantholytic cells.

The usual treatment of pemphigus is with corticosteroids plus azathioprine to reduce the amount of corticosteroids that is needed in some cases. Even with 100–150 mg daily of azathioprine, 40–80 mg daily of prednisolone may be required. Cyclophosphamide, methotrexate or gold may be used instead of azathioprine.

With current methods of treatment the mortality may be about 8 per cent, usually secondary to immunosuppression. Long-term remission of pemphigus has been reported in some patients following high-dose immunosuppressive treatment.

Other clinical aspects: Variants of pemphigus which are considerably less common and of less serious prognosis include pemphigus vegetans, foliaceus and erythematosus.

As with other autoimmune diseases, related disorders may be present and pemphigus may be associated, for example, with lupus erythematosus or thymoma and myasthenia gravis, but this is uncommon. Rarely pemphigus is associated with cancer in another part of the body or is induced by a drug (such as rifampicin, Chapter 19).

Mucous Membrane Pemphigoid (Cicatricial or Ocular Pemphigoid)

Mucous membrane pemphigoid, often called 'benign', is a bullous disease. It results from loss of attachment of the epithelium to the connective tissue. The underlying mechanism appears to be the production of autoantibodies to some component of the epithelial basement membrane.

Unlike pemphigus vulgaris, circulating autoantibodies are demonstrable in relatively few patients. Localization of immunoglobulins along the line of the epithelial basement membrane can be shown in fewer than 50 per cent but complement components may be demonstrable in about 80 per cent.

Clinically, mucous membrane pemphigoid usually affects older patients than those with pemphigus vulgaris and women between 50 and 70 are predominantly affected.

Intact vesicles or bullae are more likely to be seen in mucous membrane pemphigoid than in pemphigus vulgaris. The distribution of these lesions is often characteristic in that the gingivae are particularly affected. Mucous membrane pemphigoid is therefore an important cause of so-called 'desquamative gingivitis'. Sometimes the blisters fill with blood and then must be distinguished from generalized or localized oral purpura (Chapter 3). Scarring after healing of the bullae is rare in the mouth but in other sites, particularly the eyes or larynx, is a serious complication.

The progress of the disease is typically indolent and lesions may remain restricted to one site, such as the mouth, for several years or possibly never develop elsewhere. However, ocular involvement is the most dangerous manifestation since it can impair or destroy sight. Laryngeal or oesophageal-stenosis secondary to scarring can also develop.

Management

The diagnosis must be confirmed by biopsy. The section should be halved and a frozen section should be tested for localization of immunoglobulins or complement components along the basement membrane (*see Table 16.15*). The paraffin sections show separation of the epithelium from the underlying connective tissue which is often infiltrated by inflammatory cells.

The danger of ocular involvement is regarded by some as an indication for giving systemic corticosteroids to all patients having mucous membrane pemphigoid. However, it is by no means certain that any individual patient will develop ocular lesions, or if they do, it may be some years after the appearance of oral lesions. Regular observation is, however, essential and if there is any suspicion of ocular involvement, referral to an ophthalmologist is essential. Oral lesions can often be adequately controlled by potent topical corticosteroids such as a beclomethasone spray and this avoids the complications of systemic corticosteroid treatment.

Oral pemphigoid-like lesions have occasionally been reported in association with internal cancers (Chapter 5) or the use of certain drugs (Chapter 19).

Bullous pemphigoid is essentially a skin disease. It rarely affects the mouth but immunologically and histologically does not appear to differ from mucous membrane pemphigoid.

The Connective Tissue Diseases

This uninformative term is used to include a variety of disorders of which rheumatoid arthritis is the most common. Most of these disorders share, to a variable degree, multiple auto-antibodies and immune complex reactions probably form the basis of the pathological changes. Another feature in common is that Sjögren's syndrome may develop in association with any of them. Alternative terms are 'rheumatoid' diseases, 'collagen vascular' diseases or simply and most confusingly 'collagen diseases'.

The connective tissue diseases are generally regarded as including:

1. Rheumatoid arthritis (Chapter 11).
2. Sjögren's syndrome (Chapter 7).
3. Lupus erythematosus.
4. Systemic sclerosis (scleroderma).
5. Mixed connective tissue disease.
6. Polymyositis and dermatomyositis (Chapter 11).

One of the main features that these disease have in common is that Sjögren's syndrome may be associated with any of them. Polyarteritis nodosa and a few other diseases are sometimes also included in this group but the justification is questionable.

Systemic Lupus Erythematosus (SLE)

Lupus erythematosus is regarded as the archetypal auto-immune disease. The cause is unknown but it is believed that genetic factors are contributory and, possibly, a viral infection may initiate the disease. Some drugs (particularly hydralazine and procainamide) can also precipitate a lupus-like disease. The main immunological feature of SLE is the formation of antibodies to DNA which may initiate immune complex reactions, in particular vasculitis (*Table 16.17*).

Lupus erythematosus can produce a wide variety of clinical pictures depending on the organs which are predominantly affected.

The classic picture is that of a young woman with fever, malaise, anaemia, joint pains and a rash. The well-known rash with a butterfly pattern extending over both cheeks and the bridge of the nose is relatively uncommon, however, and not specific to lupus erythematosus. The rashes are variable in character but the butterfly rash is erythematous, often with raised margins and scaling, and photosensitivity rashes are common.

Renal involvement is present in about 75 per cent of cases coming to autopsy. Clinically, proteinuria and haematuria, often associated with hypertension, are common. Renal disease usually responds to immunosuppressive treatment but membranous glomerulonephritis produces a nephrotic syndrome with gradual progress to renal failure.

Ocular lesions may affect 20–25 per cent of patients, while involvement of the central nervous system is potentially lethal. Relatively minor disturbances of mood and depressive or hysterical behaviour are more common.

Table 16.17. Manifestations of systemic lupus erythematosus

1. Joints	Polyarthralgia
	Arthritis
2. Skin and mucous membranes	Rashes
	Stomatitis
3 . Serous membranes	Pleurisy
	Pericarditis
4. Heart	Myocarditis
	Endocarditis (Libman–Sacks)
5. Lungs	Pneumonitis
6. Kidney	Nephritis
7. Neurological	Neuroses
	Psychoses
	Strokes
	Cranial nerve palsies
8. Eye	Conjunctivitis
	Retinal damage
9. Gastrointestinal	Sjögren's syndrome
	Pancreatitis
	Hepatomegaly
10. Blood	Anaemia
	Purpura

Serositis can cause pleurisy or occasionally pericarditis and peritonitis (polyserositis).

Cardiac lesions typically cause myocarditis which leads to cardiac failure. A characteristic (Libman–Sacks) endocarditis can also develop and renders the patient susceptible to infective endocarditis. Otherwise it is frequently not recognized until autopsy. Murmurs are more often caused by anaemia.

General management

Haematological investigation shows a normochromic anaemia in most patients and often leucopenia, also caused by marrow depression.

Immunological abnormalities are shown in *Table 16.18.* Autoantibodies may cause thrombocytopenia and purpura or, less often, haemolytic anaemia. The titre of anti-DNA antibodies correlates well with the severity of the disease but only anti-double-stranded DNA is peculiar to SLE. About 70 per cent of patients with SLE also form antibodies against double-stranded RNA (anti-dsRNA) which is relatively specific to SLE, or against hybrid RNA/DNA molecules.

Corticosteroids and other immunosuppressive agents have been for some time the mainstay of treatment but there is increasing doubt as to their value for long-term management. Corticosteroids are probably most useful to control early acute manifestations and, together with immunosuppressive agents such as azathioprine, for the potentially lethal lesions such as renal involvement. Otherwise most patients appear to do well in the long term

Table 16.18. Immunological findings in systemic lupus erythematosus

---

1. Hypergammaglobulinaemia and raised ESR
2. Hypocomplementaemia
3. Antinuclear antibodies (90%)
   I.   Anti-DNA antibodies, especially anti-double-stranded DNA (Crithidial)
   II. Anti-RNA antibodies
4. Rheumatoid factor (30%)
5. LE cell phenomenon
6. False-positive serology for syphilis
7. Circulating antibodies to platelets and other blood cells

---

either with non-steroidal anti-inflammatory agents or, if these are ineffective, on very low doses of corticosteroids taken on alternate days. Antimalarials such as chloroquine also appear to be effective, especially for skin and joint lesions.

The prognosis for SLE is less gloomy than was at one time thought and a 5-year survival rate of more than 90 per cent should be expected.

Dental aspects

Oral lesions, which typically consist of erythematous areas, erosions or white patches fairly symmetrically distributed, may be seen in 10–20 per cent of patients with SLE but are rarely an early feature. The lesions often resemble those of oral lichen planus. Slit-like ulcers may also be seen near the gingival margins. SLE may also be complicated by Sjögren's syndrome in 10–30 per cent of cases. Antimalarials sometimes used to control SLE can cause lichenoid oral lesions or occasionally oral pigmentation.

Erosive lesions of SLE in the oral mucosa can be difficult to manage. The best management is uncertain but corticosteroids, often in unacceptably high doses, may be the only effective treatment.

Biopsies of oral lesions show irregular epithelial thinning and acanthosis, basement membrane thickening, liquefaction degeneration of the basal cell layer and an irregularly distributed chronic inflammatory infiltrate. Vasculitis is inconstant. Immunofluorescent staining shows lumpy deposits of immunoglobulins and complement perivascularly and along the basement membrane of lesions, and under normal skin or mucosa in up to 90 per cent of patients with SLE.

The chief problems of management include:

1. Anaemia.
2. Bleeding tendencies caused by thrombocytopenia: circulating anticoagulants rarely cause a bleeding tendency—they predispose to thrombosis.
3. Cardiac disease: cardiac failure and a susceptibility to infective endocarditis if there is Libmann–Sacks endocarditis.
4. Renal disease.

5. Corticosteroid or other immunosuppressive therapy.

6. Drug reactions: tetracyclines may cause photosensitivity rashes; sulphona-mides or penicillins may cause deterioration in SLE.

Discoid Lupus Erythematosus

Discoid lupus erythematosus is essentially a mucocutaneous disorder in which the rashes may be indistinguishable from those of SLE but serological abnor-malities are typically absent or minor, and there are no significant systemic effects. It has been suggested that discoid and systemic lupus erythematosus are different diseases but occasionally discoid disease may transform into SLE.

Oral mucosal lesions can be a feature of discoid LE and may also simulate lichen planus. In discoid LE, however, the lesions are less often symmetrically distributed and the pattern of striae is typically less well-defined or conspicu-ous. Nevertheless, differentiation can be difficult and biopsy is essential. Even this may not be diagnostic and occasionally, histological appearances interme-diate between lichen planus and lupus erythematosus are seen. Management is as for the oral lesions of SLE.

Systemic Sclerosis (Scleroderma)

Systemic sclerosis is an uncommon disease characterized by fibrosis of the subcutaneous tissues and viscera, and has a poor prognosis. Diseases with somewhat similar features but with sclerosis limited to the skin, such as CRST (calcinosis, Raynaud's, sclerodactyly and telangiectasia) may be benign variants or different entities (*Fig. 16.3*).

In systemic sclerosis, the most obvious feature is the progressive stiffening of the skin, but the gastrointestinal tract, lungs, heart and kidneys are frequently also affected.

The pathogenesis of systemic sclerosis is unknown and the immunological abnormalities consist only of circulating antinuclear antibodies in about 50 per cent of patients, or against centromeres and RNA. Their contribution to the disease process is unknown. Other laboratory findings are a normochromic anaemia and a raised ESR.

Clinically, women are predominantly affected and Raynaud's phenomenon is the most common manifestation, often associated with joint pains (polyarthral-gia). Visceral disease sometimes, however, causes the initial symptoms. The skin becomes thinned, stiff, tethered, pigmented and marked by prominent fine blood vessels (telangiectases or spider naevi). Eventually movement becomes limited. Involvement of the face causes characteristic changes in appearance, notably narrowing of the eyes and mask-like restriction of facial movement (Mona Lisa face).

Dysphagia and reflux oesophagitis are common. Pulmonary involvement leads to impaired respiratory exchange and, eventually, dyspnoea and pulmonary hypertension which is the main cause of serious cardiac disease.

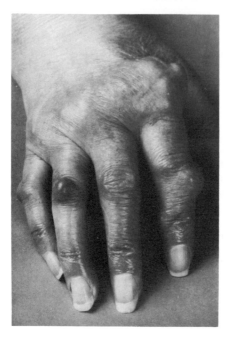

Fig. 16.3. CRST syndrome: calcinosis is shown here.

Renal disease secondary to vascular disease is typically a late feature leading to hypertension and is an important cause of death. No specific treatment is available. Penicillamine may be used but immunosuppressive drugs appear to be ineffective. Symptomatic measures are important and complications such as renal failure are managed along conventional lines. The 5-year survival rate is about 50 per cent.

Dental aspects

Some 80 per cent of patients have manifestations in the head and neck region; in 30 per cent the symptoms start there. Constriction of the oral orifice can cause progressively limited opening of the mouth (fish-mouth). The submucosal connective tissue may also be affected and the tongue may become stiff and less mobile (chicken tongue). In spite of essentially the same histological changes as those in the skin, the clinical effects on the mouth are typically relatively slight though telangiectasia may be seen.

A recognized but uncommon feature seen in fewer than 10 per cent of cases of systemic sclerosis is widening of the periodontal membrane space without tooth mobility. The mandibular angle may be resorbed or rarely there is gross extensive resorption of the jaw. Sjögren's syndrome also develops in a significant minority, but very frequently when systemic sclerosis is associated with primary biliary cirrhosis.

Occasionally, involvement of the peri-articular tissues of the temporo-mandibular joint together with the microstomia so limit access to the mouth as to make dental treatment more or less impracticable.

The main problems of systemic sclerosis are caused by dysphagia and pulmonary, cardiac or renal disease as potential contraindications for general anaesthesia.

Penicillamine therapy may cause loss of taste, oral ulceration, lichenoid reactions and other complications.

Localized Scleroderma (Morphoea)

Morphoea is characterized by the tissue changes of scleroderma, but local-ized to a single area of skin and without visceral disease or systemic effects. It was for long regarded as a variant of systemic sclerosis but more proba-bly is a distinct entity. A typical manifestation is involvement of the side of the face causing an area of scar-like contraction aptly described as *coup de sabre.* Morphoea in childhood is believed to be a cause of facial hemiatrophy.

Mixed Connective Tissue Disease

Mixed connective tissue disease (MCTD) is a multi-system disorder with two or more of the following features: SLE, scleroderma and polymyositis. Sjögren's syndrome is the main complication of dental interest.

Raynaud's disease and Raynaud's phenomenon

Raynaud's phenomenon is a common feature of many of the connective tissue diseases but is also seen in otherwise normal persons when it is termed 'Raynaud's disease'. These disorders are caused by vasomotor instability of the extremities. Cooling, or sometimes emotional disturbances, precipitate vasocon-striction, which is usually worst at the tips of the fingers. The disease tends to be slowly progressive with more frequent and prolonged episodes of spasm and, in its most severe form, ischaemia can cause atrophy of the fat pads at the fingertips or ulceration (*Fig.* 16.4).

Discomfort, aching pain or numbness and stiffness of the fingers. which become pale or cyanotic, accompany an attack. Recovery is accompanied by redness, tingling and slight oedema of the fingers.

In Raynaud's phenomenon only a few fingers of each hand are usually affected but Raynaud's disease spares only the thumb.

The main measure is the wearing of warm clothing and particularly protec-tion of the wrists and hands from chilling.

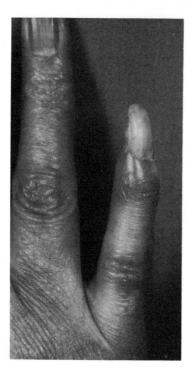

Fig. 16.4. Atrophy of the distal phalanx in severe Raynaud's syndrome in a patient with scleroderma.

Auto-immune Thrombocytopenia

Acute auto-immune thrombocytopenia is relatively common in childhood, especially between 2–5 years of age, usually following a viral infection, and subsiding spontaneously within about 3 weeks. Chronic auto-immune thrombocytopenia is mainly seen in females aged 20–50 years (*see* Chapter 3) and in AIDS.

DISEASES OF POSSIBLE IMMUNOPATHOGENESIS

RECURRENT APHTHAE STOMATITIS (CHAPTER 7)

BEHÇET'S SYNDROME

Behçet described a clinical triad of oral and genital ulceration, and uveitis. A clinical diagnosis is usually made on the presence of any two of these features, but Behçet's syndrome is a multisystem disease with a wide variety of manifestations including thrombophlebitis, rashes, arthritis, cardiovascular disease and CNS involvement (*Table 16.19*). Recently recognized variants include the MAGIC syndrome (Mouth And Genital Ulcers and Interstitial Chondritis). Behçet's syndrome mainly affects young adult males and there may be a positive family history.

Table 16.19. Behçet's syndrome: clinical features
and possible complications

1. Oral
   Aphthous stomatitis
2. Ocular
   Uveitis and hypopyon
   Retinal vasculitis
   Optic atrophy
   Blindness
3. Genital
   Ulcers
4. Neurological
   Syndromes resembling multiple sclerosis
   Syndromes resembling pseudobulbar palsy
   Benign intracranial hypertension
   Brain stem lesions
5. Cutaneous
   Pustules
   Erythema nodosum
6. Psychiatric
   Depression
7. Joints
   Arthralgia (large joints)
8. Vascular
   Aneurysms
   Thromboses of vena cavae
9. Renal
   Proteinuria
   Haematuria

Features such as arthralgia and vasculitis are suggestive of an immune-complex mediated disease, which is supported by finding circulating immune complexes. The antigen responsible for immune complex formation is unidentified but there is some evidence for a viral aetiology.

Findings such as raised serum immunoglobulin levels (especially IgA) and, in the acute stages, a raised ESR and mild leucocytosis, provide little information about the pathogenesis, which remains speculative. Indeed, since the clinical manifestations are so protean and diagnostic criteria are lacking, it is by no means certain that the many different laboratory findings that have been reported necessarily refer to the same disease.

The oral ulceration of Behçet's syndrome is indistinguishable from the common types of recurrent aphthae (Chapter 7). Similar oral ulceration may also develop in other diseases which have multisystem involvement and must be excluded when making the diagnosis (see below).

Management

Behçet's syndrome must enter into the differential diagnosis of recurrent aphthae but the diagnosis may be difficult to confirm for reasons given earlier. Oral and genital ulceration may also result from folate deficiency, when other features characteristic of Behçet's syndrome are lacking. Recurrent oral, ocular and genital lesions may also be seen in erythema multiforme and sometimes in ulcerative colitis and other conditions.

Reliable diagnostic tests for Behçet's syndrome are not available but the possibility should be considered, particularly if aphthae are associated with genital lesions and uveitis. Skin hyper-reactivity after venepuncture (pathergy) may be detectable. Patients should be screened similarly to those with aphthae to exclude underlying deficiencies and, if Behçet's syndrome is suspected, HLA typing may be of value since ocular involvement is associated with HLA-B5. An ophthalmological opinion should be obtained in any patient, since ocular involvement often culminates in impaired sight. All patients should also be examined by a physician.

Oral lesions can be symptomatically managed like common aphthae. A variety of treatments including immunosuppressive drugs such as cyclosporin, and dapsone have been tried for those with multisystem lesions, but results have been inconclusive especially as the disease is subject to spontaneous transient remissions. Colchicine may be of value and thalidomide may be the most effective treatment for otherwise intractable oral ulceration.

ERYTHEMA MULTIFORME

Erythema multiforme primarily affects young males and is characterized by recurrent mucosal and/or cutaneous lesions. Ocular, genital or oral mucous membranes may be involved together or in isolation. The typical skin lesion is the target or iris lesion (*Fig.* 16.5) in which there are concentric erythematous rings affecting particularly the hands and feet. However, virtually any type of rash can develop (hence erythema *multiforme*) and bullae may cause confusion especially with pemphigoid. Severe cases with multiple mucosal involvement and fever are termed *Stevens–Johnson syndrome*.

The aetiology of erythema multiforme is unclear but it has been suggested that it may be an immune complex disorder in which the antigens can be as diverse as various micro-organisms, particularly herpes simplex, or drugs (*Table 16.20*). Although drugs have for long been said to be an important precipitating cause, mere coincidence is difficult to exclude and it is not easy in reported cases to be certain whether the drug was given before the onset of the disease or in an attempt at treatment. However, Stevens–Johnson syndrome as a reaction to sulphonamides appears to be a well-authenticated although rare complication of the use of this group of drugs. In many instances, however, a triggering agent cannot be identified.

Management

Diagnosis can be difficult when the disease is limited to the mouth. Typical features are grossly swollen, crusted and blood-stained lips, and widespread oral ulceration with ill-defined margins. Vesicles or bullae, though rarely seen in the mouth, may be obvious on the skin. When these oral lesions are associated with ocular and dermal lesions the diagnosis can be made largely on clinical grounds.

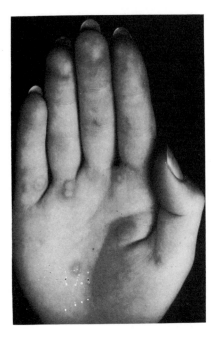

Fig. 16.5. Erythema multiforme: classic target or iris lesions.

Table 16.20. Erythema multiforme: possible causes

1. *Micro-organisms*
    Herpes simplex
    Mycoplasma
2. *Drugs*
    Barbiturates
    Carbamazepine
    Chlorpropamide
    Codeine
    Hydantoins
    Penicillins
    Phenylbutazone
    Salicylates
    Sulphonamides
    Tetracyclines
    Thiazides
3. *Pregnancy*
4. *Irradiation*
5. *Internal malignancy*

Other suggestive features are recent infections, particularly by herpes simplex or *Mycoplasma pneumoniae.* The latter may result in formation of cold agglutinins which have been reported in erythema multiforme.

Biopsy can be useful, particularly to exclude other more serious diseases such as early-onset pemphigus, but otherwise the histological features, though said to be diagnostic, are variable.

Treatment is unsatisfactory. An ophthalmological opinion should be obtained if the conjunctivae are involved. Oral lesions can be symptomatically managed with topical corticosteroids, chlorhexidine (0.2 per cent) or lignocaine gel to ease the pain. Healing usually takes 10–14 days. Severe erythema multiforme may necessitate hospital admission as feeding may be difficult. Systemic corticosteroids are frequently given but may not give anything more than symptomatic relief.

POLYARTERITIS NODOSA

Polyarteritis nodosa (periarteritis nodosa, PAN) is a multisystem disease characterized by necrotizing vasculitis affecting mainly small and medium-sized arteries. It most frequently affects middle-aged men.

PAN appears to be an immune-complex disorder. Circulating immune complexes are found which, in up to 40 per cent of patients, contain hepatitis B antigens. In some cases drugs may be responsible (especially thiouracil, iodides and sulphonamides) but in many patients no precipitating factor can be identified.

Polyarteritis has protean manifestations as a result of the capricious distribution of the lesions. Fever, anorexia, weight loss, myalgia, arthralgia and peripheral neuropathies are common but non-specific. Over 60 per cent have abdominal involvement with pain, nausea, vomiting or diarrhoea. Hypertension and angina (coronary artery disease) are common and 50 per cent have renal disease. A closely related disease (allergic granulomatosis) is distinguished by fever, asthma and eosinophilia.

General management

There are no specific laboratory investigations for PAN: histological examination of clinically involved tissue is needed to confirm the diagnosis. Leucocytosis, eosinophilia, raised ESR, hypergammaglobulinaemia and sometimes a false-positive test for rheumatoid factor may be found. Albuminuria or haematuria is common and angiography is useful to demonstrate arterial aneurysms (early PAN) or vascular occlusions (late PAN).

The prognosis is poor in untreated disease: up to 60 per cent die within a year. Systemic corticosteroids are the drugs of choice, giving a 5-year survival of over 40 per cent. Cyclophosphamide may also be of value.

Dental aspects

Submucosal nodules, haemorrhage or oral ulcers are rare manifestations. Occasionally facial palsy or other cranial neuropathies may be complications.

Dental management may be complicated by:

1. Corticosteroid therapy and immunosuppression.
2. Hepatitis B antigen carriage.
3. Hypertension.
4. Renal disease.
5. Cardiac disease.

MIDLINE GRANULOMA SYNDROME (LETHAL MIDLINE GRANULOMA)

This group of diseases has been given a variety of names as a result of the different clinical pictures presented and the varied microscopic appearances. However, the term is best reserved for diseases of, or starting in, the nasal or paranasal tissues and resulting in midfacial destruction, sometimes of hideously disfiguring degree (so–called Stewart-type granuloma) and often with a fatal outcome. More readily definable diseases such as tuberculosis, deep mycoses or neoplasms of this region should be excluded. Nevertheless, it has become apparent that these 'idiopathic' diseases are in most cases, T-cell lymphomas, which can produce microscopic pictures which are highly pleomorphic and not obviously lymphomatous. The causes of midline granuloma syndrome are shown in *Table 16.21*.

Table 16.21. Important causes of midline granuloma syndrome

1. Infections
    Tuberculosis*
    Syphilis*
    Deep mycoses
2. Idiopathic
    Wegener's granulomatosis
    Peripheral T-cell lymphomas†
    B-cell lymphomas (rarely)

*Unlikely to be seen as a cause of this syndrome now.
† Previously called lymphomatoid granulomatosis, polymorphic reticulosis,   ·
midline malignant reticulosis, Stewart-type granuloma etc.

The two main forms of midline granuloma syndrome can be identified as Wegener's granulomatosis and T-cell lymphomas (the so-called, Stewart-type granuloma) but are not reliably distinguishable clinically. They mainly affect adults between 40 and 50 years of age, and males more than females. The most common upper respiratory tract symptoms are nasal stuffiness and crusting, and often discharge, which can be bloody.

Wegener's granulomatosis

Wegener's granulomatosis is an uncommon disease characterized by granulomatous lesions in the respiratory tract and widespread vasculitis associated with giant cells. It typically terminates in a focal necrotizing glomerulonephritis and may be an immune-complex disease. Biopsy shows inflammatory changes with characteristic giant cells, though these may be few and difficult to find. A necrotizing vasculitis is the main pathological feature but is not seen in gingival biopsies where small arteries are lacking. This arteritis may, however, be seen in palatal lesions as a result of downward spread of the disease from the nasopharynx.

Wegener's granulomatosis can produce a characteristic and apparently pathognomonic form of gingivitis as its initial manifestation. The gingivae are swollen, red and have a strawberry–like texture. The chief importance of the gingival lesions of Wegener's granulomatosis is that they may allow exceptionally early recognition of the disease, when early cytotoxic treatment may be successful. The finding of leucocyte anticytoplasmic auto-antibodies (anti-neutrophil cytoplasmic antibodies: ANCA) may assist the diagnosis.

Non-specific lesions, particularly mucosal ulceration or delayed healing of extraction sockets, are complications of the later stages of disease, particularly if renal failure develops. Of the patients that have been recognized because of gingival lesions, most have died from renal complications, although early immunosuppressive therapy now appears to offer hope. Cyclophosphamide appears to be effective.

Dental management may be complicated by:

1. Renal failure.
2. Respiratory disease.
3. Corticosteroid or other immunosuppressive therapy.

T-cell lymphomas. These, if allowed to progress, can cause midfacial destruction which may be so severe as to open the cranial cavity to the exterior, though this is nowadays unlikely to be seen. In such cases death is likely to follow as a result of intercurrent infection.

As with Wegener's granulomatosis downward spread of the disease from the nasal cavity can lead to palatal necrosis and ulceration. In such cases, superimposed infection from the oral cavity can seriously confuse the microscopic picture and make diagnosis even more difficult.

In uncomplicated cases the microscopic picture is highly pleomorphic but sometimes characterized by angiocentric and angiodestructive changes, which mimic vasculitis. Wide dissemination follows sooner or later. Such changes are characteristic of diseases known as *lymphomatoid granulomatosis* and *polymorphic reticulosis,* but increasing evidence suggests that these are also T-cell lymphomas.

From the viewpoint of treatment and prognosis, T-cell lymphomas can have a highly variable course, sometimes with prolonged survival or even apparently spontaneous remissions. The optimal form of treatment is therefore uncertain but there have been reports of successful treatment with radiotherapy and cytotoxic chemotherapy if the disease is not advanced and too widely disseminated.

MIDLINE GRANULOMA SYNDROME: SUMMARY

Though these diseases are rare, they are a possible cause of oral lesions, particularly a characteristic form of proliferative gingivitis (Wegener's granulomatosis) or palatal ulceration (any type of midline granuloma). The main types are summarized in *Table 16.22,* but the point is that they are potentially lethal diseases and adequate oral biopsy may sometimes permit early diagnosis where there is palatal mucosal necrosis. The biopsy must be deep enough to reach lesional tissue that has not had its appearance changed by secondary infection.

Table 16.22. Features of the main types of midline granuloma syndrome

	Wegener's granulomatosis	*Peripheral T-cell lymphomas*
Destruction facial skeleton and soft tissues	±	+++
Systemic involvement	Pulmonary cavitation Glomerulonephritis	Predominantly lymphatic spread Liver, kidneys or other viscera may become involved
Biopsy findings	Necrotizing vasculitis, fibrinoid necrosis, multiple giant cells, ill-formed granulomas	Highly pleomorphic cellular picture, T-cells recognizable by immuno-cytochemistry. Sometimes angiocentric and angiodestructive changes
Suggested treatment	Cyclophosphamide or azathioprine + prednisolone	Radiotherapy ? + cytotoxic chemotherapy

Bibliography

Almeida O. and Scully C. (1991) Oral lesions in the systemic mycoses. *Curr. Opinion Dent.* 1, 423–8.

Anderson J. A. et al. (1986) Candidiasis hypersensitivity syndrome. *J. Allergy Clin. Immunol.* **78**, 271.

Asherson G. L. and Webster A.D. B. (1980) *Diagnosis and Treatment of Immunodeficiency Diseases.* Oxford, Blackwell Scientific.

Assem E. S. K. and Punnia–Moorty A. (1988) Allergy to local anaesthetics: an approach to a definitive diagnosis. *Br Dent J;* **164**, 44–7.

Basker R. M., Hunter A. M. and Highe A. S. (1990) A severe asthmatic reaction to polymethylmethacrylate denture base resin. *Br Dent J.* **169**, 250–1.

Beacham B. E., Kurgansky D. and Gould W. M. (1990) Circumoral dermatitis and cheilitis caused by tartar control dentifrices. *J. Acad. Dermatol.* **22**, 1029–32.

Buckley R. H. (1986) Advances in the diagnosis and treatment of immunodeficiency diseases. *Arch. Intern. Med.* **146**, 177–84.

Cawson R. A. (1963) Denture sore mouth and angular cheilitis: oral candidiasis in adults. *Br. Dent. J.* **115**, 441.

Cawson R. A. (1965) Thrush in adult out-patients. *Dent. Pract.* **15**, 361.

Cawson R. A. (1965) Gingival changes in Wegener's granulomatosis. *Br. Dent. J.* **118**, 30.

Cawson R. A. (1966) Chronic oral candidiasis and leukoplakia. *Oral Surg.* **22**, 582.

Crosher R. (1987) Intravenous tranexamic acid in the management of hereditary angio–oedema. *Br. J Oral Maxillofac. Surg.* **25**, 500–6.

Curley R. K., Macfarlane A. W. and King C. M. (1986). Contact sensitivity to the amide anesthetics lidocaine, prilocaine and mepivicaine. *Arch Dermatol.* **122**, 924–6.

Greenspan J. S. and Chisholm D. M. (1980) Connective tissue disease of doubtful origins In: Jones J. H. and Mason D. K. (eds) *Oral Manifestations of Systemic Disease.* Philadelphia, Saunders, pp.191-210.

Holgate S. T. (1988) Penicillin allergy; how to diagnose and when to treat. *Br. Med. J.* **296**, 1213–14.

Lamey P–J. and Lamb A.B. (1988) Prospective study of aetiological factors in burning mouth syndrome. *Br. Med. J.* **296**, 1243–6.

Lamey P–J., Lewis M. A. O., Rees T. D. et al. Sensitivity reaction to the cinnamonaldehyde component of toothpaste. *Br Dent J.* **168**, 115–18.

Leading Article (1985) Cyclosporin in autoimmune disease. *Lancet* **i**, 909–11.

Lichtenstein L. M. and Franci A. S. (1985) *Current Therapy in Allergy Immunology and Rheumatology.* Burlington. Ont., B.C. Decker.

Loriaux D. L. (1985) The polyendocrine deficiency syndromes. *N. Engl. J. Med.* **312**, 1568.

Mathe G. and Abitol J. (1988) From Fernand Widal rhinitis syndrome and chronic sinusitis to total mucociliary disease. *Biomed. Pharmacother.* **42**, 489–492.

McCarthy N. R. (1985) Diagnosis and management of hereditary angio-oedema. *Br. J. Oral Maxillofac. Surg.* **23**, 123–7.

Melbye M., Schonheyder H. and Kestens L. (1985) Carriage of oral *Candida albicans* associated with a high number of circulating suppressor T-lymphocytes. *J. Infect. Dis.* **152**, 1356.

Oxelius V. A. et al. (1981) IgG subclasses in selective IgA deficiency. *N. Engl. J. Med.* **304**, 1476.

Peterson D. S. and Klein D. R. (1980) Dental implications for systemic lupus erythematosus. *J. Oral Med.* **35**, 72–5.

Porter S. R., Cox M. and Scully C. (1986) Immunology for dental hygienists. *Dent. Health* **25**, 4–9.

Porter S. R. and Scully C. (1992) Orofacial manifestations of immunodeficiency. *J. Immunodef.* (in press).

Porter S. R., Scully C. and Cawson R. A. (1987) AIDS: update and guidelines for general dental practice. *Dent. Update* **14**, 9–17.

Rosen F.S., Wedgewood R. J. and Auiti F. (1983) Primary immunodeficiency diseases—Report prepared for WHO by a scientific group on immunodeficiency. *Clin. Immunol. Immunopathol.* **28**, 450–75.

Schreiber R. A. and Walker W. A. (1989) Food allergy; facts and fiction. *Mayo Clin Proc.* **64**, 1381–91.

Scully C. (1979) Orofacial manifestations of disease. 3, Skin, collagen and bacterial disease. *Hosp. Update* **5**, 969; *Dent. Update* **7**, 53.

Scully C. (1981) Orofacial manifestations in chronic granulomatous disease of childhood. *Oral Surg.* **15**, 148.

Scully C. (1986) Chronic atrophic candidosis. *Lancet* **ii**, 437–8.

Scully C. (1988) Is AIDS a problem in dentistry? *Microbial Ecol.* **1**, 142–4.

Scully C., Larkaris G., Findborg J. et al. (1991) Oral manifestations of HIV infection and their management. *Oral Surg.* **71**, 158–171.

Scully C., MacFadyen E. and Campbell A. (1982) Orofacial manifestations in cyclic neutropenia. *Br. J. Oral Surg.* **20**, 96–101.

Scully C. and Porter S.R. (1986) Immunodeficiency. In: Ivanyi L. (ed.) *Immunology of Oral Diseases.* Lancaster, MTP Press, pp. 235–56.

Scully C. and Porter S.R. (1990) Disorders of immunity. In: Jones J. H. and Mason D. K. (eds) *Oral Manifestations of Systemic Disease*, 2nd ed. Philadelphia, Saunders.

Scully C. and Porter S. R. (1991) The level of risk of transmisssion of HIV between patients and dental staff. *Br. Dent. J.* **170**, 97–100.

Sim T. C. and Grant J. A. (1990) Hereditary angioedema: its diagnosis and management perspectives. *Am. J Med.* **88**, 656–65.

Strains S. E. (1982) Acyclovir for chronic mucocutaneous herpes simplex virus infection in immuno-suppressed patients. *Ann. Intern. Med.* **96**, 270–7.

Strains S. E. (1984) Oral acyclovir to suppress recurring herpes simplex virus infections in immunodeficient patients. *Ann. Intern. Med.* **100**, 522–1.

Umetsu D. T., Ambrosino D. M. and Quinti I. (1985) Recurrent sinopulmonary infection and impaired antibody response to bacterial capsular polysaccharide antigen in children with selective IgG-subclass deficiency. *N. Engl. J. Med.* **313**, 1247–51.

Vervloet D. (1985) Allergy to muscle relaxants and related compounds. *Clin. Allerg.* **15**, 501–8.

Appendix to Chapter 16

AUTOANTIBODIES AND ASSOCIATED DISEASES

Autoantibody directed against—	*Main associated diseases*
Epithelial intercellular cement	Pemphigus
Epithelial basement membrane	Pemphigoid
Gastric parietal cell	Pernicious anaemia
Intrinsic factor	Pernicious anaemia
Acetylcholine receptor	Myasthenia gravis
Thyroglobulin	Autoimmune thyroiditis
Thyroid microsomes	Autoimmune thyroiditis
Thyroid-stimulating hormone receptor	Thyrotoxicosis
DNA	Systemic lupus erythematosus
Nucleoprotein	Scleroderma
Centromere	Scleroderma
Non-histone protein	Sjögren's syndrome
Salivary duct cells	Sjögren's syndrome
SS-A (Ro)	Sjögren's syndrome
SS-B (La)	Sjögren's syndrome
IgG	Rheumatoid arthritis
Smooth muscle	Chronic active hepatitis
Mitochondria	Primary biliary cirrhosis
Platelets	Auto-immune thrombocytopenia
Cytoplasm of neutrophils	Wegener's granulomatosis

Chapter 17

Some Skin Diseases and Infections with Oral Manifestations

Many skin diseases and infections can involve the mouth or may influence dental treatment. Several of the diseases are discussed elsewhere in this text (especially in Chapters 8 and 16) and only the other conditions with oral manifestations or those relevant to dental management are included here.

SKIN DISEASES

Oral lesions maysometimes herald the onset of some skin diseases or may be the main manifestation. The most serious diseases, pemphigus and mucous membrane pemphigoid are discussed in Chapter 16. This section covers several genetically determined disorders and a few conditions such as lichen planus that cannot at present be easily categorized.

Various skin diseases are treated with topical corticosteroids. These may, if used for prolonged periods, cause adrenocortical suppression (Chapter 10).

Ectodermal Dysplasia

Ectodermal dysplasia is a relatively common sex-linked dermatosis characterized by hypoplasia or agenesis of a wide variety of dermal appendages, including the teeth. Sweat glands may fail to form and heat control is then defective (hypohidrotic ectodermal dysplasia). The nails may also be defective and the skin somewhat fragile. Either, or in extreme cases both, the deciduous and permanent dentition may fail to form (anodontia) and as a consequence there is hypoplasia of the jaws. Teeth are more often reduced in number (hypodontia) and those present may be of simple conical form. The minor salivary glands may fail to form. There are many variants described.

In typical cases, the hair is fine, blond and scanty (hypotrichosis) especially in the tonsural region, and the eyelashes and eyebrows may be absent.

The facies is sometimes characterized by frontal bossing, a depressed nasal bridge and, if the teeth are absent, a prematurely senile (nutcracker) profile with protuberant lips. Ectodermal dysplasia rarely causes management problems apart from those related to the oral manifestations of the disease.

Table 17.1. The main types of epidermolysis bullosa

	Onset	Main sites of lesions*	Oral mucosal lesions	Dental defects	Nail defects	Scarring	Inheritance
I. Non-scarring types							
Simplex†	Neonatal onwards	Hands and feet and elbows	Rarely	No	No	No	AD
Letalis‡	Birth	Widespread	Yes§	Yes	Severe	No	AR
II. Scarring types							
Dermolytic dominant (Dystrophic)‖	Childhood	Extremities; may be haemorrhagic	Uncommon	No	Yes	Yes Soft scars	AD
Dermolytic recessive (Polydysplastic)‡‡	Birth or infancy	Widespread	Severe, mutilating	No¶	Destruction	Mutilating††	AR

AD, Autosomal dominant; AR, autosomal recessive.
* Usually also any site of trauma.
† May improve by puberty: commonest type.
‡ Usually fatal in neonatal period or childhood. Also known as Herlliz disease.
§ Vermilion border of lips spared: lesions are perioral and perinasal. May be corneal lesions.
¶ May improve by puberty.
‖ A cemental defect has been reported but destruction and loss of teeth from caries and periodontal care is a typical result of inability to brush the teeth.
†† Typically leads to destruction of hands and feet. Oesophageal stricture may lead to aspiration into airway.
‡‡ Rare and lethal.

Epidermolysis Bullosa

Epidermolysis bullosa is an uncommon bullous disease affecting skin and mucosae. Vesicles and bullae form in response to mild or insignificant trauma and lead to disabling scarring. One characteristic effect is to transform the hands into finger-less stumps in severe cases. There are several forms of epidermolysis bullosa which show different patterns of inheritance and vary greatly in severity. The severe form appears soon after birth; milder forms do not become apparent until adolescence or later (*Table 17.1*). Potent steroids may, however, help to prevent blister formation and some success has been reported with vitamin E and with phenytoin.

Dental aspects

Within the mouth the buccal sulcus may become obliterated by scar tissue with the tongue bound down to the floor of the mouth. Scarring can also obliterate the normal papillated surfaces of the tongue. Enamel hypoplasia may be seen and dental diseases such as caries and periodontal disease may become rampant. Since even 'normal' tooth-brushing can cause ulceration, adequate oral hygiene is almost impossible to achieve and a dental clearance may become necessary. Rarely, squamous cell carcinoma can complicate the oral lesions of epidermolysis bullosa.

Management problems include:

1. Oral scarring and severe microstomia.
2. Blistering after dental treatment.
3. Bullae on the face or in the airway if intubation is attempted.

Hypertension secondary to renal disease is common. General anaesthesia should therefore be avoided where possible, but, if it must be used, the face should be protected with petroleum jelly gauze and intubation should be oral rather than nasal. Iron deficiency anaemia is common and may need correction before general anaesthesia is given (Chapter 4).

Intravenous ketamine has proved a useful anaesthetic in these patients. Atropinics are often needed to control the excessive salivation seen in many of these patients. Intramuscular injections can cause sloughing and adhesive tapes easily traumatize the epidermis; these should therefore be avoided.

Dental treatment may be exceedingly difficult as a consequence of bulla formation; early preventive care is extremely important therefore. Erosions and aggravation of scarring following dental treatment (however carefully it is carried out) may possibly be reduced by giving a short course of corticosteroids. A possible regimen would therefore be to give 30 mg of prednisolone orally an hour before treatment, on the following day, and then tapered off over the next 3 days. A larger dose may be needed, but if the duration of administration is short the steroid should cause no complications.

Some suggest the use of antimicrobials to cover surgery in these patients.

Multiple Basal Cell Naevi Syndrome

The multiple basal cell naevi syndrome (Gorlin–Goltz syndrome) consists of multiple basal cell naevoid carcinomas, odontogenic keratocysts, anomalies of the vertebrae and ribs and a variety of other abnormalities.

The syndrome is inherited as an autosomal dominant trait with poor penetrance. Multiple naevoid basal cell naevi over the nose, eyelids, cheeks and elsewhere are often an early sign and there may also be pitting of the palms or soles. Skin lesions appear in childhood or adolescence. Multiple odontogenic keratocysts develop. The facial appearance is characterized by frontal and temporoparietal bossing, a broad nasal root, prominent supra-orbital ridges and a degree of mandibular prognathism (*Fig.* 17.1). Bifid ribs, vertebral defects with kyphoscoliosis and short fourth metacarpals may be noted. Other associated abnormalities may include calcification of the falx cerebri, mental handicap or cerebral tumours.

Pseudohypoparathyroidism has been described in some patients and there is also a slight increase in the incidence of diabetes mellitus. Cardiac lesions may be present.

Gardner's Syndrome (Familial Adenomatous Polyposis Coli)

Gardner's syndrome is an autosomal dominant trait of poor penetrance characterized by the association of multiple osteomas, skin fibromas and epidermoid cysts, and pigmented ocular fundus lesions with colonic polyposis.

The skin lesions, which affect any part, include fibromas, desmoid tumours, epidermoid cysts or lipomas. Multiple osteomas appear in adolescence and

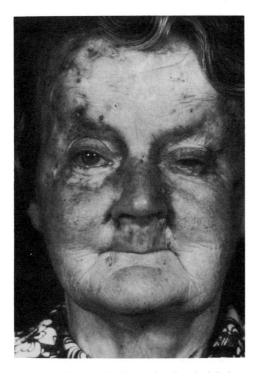

Fig. 17.1. Gorlin's syndrome: multiple basal cell naevi and typical facies.

characteristically involve the jaws, facial skeleton or frontal bone but can affect any bone. Compound odontomes and dental anomalies may be found.

Multiple polyps of the colon and rectum almost invariably undergo malignant change. Colonic resection is usually required; desmoid tumours often arise in the abdominal wall scar.

Thyroid, adrenal and biliary carcinomas may also develop.

THE PHAKOMATOSES

The phakomatoses (neurodermatoses) are four hereditary hamartomatous disorders affecting the skin and nervous system. The fourth member of this group, cerebroretinal angiomatosis, is not discussed here.

Neurofibromatosis, type I (von Recklinghausen's Disease)

Neurofibromatosis type I is a simple autosomal dominant condition in which there are tumours of the nerve sheath (neurilemomas or neurofibromas), sometimes in vast numbers, and often patches of skin hyperpigmentation (café-au-lait spots). The nerve sheath tumours may be disfiguring but are often asymptomatic unless pressure effects develop. When the tumours involve the spinal nerve roots and compress the spinal cord, pressure effects can be serious. In addition, there is an increased frequency of cerebral gliomas.

Neurofibromatosis type II is characterized by bilateral acoustic neuromas, which can cause deafness and any of the symptoms of cerebellopontine angle lesions (*see* Chapter 12) but the skin lesions of type I are lacking.

Oral mucosal neurofibromatosis is uncommon and more typically associated with endocrine disorders (MEA type III, *see* Chapter 10). Complications may include mental handicap and epilepsy in a minority. Sarcomatous change may develop in about 10 per cent of severely affected patients.

Tuberous Sclerosis (Bourneville's Disease; Epiloia)

Tuberous sclerosis is a simple autosomal dominant trait characterized by epilepsy, mental defects, adenoma sebaceum and leaf-shaped depigmented naevi. The skin lesions are not adenomas but fibromas which are characteristically distributed in a butterfly pattern across the cheeks, bridge of the nose and forehead. Oral lesions include hyperplastic gingivitis and pit-shaped defects in the teeth of both dentitions. Dental management may be complicated by cardiac or renal involvement, or by endocrinopathies—particularly diabetes mellitus—in addition to mental handicap and epilepsy.

Sturge–Weber Syndrome

Sturge–Weber syndrome (encephalotrigeminal angiomatosis) is characterized by an angiomatous defect (hamartoma) which is usually in the upper part of the face and also within the skull. The occipital lobe of the brain is then usually involved but the parietal and frontal lobes of the brain may be affected if the lower face is affected by the angioma.

Clinically, there are convulsions, hemiplegia and often mental defect. When the vascular naevus involves the face it usually extends to the underlying oral mucosa and gingivae which are red and sometimes hyperplastic, and alsoto the alveolar bone. Dental surgery in the area affected by the haemangioma may be complicated by profuse haemorrhage and should therefore only be attempted in hospital.

LICHEN PLANUS

Lichen planus is a common skin disease which frequently involves the oral mucosa. It affects up to 2 per cent of the population, mainly those over 40 years of age. The aetiology of lichen planus is unknown but lesions similar or identical to lichen planus (lichenoid lesions) can be drug reactions, particularly to gold, antimalarials, non-steroidal anti-inflammatory agents and methyldopa. Other drugs responsible for lichenoid lesions are shown in Appendix to Chapter 19. There is little evidence for an immunopathogenesis in lichen planus although there is a dense T-lymphocyte infiltrate and lichenoid lesions frequently complicate graft-versus-host disease (Chapter 16). Reported associations of oral lichen planus with diabetes mellitus, hypertension, and liver disease, have not been confirmed and there is doubt whether the so-called Grinspan syndrome of lichen planus, diabetes mellitus and hypertension is an entity or is simply aleatoric, or related to drug treatment.

Up to 70 per cent of patients with skin lesions of lichen planus have demonstrable oral lesions but only about 10 per cent of patients presenting with oral lichen planus have skin involvement. Skin lesions characteristically are small polygonal purplish or violaceous itchy papules particularly affecting the flexor surfaces of the wrist, and also elsewhere such as on the shins or periumbilically but rarely, if ever, on the face. Examination with a lens may show a fine lacy white network of striae (Wickham's striae) on these papules.

Dental aspects

Oral lesions in lichen planus include macroscopic striae, papules, white plaques, atrophic areas or erosions. The latter are sore. Oral lesions characteristically are bilateral and affect particularly the posterior part of the buccal mucosa, but may also involve the tongue, gingivae or other sites. Gingival lesions may be atrophic ('desquamative gingivitis') and need to be differentiated from somewhat similar lesions seen in mucous membrane pemphigoid. Oral lesions can persist for years although the skin lesions frequently resolve within a few months.

A drug history should be taken in order to exclude possible drug reactions. Clinical examination may show typical oral lesions but if there is any doubt about the diagnosis an oral biopsy is needed, particularly to differentiate lichen planus from lupus erythematosus or keratosis.

Oral lesions need no treatment if they are asymptomatic but topical corticosteroids such as hydrocortisone hemisuccinate pellets (Corlan), betamethasone mouthwashes (such as Betnesol) or beclomethasone sprays such as Becotide can be useful in symptomatic lichen planus, especially for severe erosive lesions. Exceptionally severe lichen planus sometimes responds only to intralesional or systemic corticosteroids. Other drugs such as vitamin A analogues (e.g. etretinate), dapsone, or cyclosporin are used rarely. The evidence that lichen planus is premalignant is slender; carcinoma can develop in patients with lichen planus, as in any other patient, and may be more likely in erosive than other forms of lichen planus.

Mercury–associated oral lesions

Some studies have shown an association between oral lichenoid lesions and dental amalgams and suggest that replacement of this material with non–metallic alternatives may cause the lesions to resolve. Other studies have failed to confirm these findings or have found that lichenoid reactions may be associated with composite restorations.

Trace amounts of mercury are absorbed and can be detected in the oral mucosa, but do not cause any local reaction and are too small in amount to have any systemic effect (Chapter 12). Larger amounts of dental amalgam can become embedded in the mucosa to produce a pigmented patch (amalgam tattoo). These may provoke a localized foreign body reaction, but in 40 per cent of cases there is no reaction. Though it is usual to regard these pigmented patches as amalgam tattoos on the basis of their clinical and microscopic appearances, X–ray energy spectroscopy shows that a variety of other materials from endodontic preparations, toothpastes and even impression media may be responsible.

Possible systemic toxic effects of mercury have been discussed in Chapter 12 and possible risks to a fetus in Chapter 10.

ORAL SUBMUCOUS FIBROSIS

Oral submucous fibrosis (OSMF), though not regarded as a connective tissue disease, has pathological changes closely similar to those of scleroderma (Chapter 16). Unlike the latter, which has severe effects on the skin but minimal effects on the oral mucosa, OSMF causes severe and often disabling fibrosis of the oral tissues alone.

Oral submucous fibrosis affects virtually only those from the Indian subcontinent. Serum immunoglobulin IgG, IgA and IgM levels are raised. No consistent specific immunological abnormalities appear to be associated, although there is an increased prevalence of connective tissue diseases. The condition appears to be related to the chewing of areca (betel) nut.

Iron deficiency anaemia may be present but this is not uncommon in Asians in the absence of submucous fibrosis. It is suggested by some that submucous fibrosis is premalignant.

Clinically, OSMF causes symmetrical fibrosis of such sites as the cheeks, soft palate or inner aspects of the lips. The fibrosis is often so severe that the affected area is almost white and so hard that it literally cannot be indented with the finger. Frequently the buccal fibrosis causes such severe restriction of opening that dental treatment becomes increasingly difficult and finally impossible. Ultimately tube feeding may become necessary.

Intra-lesional corticosteroids and regular stretching of the oral soft tissues with an interdental screw may delay fixation in the closed position. Failing this, operative treatment may become necessary.

OTHER SKIN DISORDERS

These are discussed elsewhere in the text (Chapter 16).

INFECTIOUS DISEASES WITH ORAL MANIFESTATIONS

Many infectious diseases, particularly viral infections, affect the mouth or perioral area. Most cause oral lesions of limited duration, and have little influence on dental treatment. Others, especially viral hepatitis and HIV infection, can significantly influence dental management (Chapters 8 and 16). *Table 17.2* summarizes the incubation periods; *Table 17.3* summarizes the features of many

Table 17.2. Infective diseases: incubation times and period of infectivity

Incubation period	Disease	Incubation period	Period of infectivity
< 1 wk	Diphtheria	2–5 d	Until treated
	Gonorrhoea	2–5 d	Until treated
	Scarlet fever	1–3 d	3 weeks after onset of rash
1-2 wk	Measles	7–14 d	4 days after onset of rash
	Pertussis	7–10 d	21 days after onset of symptoms
2-3 wk	Chickenpox	14–21 d	Until all lesions scab
	Mumps	12–21 d	7 days after onset of sialadenitis
	Rubella	14–21 d	7 days after onset of rash
> 3 wk	Hepatitis A	2–6 wk	Usually non-infective at diagnosis
	Hepatitis B	2–6 mth	About 3 mth after jaundice resolves*
	Hepatitis non-A, non-B†	?	?*
	HIV	Up to 5 yr	?*
	Infectious mononucleosis	30–50 d	?*
	Syphilis	10–90d	Until treated*

* Carrier states exist.
† Several viruses responsible, including hepatitis C, E and F viruses.

Table 17.3. Synopsis of infectious diseases*

Disease	Cause	Major manifestations	Main oral manifestations	Laboratory diagnosis	Specific treatment used†	Specific management problems
AIDS	HIV	Opportunistic infections Tumours Encephalopathy	Cervical lymphadenopathy Candidosis Hairy leukoplakia Kaposi's sarcoma	Lymphopenia HIV serology	Zidovudine (AZT) may help	Cross-infection Bleeding tendency Immune defect
Catscratch disease	Gram-negative bacterium	Tender papule, regional lymph nodes enlarge, mild fever	Cervical lymphadenopathy	Leucocytosis, ESR raised. Skin test	—	—
Chickenpox (varicella)	Varicella zoster virus	Rash evolves through macule, papule, vesicle and pustule: rash crops and is most dense on trunk	Oral ulcers	Complement fixation antibody titres (not usually needed)	Zoster immune globulin in high-risk patients	Problems of dissemination in immunologically compromised patient
Diphtheria	Corynebacterium diphtheriae	Tonsillar or pharyngeal exudate; cervical lymph nodes enlarged	Tonsillar exudate, palatal palsy	Culture	Antitoxin: penicillin	Respiratory obstruction myocarditis, palatal paralysis
Erysipelas	Streptococcus pyogenes	Rash (confluent erythema and oedema)	—	Culture	Penicillin	Cross-infection
Hand-foot-and-mouth disease	Coxsackie virus A strains	Rash, stomatitis, minor malaise	Oral ulceration (usually mild)	Serology	None	Highly infective: myocarditis rarely
Hepatitis	Hepatitis A,B and non-A non-B viruses	Jaundice, malaise, pale stools, dark urine	—	Serology	Immune globulin	Cross-infection, liver damage. (see Chapter 8)
Herpangina	Usually Coxsackie virus A strains	Fever, sore throat, enlarged cervical lymph nodes	Vesicles and ulcers on soft palate	Serology	None	Differential diagnosis from herpes simplex: myocarditis rarely
Herpes simplex	Herpes simplex virus Type I or 2	Fever, oral ulceration, cervical lymph node enlargement	Gingivostomatitis, herpes labialis, erythema multiforme	Serology	Acyclovir may help	Dissemination in immunologically compromised patient
Herpes zoster (shingles)	Varicella zoster virus	Rash like chickenpox but limited to dermatome	Oral ulceration in zoster of maxillary or mandibular division of trigeminal nerve. Ulcers in palate and pinna of ear in Ramsay-Hunt syndrome	Not needed	Acyclovir plus zoster immune globulin in high-risk patients	Severe pain during and after attack Eye involvement in ophthalmic zoster: may be underlying neoplasm

Disease	Cause	General features	Oral/mucosal features	Diagnosis	Treatment	Complications/remarks
Impetigo	Streptococci and/or staphylococci	Rash (bullous) spreading to other areas rapidly	Lesions on lips may resemble recurrent herpes labialis	Culture	Topical chlortetracycline or oral flucloxacillin	Cross-infection or dissemination: acute nephritis
Infectious mononucleosis	Epstein–Barr virus	Fever, lymph node enlargment, pharyngitis	Tonsillar exudate, palatal petechiae, oral ulceration	Blood film, Monospot test, Paul–Bunnell test	—	Airway obstruction
Lymedisease	Borrelia burgatorferi	Arthritis, neurological and rash	Facial palsy	Serology	Tetracycline	Heart block in some
Measles	Measles virus	Rash (maculopapular), fever, acute respiratory symptoms	Koplik's spots, pharyngitis	Not usually needed	Immune globulin in high-risk patients	Pneumonia especially in immunologically compromised patient
Mucocutaneous lymph node syndrome	Not known	Rash – hands and feet, desquamation, lymph node enlargement	Strawberry tongue, labial oedema pharyngitis		—	Myocarditis or infarction
Mumps	Mumps virus	Fever, malaise, parotitis	Sialadenitis, trismus, papillitis at salivary duct orifices	Complement fixing antibody titres to S and V antigens rise: not usually needed	—	Differential diagnosis of salivary swelling: rarely myocarditis
Mycoplasmal pneumonia (atypical pneumonia)	Mycoplasma pneumoniae (Eaton agent: PPLO)	Sore throat, fever, pneumonia	Erythema multiforme occasionally later	Culture, complement fixing antibodies, cold agglutinins	Erythromycin or tetracycline	Respiratory complicatons
Whooping cough (pertussis)	Bordetella pertussis	Cough, fever	Occasionally ulceration of lingual fraenum	Culture	Amoxycillin or for secondary infection	Respiratory complications
Poliomyelitis	Poliovirus	Paralyses		Serology	—	Respiratory involvement
Rubella	Rubella virus	Rash (mainly macular), fever, enlarged posterior cervical lymph nodes	Pharyngitis ± palatal petechiae	Serology	—	Pregnant staff (see p. 538), Congenital rubella (see p. 538)
Scarlet fever	Streptococcus pyogenes	Sore throat, fever, rash (macular), enlarged cervical lymph nodes, desquamation	Tonsillar exudate, strawberry tongue	Culture, antistreptolysin O titre	Penicillin	Rheumatic fever, acute glomerulonephritis, cross-infection
Toxoplasmosis	Toxoplasma gondii	Glandular fever type of syndrome	Sore throat	Sabin–Feldman dye test	Sulphonamide plus pyrimethamine	Differential diagnosis of cervical lymphadenopathy

*Infections discussed elsewhere include tuberculosis (Chapter 6), AIDS (Chapter 16), gonorrhoea and syphilis (Chapter 17).
† See page 534 for details of supportive care.

of the more common diseases. A few are characterized mainly by oral features or significantly influence dental care and these are discussed here. Further details of many of these diseases are found in textbooks of oral medicine.

HERPES SIMPLEX

Primary infection with herpes simplex virus (HSV) typically causes acute gingivostomatitis, fever, cervical lymph node enlargement and irritability. This is a common infection of young children but may be misdiagnosed as 'teething', or may be subclinical. The virus is usually Type I herpes simplex virus which apparently thereafter remains latent, often in the trigeminal ganglia. An increasing proportion of infections appear to be caused by Type 2 herpes simplex virus, which traditionally causes genital infections.

The virus can be spread by saliva and occasionally causes painful whitlows in dental staff not previously exposed to it (*Fig.* 17.2).

Primary herpetic gingivostomatitis is limited to the mouth and resolves within about 10 days but, in immunosuppressed patients or in those with eczema, more widespread infection may result. Acyclovir (Zovirax) is an antiviral agent effective against HSV but many patients present with disease too far advanced to benefit from treatment. Acyclovir is, however, essential to control infection in immunocompromised patients. In other patients, treatment is usually limited to supportive care such as adequate fluid intake, antipyretics and analgesics (paracetamol usually) and good oral hygiene by mouth cleansing and the use of aqueous chlorhexidine (0.2 per cent) mouthwashes.

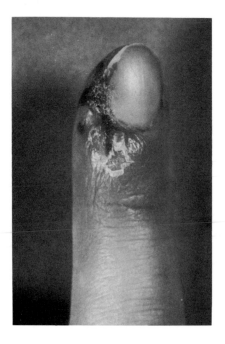

Fig. 17.2. Herpetic whitlow (herpes simplex infection) in a dental surgeon.

Many patients suffer no consequence once the primary infection resolves. Recurrent infections occur subsequently in up to 30 per cent of patients and affect the mucocutaneous junction of the lip (cold sores). Recurrences, which are often precipitated by factors such as exposure to systemic infections, sunlight, trauma, stress or menstruation respond well to 5 per cent acyclovir cream applied early. Intraoral recurrences appear to be more likely in immuno-compromised patients (such as in AIDS).

Herpetic infection is by no means exclusively a disease of childhood and adults are quite often affected since immunity may not have been acquired in early life. Those who develop herpetic infection in adult life may have particu-larly severe and prolonged systemic illness.

VARICELLA AND ZOSTER

Primary infection with the varicella-zoster virus causes chickenpox—usually a trivial illness but often with oral ulceration. The characteristic rash differen-tiates chickenpox from other causes of oral ulceration. The virus remains latent within dorsal root ganglia and usually causes no further problems. However, reactivation may lead to shingles (zoster), which involves the dermatome supplied by the sensory nerve affected. Severe pain and a rash similar to chickenpox characterize zoster; the pain may persist after the rash heals (post-herpetic neuralgia, Chapter 12). Zoster of the maxillary or mandibular divisions of the trigeminal nerve may cause facial pain (sometimes simulating toothache) and oral ulceration—unilateral and in the distribution of the nerve involved. Those with ophthalmic zoster should have an urgent ophthalmological opinion. In some 8–10 per cent of cases zoster reflects an underlying immunodeficiency state, sometimes as result of AIDS or a neoplasm, particularly a lymphoma. In most patients no precipitating factor is identified—apart from old age. Zoster is well recognized occasionally also to affect younger and immunocompetent adults. Treatment is with acyclovir by mouth, but intravenous administration is needed in immunodeficient patients particularly in those with HIV infection for whom it can be a life–threatening disease.

GLANDULAR FEVER (INFECTIOUS MONONUCLEOSIS)

Glandular fever is a syndrome characterized by fever, malaise and lymph node enlargement. Several infectious agents (HIV, cytomegalovirus,*Toxoplasma gondii*) can cause a similar syndrome (*Table 17.4*) but the most frequent is the Epstein–Barr virus (EBV), which also has epidemiological associations with Burkitt's and some other lymphomas and nasopharyngeal carcinoma. EBV is found in saliva during infectious mononucleosis and for several months there-after. Infection appears to be spread by close oral contact, such as kissing, but the infectivity is low. The disease is common among young adults and is often subclinical or unrecognized, especially in children.

Table 17.4. Causes of glandular fever syndrome

1.	Infectious mononucleosis
2.	Cytomegalovirus infection
3.	Toxoplasmosis
4.	Infectious lymphocytosis
5.	HIV infection
6.	Rarely: acute leukaemia; brucellosis)

Infectious mononucleosis (IM) is protean in its manifestations. Children suffer mainly from lymphadenopathy, sore throat and fever, while adolescents often have a vague illness with malaise and a low fever but little lymphadenopathy. A high fever with rubelliform rashes and occasionally jaundice characterizes the febrile type of IM. In the anginose type, the throat is sore with soft palate petechiae and a whitish exudate on the tonsils, and pharyngeal oedema may threaten the airway. The glandular type of IM is characterized by general, especially cervical, lymph node enlargement and splenomegaly.

Complications of infectious mononucleosis include persistent fatigue, mild liver dysfunction, EGG changes, depression, various neurological syndromes, oral ulceration and, rarely, nephritis, pancreatitis or lung infiltration. Ampicillin and amoxycillin very frequently cause a maculopapular rash which is not a manifestation of penicillin allergy, affecting the extensor surfaces of the limbs (*Fig.* 17.3).

Characteristic of IM are an excess of atypical lymphocytes in the blood: these may cause confusion with leukaemia but for the absence of other features of leukaemia such as anaemia. These cells may also be seen in, for example, viral hepatitis or chickenpox. Occasionally in IM there is mild neutropenia or thrombocytopenia.

A wide variety of serological changes characterize IM, including transient heterophil antibodies, persistent EBV antibodies and a false-positive Wassermann reaction

Heterophil antibodies are IgM antibodies that agglutinate sheep and horse red blood cells: the Paul–Bunnell test employs sheep erythrocytes but rapid methods are available to detect heterophil antibodies to horse red blood cells by detecting agglutination on a glass slide (Monospot test).

Heterophil antibodies usually develop during the first or second week of the illness (60 per cent of patients), and by 4 weeks up to 90 per cent of patients have a titre before absorption of 224 (or 28 after absorption). The titre then declines and disappears over 3–6 months.

EBV antibodies: Although several antibodies against EBV appear during the course of IM, the one most frequently tested for is the antibody to viral capsid antigen. This antibody is produced early and the titre reaches a peak at about 4 weeks. The viral capsid antibody persists for many years.

General management

No specific treatment is available but as there frequently is malaise and fatigue the patient may benefit from bed rest. Systemic corticosteroids are required if

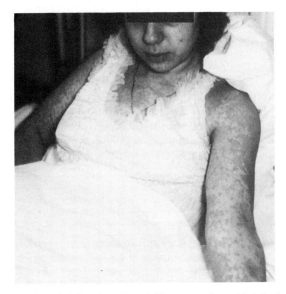

Fig. 17.3. Rash following the administration of ampicillin to a patient with infectious mononucleosis.

there is severe pharyngeal oedema which hazards the airway. Some also advise the use of penicillin since nearly 20 per cent of patients have concurrent beta-haemolytic streptococcal pharyngeal infection. Tinidazole reduces the sore throat.

Dental aspects of infectious mononucleosis

Infectious mononucleosis is an important cause of enlarged cervical lymph nodes which must be distinguished particularly from those caused by local infections, HIV, leukaemia or lymphomas. Rarely, infectious mononucleosis is clinically atypical and enlarged lymph nodes have been removed for biopsy. Unfortunately, the lymph node histopathological changes in infectious mononucleosis closely resemble those in lymphomas and an expert opinion is needed. A useful precaution in such cases is to undertake haematological examination and test for heterophil antibodies.

Within the mouth the most typical manifestation of infectious mononucleosis is a confluent creamy exudate in the fauces (to be distinguished from diphtheria) and fine petechiae at the junction of the hard and soft palate. The latter are occasionally seen in other viral infections such as rubella and HIV. Occasionally there is mucosal or gingival ulceration. EBV may also cause sialadenitis (*see below*).

CHRONIC EPSTEIN–BARR VIRUS (EBV) DISEASE

It is now recognized that EBV infection is not invariably an acute self-limiting infection. Some patients have persistent symptoms for months or years, which may be related to chronic EBV infection because of inadequate antibody production against nuclear antigen, and reduced ability to generate EBV-specific cytotoxic T-lymphocytes, with weak lymphoproliferative responses. This infection mostly affects women aged 25–40, symptoms are vague—such as malaise, fatigue and fever—and most have a negative Paul–Bunnell test. There may be an association with HLA-D7 and with atopic allergy. Treatment is not satisfactory, but intravenous gammaglobulin, and acyclovir, are under trial.

Caution must be exercised before assigning this diagnosis since several patients have eventually been shown to have other diagnoses such as SLE, ankylosing spondylitis or lymphoma, and the syndrome resembles multiple sclerosis and epidemic neuromyasthenia (chronic fatigue syndrome) in many respects.

Duncan's Disease

A rare group of patients, with specifically demonstrable defects in antibodies to EBV nuclear antigens, have Duncan's disease (sex-linked lymphoproliferative syndrome, Chapter 16), characterized by severe mononucleosis, immunoblastic sarcoma or lymphoma.

RUBELLA (GERMAN MEASLES)

Rubella is a highly infectious viral disease that causes a fairly trivial illness characterized by a macular rash starting on the face and behind the ears, mild fever, sore throat and enlarged lymph nodes (including the posterior cervical nodes). Because of the danger to the fetus, pregnant patients exposed to, or developing, rubella should have serological investigation (*see below*).

Congenital Rubella

Infection during the first trimester of pregnancy causes damage to the fetus ranging from deafness to death. If the fetus survives, mental handicap, retinopathy and cataracts, cardiac malformations and deafness may result (major rubella syndrome). The affected infant may also have liver damage, bone defects and thrombocytopenic purpura and is also infective as virus is excreted, particularly in the urine, for months after birth. Similar lesions result from fetal infection with toxoplasma, rubella, cytomegalovirus or herpes simplex (TORCH syndrome).

Prevention of congenital rubella

Immunization of non-immune prepubertal females against rubella is the most effective prophylaxis. Antibody titres (HAI test, *see below*) should be measured and immunization given only to those who are seronegative, not pregnant and

Table 17.5. Management of pregnant patient after contact with rubella

Suspected rubella	Suspected contact with rubella
1. Test acute serum for HAI antibody to rubella	1. Test acute serum for HAI antibody to rubella
2. If HAI positive in acute serum, reassure If HAI continues negative, reassure If HAI negative but then rises, then termination or rubella immuno-globulin offered	2. Test serum of the contact for rubella—this may be negative—then reassure
	3. If pregnant woman has rubella antibodies already, reassure
	4. If pregnant woman has no immunity and contact is rubella or suspected, re-test patient's sera for HAI If HAI continues negative, reassure If HAI becomes positive, offer termination or rubella immunoglobulin

HAI = haemagglutination inhibition.

not likely to become pregnant within the following 2 months. Immunity is long-lasting.

The haemagglutination inhibition (HAI) test for rubella antibodies is rapid, reliable, rises within 48 hours of illness or immunization and persists for years. The HAI test is useful to differentiate past infection from acute illness. Serum should be obtained within 2 days of the onset of the illness or within 2 weeks of exposure to the virus. If this acute serum is not available, complement fixation tests or assay of rubella-specific IgM antibody is required (*Table 17.5*).

Acquired Rubella

Rubella has little oral significance. Enlarged cervical lymph nodes including posterior cervical nodes, facial rash and occasionally oral petechiae are the orofacial manifestations. There is a risk of cross-infection to female dental staff who are non-immune and, in cases of suspected contact of a non-immune pregnant woman with rubella, expert medical advice should be sought (*Table 17.5*). Unfortunately, rashes resembling rubella (rubelliform rashes) are not uncommon, particularly with enterovirus infections, and a clinical diagnosis of rubella may not always be accurate unless supported by serological data. Females who imagine they have had rubella (and should therefore now be immune) may in fact be non-immune and are therefore at risk if pregnant.

MUMPS

Mumps is a common viral infection involving particularly the major salivary glands—usually the parotids. It is usually caused by the mumps virus, occasionally by adenoviruses or echoviruses. One or both parotids become enlarged and tender, with trismus, and oedema and erythema of the orifice of the parotid duct (papillitis). The other major salivary glands may be affected in addition to the parotids but, rarely, in the absence of parotitis. Complications of mumps are uncommon but include particularly pancreatitis, orchitis, oophoritis and meningo-encephalitis. Mumps should always be considered in the differential diagnosis of swellings of acute salivary glands, particularly in the young (*Table 7.3*).

OTHER FORMS OF INFECTIOUS SIALADENITIS

Parotitis is now a recognized manifestation of AIDS especially in children (Chapter 16). Recurrent parotitis in other children and adolescents may also be caused by cytomegalovirus, or may be associated with EBV or other agents. Bacterial sialadenitis is normally an ascending infection secondary to a dry mouth (Chapter 7).

DIPHTHERIA

Diphtheria, although preventable by active immunization, continues to be seen from time to time mainly where immunization has been neglected (Appendix 17).

Corynebacterium diphtheriae multiplies mainly on the pharyngeal mucous membranes to produce an inflammatory reaction, surface necrosis and exudate (pseudomembrane). It also produces exotoxin which when absorbed causes myocardial and neurological damage.

Tonsillar or pharyngeal diphtheria produces a faucial pseudomembrane which may spread to the palate or rarely on to the oral mucosa. The membrane is creamy-yellow or grey, firmly attached and associated with faucial oedema. There is a mild sore throat but disproportionate cervical lymph node enlargement which in severe cases produces a bull-neck appearance. Nasal, laryngeal or tracheal diphtheria are variants. Palatal paralysis is one of the earliest neuropathies and develops during the third week of the illness. Any suggestion of diphtheria must be taken seriously and medical advice immediately obtained. Swabs should be taken for bacterial culture, the immunity to diphtheria established and antibiotics (usually penicillin) given. Diphtheria antitoxin is needed if the patient has not been actively immunized against diphtheria.

BUCCAL CELLULITIS

Buccal cellulitis is an uncommon but distinctive infection characterized by swelling, tenderness, induration and warmth of the cheek soft tissues in the absence of an adjacent oral or skin lesion. Almost invariably seen in children under the age of 5 years, most infections are caused by *Haemophilus influenzae* type B which may spread by bacteraemia, by lymphatics from for example, otitis media, or more probably from direct invasion through the oral mucosa.

SOME SKIN DISEASES AND INFECTIONS WITH ORAL MANIFESTATIONS 541

A minority develop meningitis. Blood and cerebrospinal fluid cultures should be taken and treatment with intravenous cefuroxime started.

SEXUALLY TRANSMITTED DISEASES

There is a rising incidence of sexually transmitted (venereal) diseases,with oral lesions in some cases. Some groups are at especially high risk (*Table 17.6*), especially sexually promiscuous young adults. More than one of these diseases, or other communicable diseases such as viral hepatitis or infection with herpes simplex or HIV, may be associated in the same patient.

Table 17.6. High risk groups for sexually transmitted diseases

Homosexuals, bisexuals and promiscuous heterosexuals
Prostitutes
Armed forces
Merchant seamen
Aircrews
Frequent business travellers overseas
Drug addicts and alcoholics
Educationally subnormal
Sexual partners of the above groups

SYPHILIS

Syphilis is a serious sexually transmitted disease as it may damage the cardio-vascular or nervous systems and can be fatal if untreated.

Primary Syphilis

The incubation period of syphilis is about 3 weeks (range 10–90 days). Over 80 per cent of cases are in homosexual men. Primary infection with *Treponema pallidum* causes a chancre (primary or Hunterian chancre) which begins as a small, firm, pink macule (usually on the glans penis or vulva), changes to a papule and then ulcerates to form a painless round ulcer with a raised margin and indurated base. Untreated chancres heal in 3–8 weeks but are highly infectious and are associated with enlarged painless regional lymph nodes. Primary chancres may involve the lips or tongue.

Management

Diagnosis of syphilis is by dark-ground microscopy and serology. Exudate from the chancre should be examined for treponemes by dark-ground microscopy. In

Table 17. 7. Serological tests for syphilis*

| | Stage of disease | | | | | |
| | Primary | | Secondary | | Tertiary | |
Test	U	T	U	T	U	T
Non-specific tests						
VDRL	Become +ve late	—ve	+ ve	—ve	Usually +ve	± ve
Specific tests						
RPCFT	Become + ve early	+ ve	+ ve	+ ve	+ ve	± ve
FTA-Abs						
TPHA						
TPI						

U, Untreated; T, treated.
* For explanation of abbreviations see p.543. .

oral lesions, the diagnosis is frequently confused by oral commensal treponemes. To minimize confusion therefore, oral lesions should be thoroughly swabbed with sterile gauze or cotton wool to remove as many contaminating oral bacteria as possible, then gently but thoroughly scraped with an instrument such as a sterile plastic spatula. The scraping is then transferred to a slide, covered with a coverslip and examined as quickly as possible by dark-ground microscopy. If the lesion is a chancre, many large but slender, regular, helical forms with a leisurely rotational movement across the field should be seen. This investigation is important as serology is usually negative at this stage (*Table 17.7*). Biopsy may be uninformative and is unlikely to be diagnostic.

Procaine penicillin 600 000 units intramuscularly daily for 10 days (or tetracycline or erythromycin for 14 days) should be given. Patients must be followed up clinically and serologically for 2 years and contacts traced.

Secondary Syphilis

Secondary syphilis follows the primary stage after 6–8 weeks but a healing chancre may still be present. It is this stage that classically causes oral lesions but these appear in only about one-third of patients. As in the primary stage, the mucosal lesions are highly infectious.

The typical signs and symptoms of secondary syphilis are fever, headache, malaise, a rash (characteristically, symmetrically distributed coppery maculopapules on the palms) and generalized painless lymph node enlargement. Painless oral ulcers (mucous patches and snailtrack ulcers) are the typical oral lesions at this stage.

Management

Mucosal lesions should be examined for *T. pallidum* as described above. Blood should be taken for serological examination and is often positive (*see below* and *Table 17.7*). Treatment is as for primary syphilis (*see below;* Herxheimer reaction).

Tertiary Syphilis

If untreated, syphilis progresses to a tertiary stage 3–10 or more years after infection in about 30 per cent of patients. The remaining patients are, however, serologically reactive and are said to have latent syphilis. The characteristic lesion is the gumma, a localized granuloma varying in size from a pin head to several centimetres. Gummas breakdown to form deep punched-out ulcers affecting skin or mucosa. Skin gummas heal with depressed shiny scars (tissue-paper scars). Mucosal gummas may destroy bone, particularly the palate, or involve the tongue. Bone gummas may affect the long bones (especially the tibia–'sabre tibia') or skull, producing lytic lesions and periostitis with new bone formation. Gummas are non-infectious.

The main oral manifestation of late stage syphilis is, however, leukoplakia, particularly of the dorsum of the tongue, which has a high potential for malignant change.

Cardiovascular syphilis, which affects only about 10 per cent of patients, is a late complication and causes aortitis, coronary arterial stenosis or aortic aneurysms (Chapter 2). A similar number of patients develop neurosyphilis (Chapter 12).

Management

The diagnosis of tertiary syphilis is confirmed by serology. Treatment is with procaine penicillin, 600 000 units daily for 3 weeks, and lifelong follow-up. Systemic corticosteroids are given at the start of antibiotic therapy in order to reduce the possibility of a Jarisch–Herxheimer reaction (febrile reaction often with exacerbation of the local syphilitic lesions).

Congenital Syphilis

Syphilis in the pregnant patient (after the fifth month) may result in infection of the fetus. Congenital syphilis is now almost unknown in Great Britain but is a rare cause of mental handicap, deafness and blindness. Affected children are highly infectious until about 2 years of age. Penicillin is the usual treatment.

Serological Tests for Syphilis

Non-specific tests: The test usually used is the VDRL (Venereal Disease Research Laboratory) test—a flocculation test which is positive in all treponematoses (e.g. yaws, bejel, pinta). A positive VDRL appears towards the end of primary syphilis and remains positive in untreated secondary or tertiary syphilis. The VDRL usually becomes negative in treated syphilis (*see Table 17.7*).

False-positive VDRL results can be caused technically or by several diseases (*Table 17.8*), but the VDRL is useful as a simple screening test.

Newer non-specific tests include the rapid plasma reagin (RPR) test and the automated reagin test (ART). The Wassermann reaction and the Kahn test are rarely used now.

Table 17.8. Causes of false-positive VDRL tests

1. Technical faults
2. Acute infections such as viral pneumonia, malaria, leptospirosis
   (VDRL +/ve for 6 months)
3. After immunizations
   (VDRL +/ve for 6 months)
4. Chronic infections such as tuberculosis
   (VDRL +/ve for more than 6 months)
5. Connective tissue disease
   (VDRL +/ve for more than 6 months)

Specific tests: Specific tests overcome the problem of the false-positive results found in the VDRL caused by non-related diseases, but still cannot differentiate syphilis from other treponemal diseases such as yaws or bejel in those from tropical and semi-tropical countries.

Specific tests include the Reiter protein complement fixation test (RPCFT), the fluorescent treponemal antibody (absorbed) (FTA-Abs) test, the treponemal haemagglutination (TPHA) test and the treponemal immobilization (TPI) test.

Specific tests become positive during primary and remain positive through untreated secondary or tertiary syphilis, as does the VDRL. However, in contrast to the VDRL, most of the specific tests remain positive even in treated syphilis.

Both specific and non-specific tests are therefore used in each case to distinguish those with active syphilis from those who have had syphilis which has been effectively treated (*see Table 17.7*).

GONORRHOEA

Gonorrhoea is about 15 times as common as syphilis but is less common than other sexually transmitted diseases such as non-specific urethritis. Gonorrhoea is caused by *Neisseria gonorrhoeae* and usually causes urethritis or proctitis in males, and urethritis or endocervicitis in females. Dysuria and urethral or vaginal discharge are the common symptoms, and an important complication is urethral stenosis. However, gonorrhoea in all sites is frequently asymptomatic, a fact that increases the chances of spread.

General management

Diagnosis depends on laboratory tests including Gram-stained smears (to show the Gram-negative diplococci within leucocytes), bacterial culture and sensitivity tests. Repeated smears or culture may be required, particularly in female contacts. Serological tests are uninformative.

Penicillin is usually still the drug of choice in the UK and is often given as 2 g ampicillin plus 1 g probenecid as a single oral dose. Patients hypersensitive to penicillin can be treated with co-trimoxazole, 4 tablets 12-hourly for 2 days.

Penicillin-resistant strains of *N. gonorrhoeae* may be resistant also to many other antibiotics: spectinomycin 2–4 g i.m. should then be used.

Dental aspects of gonorrhoea

In contrast to the high incidence of urethral gonorrhoea, oropharyngeal lesions appear to be rare. Fellatio is probably the main cause of such infections but it has been shown that saliva normally strongly inhibits the growth of *N. gonorrhoeae* and there is no direct evidence for pharyngeal-to-pharyngeal or for pharyngeal-to-genital transmission.

The oropharynx seems to be the most frequently affected oral site, especially perhaps in male homosexuals. The tonsils become red and swollen with a greyish exudate and there is regional lymphadenitis. Lesions in other parts of the oral mucosa are described as showing fiery erythema and oedema, sometimes with painful superficial ulceration. The inflamed mucosa may also be covered with a yellowish or greyish exudate, which when detached may leave a bleeding surface. The severity of the symptoms may vary widely and in extreme cases there may be painful oral or pharyngeal ulceration, cervical lymphadenitis, fever and malaise. However, the infection may be asymptomatic, and the throat appear normal.

Though a rarity, gonococcal stomatitis may be suspected when there is acute stomatitis and/or pharyngitis (*a*) without features ascribable to other oral diseases; (*b*) with severe but ill-defined inflammation or painful ulceration; (*c*) in a young adult; and especially (*d*) with a history of recent sexual contact.

A throat swab should be taken in suspected cases and Gram-staining should show polymorphs containing Gram-negative diplococci. Confirmation is by culture and identification of *N. gonorrhoeae,* as saprophytic neisseriae are common in the mouth. Penicillin is effective in 97 per cent of oropharyngeal infections. There is no evidence that oral gonococcal infections can be transmitted by coughing and droplet infection, or by saliva to the dentist (especially if normal cross-infection control is practised), except if the dentist works with ungloved hands or has a needle-stick injury. Furthermore, dental procedures on an infected patient will not produce haematogenous spread or deep infection.

GENITAL WARTS (CONDYLOMATA ACUMINATA)

The incidence of human papillomavirus (HPV) infections is increasing in the UK. Some 65 per cent of sexual contacts of patients with genital warts (condylomata acuminata) develop genital warts after an incubation period that may exceed 2 years. Genital warts may be found on the penis, vulva or vagina or perianally, or may be unseen in the meatus of the urethra. Oral and perioral lesions may occur and are infectious. Oral condylomata acuminata can be a manifestation of AIDS and related disorders. HPV also cause focal epithelial hyperplasia (Heck's disease)—predominantly seen in Eskimos and American Indians—common warts and papillomas.

MOLLUSCUM CONTAGIOSUM

This viral infection may be sexually transmitted and the characteristic umbilicated papules may be seen on the face and, rarely, intraorally. Oral molluscum contagiosum can be a manifestation of AIDS and related disorders.

NON-SPECIFIC URETHRITIS

Non-specific urethritis (NSU) is of relevance to dentistry in that it may be a feature of Reiter's disease (Chapter 11).

AIDS (SEE CHAPTER 16)

VIRAL HEPATITIS (SEE CHAPTER 8)

Bibliography

Block M. S. and Gross B. D. (1982) Epidermolysis bullosa dystrophica recessive. *J. Oral Maxillofac. Surg.* **40**, 753–8.

Borysiewicz L. K., Haworth S. J., Cohen.J et al. (1986) Epstein–Barr virus specific immune defects in patients with persistent symptoms. *Q. J. Med.* **58**, 111–21.

Catterall R. D. (1981) Biological effects of sexual freedom. *Lancet* **i**, 315–19.

Cawson R. A. (1968) Treatment of oral lichen planus with betamethasone. *Br. Med. J.* **1**, 86.

Cawson R. A. and McSwiggan D. A. (1969) An outbreak of hand-foot-and-mouth disease in a dental hospital. *Oral Surg.* **27**, 451.

Cawson R.A. and Spector R.G. (1989) *Clinical Pharmacology in Dentistry.* 5th edn. Edinburgh, Churchill Livingstone.

Chartrand S. A. and Harrison C. J. (1986) Buccal cellulitis revisited. *Am. J. Dent.* **140**, 891.

Editorial (1980) Tests for infectious mononucleosis. *Br. Med. J.* **1**, 1153–4.

Finegold S.M. (1988) Legionnaire's disease—still with us. *N. Engl. J. Med.* **318**, 571-3.

Fiumara N. J. (1978) *The Sexually Transmissible Diseases.* Chicago, Year Book.

Fotos P. G., Westfall H. N., Snyder I. S. et al. (1985) Prevalence of Legionella-specific IgG and IgM antibody in a dental clinic. *J. Dent. Res.* **64**, 1382–5.

Giunta J. L. and Fiumara N. J. (1986) Facts about gonorrhea and dentistry. *Oral Surg.* **62**, 529.

Grattan C. E. H., Small D., Kennedy C. T. C. et al. (1986) Oral herpes simplex infection in bullous pemphigoid. *Oral Surg.* **61**, 40–3.

Guess H. A., Broughton D. D., Metton L. J. et al. (1985) Epidemiology of herpes zoster in children and adolescents. *Pediatrics* **76**, 512–17.

Harris S. A. and Large D. M. (1984) Gorlin's syndrome with a cardiac lesion and jaw cysts with some unusual histological features. *Int. J. Oral Surg.* **13**, 59–64.

Iwu, C.O. (1990) Ludwig's angina: report of seven cases and review of current concepts in management. *Br. J. Oral Maxillofac. Surg.* **28**, 189-93.

Kalman C. M. and Laskin O. L. (1986) Herpes zoster and zosteriform herpes simplex virus infections in immunocomptent adults. *Am. J. Med.* **81**, 775.

Ogden G.R. and Kerr M. (1989) Mucocutaneous lymph node syndrome (Kawasaki disease). *Oral Surg.* **67**, 569-72.

Pindborg J. J. (1980) Diseases of the skin. In: Jones J. H. and Mason D. K. (ed.) *Oral Manifestations of Systemic Disease.* London, Saunders.

Pindborg J. J., Murti P. R., Bhonsle R. B. et al. (1984) Oral submucous fibrosis as a precancerous condition. *Scand. J. Dent. Res.* **92**, 224–9.

Porter S. R., Malamos D. and Scully C. (1986) Mouth-skin interface. *Update* **32**, 94–6.

Samaranayake L.P. and Scully C. (1988) Oral disease and sexual medicine. *Br. J. Sexual Med.* **15**, 138–43 and 174–80.

Scully C. (1980) Oral mucosal lesions in association with epilepsy and cutaneous lesions: Pringle-Bourneville syndrome. *Int. J. Oral Surg.* **10**, 68.

Scully C. (1980) The orofacial manifestations of the neurodermatoses. *J. Dent. Child.* **47**, 255.

Scully C. (1982) Serum IgG, IgA, IgM, IgD and IgE in lichen planus: no evidence for a humoral immunodeficiency. *Clin. Exp. Dermatol.* **7**, 163–7.

Scully C. (1985) Ulcerative stomatitis, gingivitis and rash: a diagnostic dilemma. *Oral Surg.* **59**, 261–3.

Scully C., Eckersall D., Emond R. T. D. et al. (1981) Serum amylase isoenzymes in mumps: estimation of salivary and pancreatic isozymes byisoelectric focussing. *Clin. Chim. Acta* **113**, 281.

Scully C. (1988) Viruses and salivary gland disease. *Oral Surg.* **66**, 179–82.

Scully C. (1989) Orofacial herpes simples virus infections. *Oral Surg.* **68**, 701–10.

Scully C., Cox M., Prime S.S. et al. (1988) Papilloma viruses: the current status in relation to oral disease. *Oral Surg.* **65**, 526–32.

Scully C. and Elkom M. (1985) Lichen planus: review and update on pathogenesis. *J. Oral Pathol.* **14**, 431–58.

Scully C. and Porter S. R. (1987) The mouth and the skin. In: Verbov J. (ed.) *Relationships in Dermatology,* Vol. 8. MTP Press, Lancaster.

Scully C., Prime S. and Maitland N. (1985) Papillomaviruses: their possible role in oral disease. *Oral Surg.* **60**, 166-74.

Scully C. and Samaranayake L.P. (1990) *Clinical Virology in Dentistry and Oral Medicine.* Cambridge, Cambridge University Press.

Scully C. and Williams G. (1978) Oral manifestations of communicable diseases. *Dent. Update* **5**, 295–311.

Smith O.P., Prentice H.G., Madden G.M. et al. (1990) Lingual cellulitis causing upper airways obstruction in neutropenic patients. *Br. Med. J.* **300**, 24.

Sondergaard J. O., Bulow S., Jarvinen H. et al. (1987) Dental anomalies in familial adenomatous polyposis coli. *Acta Odontol. Scand.* **45**, 61–3.

Tabi M. and Strauss E. (1985) Chronic Epstein-Barr virus disease: a workshop held by the National Institute of Allergy and Infectious Diseases. *Ann. Intern. Med.* **103**, 951–4.

Traboulisi E. I., Krush A. J., Gardner E. F. et al. (1987) Prevalence and importance of pigmented ocular fundus lesions in Gardner's syndrome. *N. Engl. J. Med.* **316**, 661–7.

Weits-Binnerts J. J., Hoff M. and van Grunsven M. F. (1982) Dental pits in deciduous teeth; an early sign in tuberous sclerosis. *Lancet* **ii**, 1344–5.

Welliver R. C. (1986) Allergy and the syndrome of chronic Epstein-Barr virus infection. *J. Allergy Clin. Immunol.* **78**, 278.

Wray D., Scully C., Rennie J. S. et al. (1980) Major and minor salivary gland involvement in *Mycoplasma pneumoniae* infection. *Br. Med. J.* **1**, 1421.

Wright J.E. (1989) Cervical lymphadenitis in childhood: which antibiotic agent? *Med. J. Aust.* **150**, 150-1.

Appendix to Chapter 17

IMMUNIZATION SCHEDULES

Age	Immunization against
3-6 months 6 weeks later 6 months later	Diphtheria, pertussis, tetanus (DPT); polio
2 years	Measles (optional)
5 years	Diphtheria, tetanus, polio
11–13 years	BCG (those exposed to tuberculosis); rubella (non-immune girls and women)
16 years	Tetanus, polio, hepatitis B (high-risk groups)

Chapter 18

Management of Emergencies in the Dental Surgery

Life-threatening emergencies in the dental surgery are fortunately rare but their very rarity makes it likely that the dental surgeon may be caught by surprise, if not totally unprepared. There is also little chance of practising the technique of cardiopulmonary resuscitation, which can be life-saving only if carried out immediately and efficiently.

Emergencies are most likely to arise during general anaesthesia, when the dentist must be particularly alert for the slightest signs of complications. The elderly and medically handicapped are also particularly at risk.

Only a few emergencies can be treated definitively in the dental surgery. Suggestions in some texts that 20 or more drugs should be kept for the management of emergencies are not practical, as so large a number of drugs could be a source of confusion and, if incorrectly used, dangerous. However, all dentists should know how to clear and maintain the airway, and how to carry out cardiopulmonary resuscitation. They should also be able to perform venepuncture.

The collapse of a patient in the dental surgery is a disturbing experience for all concerned—even if the outcome is complete recovery. Emergencies should be prevented wherever possible by careful assessment of the patient and care in treatment, particularly when general anaesthesia is used. *Forewarned is forearmed* applies especially to emergencies.

Confidence and satisfactory management of emergencies can be increased by:

1. Always having readily available a telephone and the number of the local hospital and patient's general medical practitioner (or another helpful local practitioner).
2. Training ancillary staff in emergency procedures.
3. Having a readily available emergency kit that is frequently checked and working, as suggested in *Table 18.1*. Unfortunately, recent surveys have shown that many practitioners have woefully inadequate emergency facilities.

The chief emergencies are as follows:

1. Fainting and other causes of sudden loss of consciousness.
2. Anaesthetic emergencies (particularly respiratory obstruction or arrest).
3. Acute chest pain, particularly myocardial infarction.
4. Cardiac arrest.
5. Anaphylactic shock.

Table 18.1. Suggested emergency kit

Portable apparatus for administering oxygen
  British Oxygen Company or Medical and Industrial Equipment Ltd
or for administering air
  Air-viva resuscitator (B.O.C.)
Oral airway
  Portex disposable Guedel airways sizes 1–4
Aspirator
  Any high vacuum aspirator
Tourniquet
  Any
Disposable syringes
  2 ml and 10 ml sizes
Disposable needles
  Size 19 and 21
Adrenaline
  Adrenaline injection BP (0.5 ml ampoules of 1 in 1000 solution)
Corticosteroid
  Hydrocortisone sodium succinate injection BP (or Efcortelan soluble or Solu-Cortef) or hydro-
  cortisone sodium phosphate (Efcortesol) (100 mg vials)
Diazepam
  Diazepam for injection (10 mg vials)
Glucose
  Dextrose injection BPC (20% or 50% solution)
Nitrous oxide/oxygen
  Anaesthetic machine, relative analgesia machine or Entonox
Flumazenil

6. Collapse in a patient with history of corticosteroid therapy.
7. Strokes.
8. Fits.
9. Asthmatic attacks.
10. Drug reactions and interactions.
11. Maxillofacial injuries.
12. Psychiatric emergencies.
13. Haemorrhage.
14. Inhaled foreign body.

Fuller discussion of these conditions can be found in the relevant chapters; this section is limited to the tabulation of the main diagnostic and management points in these emergencies for easy reference.

SUDDEN LOSS OF CONSCIOUSNESS

Fainting

Fainting is the most common cause of sudden loss of consciousness. Up to 2 per cent of patients faint before or during dental treatment. Predisposing factors include:

1. Anxiety.
2. Pain.
3. Fatigue.
4. Fasting (possibly).
5. High temperature and relative humidity.

Young fit adult males in particular are prone to faint in the dental surgery, especially after injections.

Signs and symptoms

1. Premonitory dizziness, weakness or nausea.
2. Pallor.
3. Cold moist skin.
4. Pulse initially slow and weak, then rapid and full.
5. Loss of consciousness: limp patient.

Management

1. Lower the head (preferably by laying patient flat or putting head between knees).
2. Clothing if tight, should be loosened at the neck but smelling salts are of no value unless the patient is already recovering.
3. Recovery is usually rapid and the patient should be reassured: if there is no recovery consider other causes of collapse—especially anaphylaxis, bradycardia, myocardial infarction or hypoglycaemia (diabetic). Monitor the pulse.
4. Defer further treatment where possible.

Differential diagnosis.   Fainting often simulates the early stages of more serious emergencies such as:

1. Myocardial infarction.
2. Stroke.
3. Corticosteroid insufficiency.
4. Epilepsy.
5. Drug reactions.
6. Hypoglycaemia.
7. Bradycardia or heart block.

The cause of sudden loss of consciousness may be suggested by the patient's history. Collapse of a diabetic at lunchtime, for example, is likely to be caused by hypoglycaemia. Collapse of a patient with angina or previous myocardial infarction is likely to be caused by a myocardial infarct. Collapse at the sight of a needle or during an injection is likely to be a simple faint, but if it follows some minutes after an injection of penicillin, is likely to be anaphylaxis. The simple precaution of laying patients flat before giving injections will prevent fainting. The clinical features of the episode, for example severe chest pain, may also aid the diagnosis.

Collapse of Uncertain Cause

In the absence of an obvious diagnosis of the cause of sudden loss of consciousness:

1. The patient should be laid flat. Recovery is almost instantaneous if the patient has simply fainted. If there is not immediate recovery, then take the pulse: an absent pulse means cardiac arrest.
2. If the pulse is palpable, give glucose, orally (4 sugar lumps) if the patient has not completely lost consciousness; or 20 ml of 20–50 per cent sterile glucose intravenously if unconscious. A hypoglycaemic patient will rapidly improve with this regimen. If there is still no improvement, medical assistance should be summoned.
3. In the meantime, maintain the airway and give oxygen.
4. Give hydrocortisone sodium succinate 200 mg intravenously.

Collapse of a Diabetic Patient

Hypoglycaemia is the most dangerous complication of diabetes since the brain is starved of glucose. Glucose but *not insulin* should be given to the diabetic who collapses, unless it is certain that the cause is hyperglycaemia. Remember also that collapse may be caused by other disease, for example myocardial infarction, since ischaemic heart disease is a common complication of longstanding diabetes.

Diagnosis

Increasing drowsiness, disorientation, excitability or aggressiveness in a diabetic, especially if it is known that a meal has been missed, suggests hypoglycaemia.

Management

1. Lay the patient flat.
2. If conscious, give glucose orally (at least 4 sugar lumps). If unconscious, give sterile glucose intravenously (20 ml of 20–50 per cent solution) or intramuscular glucagon 1 mg.
3. Call ambulance.

The differences between hypo- and hyperglycaemic coma, discussed in Chapter 10 are summarized again here:

Hypoglycaemia	*Hyperglycaemia*
Rapid onset	Slow onset
Irritability or aggressiveness	Drowsiness or disorientation
Moist skin	Dry skin, dry mouth, deep breathing, hypotension
Pulse full and rapid	Pulse weak
Blood sugar low	Blood sugar increased
Urine sugar absent	Urine sugar usually present

ANAESTHETIC EMERGENCIES

Anaesthetic emergencies include:

1. Respiratory failure.
2. Respiratory obstruction.
3. Anaesthetic overdose, or drug interactions.
4. Cardiac arrest.
5. Anaphylaxis (intravenous agents).
6. Circulatory failure in corticosteroid-treated patient.

Respiratory Failure

Causes

Anaesthetic overdose or hypoxia.

Diagnosis

1. Breathing stops.
2. Ashen cyanosis.
3. Pulse initially rapid and weak: later irregular or impalpable.
4. Cardiac arrest follows.

Management

1. Stop anaesthetic.
2. Inspect and clear airway and give oxygen.
3. Lay patient flat.
4. Inflate chest rhythmically with oxygen or by mouth-to-mouth resuscitation (1 inflation about every 5 seconds).
5. Call ambulance.

Respiratory Obstruction

Causes

Laryngeal spasm or foreign material in the airway.

Diagnosis

1. Breathing stops or is irregular with crowing or croaking on inspiration.
2. Violent respiratory efforts.
3. Increasing cyanosis.

Management

1. Stop anaesthetic: give oxygen.

2. Inspect and clear airway by suction; if obstruction is not in the pharynx but lower in respiratory tract, laryngotomy or tracheostomy may be needed.

3. After recovery, if a foreign body is lost, refer for a chest radiograph. If foreign body in chest, refer immediately to a casualty unit and then a chest surgeon.

Anaesthetic Overdose or Drug Interaction

Diagnosis

1. Pallor

2. Bradycardia (halothane) or tachycardia (other anaesthetic agents).

3. Hypotension.

4. Respiratory depression (barbiturates especially).

Management

1. Stop anaesthetic; give oxygen and ventilate artificially if necessary.

2. Give cardiopulmonary resuscitation if necessary.

3. Call ambulance.

ACUTE CHEST PAIN

Acute severe chest pain is usually caused by angina or myocardial infarction.

Diagnosis

1. Severe crushing retrosternal pain.

2. Breathlessness, vomiting and loss of consciousness if there is an infarct.

3. Pulse may be weak or irregular if there is an infarct.

Management

1. If the patient has a history of angina give anti-anginal drugs if he has them (glyceryl trinitrate 0.5 mg sublingually) If no relief of pain in 3 minutes—probably an infarct.

2. Summon assistance.

3. Do not lay patient flat if this increases breathlessness.

4. Give nitrous oxide and oxygen (50/50) to relieve pain and anxiety.

5. Reassure patient.

6. Call ambulance.

CARDIAC ARREST

Recognition is difficult in the anaesthetized patient unless the pulse is continuously monitored. Suggestive features are sudden pallor and respiratory arrest: only later do the pupils dilate. Asystole and ventricular fibrillation account for most cardiac arrests.

Causes

Myocardial infarction, hypoxia, anaesthetic overdose, anaphylaxis or severe hypotension.

Diagnosis

1. Loss of consciousness.
2. Absence of arterial pulses (feel carotid artery, anterior to sternomastoid).

Other signs too late to be of use include:

1. Respiratory arrest and eventual cyanosis.
2. Pupil dilatation and absence of light reaction.
3. No measurable blood pressure.

Management

Cardiopulmonary resuscitation:

1. Summon assistance* and note the time.
2. Lay patient on floor.†
3. Give two firm sharp blows to the mid sternum with the side of the closed fist, this occasionally restarts the heart in normal rhythm but may alternatively precipitate ventricular fibrillation.
4. Clear the airway.
5. Give external cardiac compression at 60/minute. Depress sternum 2 inches at each compression.
6. Artificially ventilate once every five chest compressions, if 2 operators are present. Use airway with face mask and oxygen, or mouth-to-mouth.
7. If a competent person is present, instruct him to set up a drip and infuse 100 ml of 8.4 per cent sodium bicarbonate, continued at 10 ml/min.Defibrillation may also be indicated if there is ventricular fibrillation or asystole.
8. Persist until there is restoration of good spontaneous pulse, of blood pressure, purposive movements (not twitches), reflex activity or of consciousness. If the patient recovers he should be admitted to hospital.

---

* Call members of the surgery staff for immediate assistance, and also an ambulance.
† It may be difficult and cause serious delay to move a heavy patient out of a dental chair on to the floor. If the dental chair allows the patient to be laid flat with the legs at least level with the head, then it may be preferable to carry out resuscitation there with the operator standing beside the chair.

If the patient is not resuscitated after 15 minutes, recovery is unlikely. The duration of resuscitation should not be assessed subjectively as, in these alarming circumstances, a few seconds may seem like minutes or hours.

ANAPHYLACTIC SHOCK

Causes
Usually penicillin but also (rarely) methohexitone.

Diagnosis*
1. Patient may complain of facial flushing, itching, paraesthesiae or peripheral coldness.
2. Wheezing, abdominal pain, nausea.
3. Loss of consciousness.
4. Pallor going on to cyanosls.
5. Cold clammy skin.
6. Rapid weak or impalpable pulse.
7. Facial oedema or sometimes urticaria.

Management
1. Lay patient flat with legs raised.
2. Give 1 ml of 1 in 1000 adrenaline intramuscularly (adult). Repeat after 15 minutes until recovery starts.
3. Give 10–20 mg chlorpheniramine slowly intravenously.
4. Give 200 mg of hydrocortisone sodium succinate intravenously.
5. Give oxygen.
6. Call ambulance.

COLLAPSE OF A PATIENT WITH A HISTORY OF CORTICOSTEROID THERAPY

Causes
Adrenal insufficiency in general anaesthesia, trauma, infections or other stress.

---

*Reaction normally starts some minutes after an injection, not immediately as in the case of fainting. In general, however, the quicker the onset the more severe the reaction is likely to be.

Diagnosis

1. Pallor.
2. Pulse: rapid, weak or impalpable.
3. Loss of consciousness.
4. Rapidly falling blood pressure.

Management

1. Lay patient flat and raise legs.
2. Give at least 200 mg hydrocortisone sodium succinate intravenously.
3. Call ambulance.
4. Give oxygen.
5. Consider other possible reasons for collapse.

STROKES

Patients usually hypertensive.

Diagnosis

Varies with size and site of brain damage.

1. Loss of consciousness.
2. Weakness of arm and leg on one side.
3. Side of face may droop.

Management

1. Maintain clear airway.
2. Call ambulance.

FITS

Causes

1. In a known epileptic, starvation, menstruation and some drugs such as methohexitone, tricyclics or alcohol may precipitate a fit.
2. Fits may also follow loss of consciousness for other reasons—especially a deep faint.

Diagnosis of grand mal attack

1. Loss of consciousness with rigid, extended body. Sometimes preceded by brief cry.
2. Widespread jerking movements.
3. Incontinence sometimes.
4. Slow recovery with the patient sometimes remaining dazed.

Management

1. Put patient prone in head-injury ('recovery') position. Most fits terminate spontaneously. All that is needed is to stop the patient damaging himself.
2. If the convulsions do not stop within 5 minutes, or if another attack starts, give adult 10–20 mg diazepam intravenously (or intramuscularly, but absorption is slow and unpredictable). Maintain airway and give oxygen.
3. Call an ambulance.
4. Repeat diazepam if no recovery within 5 minutes.

ASTHMATIC ATTACKS

Causes

Anxiety, infection or exposure to allergen.

Diagnosis

1. Breathlessness.
2. Expiratory wheezing, but may not be apparent because of shallow breathing.
3. Accessory muscles of respiration in action.
4. Rapid pulse (usually over 110 per minute).

Management

1. Reassure patient.
2. Do not lay patient flat.
3. Give the anti-asthmatic drugs normally used (such as salbutamol nebulizer) and then immediately,
4. Give hydrocortisone sodium succinate 200 mg intravenously.
5. Give oxygen.
6. If no response within 2–3 minutes, give salbutamol or terbutaline rather than aminophylline, by slow i.v. injection
7. Call ambulance.

DRUG REACTIONS AND INTERACTIONS

These include particularly:

1. Anaphylaxis (*see above*).
2. Reactions to local anaesthetics (rarely).
3. Overdose of intravenous barbiturates.
4. Hypotension resulting from interaction of intravenous barbiturates with antihypertensive drugs.
5. Hypertension from interaction of pethidine with monoamine oxidase inhibitors.

Local Anaesthetic Reactions

These include:

1. Fainting (unrelated to the anaesthetic agent).
2. Intravascular injection of local anaesthetic.
3. Temporary facial palsy or diplopia.
4. Local anaesthetic allergy.
5. Cardiovascular reactions.

All, except minor reactions such as fainting, are exceedingly rare.

Intravascular injection of local anaesthetic*

Cause.
1. Failure to use aspirating syringe.
2. Rapid injection.

Diagnosis.
Possible effects may include agitation, confusion, drowsiness, fits or loss of consciousness.

Management.
1. Lay patient flat.
2. Reassure.
3. Maintain airway.

Most patients recover spontaneously within half an hour.

---

* Experiments have suggested that at least 10 per cent of injections for mandibular blocks enter a blood vessel. If the whole injection entered the vein there would be (*a*) total failure of any local anaesthetic effect and probably also (*b*) severe systemic symptoms. In practice both these mishaps are rarities and certainly do not follow 10 per cent of mandibular blocks. The use of an aspirating syringe is of little more than theoretical value.

Temporary facial palsy, diplopia or localized facial pallor

These can occasionally result when the anaesthetic tracks towards the facial nerve or orbital contents but they will wear off with the anaesthetic. The eyelids should be closed and a protective dressing worn until the anaesthetic abates.

Local anaesthetic allergy

Allergy to local anaesthetics, if it exists, is managed as for anaphylaxis.

Cardiovascular reactions

Management. Usually only palpitations. Reassure. Await natural subsidence of symptoms. If reaction is severe, such as myocardial infarction (probably coincidental), treat as above.

Overdose of Intravenous Barbiturates

1. Clear airway, lay patient flat and artificially ventilate.
2. Summon assistance.

Hypotension Resulting from Interaction of Intravenous Barbiturates with Antihypertensive Drug

1. Clear airway, lay patient flat and artificially ventilate if necessary.
2. Summon assistance.

Hypertension Resulting from Interaction of Pethidine with Monoamine Oxidase Inhibitors

This reaction is difficult to manage (but an alpha-blocker such as phentolamine should be given if there is severe hypertension). Medical help is needed.

MAXILLOFACIAL INJURIES

Management (*see* Chapter 13)

1. Lay patient in head-injury position.
2. Establish and maintain a clear airway.
3. Check for head injury.

4. Check for chest injury or damage to limbs, spine, liver, spleen or kidneys.
5. Check for ocular injuries.
6. Call ambulance.

PSYCHIATRIC EMERGENCIES

May be caused by psychiatric disorders or

1. Drugs: especially barbiturates or other drugs of addiction, or corticos- teroids.
2. Pain or discomfort.
3. Infections, particularly in the elderly.
4. Hypoglycaemia.
5. Temporal lobe epilepsy.
6. Cerebral tumours.

Management

1. Summon psychiatric assistance or call ambulance.
2. Do not sedate the patient; this may confuse the diagnosis and may occasionally be fatal. Diazepam is likely also to worsen the excitement of a psychotic patient.
3. If the patient is violent and uncontrollable, call the police.
Emergency admission procedures are shown in Appendix to Chapter 14.

Hyperventilation Syndrome

The textbook picture of hyperventilation syndrome is that of an anxious or hysterical young woman overbreathing until carbon dioxide washout results in tetany and paraesthesia. However, the clinical features vary widely (*Table 18.2*)

Table 18.2. Hyperventilation syndrome: symptoms

Neurological and psychological
  Anxiety
  Weakness
  Lightheadedness
  Dizziness
  Disturbed consciousness
  Paraesthesia
  Tetany
  Muscle pain or stiffness
Cardiovascular and respiratory
  Palpitations
  Chest pain
  Breathlessness
Others
  Dry mouth

and males are often affected. Organic causes include pain and cardiovascular or nervous system disease. Hyperventilation is also a response to acidosis (either metabolic or drug-associated) and to poor respiratory exchange, but in this case hyperventilation is a compensatory physiological response.

The common denominator underlying hyperventilation syndrome is usually anxiety but this in turn can either cause or result from cardiovascular symptoms such as extra-systoles or tachycardia.

Management

The diagnosis is obvious in typical cases as described above, but in less well-defined cases patients should be reassured and then encouraged to rebreathe into a paper bag to overcome the alkalosis. Patients should later, between attacks, be encouraged to overbreathe to show them how the symptoms develop. Any underlying cause should be investigated and if necessary treated. Otherwise the most important aspect of treatment, if reassurance is ineffective, is sedation, usually with diazepam. If, however, there is obvious sympathetic overactivity as shown particularly by tachycardia or dysrhythmias, a cardiologist's opinion should be obtained as treatment with a beta-blocker may be necessary. In patients with hysterical personalities, however, the response to treatment may be poor.

HAEMORRHAGE

Causes

Usually local, particularly traumatic extractions. Uncommonly caused by haemorrhagic disease, but this must always be considered (Chapter 3). Post-extraction bleeding often worries the patient excessively because a little blood makes a lot of mess.

Management

1. Reassure patient.
2. Get fussing relatives out of the way.
3. Gently clean the mouth and locate the source of bleeding.
4. Suture the socket under local anaesthesia.
5. Inquire into history, especially family history.
6. If bleeding is persistent or severe and there has been loss of more than about 500 ml, or if the patient is severely anaemic or debilitated, then admit to hospital. Tranexamic acid (500 mg in 5 ml, by slow intravenous injection) may be effective in the interim.
7. Call ambulance if bleeding is uncontrollable.

INHALED FOREIGN BODIES

Prevention of inhalation of a foreign body such as a tooth or endodontic instrument is far better than cure: at the least there is great embarrassment, at worst respiratory obstruction, lung abscess or death. If the patient cannot cough the object out, do not slap him on the back, rather use the Heimlich manoeuvre to clear the airway. Failing this, endoscopy may be required as an emergency.

If a foreign body is lost and its location unknown:

1. Check the mouth and immediate area around the patient.

2. Take plain radiographs—two views at right-angles—of abdomen and of chest.

3. Bronchoscopy may well be required as the object may not be visible on X-ray.

Bibliography

Cawson R.A. and Spector R.G. (1989) *Clinical Pharmacology in Dentistry*. 5th edn. Edinburgh, Churchill Livingstone.

Chamberlain D.A. and Williams J.M. (1976) Immediate care of cardiac emergencies. *Anaesthesia* **31**, 760.

Donaldson D. and Wood W.W. (1975) Recognition and control of emergencies in the dental office. *J. Can. Dent. Assoc.* **41**, 228–32.

Drug and Therapeutics Bulletin (1989). Drugs for the Doctor's Bag. **29**, 17–19.

Editorial (1981) Treatment of anaphylactic shock. *Br. Med. J.* **282**, 1011.

Editorial (1981) Inhaled foreign bodies. *Br. Med. J.* **282**, 1649–51.

Edmondson H.D. and Frame J.W. (1986) Medical emergencies in general practice. *Dent. Update* **11**, 263–73.

Edmondson H.D., Gordon P.H., Lloyd J.M. et al. (1978) Vasovagal episodes in the dental surgery. *J. Dent.* **6**, 18–5.

McGimpsey J.G. (1977) Fainting in the dental surgery. *Br. Dent. J.* **143**, 53–7.

Perks E.R. (1977) The diagnosis and management of sudden collapse in dental practice. Part 1. The incidence of emergencies. *Br. Dent. J.* **143**, 196–200.

Perks E.R. (1977) The diagnosis and management of sudden collapse in dental practice. Part 2. Collapse under general anaesthesia. *Br. Dent. J.* **143**, 235–7.

Perks E.R. (1977) The diagnosis and management of sudden collapse in dental practice. Part 3. Collapse in the dental chair under local anaesthesia. *Br. Dent. J.* **143**, 307–11.

Rowlands D.J. (1976) Cardiac arrest. *Br. J. Hosp. Med.* **15**, 310–19.

Scully C. (1987) *The Mouth in Health and Disease*. London, Heinemann.

Shirlaw P. J., Scully C., Griffiths M.J. et al. (1986) General anaesthesia, parenteral sedation and emergency drugs and equipment in general dental practice. *J. Dent.* **14**, 247–50.

Whitwam J.G. (1978) Adverse reactions to i.v. induction agents. *Br. J. Anaesth.* **50**, 677–87.

Appendix to Chapter 18

ADVICE CONCERNING POISONS OR DRUGS

Drug Information Units operate in many areas, or hospital pharmacies can be consulted. The following also give specialist advice on the management of poisoning or adverse drug reactions.

Centre	Telephone	
London	Guy's Hospital	071-955 5000
Edinburgh	Royal Infirmary	031-229 2477
Cardiff	Royal Infirmary	0222-492233
Belfast	Royal Victoria Hospital	0232-240503
Birmingham	General Hospital	021-2368611
Bristol	Royal Infirmary	0272-230000
Manchester	Booth Hall Children's Hospital	061-7957000
Newcastle	Royal Victoria Infirmary	0632-325131
Leeds	General Infirmary	0532-432799
Dublin	Infirmary	0001-972844

Chapter 19

Drug Problems in Dental Practice

As discussed in Chapter 1, many dental patients—possibly 10 per cent overall—are having drug treatment for a variety of diseases or are taking other medication. Many of these drugs have a potential for or may cause interactions with drugs used for dental purposes (Appendix to this chapter).

By contrast, drugs used routinely in dentistry rarely cause significant adverse effects unless used recklessly. The chief dangers are those of general anaesthesia, particularly with intravenous agents, and occasionally of allergic reactions, particularly to penicillin (Chapters 1, 16 and 18). Local anaesthetic agents, such as lignocaine with adrenaline, the most widely used drugs in dentistry, have proved in practice to be remarkably safe. However, *noradrenaline* is dangerous and able to cause potentially lethal hypertension.

Dental amalgams and other dental materials have few proven toxic effects if used appropriately. Possible toxic effects of mercury on the nervous system have been discussed in Chapter 12 and possible local effects have been discussed in Chapter 17.

The main problems caused by drugs in dentistry may therefore be summarized as follows:

1. Oral side-effects of drugs.
2. Drug reactions and interactions in dental practice.
3. Adverse effects of drugs used in dentistry in the medically compromised patient.
4. Drug dependence and abuse.

ORAL SIDE-EFFECTS OF DRUGS

Oral side-effects caused by drugs are relatively uncommon but important. The most common drug-induced oral disorders are candidosis (usually caused by tetracyclines, ampicillin or corticosteroids), phenytoin-induced gingival hyperplasia and dry mouth caused by many drugs with an atropinic action. Some drugs almost invariably cause oral side-effects, for example oral ulcers with some of the cytotoxic agents, while other drugs have few reported oral complications. Some newer habits such as the use of oral snuff (smokeless tobacco) can cause gingival recession and leukoplakia and probably predispose to oral cancer. Some drugs that may occasionally cause oral complications are tabulated in the Appendix to this chapter.

DRUG REACTIONS OR INTERACTIONS IN DENTAL PRACTICE

Few of the drugs commonly used in dental practice cause significant adverse reactions. The extreme rarity of reactions to local anaesthetics—even in patients with cardiac disease—the lack of evidence of interactions with tricyclic or other antidepressants, and the rarity of hypersensitivity reactions have been stressed (Cawson, Curson and Whittington, 1983). Furthermore, the introduction of parabens-free local anaesthetics is likely further to reduce side-effects. The use of general anaesthetic or sedative techniques, however, is more likely to produce adverse reactions (Appendix to this Chapter and Chapter 18).

Drug interactions are rare in general dental practice because few drugs are routinely used in dental treatment. If, however, general anaesthesia is used, drug interactions are more likely. Drug interactions are also more common in the elderly or medically handicapped patient. Some possible drug interactions are shown in the Appendix to this chapter.

ADVERSE EFFECTS OF DRUGS USED IN DENTISTRY IN THE MEDICALLY COMPROMISED PATIENT

Possible contraindications to the main drugs prescribable by the dental surgeon are tabulated in the Appendix to this chapter. Dental surgeons will encounter some of the conditions rarely, if at all, but the danger of adverse reactions is much increased where general anaesthesia is used. Any suggestion of previous drug reaction or allergy, and particularly any adverse reaction during anaesthesia, should be taken seriously. Patients with allergy to one drug, those who suffer from atopic disease (eczema, asthma or hay fever) and patients with Sjögren's syndrome or HIV disease may be particularly liable to drug allergies. Other patients who are at particular risk from drug reactions are those with cardiovascular, hepatic or renal disease.

The pharmacology, advantages and disadvantages of anaesthetic agents and other drugs used in dentistry and the legal aspects of prescribing are discussed more fully in texts of dental pharmacology (see Bibliography).

SUBSTANCE DEPENDENCE AND ABUSE

Many drugs and chemicals can cause central nervous system stimulation, depression or hallucinations, or distort perception, thinking or judgement. Abuse of such drugs is increasingly common and presents management difficulties in dentistry, particularly because of behavioural disorders, drug resistance or interactions, hepatitis, AIDS or social problems. Of extreme concern is the high level of psychoactive drug use in the medical and allied professions. A study of medical personnel in the USA in 1986 showed that over half the respondents had used marijuana or cocaine recreationally, or opioids or tranquillizers for self-treatment.

Abuse of a drug is defined as self-administration in a manner that deviates from the cultural norm; the term is therefore not precise and alcohol in particular is often not thought of as a drug of dependence.

Drugs are abused *experimentally* on only one or two occasions because of curiosity; for *recreation*, when they are used in a relatively controlled way; or *in special circumstances*, for example to relieve anxiety or fatigue. *Compulsive drug abuse* is what is generally known as addiction: the drug is taken without any medical indication and despite adverse medical and social consequences. There is intense dependence upon the drug and there are severe physical or psychological effects if it is stopped (withdrawal syndrome). Numerous drugs and chemicals are abused.

It must be pointed out that the following description of the relative frequency and adverse effects of drug abuse is only a glimpse of a frequently changing scene. The changing factors are the price and availability of different drugs as well as the introduction of various home-produced drugs.

Dental Aspects

Those who abuse drugs not uncommonly abuse several, including alcohol and tobacco. Common oral problems include a high incidence of oral neglect, caries, periodontal disease, smokers' keratoses, gingival and/or buccal pigmentation and facial trauma. Common management problems are hazards of cross-infection with hepatitis viruses and HIV; anxiety and dental fear; and behavioural problems including a craving for sweets and irregular dental attendance.

Alcohol

The consumption of alcohol is steadily increasing throughout the world and alcohol abuse is the most common form of drug abuse.

Alcoholism causes the most serious drug-related effects in many countries, since both affected individuals and others are involved, particularly as a result of road traffic accidents. Up to 5 per cent of British adults may be alcohol-dependent and 15 per cent of American adults have abused or continue to abuse alcohol.

The causes of alcoholism are obscure and one eminent psychiatrist has stated that nothing useful is known about this aspect of the disease. The probability of developing alcoholism is greater in several groups, especially those to whom alcohol is freely available (*Table 19.1*).

Two major difficulties are to define and detect alcoholism. A loose definition is *consumption of alcohol to such a degree as to cause deterioration in social behaviour, or physical illness, and the development of dependence, from which withdrawal is difficult or causes adverse effects.*

Table 19.1. Risk factors for and findings suggestive of alcoholism

1. Occupation	Publicans and other workers in the drink industries
	Entertainers
	Commercial travellers
	Bored housewives
	Bachelors over 40
	Armed forces
	Doctors
2. Social problems	Marital disharmony
	Absenteeism
	Frequent changes of job
	Convictions for offences associated with alcohol
3. History of accidents	
4. Family history of alcoholism	
5. Alcohol-associated disease, especially	Macrocytosis
	Cirrhosis

Detection of alcoholism

Signs or symptoms of recent excessive drinking include slurred speech, smell of alcohol on the breath, signs of self-neglect whether of the mouth or shabbiness of clothes, an evasive, truculent, over-boisterous or facetious manner, indigestion (particularly heartburn), anxiety (often with insomnia), or tremor of the hands. Later there may be palpitations (and tachycardia) and signs of liver disease, malnutrition, cardiomyopathy or hypoglycaemia. No social class or profession seems to be immune, not only is there a high prevalence of alcoholism amongst vagrants but also among doctors.

The difficulties in recognising whether a patient has been taking alcohol are shown by a survey in a British teaching hospital where it was found that over 30 per cent of patients attending the casualty department had blood alcohol levels over 80 mg/100 ml. Medical staff, who at the same time were attempting to detect inebriation clinically, underestimated the true extent of the problem by 19 per cent. Recognition of the alcoholic is notoriously difficult and even if the disorder is suspected the history is often a hopelessly unreliable guide to the amount of alcohol consumed. Women are traditionally even more evasive about their drinking habits, but it is important to bear in mind that women are almost as frequently alcoholic as men. In Great Britain alcoholic cirrhosis is as common in women as in men.

The CAGE questionnaire may be helpful: a positive response to any of the following questions suggests a diagnosis of alcoholism:

1. Have you ever felt the need to **C**ut down on drink?
2. Have you ever felt **A**nnoyed by criticism of your drinking?
3. Have you ever felt **G**uilty about drinking?
4. Do you drink a morning **E**ye opener?

Laboratory investigations that may be helpful include raised blood levels of alcohol, γ-glutamyl transpeptidase and other hepatic enzymes. However, raised liver enzyme values can also be found with socially acceptable alcohol consumption. Folate deficiency of no obvious cause is also suspicious. Macrocytosis alone is one of the earliest signs of alcoholism and later there may be macrocytic anaemia.

Laboratory investigations must therefore be interpreted in the light of clinical findings and are of value mainly in the preoperative assessment of patients, or the interpretation of clinical signs.

Many diseases can be caused or aggravated by alcohol. There is a high incidence of alcohol-associated accidents and disease and some 20-30 per cent of those seeking acute medical or surgical attention may be alcoholics.

Complications of alcoholism include:

1. Injuries, including maxillofacial, from accidents or assaults.
2. Social problems.
3. Liver disease.
4. Nutritional defects.
5. Pancreatitis.
6. Alcohol gastritis and peptic ulcer.
7. Predisposition to infections, especially pneumonia and tuberculosis.
8. Cardiomyopathy.
9. Myopathy.
10. Brain damage and epilepsy.

In one British study of alcoholics, the mortality rate over 15 years was about 300 per cent above the norm.

Alcohol is an important, if not the main, causal factor in over 25 per cent road traffic accidents and also in many other accidents or assaults. Many patients with maxillofacial or head injuries have been drinking.

Common social problems include marital difficulties, aggressive behaviour, crime, absenteeism and financial embarrassment. Alcohol is often a factor in violent or sexual crimes and suicides and also contributes to the spread of sexually-transmitted diseases including HIV.

Acute alcoholic hepatitis may follow binge drinking and cirrhosis commonly results from chronic alcoholism. The inadequate diet of many alcoholics causes various nutritional defects which can cause peripheral polyneuropathies (burning hands and feet), pellagra, amblyopia (visual defects) and various organic brain disorders (Wernicke's encephalopathy and Korsakoff's psychosis) or epilepsy. Alcoholism in pregnancy may lead to the fetal alcohol syndrome.

The features of alcohol withdrawal are similar to, but usually less severe than, the barbiturate withdrawal syndrome (p. 573). During the first 24 hours there is tremor, anxiety, sweating, weakness, nausea and insomnia. This is followed by vomiting, abdominal cramps and hallucinations and, in severe cases, convulsions (delirium tremens, DTs, rum fits). Hyperthermia is common and there may be exhaustion or cardiovascular collapse. The whole withdrawal syndrome lasts about a week and requires medical supervision and the use of benzodiazepines or chlormethiazole.

The chronic alcoholic needs medical treatment including:

1. Admission to manage rehabilitation and ensure abstinence.
2. Use of drugs that cause unpleasant side-effects if alcohol is taken (disulfiram—Antabuse).

Dental aspects of alcoholism

The most common oral effect of alcoholism is neglect leading to advancedcaries and periodontal disease, and there is sometimes dental erosion. There may be folate deficiency or other anaemia, with glossitis and sometimes angular stomatitis or recurrent aphthae. Alcoholic cirrhosis may cause a bleeding tendency and a rare manifestation is bilateral painless swelling of the parotids or other major salivary glands (sialosis, Chapter 7).

Orofacial features include a smell of alcohol on the breath, telangiectases and possibly rhinophyma ('grog blossom').

Spirit drinking was thought to be a cause of leucoplakia, but this may have applied to the nineteenth century, when alcohol was heavily adulterated, or associated factors operated. By contrast, the increasing consumption of alcohol in recent years has not been associated with any increase in oral cancer; indeed oral cancer has declined until recently in men and not increased in women.

One of the most important dental complications of excessive alcohol intake is maxillofacial trauma and head injuries (Chapter 13) and unconsciousness in such patients may be due at least in part to the alcohol itself.

Wound healing may also be impaired in the severe chronic alcoholic and in a series reported in the USA alcoholism was found to be a common factor in 22 patients with osteomyelitis following mandibular fractures.

Many alcoholics present no dental management problems but complications may include:

1. Erratic attendance for dental treatment.
2. Aggressive behaviour.
3. Liver disease.
4. Cardiomyopathy.
5. Drug interactions (Appendix to this chapter).

Cirrhosis delays the metabolism of many drugs and there may be a bleeding tendency and possibly anaemia. General anaesthesia is therefore best avoided especially if the patient has premedicated himself with alcohol, which increases the risk of vomiting and inhalation of vomit. Alcoholics are especially prone to aspiration lung abscess. Alcoholic heart disease is also a contraindication to general anaesthesia.

Drug interactions with alcohol which may be important in dental management include:

Anaesthetics and sedatives: General anaesthetic agents, sedatives or hypnotics generally have an additive effect with alcohol, although these interactions are not entirely predictable. Heavy drinkers, however, become tolerant not only of alcohol but also of other sedatives. Alcoholics are also notoriously resistant to general anaesthesia. Once liver disease develops the position is reversed and drug metabolism is then impaired (Chapter 8) and drugs have a disproportionately greater effect.

Analgesics: Aspirin should be avoided since it is more likely in the alcoholic patient to cause gastric erosions and bleeding, and to precipitate bleeding. The hepatotoxic effects of paracetamol are not enhanced and it is probably a safe analgesic in this group (Appendix to this chapter).

Metronidazole: Metronidazole and alcohol interact to cause widespread vasodilatation, nausea, vomiting, sweating and palpitations similar to the Antabuse reaction. The effects are unpleasant or alarming but rarely dangerous.

Fetal alcohol syndrome

Alcohol is now the most common teratogen apart from smoking to which the fetus is exposed. Chronic ingestion may cause spontaneous abortion or birth defects (fetal alcohol syndrome, FAS). The prevalence of FAS is similar to that of Down's syndrome.

FAS affects growth, CNS and orofacial features. Most affected children are of short stature. Microcephaly is common and associated with a low IQ, difficulties in eating and speech and muscular incoordination. The FAS patient is irritable as an infant, hyperactive as a child and highly unsociable as an adult.

Facial features include hypoplastic maxillae, low nasal bridge, indistinct philtrum with a hypoplastic upper lip and other features, including small teeth with dysplastic enamel.

Nicotine and Tobacco

Cigarette smoking is a major hazard to health and contributes to the development of many diseases (*Table 19.2*). Combustion of tobacco gives rise not only to nicotine, tar and carbon monoxide but also about 4000 other compounds, including nitrosamines and aromatic amines, which are known carcinogens.

There appears to be dependence upon nicotine in chronic smokers. Heavy smokers appear to require a stable blood concentration of nicotine—if they change to a different type of cigarette they also change the pattern of smoking to keep their nicotine levels constant. Smokers metabolize some other drugs

Table 19.2. Diseases associated with cigarette smoking

Cardiovascular disease	Respiratory disease
Ischaemic heart disease	Carcinoma of bronchus
Cerebrovascular disease	Chronic obstructive airways disease
Peripheral vascular disease	Fetus
Buerger's disease	Increased prevalence of abortion
Carcinoma of	Low birthweight
Bronchus and possibly also	Increased risk of perinatal death
Larynx	Increased risk of sudden infant death
Bladder	Peptic ulcer
Pancreas	Alcoholism

more rapidly and require, for example, higher doses of benzodiazepines than nonsmokers. Withdrawal leads to nausea, headache, constipation or diarrhoea, irritability, insomnia, poor concentration and increased appetite.

Dental aspects of smoking and smokeless tobacco

Smoking may cause mucosal keratinization and pigmentary incompetence. Smoker's keratosis, in which there is diffuse hyperkeratosis of the palate, is typically caused by pipe smoking. The hyperkeratosis itself is benign and rapidly reversible even after many years of pipe smoking. However, there is some epidemiological evidence of an association between pipe smoking and oral cancer, but when cancer develops in a pipe smoker it is likely to be in the lower retromolar region and not in the area of keratosis.

Oral snuff dipping and chewing tobacco predispose to leukoplakia and oral cancer. Up to 46 per cent of regular users develop leukoplakia. Currently there is particular concern over the mucosal reactions and the carcinogenic potential of the widespread use of smokeless tobacco by children and adolescents, especially in the USA. By contrast, increased cigarette smoking had been associated with an overall *decline* in the incidence of cancer in the mouth in Great Britain, but a great increase in lung cancer. Oral cancer is, however, now increasing.

Cigarette smoking is the most common cause of extrinsic staining of teeth. Stopping smoking is not merely difficult but may bring other problems. Aggravation or the onset of recurrent aphthae is noted by some, while others take to eating sweets as a substitute for smoking and may then have increased caries activity, or put on weight.

Difficulties in dental management may include:

1. Chronic obstructive airways disease.
2. Ischaemic heart disease.
3. Resistance to sedation.
4. Associated disorders such as alcoholism or peptic ulcer.

Intravenous drug abuse

Intravenous injection is frequently used by those who abuse drugs. Frequently, injection technique is filthy and even water from a lavatory pan may be used to dissolve the drug. The life–style of these addicts is such that sexually transmitted disease is also common among them. Serious infections are therefore a major complication of intravenous drug abuse, irrespective of the nature of the drug itself. Another consequence of this life style is the frequent risk of maxillofacial injuries Common complications of intravenous drug abuse therefore include the following:

1. Viral hepatitis (particularly B, C and D) or chronic liver disease.
2. Infective endocarditis and consequent cardiac lesions.
3. Maxillofacial injuries.
4. HIV infection.
5. Sexually transmitted diseases.

6. Tetanus.
7. Venous thromboses making intravenous injection difficult.

Infective endocarditis among intravenous drug abusers

It should be noted that infective endocarditis among drug abusers is common but usually a consequence of infected injections—not dental treatment. However, those drug addicts who have had endocarditis as a result of their habits also become susceptible to the disease as a consequence of dental treatment and will need appropriate prophylaxis.

Hypnotics and Sedatives

Dependence can follow the use of virtually any hypnotic or sedative, but especially barbiturates. Dependence on benzodiazepines is becoming common but the effects are considerably less severe than with most other sedatives.

The pattern of dependence on sedatives varies widely and often neither patient nor doctor realizes that it has developed, since the anxiety, tremor and insomnia that follow the drug's withdrawal are incorrectly attributed to the return of the original anxiety state.

Barbiturate addiction usually develops in patients who have been prescribed barbiturates for insomnia or anxiety. Two main types of barbiturate addict are recognized and either may also abuse other drugs:

1. Middle-aged women, often living alone, taking large quantities of barbiturates orally and living in a dream world, form the largest group of barbiturate addicts. Chronic toxicity such as rashes and ataxia often develop.

2. Young addicts, who take barbiturates (`sleepers') for immediate effect, by injection, can develop multiple abscesses, gangrene, hepatitis, AIDS, infective endocarditis and occasionally tetanus, as discussed earlier. Most of these complications are caused by filthy injection technique.

Barbiturates are also responsible for many of the lethal overdoses taken by addicts to any drugs, since barbiturates are often used to adulterate more expensive drugs such as heroin.

With chronic use, the addict begins to think slowly, has increasing emotional lability and shows signs of self-neglect. Concentration and judgement are increasingly impaired and the barbiturate addict becomes irritable. Although tolerance to barbiturates increases remarkably, the lethal dose remains the same, and accidental overdose is a relatively common cause of death, especially if alcohol is also taken. Should barbiturates be withdrawn from an addict, the patient initially improves and any ataxia disappears. However, within 12–16 hours a dangerous withdrawal syndrome can develop. Nausea, anxiety, tremor, insomnia,weakness and postural hypotension, are followed by abdominal pain. After 36–48 hours there is loss of consciousness and often fits and sometimes death. The syndrome has a slower onset in those who have been using long-acting barbiturates. Barbiturates must only be withdrawn under strict medical supervision. Barbiturates are Controlled Drugs.

Dental aspects of barbiturate abuse

Oral complications of barbiturate abuse are rare. A bullous mucosal reaction has been reported but, more common, are manifestations such as atypical facial pain, related to the underlying condition for which the drug was prescribed.

Dental management may be complicated by:

1. Altered drug metabolism.
2. Hepatitis B and non-A non B hepatitis.
3. Infective hepatitis.
4. Sexually transmitted disease.
5. Epilepsy.
6. Maxillofacial injuries.
7. Tetanus.
8. HIV infection.

Barbiturates induce liver drug-metabolizing enzymes and cause resistance to anaesthetics, but also enhance the sedative effects of some drugs.

Benzodiazepines

Benzodiazepines are very widely prescribed but despite concern about the problem, abuse is relatively uncommon. Fewer than 1 per cent of the population claim to use these sedatives non–medically and then usually infrequently. However, benzodiazepines may be one component of multiple drug abuse. Some patients, mainly housewives, also claim to have become dependent as a result of having been prescribed benzodiazepines for chronic anxiety.

Mild physical and psychological dependence on benzodiazepines can develop. Withdrawal symptoms are frequently delayed in onset compared with the barbiturates but may last 8–10 days. Typical effects include insomnia, anxiety, loss of appetite, tremor, perspiration and perceptual disturbances. Sudden withdrawal particularly of short–acting benzodiazepines can cause confusion, fits, toxic psychosis or a condition resembling delirium tremens.

Benzodiazepines should therefore only be prescribed for short periods (not more than 2 weeks). In those that have become dependent, withdrawal should be gradual. The benzodiazepine should be changed to diazepam and this should be reduced by fortnightly decrements of 2.5 mg or less. Complete withdrawal may take several weeks or even months.

Unlike other drugs of abuse, benzodiazepines are not, at the time of writing, Controlled Drugs and are virtually harmless in overdose.

Opioids (narcotics)

Morphine, heroin and pethidine are the main examples, but many synthetic analogues or derivatives are also abused. These powerful analgesics appear to act by mimicking the natural brain peptides—enkephalins and endorphins. Opioid abuse is widespread in some communities, especially in the USA. Nearly 40 per cent of US army conscripts used narcotics at some time during their year in Vietnam and one-half of these became physically dependent. In the USA some 6 per cent of all hospitalized patients abuse drugs other than alcohol. Abuse of opioids in the UK is mainly in urban areas, particularly the new towns and the major cities such as London and Edinburgh. The enormous use of intravenous heroin is a major drug problem in Great Britain.

Opioid abuse is particularly troublesome to the community because of the amount of crime committed to obtain money to buy drugs, and the frequency of HIV infection.

Opioid abuse develops in three main ways:

1. Use by adolescents in an experimental or recreational way, or as part of a life-style.
2. As a sequel to their medical use for severe pain.
3. Dependence on methadone used for treatment of established dependence.

In practical terms addicts fall into several groups:

Junkies: These are often unemployed, buy illicit heroin (frequently obtaining the money by crime or prostitution) and typically associate with other addicts.

Stables: These addicts are in most ways the opposite of junkies and appear to be respectable members of society.

Loners: Loners are usually not criminals, do not associate with other addicts but use various non-prescribed drugs.

Two-worlders: These addicts may be in fairly steady employment, like stables, but associate with other addicts, often engage in criminal activities and use both prescribed and illicitly obtained drugs.

Detection of opioid abuse

Early signs of opioid abuse can be difficult or impossible to detect and may remain unsuspected until needle marks are seen, syringes found, or medical complications develop. However, lack of concentration, poor performance at work, irritability, desire to be left alone, absences from home or self-neglect are suggestive of abuse. Loss of weight and emaciation, pupil constriction and chronic constipation are more specific signs. Needle marks or thromboses of veins, particularly in the forearms and legs, are common, but addicts are now remarkable adept at finding veins, even lingual or penile veins, that escape casual inspection. Opioids may also be used subcutaneously (skin popping), as snuff or as cigarettes. Many narcotic addicts also abuse alcohol or cocaine.

Complications of opioid abuse

Illegal intravenous drugs are often adulterated with talc, sucrose, baking soda, quinine or starch, and often suspended in dirty water. Syringes and needles are often re-used or shared by several addicts. Infective complications such as septicaemia and pneumonia are therefore common and an acute right-sided endocarditis can be rapidly fatal or may leave substantial cardiac damage. Hepatitis B, C and D are frequently the result of using contaminated injection equipment and indulging in associated activities such as sexual promiscuity or homosexuality (Chapter 8). In some areas addicts are the group at greatest risk from viral hepatitis. Infection with HIV is an increasing problem and in certain areas, such as the east of Scotland, well over 50 per cent of heroin addicts were HIV antibody-positive by early 1987, and intravenous drug abuse is now a major cause of spread of the infection in the USA. Sexually transmitted diseases are also prevalent.

The mortality among opioid addicts is 2–6 per cent per annum: deaths are usually from overdose. This is often accidental as a result of impure drugs or the combination with another CNS depressant such as alcohol. Less often, there may be an anaphylactoid reaction to the opioid or impurities in the preparation. Suicide and assaults are other common causes of death, as will probably be AIDS. The morbidity is also high from other infective complications, violence or malnutrition.

Withdrawal of narcotics leads to a withdrawal syndrome within about 8 hours (*cold turkey*). Early features include lacrimation, rhinorrhoea, sweating and persistent yawning. After about 12 hours the addict enters a phase of restless tossing sleep (*yen*) when there is pupil dilatation, tremor, gooseflesh, anorexia, nausea, vomiting, muscle spasms, orgasms,diarrhoea and abdominal pains. Pulse rate and blood pressure also rise.

Although the withdrawal syndrome subsides within about a week, the addict is, for a few weeks thereafter, intolerant of stress and pain. The respiratory response to carbon dioxide is reduced and general anaesthesia may be hazardous.

Medical supervision and the use of oral methadone are needed in the management of opioid dependence.

In spite of widespread belief to the contrary, pentazocine is also used as a drug of dependence, particularly amongst medical and paramedical personnel in the USA. Pentazocine is therefore a Controlled Drug in Great Britain. Pentazocine tablets together with an antihistamine (Ts and Blues, Appendix to this chapter) have been used intravenously as an alternative to the more expensive heroin. Distalgesic and co-proxamole (because of the dextropropoxyphene) and dipipanone are also used as drugs of addiction.

Dipipanone is less sedating than morphine and may therefore be abused, but is available only in tablet form and in combination with an anti–emetic (Diconal).

Use of an illicitly manufactured pethidine–like drug (MPDP) which caused specific damage to the substantia nigra of the basal ganglia and extreme parkinsonian rigidity has incidentally led to more detailed understanding of Parkinson's disease and a search for other environmental causes.

Dental aspects of opioid dependence

There are no specific oral effects of opioid dependence but there is often oral neglect, advanced periodontal disease and caries. Patients with endocarditis may have oral petechiae.

The identification of addicts is difficult especially in view of the different types described earlier. However, abnormal behaviour, persistently constricted pupils, or outlining of veins are highly suspicious features.

Few drugs prescribable by the dental surgeon under National Health Service regulations are likely to appeal to the drug addict, but this is not the case with medical practitioners who may find themselves manipulated to a remarkable degree by addicts trying to procure supplies of drugs. Simulation of pain is a common manoeuvre to obtain narcotics. Prescription pads may be stolen or drug cabinets raided. Dental drugs that may be attractive to the addict include pethidine, codeine, pentazocine and dextropropoxyphene (in co-proxamol and Distalgesic).

Dental treatment can often be given to narcotic addicts without fear of complications, but possible difficulties include:

1. Behavioural disturbances and withdrawal symptoms.
2. Cardiac lesions
3. Maxillofacial injuries.
4. Hepatitis or chronic liver disease.
5. Infective endocarditis.
6. Sexually transmitted diseases, including HIV infection.
7. Venous thromboses making intravenous injection difficult.
8. Analgesia (*see below*).
9. Tetanus.
10. Feigning pain or stealing drugs or prescription forms.

Many addicts tolerate pain poorly and complain that local anaesthesia is insufficient for operative procedures. Furthermore, those under treatment for addiction have a period of several weeks during which they are particularly hypersensitive to pain and stress.

In the established addict, non-narcotic analgesics may be ineffective in controlling dental pain, so that large doses of opioids may have to be given. Pentazocine, being a narcotic antagonist, should not be used for such patients as it may precipitate a withdrawal syndrome. Local anaesthesia is often of little value and general anaesthesia may therefore be preferred unless there are other medical contraindications. Nausea and vomiting are common if the narcotics are stopped preoperatively.

If the patient is under treatment for addiction, opioids must be avoided. Local anaesthesia is preferable at this time, since reduced sensitivity to carbon dioxide is a contraindication to general anaesthesia.

Needless to say, opioids should not be given or prescribed without first seeking expert advice (*see* The Misuse of Drugs Act), and their only indication in dentistry is for severe postoperative pain.

Amphetamines

Amphetamines are the main drugs in a group of central stimulants that also include cocaine, phenmetrazine, methylphenidate and, to a lesser extent, diethylpropion. These drugs are characterized by their ability to elevate mood.

Amphetamine addiction may develop in the following ways:

1. As a result of their medical use for slimming or for depression.
2. Following use for their euphoriant effect.
3. Following their use, for example by lorry drivers, to stave off fatigue in order to continue their work.

Amphetamines are taken orally or intravenously (*speed*). Chronic toxicity causes restlessness, hyperactivity, loss of appetite and weight, tremor, repetitive movements and picking at the face and extremities. Eventually with large doses, a paranoid psychosis may develop. There is no true withdrawal syndrome and, in this respect, amphetamine addiction is quite different from opioid or barbiturate dependence.

Dental aspects of amphetamine dependence

Bruxism may result from chronic amphetamine use and there can be xerostomia and increased caries incidence. Amphetamine addicts may be remarkably resistant to general anaesthesia and, if using intravenous drugs, may have many of the problems of opioid addicts. Monoamine oxidase inhibitors are contraindicated (Appendix to this chapter).

Other amphetamines

The current fashion is for drugs which give an instant jolt of stimulation and as a result free base cocaine (*crack, see below*) is widely abused, particularly in the USA. Pure crystalline methamphetamine (*ice*) acts, when inhaled, almost as rapidly as intravenous cocaine but has several hours duration of action.

Ecstasy (methylene–deoxymethamphetamine—MDMA) has similar properties to other amphetamines but is more potently hallucinogenic possibly because of chemical affinities with mescalin.

Amphetamines are relatively easily synthesized and the illicit manufacture of methamphetamine alone is estimated to be a *three billion dollar* industry in the USA.

Cocaine

From being a fashionable drug of abuse for wealthy, apparently respectable members of society in the USA, cocaine has become one of the most widely abused drugs, as a result of smuggling on an enormous scale mainly from South America. By 1986, almost 15 per cent of the US population had experimented with cocaine and almost 5 per cent of these had become dependent.

Cocaine is inhaled (*snorted*), smoked, or injected intravenously, intramuscularly or hypodermically. It is also taken orally, sublingually, rectally or vaginally. Free base cocaine *crack*, obtained by boiling cocaine hydrochloride with sodium bicarbonate, acts so rapidly that, when inhaled or smoked, its effects are similar to intravenous cocaine.

Abuse is characterized by feelings of well-being and heightened mental activity. The cocaine addict is garrulous, witty and the life and soul of the party, but later shows diminished activity.

The cocaine addict has been described as a 'sexed-up extrovert with dilated pupils', in contrast to the opioid addict who is 'a depressed introvert with constricted pupils'.

Toxic reactions to cocaine abuse include angina, coronary spasm, ventricular dysrhythmias, myocardial infarction, cerebrovascular accidents, convulsions and death.

Large doses of cocaine produce paranoia, visual hallucinations (*snowlights*) and tactile hallucinations. The latter are typically of insects crawling over the skin (formication, 'cocaine bugs'). On stopping cocaine, symptoms proceed through a crash phase of depression and craving for sleep, a withdrawal phase of lack of energy and then an extinction phase of recurrence of craving evoked by various external stimuli but of lesser intensity. Deaths from cocaine are becoming increasingly common as the drug becomes increasingly widely used.

As a constituent of Brompton cocktail (cocaine, heroin or morphine and alcohol), cocaine was used for the management of patients with terminal disease.

Dental aspects of cocaine addiction

Oral use of cocaine temporarily numbs the lips and tongue. The main oral effects of cocaine addiction may be a dry mouth and bruxism or dental erosion, but rarely, long-term inhalation of cocaine can cause, in addition to nasal symptoms similar to those of the common cold, perforation of the nasal septum and ulceration of the palate as a result of ischaemic necrosis. Caries and periodontal disease, especially acute necrotizing gingivitis are increased. Behavioural problems may interfere with dental treatment.

Dental treatment should not be given until 6 hours after the last dose of cocaine has been taken and it may be advisable to avoid adrenaline-containing local anaesthetics because of enhanced sympathomimetic action. However, it is not known whether this is of practical significance.

Patients who inject cocaine are at risk from the same blood–borne infections as other addicts. Children born to cocaine-using mothers are more prone to have ankyloglossia.

Cannabis

Cannabis (marijuana) is a widely abused drug. It can be taken by many routes but is often smoked as a *reefer* (Appendix to this chapter). The effects are prompt, somewhat resemble those of alcohol, but differ with dose and routeof administration. Large doses cause dreams, hallucinations, feeling of depersonalization, impaired memory and depressed motor function. Hunger, dry mouth and enhanced sense of taste, smell and hearing may develop.

Withdrawal of cannabis can cause tremor, irritability, insomnia, anorexia and fever. It is controversial whether there are serious medical effects of cannabis abuse, or that the abuse of hard drugs such as narcotics necessarily follows the use of soft drugs such as cannabis. However, the single best predictor of cocaine abuse is frequent use of cannabis during adolescence. Users of cannabis may, however, experience tachycardias and in those with ischaemic heart disease, angina can result. The only other established health risks are neurological impairment, bronchitis and possibly impaired fertility.

Dental aspects of cannabis addiction

There are no specific oral manifestations or aspects of cannabis addiction that influence dental management in most patients, but there is concern that cannabis use may predispose to oral cancer.

Psychodelics (Hallucinogens, Psychotomimetics or Psychotogens)

Psychodelic drugs induce feelings of enhanced clarity of sensation, higher awareness of sensory input and altered perception. They include:

1. Indolealkylamines such as lysergic acid diethylamide (LSD) and psilocybin.
2. Phenylethylamines such as mescaline.
3. Phenylisopropylamines.
4. Phencyclidine (PCP) and derivatives such as ethyl phenylcyclohexamine (PCE) and thiencylcyclophexyl piperidine (TCP).

In addition, as mentioned earlier, the amphetamine *Ecstasy* (methylene–deoxymethamphetamine—MDMA) is hallucinogenic as excessive doses of other amphetamines may be.

Hallucinogens are rarely used over long periods and LSD in particular can cause persistent schizophrenia–like psychosis if it is. Up to 12 per cent of adolescents are estimated to have taken hallucinogenic agents. These drugs often cause sympathomimetic effects such as pupil dilatation, tremor, nausea and a rise in blood pressure, pulse rate and temperature. *Synaesthesia*, the overflow from one sense to another when, for example, colours are heard, is common. There is often lability of mood, panic and delusions of magical powers such as being able to fly. Whilst under the influence of these drugs, deaths, accidents and assaults as a result of delusions are therefore common. There is no withdrawal syndrome when psychodelic drugs are stopped, but permanent mental disturbance can follow.

Phencyclidine (PCP) is a psychodelic frequently abused by smoking, snorting or eating—rarely intravenously. It causes a syndrome closely resembling schizophrenia and manic depressive psychosis, and may produce numbness of the extremities, facial grimacing, jaw clenching, expressive dysphasia and memory loss. Nystagmus and hypertension are also prominent features of PCP abuse.

Phencyclidine, which was originally developed as a general anaesthetic, produces a state of dissociative anaesthesia in which the subject becomes detached or dissociated from all bodily sensations and pain. The user may severely injure himself because of these dissociative effects and the psychotic reactions cause violently aggressive behaviour towards others. Phencyclidine is therefore now regarded as one of the most dangerous drugs of addiction.

Phencyclidine is easy to produce and may therefore become a frequent drug of abuse, as it has in the USA. Because of its low price and availability, it is often sold with, or as a misrepresentation of, other drugs of abuse. Addicts to the latter may therefore be unknowingly exposed to phencyclidine. The closely related anti–Parkinsonian drug, procyclidine may sometimes also be abused.

Dental aspects of psychodelic drug abuse

Grossly abnormal behaviour can develop from abuse of any of the psychodelic drugs and a psychiatric opinion should be obtained. Hallucinogen-induced crises often respond to diazepam 10–20mg orally, but intravenous diazepam or intra-muscular chlorpromazine may be needed.

Intravenous barbiturates may induce convulsions, respiratory distress or coma in these patients, and should be avoided. Opioids are also contraindicated.

Miscellaneous Agents of Abuse

Abuse can develop of a variety of drugs or chemicals, including anaesthetic agents and organic solvents.

Anaesthetic abuse

Nitrous oxide has all the properties of a drug of addiction, in that it induces impaired consciousness with a sense of dissociation and often of exhilaration (laughing gas). The reason that it has not become a widely abused drug is simply the practical problem of carrying the heavy cylinders around. However, addiction to nitrous oxide is an occupational hazard of anaesthetists and dental surgeons. Chronic abuse of nitrous oxide can lead to interference with vitamin B_{12} metabolism and neuropathy. Sixteen of a series of 18 patients with this type of polyneuropathy were dentists, most of whom had abused nitrous oxide for periods exceeding 3 months. Vague neurological symptoms have also been reported by dentists and dental staff working in environments contaminated by nitrous oxide. Occasionally patients have died as a result of drowsiness of an anaesthetist abusing nitrous oxide.

Cases of nitrous oxide abuse have been reported in the USA among dental and medical students who obtained supplies by stealing large hospital cylinders.

Abuse of halothane is a hazard, particularly in the USA. A particularly remarkable case is that of a nurse who developed skeletal fluorosis, hypertension and renal damage as a consequence of secretly sniffing another fluorinated hydrocarbon anaesthetic, methoxyflurane.

Ether and chloroform are rarely abused, as they were in the past, as other agents are more readily available.

Organic solvent abuse

Solvent sniffing is increasingly common and has led to many deaths of children and young adults. The sniffers are usually male teenagers who are predominantly glue-sniffers. Glue is squeezed into a paper or plastic bag, placed around the mouth and inhaled. Those who sniff petrol or other organic liquids inhale them from a cloth soaked in the liquid or directly from the container. Abusers of aerosol sprays often inhale through a cloth which traps the particulate matter but permits the propellant to pass, but some spray the aerosol directly into the mouth. Used in the latter way these aerosols are highly dangerous and can cause severe respiratory damage or death.

Signs of solvent abuse include slurred speech, euphoria, anorexia and a circumoral (glue sniffers') rash. Jaundice may be seen and the pulse may be irregular due to dysrhythmias.

Sniffing solvents produces an effect somewhat between that of alcohol and a psychotomimetic. Toxic effects include hypoxia, cardiac dysrhythmias and sometimes sudden death, liver damage and neurological damage and delusions. If liver function is impaired, it can interfere with drug metabolism. Specific chemicals may also have additional side-effects. Chronic abuse of petrol, for example can cause respiratory damage, anaemia, lead poisoning and cranial nerve palsies. A syndrome of mental handicap, hypotonia, scaphocephaly and high malar bones, has also been reported in children of mothers who inhaled petrol during pregnancy (fetal gasoline syndrome).

Bibliography

Note: Overall, the most up to date source of reference is the British National Formulary published by the British Medical Association and the Pharmaceutical Society (London) and revised twice a year.

Anderson H. R., Macnair R. S. and Ramsey J. D. (1985) Deaths from abuse of volatile substances; a national epidemiological survey. *Br Med J.* **290**, 304–7.

Barclay J. K., Hunter K. MacD. and Jones H. (1980) Diazepam and lorazepam compared as sedatives for outpatient third molar surgery. *Br.J. Oral Surg.* **18**, 141–9.

Barnett R. and Shusterman S. (1985) Fetal alcohol syndrome. *J. Am. Dent. Assoc.* **111**, 591–3.

Calvey T. N. (1978) *Drug Interactions of Dental Significance.* Macclesfield, Imperial Chemical Industries Ltd.

Cawson R. A., Curson I. and Whittington D. R. (1983) The hazards of dental local anaesthetics. *Br. Dent.J.* **154**, 25.

Cawson R. A. and Spector R. G. (1989) *Clinical Pharmacology in Dentistry*, 5th edn. Edinburgh, Churchill Livingstone.

Clarren S. K. (1981) Recognition of fetal alcohol syndrome. *JAMA* **245**, 2436–2439.

Cleaton-Jones P., Austin I. C., Moyes D. G. et al. (1978) Nitrous oxide contamination in dental surgeries using relative analgesia. *Br. J. Anaesth.* **50**, 1019–1024.

Committee on the Review of Medicines (1980) Systematic review of the benzodiazepines. *Br. Med. J.* **1**, 910–2.

Davies D. M. (1977) *Textbook of Adverse Drug Reactions.* Oxford, Oxford University Press.

Dodson M. E. (1982) Adverse reactions and anaesthesia. *Adverse Drug Reaction Bull.* No. 96.

Donaldson D. and Gibson G. (1980) Systemic complications with intravenous diazepam. *Oral Surg.* **49**, 126–30

Driscoll E. I., Gelfman S. S., Sweet I. B. et al. (1979) Thrombophlebitis after intravenous use of anaesthesia and sedation: its incidence and natural history. *Oral Surg.* **37**, 809-15.

Editorial (1977) Deaths due to drug treatment. *Br. Med. J.* **1**, 1492.

Ernsert V L, Grady D G, Green J C, et al. (1990) Smokeless tobacco use and health effects among baseball players. *JAMA*, **264**, 218–4.

Fortenberry I. D. (1985) Gasoline sniffing. *Am.J. Med.* **79**, 740–2.

Fridrich H. H.. Zach G. A. and Fridrich K. L. (1986) Aspirin-intolerance syndrome. *Oral Surg.* **61**, 463–5.

Friedlander A. H. and Gorelick D. A. (1988) Dental managment of the cocaine addict. *Oral Surg,* **65**, 45–48.

Friedlander A. H. Mills M.J. and Gorelick D A. (1987) Alcoholism and dental management. *Oral Surg.* **63**, 42–46.

Gawin F. H. and Ellinwood E. H. (1988) Cocaine and other stimulants. *N. Engl. J. Med..* **318**, 1173–1182.

Gerald M. C. (1978) Drug interactions in dental practice. *Dent. Clin. North Am.* **22**, 151-71.

Grogono A. W. and Seltzer I. L. (1980) A guide to drug interactions in anaesthetic practice. *Drugs* **19**, 271–9.

Harris E.F., Friend G.W. and Tolley E.A. (1992) Enhanced prevalence of ankyloglossia with maternal cocain use. *Cleft Palate Craniofac. J.* **29**, 72–76.

Haverkos H.W. and Lange W.R. (1990) Serious infections other than human immunodeficiency virus among intravenous drug abusers. *J Infect Dis.* **161**, 894–902.

Holt S., Stewart I. C., Dixon I. M. I. et al. (1980) Alcohol and the emergency service patient. *Br. Med.J.* **281**, 638–9.

Hunter A. G. W., Thompson D. and Evans I. A. (1979) Is there a fetal gasoline syndrome? *Teratology* **20**, 75–80.

Iosub S., Fuchs M., Bingo N. et al. (1981) Fetal alcohol syndrome revisited. *Pediatrics* **68**, 475-9.

Isaacs S. O., Martin P. and Washington I. A. (1986) Phencyclidine (PCP) abuse. *Oral Surg.* **61**, 126–129.

Krutchkoff D.J., Eisenberg E., O'Brient J. E. et al. (1990) Cocaine–induced dental erosions. *N. Engl. J. Med.* **320**, 408.

Leading Article (1985) Drug reactions during anaesthesia. *Lancet* **i**, 1222-3.

Mitchell J.R. (1988) Acetominophen toxicity. *N. Engl. J. Med.* **319**, 1601.

Ong T.K., Rustage K.J., Harrison K.M. et al (1988). Solvent abuse: an anaesthetic management problem. *Br. Dent. J.* **164**, 150–1.

Ratcliff J.S. and Collins G.B. (1987) Dental management of the recovered chronically dependent patient. *J. Am. Dent. Assoc.* **114**, 601–3.

Rosenbaum C. E. (1980) Dental precautions in treating drug addicts: a hidden problem among teens and preteens. *Pediatr. Dent.* **2**, 94–6.

Smiler B. A. (1975) Drugs in dentistry. *Medical Market Media* **75**, 13–14.

The Health Consequences of using Smokeless Tobacco. A report of the Advisory Committee to the Surgeon General (1986); NIH Bethesda: N086–2874

Waldman H B. (1989) Fetal alcohol syndrome and the realities of our time. *J. Dent. Child. Nov.* 435–7.

Walker D. M. (1982) Adverse reactions to drugs and materials in dentistry. *Dent. Update* **20**, 537–45.

Woods J.H., Katz J.L. and Winger G. (1988); Use and abuse of benzodiazepines. *JAMA* **260**, 3476–80.

Appendix to Chapter 19

POSSIBLE ADVERSE REACTIONS TO ANAESTHETIC, SEDATIVE AND RELATED DRUGS

Drug	Possible adverse reaction
Premedication	
Benzodiazepine	May unmask depression (weepiness and sadness)
Opioids	Vomiting, allergy, respiratory depression
Droperidol	May increase anxiety
	Extrapyramidal effects
Atropine or hyoscine	Dry mouth: worsensglaucoma
Anaesthetic and related agents	
Suxamethonium	Muscle pains—especially if patient exercises postoperatively
	Rarely—malignant hyperthermia
	Rarely—apnoea
Tubocurarine	Hypotension/bronchospasm
Halothane	Shivering
	Hepatitis
	Dysrhythmias
	Rarely—malignant hyperthermia
Nitrous oxide	Transient deafness from diffusion of gas into the middle ear (rarely)
Naloxone	Hypertension
Methohexitone	Convulsions
	Respiratory depression
Diazepam	Thrombophlebitis
	Respiratory depression (slight)
Midazolam	Respiratory depression (severe)

POSSIBLE DRUG INTERACTIONS IN DENTISTRY

Note: This is not an absolutely complete list.Many of these drug interactions are of little more than theoretical importance in dentistry, or are the result of overdose of one or both agents. However, there can be wide individual variation in response to drugs, especially sedating agents.

Drug used in dentistry	Drug	Possible effects
Adrenaline	Halothane	Dysrhythmias
	Tricyclics	Pressor response in overdose
Anaesthetics	Antihypertensives	Hypotension
	MAOI	Enhanced hypotension: anaesthetics potentiated
Antibiotics	Oral anticoagulants	Enhanced anticoagulant effect
(some only)	Oral contraceptives	Reduced contraception
Aspirin	Alcohol	Increased risk of gastric bleeding
	Corticosteroids	Increased liability of peptic ulceration
	Methotrexate	Enhanced methotrexate activity
	Metoclopramide	Potentiation
	Midazolam	Potentiation
	Oral anticoagulants	Enhanced anticoagulant effect
	Oral hypoglycaemics	Enhanced hypoglycaemic effect
	Phenylbutazone	Increased liability of peptic ulceration
	Probenecid	Uricosuric action reduced
	Sulphinpyrazone	Uricosuric action reduced

Drug used in dentistry	Drug	Possible effects
Barbiturates	Alcohol	May be increased sedation or resistance
	Antihypertensives	Hypotension
	Antihistamines	Enhanced sedation
	Corticosteroids	May precipitate hypotensive crisis
	MAOI	Enhanced sedation
	Oral anticoagulants	Reduced anticoagulant activity
	Phenothiazines	Tremor
	Tricyclics	Cardiac arrest
Carbamazepine	Contraceptive pill	Reduced efficacy of 'pill'
	Dextropropoxyphene	Enhanced effect of carbamazepine
	Diazepam	Enhanced sedation
	Doxycycline	Reduced doxycycline effect
	Lithium	Neurotoxicity
	MAOI	Possible hypertension
	Oral anticoagulants	Reduced anticoagulant effect
	Sodium valproate	Reduced effect of valproate
Cephalosporins	Oral anticoagulants	Increased bleeding tendency
	Diuretics	Increased nephrotoxicity
Codeine	MAOI	Coma
Corticosteroids	Aspirin or other analgesics	Increased liability to peptic ulceration
	Antidiabetics	Reduced effect of antidiabetic
	Antihypertensives	Reduced effect of antihypertensive
Co-trimoxazole	Methotrexate	Possible folate deficiency
	Oral anticoagulants	Increased bleeding
	Oral hypoglycaemics	Enhanced hypoglycaemia
	Phenytoin	Phenytoin toxicity
	Zidoridine	Marrow toxicity
Dextropropoxyphene	Alcohol	Central nervous system depression
	Carbamazepine	Enhanced effect of carbamazepine
	Oral anticoagulants	Enhanced anticoagulant effect
	Orphenadrine	Tremor, anxiety and confusion
Diazepam or other sedatives	Alcohol	Additive or potentiation
	Antihistamines	Enhanced sedation
	Carbamazepine	Enhanced sedation
	Cimetidine	Enhanced sedation
	Erythromycin	Enhanced sedation
	Halothane	Enhanced activity of halothane
	L-dopa	Antagonism
	Lithium	Hypothermia
	Pentazocine and other opiates	Respiratory depression
	Phenytoin	Phenytoin toxicity
	Suxamethonium	Activity of suxamethonium reduced
	Tricyclics	Enhanced sedation
Ephedrine	MAOI	Hypertension
	Tricyclics	Hypertension
	Adrenaline	Dysrhythmias
Erythromycin	Midazolam	Midazolam enhanced
	Terfenadine	Dysrhythmias
Halothane	Aminophylline	Dysrhythmias
	Antihypertensives	Hypotension
	Diazepam	Enhanced activity of halothane
	Diethylproprion	Dysrhythmias
	Fenfluramine	Dysrhythmias
	Isoprenaline	Dysrhythmias
	Levodopa	Dysrhythmias
	Lithium	Dysrhythmias

Drug used in dentistry	Drug	Possible effects
Halothane	Opiates	Respiratory depression
	Phenothiazines	Respiratory depression, hypotension
	Phenytoin	Phenytoin toxicity
Ketamine	CNS depressants	Increased sedation
	Amphetamines	Hypertensive crisis
Ketoconazole	Terfenadine	Cardiac dysrhythmias
Monoamine oxidase inhibitors*	Antihypertensives	Reduced or increased hypotensive effect
	Tyramine-containing foods	Hypertensive crisis
	Levodopa	Hypertensive crisis
	Methohexitone	Hypotension
	Opiates	Respiratory depression
	Oral anticoagulants	Enhanced anticoagulant effect
	Oral hypoglycaemics	Enhanced hypoglycaemia
	Pethidine	Hypertensive crisis
	Propranolol	Hypertensive crisis
	Tricyclics	Excitation and other interactions
Mefenamic acid	Oral anticoagulants	Enhanced anticoagulant effect
	Oral hypoglycaemics	Enhanced hypoglycaemia
Methohexitone	Alcohol	Increased sedation
	Antihypertensives	Hypotension
	MAOI	Coma
	Opiates incl. pentazocine	Respiratory depression
	Phenothiazines	Respiratory depression and/or hypotension
Metronidazole	Alcohol	Headache and hypotension
	Oral anticoagulants	Increased bleeding
Midazolam (see Diazepam)	Oral contraceptive	Decreased contraception
Noradrenaline	Tricyclics	Hypertension
Opiates	Halothane	Respiratory depression
	MAOI	Respiratory depression or coma
	Methohexitone	Respiratory depression
Paracetamol	Cholestyramine	Reduced absorption of paracetamol
	Metoclopramide	Potentiation
	Oral anticoagulants	Increased bleeding tendency
Pentazocine	Diazepam	Respiratory depression
Pethidine	MAOI	Hypertensive crisis
	Phenothiazines	Respiratory depression
Phenothiazines	Alcohol	May be increased sedation
	Antihistamines	Enhanced sedation
	Antihypertensives	Hypotension
	Barbiturates	Tremor
	Oral anticoagulants	Enhanced anticoagulant effect
	Pethidine	Respiratory depression
	Tricyclics	Convulsions
Phenylbutazone	Aspirin	Increased liability to peptic ulceration
Promethazine	Methohexitone	Increased side-effects of methohexitone
Sulphonamides**	Methotrexate	Increased methotrexate toxicity
	Oral anticoagulants	Enhanced anticoagulant effect
	Oral hypoglycaemics	Enhanced hypoglycaemia
	Phenytoin	Phenytoin toxicity
Suxamethonium	Cytotoxic drugs	Prolonged muscle paralysis
	Diazepam	Activity of suxamethonium reduced
	Diethylstilboestrol	Prolonged muscle paralysis
	Digitalis	Digitalis toxicity enhanced
	Ecothiopate	Prolonged muscle paralysis

Drug used in dentistry	Drug	Possible effects
Suxamethonium	Lithium	Onset of suxamethonium delayed, action prolonged
	Spironolactone	Plasma potassium rises—potential dysrhythmias
Tetracyclines	Antacids	Lower serum levels of tetracyclines
	Barbiturates	Reduced doxycycline blood levels
	Cimetidine	Reduced serum tetracycline levels
	Iron	Reduced serum tetracycline levels
	Methoxyflurane	Renal damage
Tetracyclines	Milk	Reduced tetracycline absorption
	Oral anticoagulants	Bleeding tendency
	Oral contraceptive	Reduced contraceptive effect
Thiopentone	Alcohol	Increased sedation
	Antihypertensives	Hypotension
	MAOI	Coma
	Opioids	Respiratory depression
	Phenothiazines	Respiratory depression
	Sulphonamides	Barbiturate potentiated
Tricyclics	Adrenaline	Hypertensive response in overdose
	Alcohol	Enhanced CNS depression
	Antihypertensives	Impaired blood pressure control
	Atropinics	Enhanced atropinic effects
	Diazepam	Enhanced sedation
	MAOI	Excitation and other interactions
	Oral anticoagulants	Enhanced anticoagulant effect
	Phenothiazine	Convulsions

* Includes selegine
** Co-trimoxazole contains a sulphonamide.

POSSIBLE DISEASE CONTRAINDICATIONS TO DRUGS THAT MAY BE USED IN DENTISTRY

Note: Many of these reactions are likely to be of more theoretical interest than clinical significance, so that reference should also be made to the appropriate chapters for particular diseases. In pregnancy avoid all drugs unless absolutely essential.

Drug	Possible contraindications	Possible reaction
Adrenaline	Hypertension	Hypertension (theoretical)
	Hyperthyroidism	Dysrhythmias (theoretical)
	Ischaemic heart disease	Dysrhythmias
	Phaeochromocytoma	Hypertension
Ampicillin,	Allergy	Anaphylaxis
or amoxycillin	Chronic lymphocytic leukaemia	Rash
or derivatives	Gout	Rash
	Infectious mononucleosis	Rash
Aspirin	Allergy to aspirin including aspirin-induced asthma	Anaphylaxis
	Bleeding disorders	Gastric bleeding
	Children	Reye's syndrome
	Diabetics on drugs	Hypoglycaemia
	Glucose 6-phosphate-dehydrogenase	Haemolysis
	Liver disease	Bleeding tendency
	Peptic ulcer	Gastric bleeding
	Renal disease	Fluid retention and gastric bleeding
	Children with fever	Reye's syndrome

Drug	*Possible contraindications*	*Possible reaction*
Atropinics	Glaucoma	Raised intraocular pressure
	Hyperthyroidism	Tachycardias
	The elderly	Confusion: urine retention
	Urinary retention or prostatic hypertrophy	Urinary retention
Carbamazepine	Glaucoma	Raised intraocular pressure
	Liver disease	Hepatotoxic
	Pregnancy	Teratogenic
	The elderly	Agitation or confusion
Carbenoxolone	Liver disease	Toxicity
Cephalosporins*	Allergy to cephalosporins	Anaphylaxis
	Allergy to penicillins	Allergy
Chloral hydrate	Cardiovascular disease	Fluid retention
	Gastritis	Gastric irritation
	Liver disease	Coma
	Renal disease	CNS depression
Clindamycin	Liver disease	Increased toxicity
	The elderly	Pseudomembranous colitis
Codeine	The elderly	Constipation
	Liver disease	Respiratory depression
	Hypothyroidism	Coma
Corticosteroids	Diabetes mellitus	Diabetes worsened
	Hypertension	Increased hypertension
	Peptic ulcer	Perforation
	Tuberculosis	Possible dissemination
Co-trimoxazole	Elderly	Agranulocytosis
	Glucose phosphate-dehydrogenase deficiency	Haemolysis
	Liver disease	Enhanced toxicity
	Porphyria	Acute exacerbation
	Pregnancy	Folate deficiency
	Renal disease	Increased toxicity
Dextropropoxyphene	Liver disease	Potentiated
	Respiratory disease	Respiratory depression
	Pregnancy	Fetal depression
Diazepam	Cerebrovascular disease	Cerebral ischaemia
	Chronic obstructive airways disease	Respiratory depression
	Glaucoma	Increased ocular pressure
	Hypothyroidism	Coma
	Neuromuscular disorders	Deterioration
	Porphyria	Acute exacerbation
	Pregnancy	Fetal depression
	Severe kidney disease	Increased diazepam effect
	Severe liver disease	Increased diazepam effect
	The elderly	Cerebral ischaemia
	Children	Increased activity
Dihydrocodeine	Hypothyroidism	Coma
	Liver disease	Increased toxicity
	Renal disease	Increased toxicity
	Respiratory disease	Respiratory depression
	The elderly	Increased toxicity
Enflurane	Epilepsy	Epileptogenic
Erythromycin estolate	Liver disease	Hepatotoxic
Halothane	Cardiac dysrhythmias	Increased dysrhythmias
	Halothane hepatitis	Hepatitis
	Malignant hyperpyrexia	Pyrexia
	Recent anaesthesia with halothane	Hepatitis

Drug	Possible contraindications	Possible reaction
Hyoscine	Children	Hallucinations
Ketamine	Adults	Hallucinations
	Epilepsy	Fits
	Hypertension	Hypertension increased
	Malignant hyperpyrexia	Hyperpyrexia
	Psychiatric disease	Psychotic reactions
	Raised intracranial pressure	Increased intracranial pressure
Ketoconazole	Liver disease	Hepatotoxic
	Renal disease	Hepatotoxic
Lincomycin	(see Clindamycin)	
Mefenamic acid	Asthma	Bronchospasm
	Bleeding disorders	Interferes with platelets
	Diarrhoea	Diarrhoea worse
	Peptic ulcer	Bleeding
	Pregnancy and lactation	Teratogenic?
	Renal disease	Renal damage
Methohexitone	Addison's disease	Coma
	Allergies	Anaphylaxis
	Barbiturate sensitivity	Anaphylaxis
	Cardiovascular disease	Cardiovascular depression
	Dystrophia myotonica	Increased weakness
	Epilepsy	Fits
	Hypothyroidism	Coma
	Liver disease	Increased respiratory depression
	Myasthenia gravis	Increased weakness
	Porphyria	Acute exacerbation
	Post-nasal drip	Laryngeal spasm
	Respiratory disease	Respiratory depression
Metronidazole	Blood dyscrasias	Leucopenia
	CNS disease	Neuropathy
	Renal disease	Increased drug effect
	Pregnancy(first trimester)	Teratogenic?
Midazolam (see Diazepam)		
Opioids	Asthma	Bronchospasm
	Carcinoid tumour	Increased toxicity
	Chronic obstructive airways disease	Respiratory depression
	Head injury	Obscures diagnosis
	Hypothyroidism	Coma
	Liver disease	Increased respiratory depression
	Pregnancy	Fetal respiratory depression
	Renal disease	Increased respiratory depression
	Urinary retention or prostatic enlargement	Urinary retention
Paracetamol	Liver disease	Hepatotoxicity
	Renal disease	Nephrotoxicity
Penicillins	Allergy to penicillin	Anaphylaxis
	Renal disease	Hyperkalaemia with i.m. benzyl penicillin
Pentazocine	Head injury	Obscures diagnosis
	Hypertension	Hypertension increased
	Kidney disease	Increased toxicity
	Liver disease	Enhanced activity
	MAOI	Coma
	Myocardial infarct (recent)	Cardiac arrest
	Narcotic addict	Withdrawal syndrome
	Pregnancy	Fetal respiratory depression

Drug	Possible contraindications	Possible reaction
Pethidine	Hypothyroidism	Coma
Promethazine	Liver disease	Coma
	Diabetes	Hyperglycaemia
Rifampicin	Liver disease	Hepatotoxic
Sulphonamides	Glucose-6-phosphate dehydrogenase deficiency	Haemolysis
Sulphonamides	Porphyria	Acute exacerbation
	Pregnancy	Fetal haemolysis
	Renal disease†	Crystalluria
Sumatriptan	Cardiac disease	Coronary vasoconstriction
Suxamethonium	Burns	Dysrhythmias
	Dystrophia myotonica	Increased muscle weakness
	Liver disease	Apnoea
	Malignant hyperpyrexia	Hyperpyrexia
	Myasthenia gravis	Increased muscle weakness
	Renal disease	Apnoea
	Suxamethonium sensitivity	Apnoea
Tetracyclines	After gastrointestinal surgery	Enterocolitis
	Children under 12	Tooth staining
	Myasthenia gravis	Increased muscle weakness
	Pregnancy	Tooth staining (fetus)
	Renal disease†	Nephrotoxicity
	Systemic lupus erythematosus	Photosensitivity rashes
Thiopentone	Addison's disease	Coma
	Barbiturate sensitivity	Anaphylaxis
	Cardiovascular disease	Cardiovascular depression
	Dystrophia myotonica	Increased weakness
	Hypothyroidism	Coma
	Liver disease	Increased anaesthesia
	Myasthenia gravis	Increased weakness
	Porphyria	Acute porphyria
	Post-nasal drip	Laryngeal spasm
	Respiratory disease	Respiratory depression
Tranexamic acid	Haematuria	Renal tract obstruction
	Thromboembolic disease	Thromboses
Triclofos	(see Chloral hydrate)	
Tricyclics	Cardiovascular disease	Postural hypotension :arrhythmias
	Epilepsy	Increased fits
	Liver disease	Increased drug effect
	The elderly	Confusion
		Hypotension
Trimeprazine	Diabetes	Hyperglycaemia

* Some cephalosporins give a false-positive reaction for glycosuria.
† Not sulphadimidine.
‡ Not doxycycline.

DRUGS THAT SHOULD BE AVOIDED OR USED ONLY IN REDUCED DOSES IN SPECIFIC CONDITIONS

Condition	Drug that may be contraindicated or dose reductions needed
Addison's disease (hypoadrenocorticism)	Any general anaesthetic, particularly - Methohexitone Thiopentone
Allergies	Aspirin Methohexitone Penicillin

Condition	*Drug that may be contraindicated or dose reductions needed*
Asthma	Aspirin
	Mefenamic acid
	Opioids
Bleeding disorders	Aspirin
	Corticosteroids
	Dextropropoxyphene
	Frusemide
	Imipramine
	Mefenamic acid
	Phenothiazines
Burns	Suxamethonium
Carcinoid syndrome	Opioids
Cardiovascular diseases	Adrenaline (in large doses)
	Chloral hydrate
	Halothane
	Methohexitone
	Pentazocine
	Thiopentone
	Tricyclics
Cerebrovascular disease	Diazepam
Children	Aspirin
	Atropine
	Dihydrocodeine
	Hyoscine
Children under 12 years	Tetracyclines
Chronic lymphocytic	Amoxycillin
leukaemia	Ampicillin
Constipation	Codeine
Diabetes mellitus	Corticosteroids
	Promethazine
	Trimeprazine
Diarrhoea	Clindamycin
	Mefenamic acid
Drug addiction	Pentazocine†
Dystrophia myotonica	Methohexitone
(Myotonic dystrophy)	Suxamethonium
	Thiopentone
Elderly	Atropinics
	Diazepam
	Dihydrocodeine
	Enflurane
	Ketamine
	Tricyclics
Epilepsy	Methohexitone
	Phenothiazines
	Tricyclics
Glaucoma	Atropinics
	Carbamazepine
	Diazepam
Glucose-6-phosphate	Aspirin
dehydrogenase deficiency	Co-trimoxazole
	Sulphonamides
Gout	Amoxycillin
	Ampicillin
	Aspirin
Head injury	Ketamine
	Opioids
	Pentazocine

Condition	*Drug that may be contraindicated or dose reductions needed*
Hypertension	Adrenaline
	Corticosteroids
	Ketamine
	Pentazocine
	Propanidid
Hyperthyroidism	Adrenaline (in large doses)
	Atropinics
Hypothyroidism	Any general anaesthetic
	Codeine
	Diazepam
	Dihydrocodeine
	Methohexitone
	Opioids
	Pethidine
	Thiopentone
Infectious mononucleosis	Amoxycillin
	Ampicillin
Liver disease	Any general anaesthetic
	Aspirin
	Carbamazepine
	Chloral hydrate
	Clindamycin
	Co-trimoxazole
	Dextropropoxyphene
	Diazepam
	Dihydrocodeine
	Erythromycin estolate
	Halothane
	Ketoconazole
	Methohexitone
	Opioids or codeine
	Paracetamol
	Pentazocine
	Phenothiazines
	Rifampicin
	Suxamethonium
	Thiopentone
	Tricyclics
Malignant hyperpyrexia	Halothane and other inhalational anaesthetics
	Ketamine
	Suxamethonium
Neuromuscular diseases	Diazepam
	Methohexitone
	Suxamethonium
	Tetracyclines
	Thiopentone
Peptic ulcer	Aspirin
	Chloral hydrate
	Corticosteroids
	Mefenamic acid
Phaeochromocytoma	Adrenaline
Porphyria	Co-trimoxazole
	Diazepam
	Methohexitone
	Sulphonamides
	Thiopentone
Pregnancy	Care with all drugs
	Co-trimoxazole

Cond ition	Drug that may be contraind icated or d ose red uctions needed
	Diazepam
	Etretinate
Pregnancy	Mefenamic acid
	Metronidazole
	Opioids
	Pentazocine
	Sulphonamides
	Tetracyclines
Psychiatric disease	Ketamine
Raised intracranial pressure	Ketamine
Renal disease	Any general anaesthetic
	Acyclovir (systemic)reduce dose only
	Aspirin
	Chloral hydrate
	Co-trimoxazole
	Dihydrocodeine
	Lincomycin
	Mefenamic acid
	Opioids
	Pentazocine
	Sulphonamides
	Suxamethonium
	Tetracyclines
Respiratory disease	Any general anaesthetic
	Dextropropoxyphene
	Diazepam
	Dihydrocodeine
	Methohexitone
	Opiates
	Thiopentone
Systemic lupus erythematosus	Tetracyclines
Thrombotic disease	Amino caproic acid
	Tranexamic acid
Tuberculosis	Corticosteroids
Urinary retention	Atropinics
(or prostatic disease)	Opioids

* Check the relevant disease for more information. This is nol a complete list.
† Pentazocine is contraindicated in narcotic addicts.
‡ Halothane on repeated administration may cause hepatitis.

ORAL SIDE-EFFECTS THAT OCCASIONALLY FOLLOW DRUG TREATMENT
Most are rare but the more common are marked*

Tooth discoloration
Chlorhexidine*
Fluorides
Iron*
Tetracyclines

Oral candidosis
Broad-spectrum antimicrobials*
Corticosteroids
Drugs causing xerostomia
Immunosuppressives

Oral ulceration
Allopurinol
Cytotoxics*
Emepromium
Gold salts
Indomethacin
Isoprenaline
Methyldopa
Pancreatin
Penicillamine
Phenindione

Oral ulceration
Potassium chloride
Proguanil

Facial pain
Phenothiazines
Stilbamidine
Vinca alkaloids

Erythema multiforme (Stevens Johnson syndrome)
Busulphan
Carbamazepine
Clindamycin
Codeine
Frusemide
Penicillin
Phenobarbitone
Phenytoin
Sulphonamides*
Tetracyclines

Angio-oedema
Aspirin
Essential oils
Penicillin*

Gingival hyperplasia
Contraceptive pill
Cyclosporin
Diltiazem
Nifedipine
Nitrendipine
Phenobarbitone
Phenytoin*
Primidone

Oral mucosal pigmentation
ACTH
Amodiaquine
Anticonvulsants
Busulphan
Chloroquine*
Contraceptive pill
Heavy metals
Mepacrine*
Phenothiazines

Lichenoid reactions
Allopurinol
Captopril
Chloroquine
Chlorpropamide*
Dapsone
Gold salts*
Labetalol
Mepacrine
Methyldopa*

Lichenoid reactions
Non-steroidal anti-inflammatory agents
Oxprenolol
Penicillamine
Phenothiazines
Practolol
Propranolol
Tetracycline
Thiazides
Tolbutamide
Triprolidine

Lupoid reactions
Gold salts
Griseofulvin
Hydralazine*
Isoniazid
Methyldopa
Penicillin
Phenytoin
Procainamide*
Streptomycin
Sulphonamides
Tetracyclines

Pemphigus-like reactions
Penicillamine
Rifampicin

Pemphigoid-like reactions
Clonidine
Frusemide
Psoralens

Salivary gland swelling
Anti-thyroid agents
Chlorhexidine
Ganglion-blocking agents
Insulin
Iodides
Isoprenaline
Methyldopa
Oxyphenbutazone
Phenothiazines
Phenylbutazone
Ritodrine
Sulphonamides

Salivary gland pain
Bethanidine
Clonidine
Cytotoxics
Guanethidine*
Methyldopa

Hypersalivation
Anticholinesterases*

Hypersalivation
Buprenorphine
Ethionamide
Haloperidol
Iodides
Ketamine
Niridazole

Xerostomia
Adriamycin
Amphetamines
Anti-Parkinsonians
Antihistamines
Atropinics*
Benzhexol
Clonidine
L-dopa
Ganglion blocking agents
Lithium
Monoamine oxidase inhibitors*
Propantheline
Tricyclics*

Red saliva
Rifampicin
Disturbed taste (can also result from
    drugs causing xerostomia)
Anti-thyroids
Biguanides
Clofibrate
Ethionamide
Gold salts
Grisefulvin
Guanoclor
Lincomycin
Lithium salts
Metronidazole
Niridazole
Penicillamine
Phenindione

Cervical lymph node enlargement
Phenytoin
Primidone

Involuntary facial movements
Butyrophenones*
Carbamazepine
Levodopa
Methyldopa
Metoclopramide
Phenyclidine
Phenothiazines*
Tetrabenazine
Tricyclics

Trigeminal paraesthesia
Acetazolamide*
Cyclosporin
Ergotamine
Hydralazine
Isoniazid
Labetalol*
Methysergide
Monoamine oxidase inhibitors
Nalidixic acid
Nitrofurantoin
Phenytoin
Propranolol
Solvent abuse
Stilbamidine
Streptomycin
Sulphonylureas
Sulthiame*
Tricyclics

Facial flushing
Chlorpropamide

SOME STREET NAMES AND OTHER TERMS FOR DRUGS OF ABUSE

Street names	Drug
Acapulco gold	Cannabis
Acid	LSD
Animal tranquillizer	Phencyclidine
Angel dust/mist	Phencyclidine
Beans	Amphetamine
Bennies	Amphetamine
Bhang*	Cannabis
Black tar	Heroin
Blanco	Heroin
Blue angel/devil/heaven	Amylobarbitone
C	Cocaine
Cadillac	Cocaine
Candy	Barbiturates

Street names	Drug
Charas	Cannabis
Charlies	Cocaine
Chip	Heroin
Christmas trees	Barbiturates
Coke	Cocaine
Co-pilot	Methamphetamine
Crack	Cocaine free base
Crystal	Methamphetamine
Crystal joints	Phencyclidine
Cubes	LSD
Dagga*	Cannabis
Dexies	Dexamphetamine
Doe	Methamphetamine
Dope	Heroin
Dot	LSD
Downers	Barbiturates
Ecstasy	Methylene deoxyamphetamine
Elephant	Phencyclidine
Freebase	Cocaine
Ganga*	Cannabis
Girl	Cocaine
Gold dust	Cocaine
Goofballs	Barbiturates
Goon	Phencyclidine
Grass	Cannabis
Gunk	Morphine
H	Heroin
Hash(hashish*)	Cannabis
Hocus	Morphine
Hog	Phencyclidine
Horse	Heroin
Horse tranquillizer	Phencyclidine
Ice	Methamphetamine
Jack up	Amylobarbitone
Junk	Cocaine
KJ	Phencyclidine
Lady	Cocaine
Lilly	Secobarbitone
Love drug	Methamphetamine
Ludes	Methaqualone
(Marihuana)* marijuana	Cannabis
Mesc	Mescaline
Mist	Phencyclidine
Monkey	Morphine
Mushroom	Psilocybin
Nebbies	Pentobarbitone
Panama gold	Cannabis
Paris	Methaqualone
PCP	Phencyclidine
Peace pills	Phencyclidine
Peaches	Amphetamine
Pink	Morphine
Pot	Cannabis
Purple haze	LSD
Purple hearts	Dexamphetamine and amylobarbitone
Quads	Methaqualone
Red devils	Secobarbital
Reefer	Cannabis

Street names	Drug
Rock	Cocaine
Rocket fuel	Phencyclidine
Scuffle	Phencyclidine
Silly putty	Psilocybin
Snow	Cocaine
Soapers	Methaqualone
Soma	Phencyclidine
Speed	Amphetamine (intravenously)
Speedball	Opioids and amphetamine (or cocaine and heroin)
T	Phencyclidine
TCP	Thiencylcyclohexyl piperidine
Tea	Cannabis
Tic tac	Phencyclidine
Ts and blues	Pentazocine and tripelannamine
Weed	Cannabis
White lightning	LSD
Yellowjackets	Pentobarbitone

* Correct name in country of origin.

Appendix Miscellaneous Uncommon or Rare Disorders of Possible Relevance to Dentistry not Included Elsewhere

Disorders	Manifestations	Oral features	Management problems
Acanthosis nigricans	Pigmented papillomatous skin lesions	Papillomatous lesions	Adenocarcinoma (usually gastrointestinal)
Acrodermatitis enteropathica zinc deficiency	Skin vesicles Hair loss Diarrhoea	Perioral or oral erosions	Malabsorption syndrome
Alstrom's syndrome	Nerve deafness Retinitis pigmentosa	—	Diabetes mellitus
Ataxia telangiectasia	Mental handicap Ataxia Immunodeficiency	Occasional telangiectasia	Mental handicap Diabetes mellitus Hypoadrenocorticism
Beckwith's syndrome	Gigantism Omphalocoele or umbilical hernia Obesity	Macroglossia	Hypoglycaemia Hyperlipidaemia Diabetes mellitus Obesity
Biemond's syndrome	Hypogonadism	Hypoplastic middle third of face	
Blackfan–Diamond syndrome	Red cell aplasia	—	Anaemia
Bloom's syndrome	Telangiectasia Depigmentation Short stature	Chronic cheilitis Carcinoma	50% Develop neoplasia, particularly lymphoreticular
Cerebrohepatorenal syndrome (Lowe)	Hypotonia Flexion contractures	Micrognathia	Bleeding tendency Epilepsy
Chondroectodermal dysplasia (Ellis-van Creveld syndrome)	Polydactyly Dwarfism Ectodermal dysplasia	Midline defect in upper lip Natal teeth Conical or bicuspid teeth	Cardiac defects Mental handicap
Cockayne's syndrome	Neuropathy Premature ageing Dwarfism Deafness	Prognathism	Deafness Mental handicap Blindness
Coffin–Lawry syndrome	Mental handicap Osteocartilaginous anomalies	Hypoplastic zygoma and maxilla	Mental handicap
Congenital indifference to pain	Self-mutilation Bone fractures and infections	Self-mutilation	Patient incapable of perceiving pain

Cowden's syndrome	Multiple hamartomas Papular skin lesions	Papillomatosis Papules Leukoplakia Carcinoma	Breast or thyroid carcinoma
Darier's disease	Skin pigmentation Alopecia Nail defects		—
Dyskeratosis congenita	Aplastic anaemia	Rarely squamous carcinoma	Pancytopenia Multiple oral carcinomas
Fabry's disease (Angiokeratoma corporis diffusum)	Angiokeratomas Extremity pain Hypertension Fever	Angiokeratomas	Hypertension Renal disease Myocardial infarction
Fanconi's anaemia	Abnormalities of radius	Dental defects	Anaemia, leukaemia Renal defects Diabetes mellitus Hypoadrenocorticism
Focal dermal hypoplasia (Goltz syndrome)	Fatty deposits in skin Anomalies of extremities Skin atrophy	Labial papillomas ± cleft lip-palate Enamel hypoplasia Large pulp horns High arched palate Cross bite Open bite	—
Fragile X syndrome	Long face Large ears		Mental handicap
Froehlich's syndrome	Obesity Hypogonadism		± Mental handicap Obesity Visual defects
Hallermann–Streiff syndrome	Hypotrichosis Cranial anomalies Micro-ophthalmia Cataracts	Mandibular hypoplasia TMJ abnormal position Dental anomalies	—
Hermansky–Pudlak syndrome	Albinism Bleeding tendency	Gingival haemorrhage	Bleeding tendency
Hyalinosis cutis et mucosae	Waxy skin nodules Hoarseness	Oral plaques and infiltration	Laryngeal involvement Epilepsy Mental handicap
Incontinentia pigmenti (Bloch–Sulzberger syndrome)	Pigmented skin lesions Skeletal defects Neurological defects	Dental hypoplasia Hypodontia Conical teeth	Epilepsy Visual defects Immunodeficiency
Kartagener's syndrome	Sinusitis Dextrocardia	—	—
Klippel–Feil deformity	Abnormalities of cervical vertebrae	—	Syringomyelia Fainting attacks

Disorders	Manifestations	Oral features	Management problems
Laurence–Moon–Biedl syndrome	Retinitis pigmentosa, Polydactyly, Obesity	—	Mental handicap, Blindness, Obesity
Maffuci syndrome	Haemangiomas, Enchondromas, 20% develop chondrosarcomas	Haemangiomas	Anaemia
Marcus–Gunn syndrome	Ptosis, Lid winking in conjunction with jaw movement	—	—
Moebius syndrome	Congenital facial palsy	Facial palsy	Facial palsy
Noonan's syndrome	Skeletal and muscular anomalies, Webbed neck, short stature	May be hypoglossal palsy, Micrognathia, Dental defects	Cardiac defects, Pulmonary stenosis, Thyroid disease
Papillon–Lefevre syndrome	Palmar and plantar hyperkeratosis	Periodontosis	—
Pierre–Robin syndrome	—	Micrognathia, Cleft palate, Glossoptosis	Cardiac defects, Airways obstruction
Prader–Willi syndrome	Mental handicap, Obesity, Hypogonadism	Dental defects	Diabetes mellitus
Progeria (Werner or Hutchinson–Gilford syndrome)	Alopecia, dwarfism, senile appearance, hydrocephalic appearance	Mandibular hypoplasia, delayed eruption crowding	Early atheroma with coronary and cerebrovascular insufficiency
Rieger's syndrome	Hypodontia, Ocular anomalies	Hypodontia, Maxillary hypoplasia	Blindness
Rothmund–Thomson syndrome	Poikiloderma, cataracts, hypogonadism, dwarfism	Microdontia, dental hypoplasia	Visual defect

Syndrome			
Ruvalcaba–Myrhe–Smith syndrome	Macrocephaly Intestinal polyps Penile pigmented macules	Tongue polyps	Mental handicap
Scurvy	Purpura	Gingival swelling and haemorrhage	Bleeding tendency
Schmidt's syndrome	Hypoadrenocorticism Hypoparathyroidism	Candidosis	Diabetes mellitus Autoimmune diseases Malabsorption syndrome
Seckel's syndrome	Microcephaly Mental handicap	Zygomatic hypoplasia Mandibular hypoplasia	Mental handicap
Sjögren–Larsson syndrome	Ichthyosis Mental handicap Cerebral palsy	Dental hypoplasia, indifference to pain	Mental handicap Cerebral palsy
Smith–Lemli–Opitz syndrome	Short stature Mental handicap Urogenital anomalies Syndactyly	Maxillary abnormalities	Mental handicap Cerebral palsy
Takayasu's disease	Pulseless large arteries from aortic arch	Pain in muscles of mastication, ulcers	Syncope Steroid therapy
Treacher–Collin's syndrome	Downward sloped palpebral fissures	Mandibulofacial dysostosis	Deafness Airways obstruction Cardiac defects
Tylosis	Palmar and plantar hyperkeratosis	—	Oesophageal carcinoma
Vitiligo	Depigmented area of skin	Rarely depigmentation	Thyrotoxicosis Hypoadrenocorticism
Waardenburg's syndrome	Deafness Heterochromia iridis White forelock		Deafness (20%)
Werner's syndrome	Cataracts Osteoporosis Thyroid cancer	Prognathism	Diabetes mellitus
Xeroderma pigmentosum	Hyperpigmentation Mental handicap	Squamous cancer of lip at early age	Tendency to skin malignancy

Index